ENVISION • DESIGN • TRAIN

A PICTORIAL HISTORY OF THE U.S. ARMY MEDICAL DEPARTMENT CENTER & SCHOOL

1920 *to* 2010

We save lives...on and off the battlefield!

Adriane Askins Neidinger
U.S. Army Medical Department Center & School
3630 Stanley Road, Bldg 2840, Fort Sam Houston, Texas 78234

www.cs.amedd.army.mil

2012

Table of Contents

Foreword

"We envision, design, and train a premier military medical force for decisive action in support of our Nation."

The Army Medical Department exists for one reason: to ensure the Soldier pictured here and his Family have access to the very best healthcare possible, on the battlefield and at home.

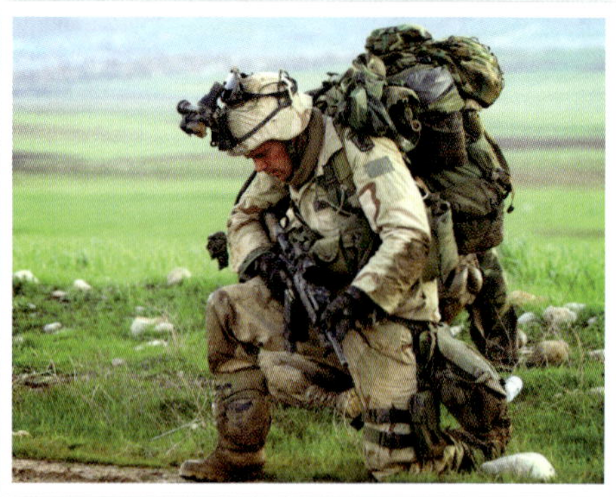

Today's mission statement for the Army Medical Department Center and School (AMEDDC&S) aptly describes what legions of professionals working here have been doing to provide and advance professional military medical education for the past 90 years. It also describes the work these professionals have done and continue to do to ensure healthcare on the battlefield and in humanitarian settings is the very best possible. This volume tells their story in pictures and words.

By virtue of its core mission of saving lives on and off the battlefield, the AMEDD has always been a unique organization within the U.S. Army. The AMEDD conserves and advances health, treats patients who become ill and injured, and provides a full range of healthcare services to Soldiers and other warriors deployed around the world.

For 90 years the Army, Navy, Air Force, Coast Guard, and Department of Veterans Affairs have looked to the AMEDDC&S for the very best in education and training to care for America's sons and daughters in dangerous places and in brick and mortar hospitals and clinics.

To be successful we rely on the competent and creative intellect of Soldiers, Sailors, Airmen, and Civilians to mold the next generation of those ensuring the success of our military healthcare system. This same professional intellect is required to envision how healthcare can best be provided in austere and dangerous settings, and then design that system.

Every Army healthcare leader since World War II is a graduate of one or more AMEDDC&S programs of instruction. No Army healthcare Soldier can deploy to conflict or combat without first attending school at the AMEDDC&S. The doctrine and organizations used to provide healthcare to America's warriors in combat are written and developed at the AMEDDC&S. Army Medical Department readiness does, indeed, start here.

Today's men and women of the AMEDDC&S carry on the very best traditions first begun at Carlisle Barracks, Pennsylvania, in 1920 and then continued on Fort Sam Houston, Texas, beginning in 1946. We are proud to share their story with you.

David A. Rubenstein, FACHE
Major General, U.S. Army,
Commanding General

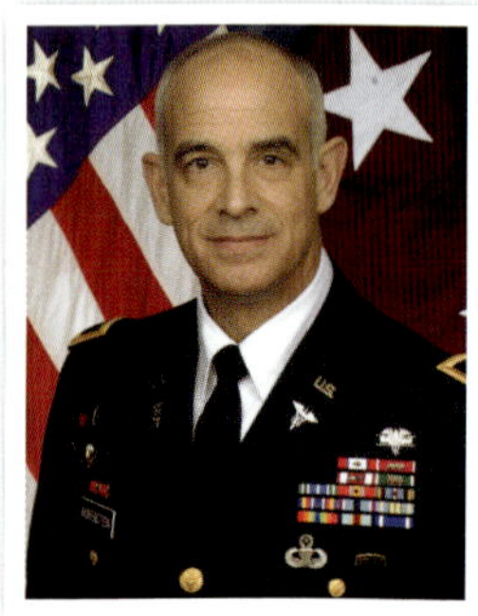

Preface

I had been in my position as the Army Medical Department Center and School's (AMEDDC&S) historian a little less than a year when I was tasked by MG David A. Rubenstein with producing the first-ever pictorial history of the AMEDDC&S. It sounded simple enough—compile and publish a collection of images that illustrated the history of the AMEDDC&S from its beginning at Carlisle Barracks, Pennsylvania, in 1920 to the present.

As I and the various contributors to this publication combed old Annual Historical Reports (AHRs), After Action Reports (AARs), scrapbooks, newspapers, journals, and museum collections, it became apparent that all years were not created equal. Content, quality, and preservation of not only photos but documentation of command events varied wildly from year to year. To verbally illustrate the years with little photographic documentation, excerpts from articles and reports were included to round out the proverbial "picture" of our past. What started off as a pictorial history has become, de facto, the first baseline history of the AMEDDC&S.

The AMEDDC&S has had several organizational name changes since 1920. It has been at various times the Medical Field Service School (MFSS) in the time periods of 1920-1946, 1947-1955, and 1960-1972; Army Medical Service School (AMSS) in 1946-1947 and 1955-1960; Academy of Health Sciences (AHS), 1972-1991; and the Army Medical Department Center and School (AMEDDC&S) from 1991 to the present. It has also been endearingly called the "Schoolhouse" by many AMEDD generations. Organizational name changes were not always recognized in official reports and/or articles; it appears that various authors continued to use organization names they were most familiar with or partial to. Schoolhouse activities were also mistakenly called Brooke Army Medical Center (BAMC) or Health Services Command (HSC) activities years after having been moved from under those commands, so readers might see two or three different organizational names for the schoolhouse used during a single year.

What readers will see in this history is that there have been many changes over time, but the mission to ENVISION • DESIGN • TRAIN has remained the same over the past 90 years of history.

– Adriane Askins Neidinger
AMEDDC&S, Command Historian

Acknowledgements

Any endeavor of this magnitude could not have been accomplished without contributions, assistance, and encouragement from many people. First and foremost, I would like to acknowledge MG David A. Rubenstein, Commander, Army Medical Department Center and School for the honor of being assigned the production of the first ever pictorial history of the AMEDDC&S. He had his choice of seasoned medical military historians in the area to choose from yet he selected me. A personal "thank you" goes directly to him for the opportunity to research this honorable organization but to also ensure that its history is documented for not only the AMEDD community, but the general public.

I would like to acknowledge my fellow historians at the AMEDDC&S Leader Training Center, Dr. Wayne Austerman and Mr. Bob Glisson, for their contributions. Readers will find the indelible watermark of Dr. Austerman's writing style on the first section dealing with the early years of the Medical Field Service School. Mr. Bob Glisson, a young officer at the Academy of Health Sciences in the 1980s, contributed most of the 1980s information. Mr. Warrington Lee Austerman receives my special thanks for volunteering to scan and annotate captions for the section his father wrote.

Contributions in the form of additional research, image scanning, and captions writing came from the following officers of CCC 11-004: CPT Gordon Briscoe, CPT Ali Salerno, CPT Travis Lloyd, CPT Danny Garrett, CPT Jack T. Alley, CPT Lauren Osinski, 1Lt Trimeka Rivers, CPT Kelly Crimmings, CPT William "Bill" Vasios, CPT Joshua Jones, CPT Shane Smith, CPT Stacy Grant, and CPT Mitzi Rivera. Their voluntary participation was due to a serendipitous conversation with Jim E. Wise III, LTC-SGL. I can't thank Mr. Wise enough for support throughout the project or the willingness and enthusiasm of our future leadership in this history project. Others who volunteered in a similar manner include: Ms. Pam Ellis, SFC Ronnie Palmer, SPC Sonia McNair, CPT Dennis Penacerrada, Ms. Blanca I. Loya, Mr. Carlos Martinez, Ms. Lori Newman, and Mr. Mike Gray.

I would like to acknowledge Ms. Norma Sellers, Ms. Joan Bares, Ms. Misty Carrillo, and Miss Kay Livingston of the Stimson Library for their assistance with this book. Much of the documentation of our organization's history would be lost if it hadn't been for the present and past staff of the Stimson Library. While the AMEDDC&S has never had an official archivist, the librarians have collected and preserved the organization's history in a series of documents referred to as the "Scrapbooks," as well as cataloged and maintained the AMEDDC&S Special Collection of historic documents. These were invaluable resources in piecing together the history.

A hearty thanks goes to the Directors and Staffs of both the AMEDD Museum and Fort Sam Houston Museum, who were always ready to assist and provide access to their photo and artifact collections. This includes, but is not limited to, Mr. Scott Schoner, AMEDD Museum Director; Ms. Paula Ussery, AMEDD Museum Curator; Mr. Chuck Franson, Registrar; Mr. John Manguso, FSH Museum Director; Mr. Martin Callahan, FSH Museum Specialist; and Ms. Mary Hope, OMH Archivist.

Ms. Liz Holder, Knowledge Management Division, deserves special recognition for having designed the initial maquette of the book layout and digital enhancement of some of the grainier images. Thanks also to Martha Waldman, AMEDDC&S Marketing, for the initial proofreading.

Last but not least I'd like to thank my sons, Rowan and Aidan Neidinger, for their patience and understanding while I worked on "THE BOOK."

– Adriane Askins Neidinger
AMEDDC&S, Command Historian

ENVISION • DESIGN • TRAIN

A PICTORIAL HISTORY OF THE
U.S. ARMY MEDICAL DEPARTMENT CENTER & SCHOOL

1920 *to* 2010

We save lives...on and off the battlefield!

Carlisle Barracks: The Early Years (1920 – 1945)

The last mutter of the guns had barely been stilled in November 1918, when it became apparent to the AMEDD's senior leadership that "the great many lessons learned... during the war should not be forgotten in the years to come, as it had been the custom of the past during the ensuing years of peace between wars." As was the usual practice, a war-weary public and a parsimonious Congress oversaw the dissolution of the magnificent medical enterprise that had mustered 152,000 medical officers, nurses and enlisted corpsmen to serve the over two million American troops deployed to Europe during the conflict.

The Emblem of the Medical Field Service School

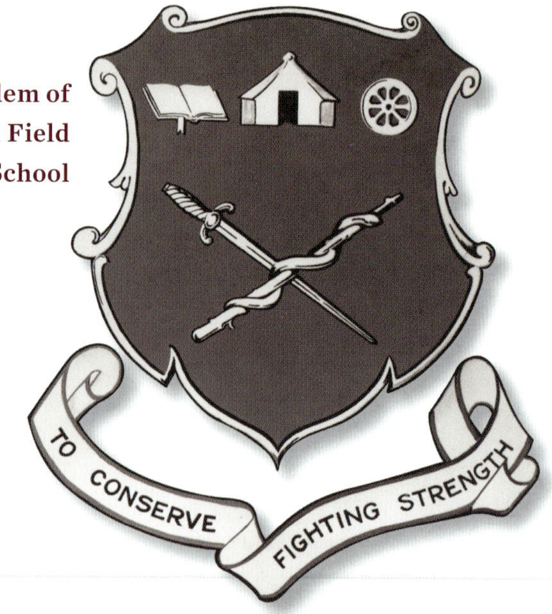

Headquarters Section of the Medical Detachment of an Infantry Regiment
The regimental surgeon, the assistant regimental surgeon, dental officer, veterinary officer and enlisted personnel. During combat they established the regimental aid station for treatment of casualties in the vicinity of regimental headquarters.

(MSFF Illustrated Album, copy 7, 1930. Stimson Library Special Collections)

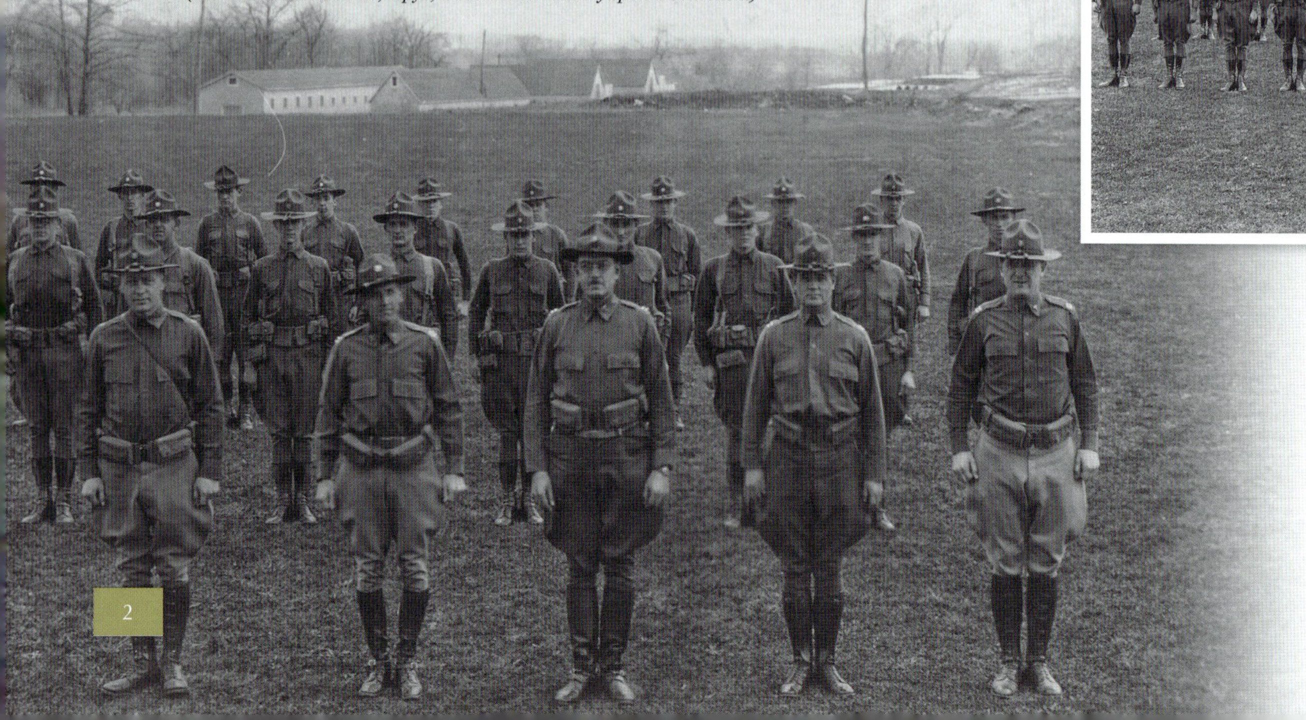

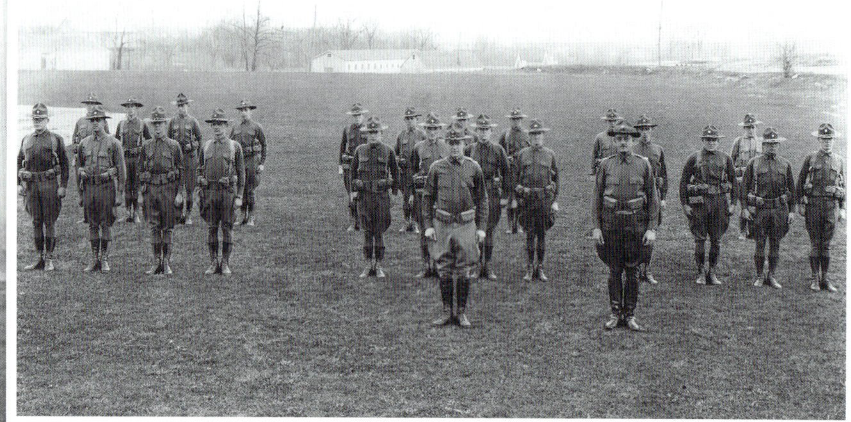

Battalion Medical Section of an Infantry Battalion
The battalion surgeon, the assistant battalion surgeon and enlisted personnel. This section was divided into three squads: (1) litter bearer squad, (2) company aid squad, (3) battalion aid station squad. They collected and treated the casualties in this battalion.

(MSFF Illustrated Album, copy 7, 1930. Stimson Library Special Collections)

The reduced AMEDD's postwar Surgeon General was Major General Merritte W. Ireland, who had headed the department's effort in wartime Europe. He had observed an appalling ignorance of military procedures and tactics among many hastily inducted medical officers and was determined to correct the situation in future conflicts. The creation of a Medical Field Service School was very much the product of Ireland's personal vision, allied to the widespread realization that the swift pace of mobilization in any future war would require all serving medical professionals to possess the requisite military skills and knowledge from the start.

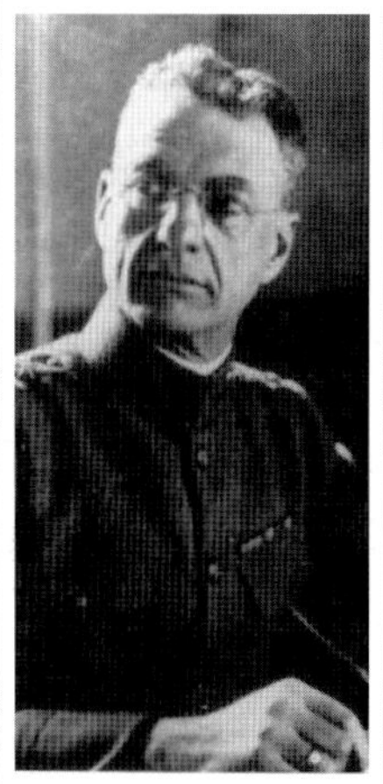

Major General Merritte W. Ireland

(U.S. Army Photo, www.history.amedd.army.mil)

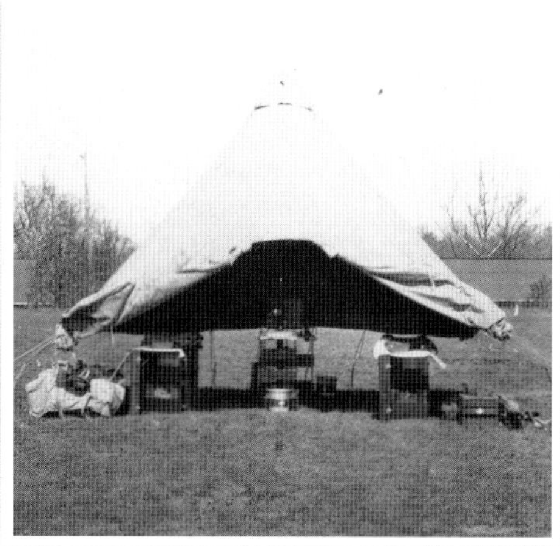

Battalion Dispensary
Established in the field, the Battalion Dispensary was similar to the Battalion Aid Station, which was established during combat. Same personnel and equipment.

(MSFF Illustrated Album, copy 7, 1930. Stimson Library Special Collections)

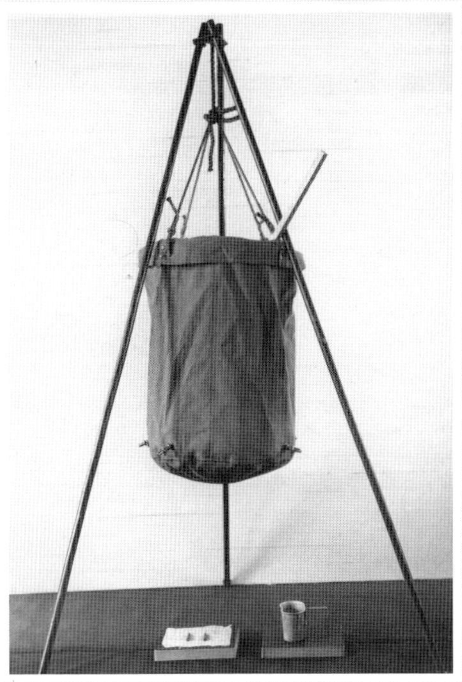

Water Sterilizing Set
Water was chlorinated in this 36-gallon Lyster bag to provide proper drinking water in the field. Calcium hypochlorite was supplied for this purpose in sealed tubes containing one gram each.

(MSFF Illustrated Album, copy 7, 1930. Stimson Library Special Collections)

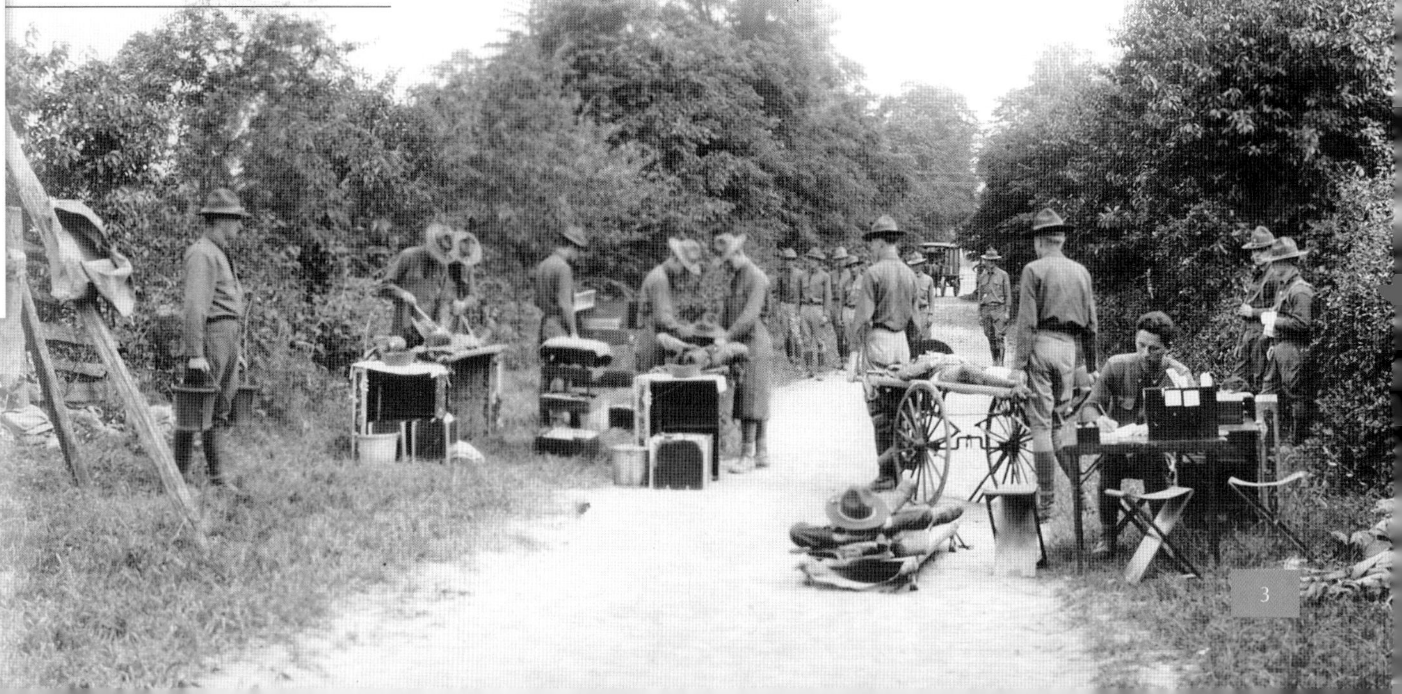

Battalion Aid Station
Casualties are collected at these stations and given emergency treatment. Patients are then removed to the Collecting Station by litter bearers from that station.

(MSFF Illustrated Album, copy 7, 1930. Stimson Library Special Collections)

So it was under Major General Ireland's visionary aegis that the Medical Field Service School was established at the old cavalry post of Carlisle Barracks, Pennsylvania, on 15 May 1920 in one of the seminal events of the AMEDD's modern history. Colonel Percy Ashburn, the school's first commandant, and his staff were charged with creating an institution that answered the need for reservists and regulars alike. On 27 May 1921, the first class of student officers reported to the school to begin its quarter-century of proud service at that location.

The Receiving Department of a Collecting Station
The wounded were collected and sorted at this point and property was exchanged to prevent depletion of supplies at stations farther forward.

(MSFF Illustrated Album, copy 7, 1930. Stimson Library Special Collections)

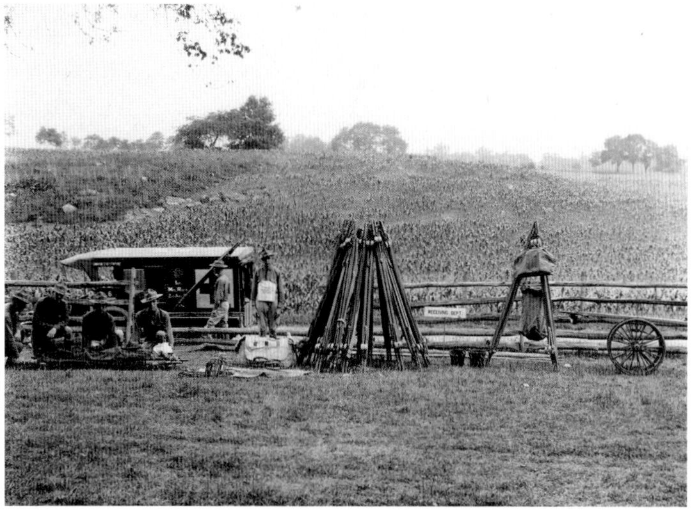

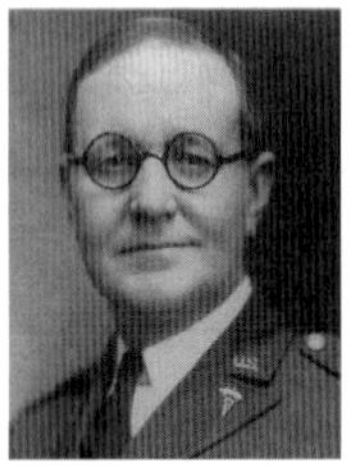

Colonel Percy Ashburn

(U.S. Army Photo, www.history.amedd.army.mil)

The Collecting Company
Each medical regiment contained three of these companies. The company was divided into a company headquarters and three platoons. The first platoon made contact with the brigade it served and also established and operated the Collecting Station. The second and third platoons were litter bearers who brought the wounded from the aid stations to the Collecting Station.

(MSFF Illustrated Album, copy 7, 1930. Stimson Library Special Collections)

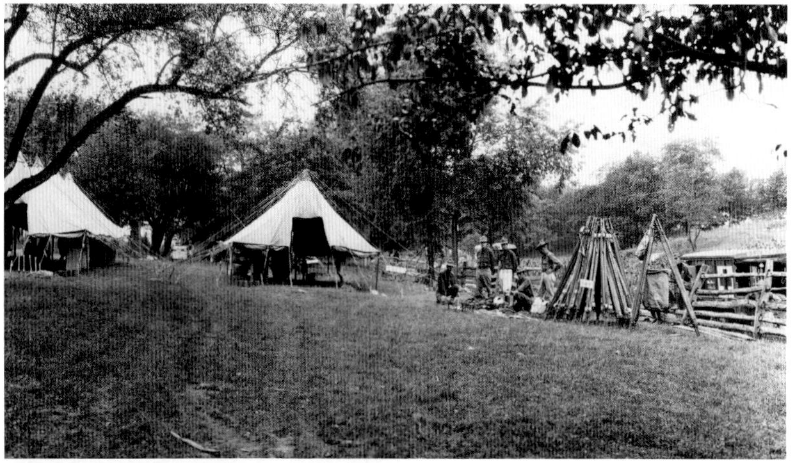

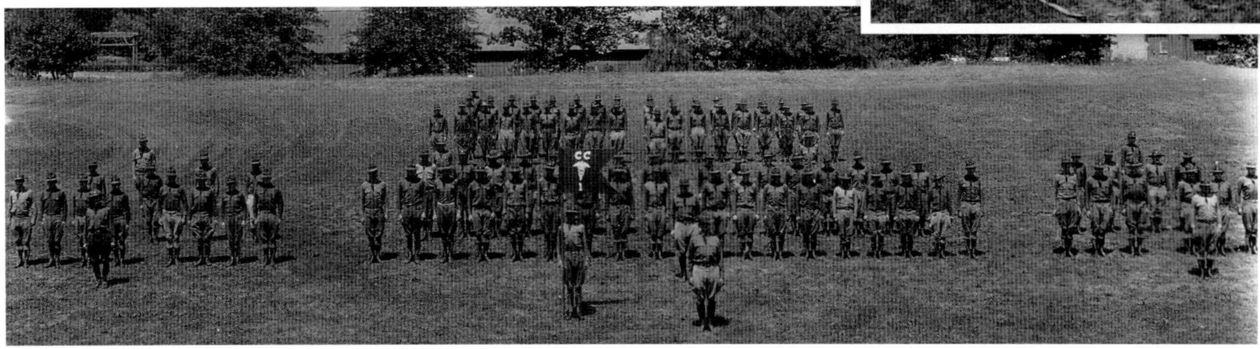

A Collecting Station
One of these collecting stations was established by the Collecting Company for each brigade in action. At this station, patients were sorted, given temporary treatment and prepared for evacuation to the Hospital Station in the rear.

(MSFF Illustrated Album, copy 7, 1930. Stimson Library Special Collections)

As sternly dedicated as they were, the Carlisle faculty were serving in a peacetime Army fielded by a nation that wanted no more of Europe's wars. Funds were sparse and resources limited. By the close of the 1930s, fewer than 2,000 members of the postwar AMEDD had attended a course of study at the Pennsylvania campus. The Medical Field Service School in many ways reflected the Army it served. "Things were held together by custom, habit, standard operating procedure, regulations, and a kind of general conspiracy among the responsible officers," noted a contemporary observer. "In the stillness of peace, the system worked." (Eugene Venable, Command Historian, U.S. Army Health Services Command, draft manuscript, "A History of the U.S. ARMY Medical Field Service School," 1977.)

The Seriously Wounded Department of the Collecting Station
Seriously wounded soldiers were prepared for further evacuation. Field surgery was limited to stabilizing to combat shock and help the patient endure transportation to larger combat hospitals in the rear.

(MSFF Illustrated Album, copy 7, 1930. Stimson Library Special Collections)

The Slightly Wounded Department of the Collecting Station
The less seriously wounded were treated in this department and prepared for further evacuation to the rear. Many of these casualties were returned to the firing line.

(MSFF Illustrated Album, copy 7, 1930. Stimson Library Special Collections)

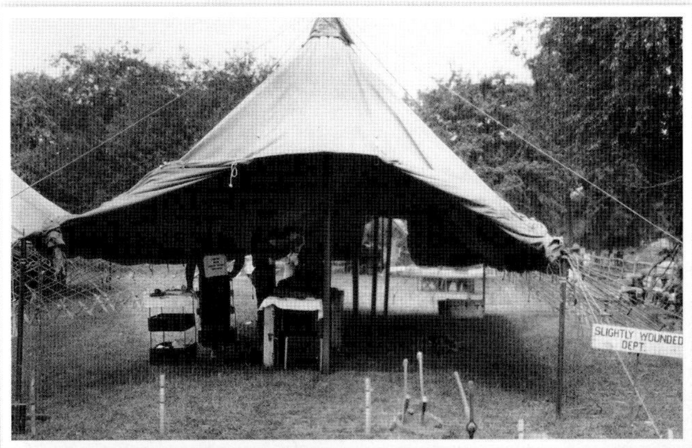

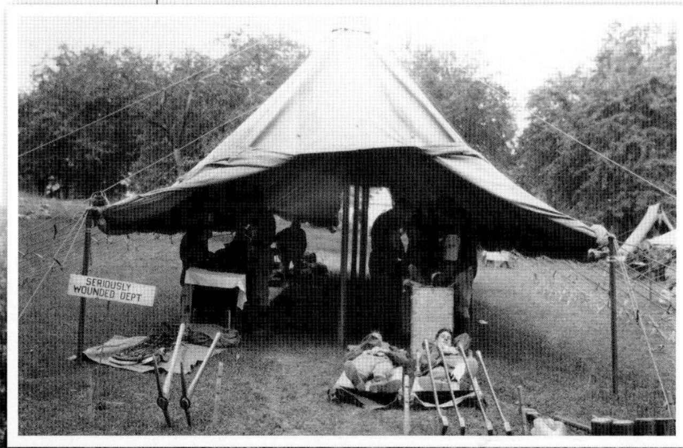

Collecting Company Headquarters, Message Center and Record of Patients
A record was made, at this point, of the number and type of casualties passing through the station. This was also an important center for messages.

(MSFF Illustrated Album, copy 7, 1930. Stimson Library Special Collections)

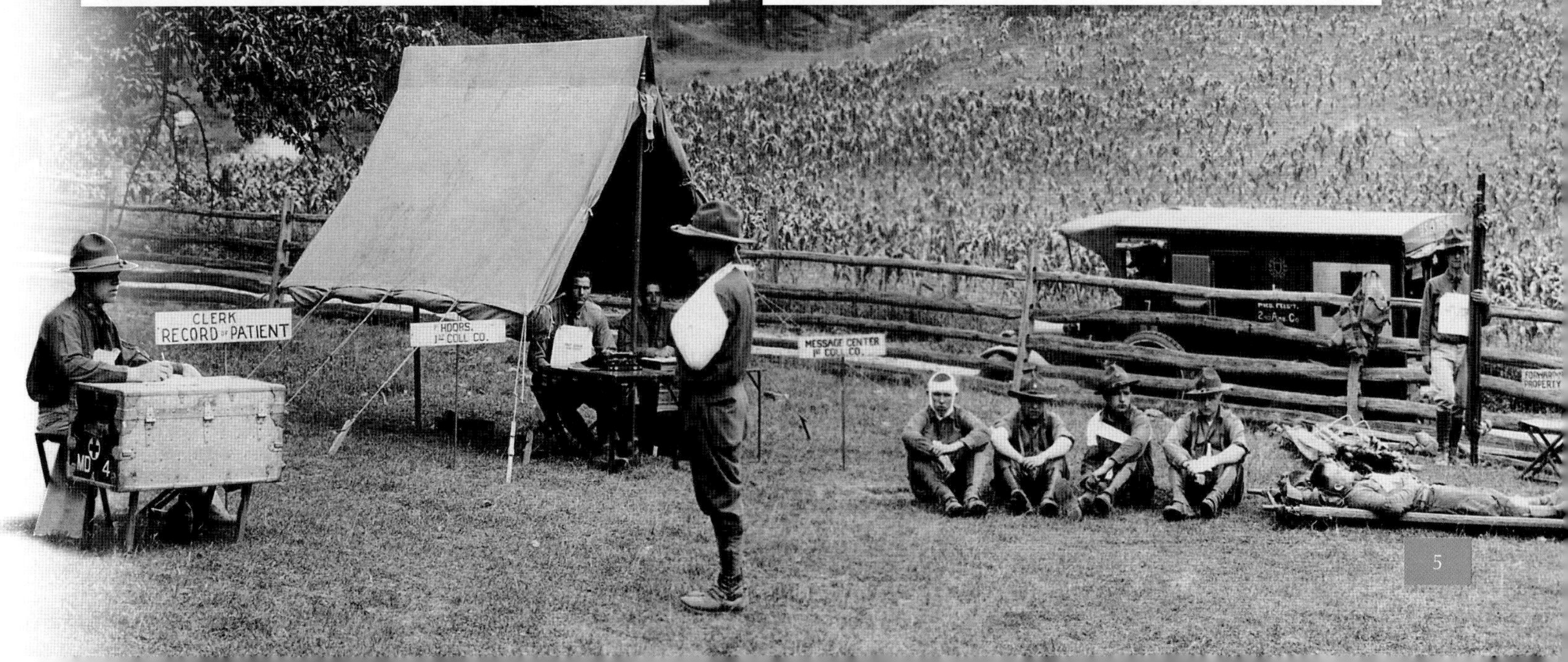

With the rise of global tensions during the 1930s, the AMEDD underwent a modest expansion while the Carlisle school remained dedicated to its mission. "...Courses conducted were many and varied with one endeavor in mind: to train the medical officer in such a manner as to equip him with the knowledge and skills required of a military officer and to enable him to function efficiently as a member of the armed forces." (Eugene Venable, Command Historian, U.S. Army Health Services Command, draft manuscript, "A History of the U.S. ARMY Medical Field Service School," 1977.) The pace and scope of operations were soon accelerated as President Roosevelt declared a limited national emergency, which became a state of war as events proceeded in Tokyo and Berlin. The period of 16 September 1940 to 7 December 1945 is known in the school's history as the "War Program."

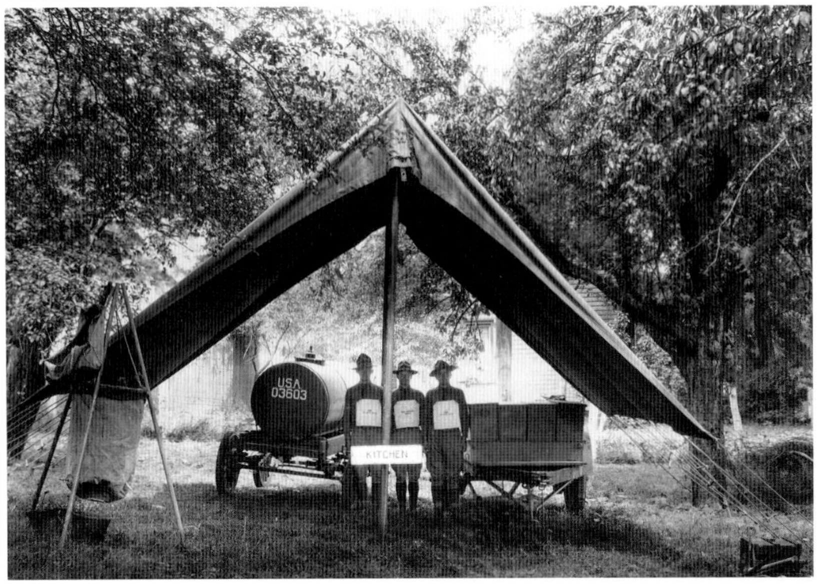

The Collecting Company Kitchen

This kitchen prepared food for the company and hot liquids for patients. A rolling kitchen and water cart were provided.

(MSFF Illustrated Album, copy 7, 1930. Stimson Library Special Collections)

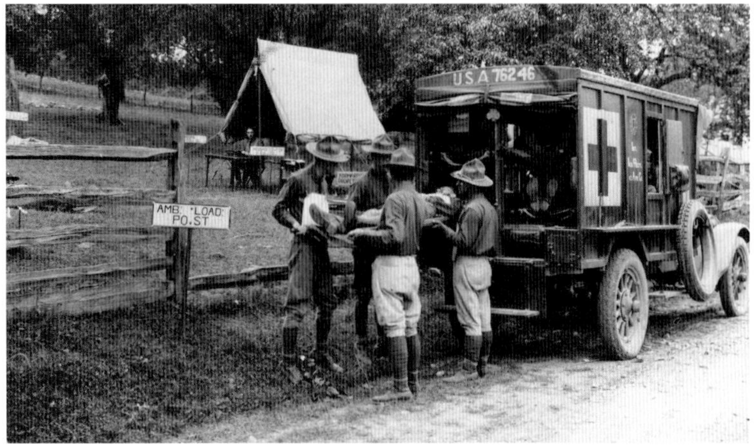

The Forwarding Department of the Collecting Station

Patients were moved to this department to await transportation to the rear. A Loading Post was established at this point by an Ambulance Company of the regiment, and patients were transported by ambulance to the Hospital Station.

(MSFF Illustrated Album, copy 7, 1930. Stimson Library Special Collections)

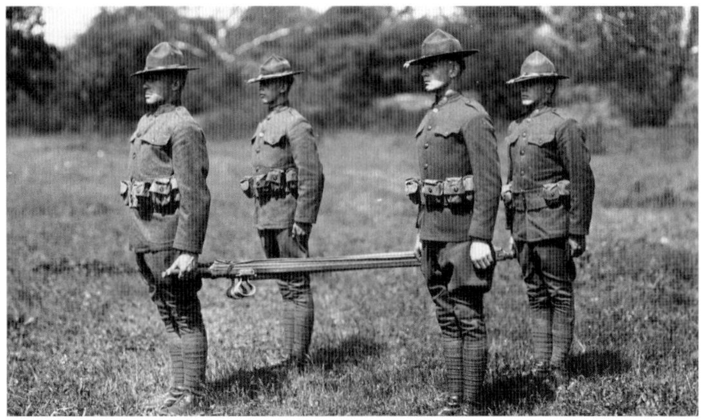

A Litter Squad

Four bearers were used for the average carrying distance. Two bearers were sufficient when using the wheeled litter or when carrying short distances.

(MSFF Illustrated Album, copy 7, 1930. Stimson Library Special Collections)

The curriculum and scale of instruction expanded along with the war effort. On 1 July 1941, the Medical Administrative Officer Candidate School opened at Carlisle. This course played a significant role throughout the conflict. Carlisle was the sole source provider for these valuable specialists until a new facility opened at Camp Barkley, Texas, in 1942.

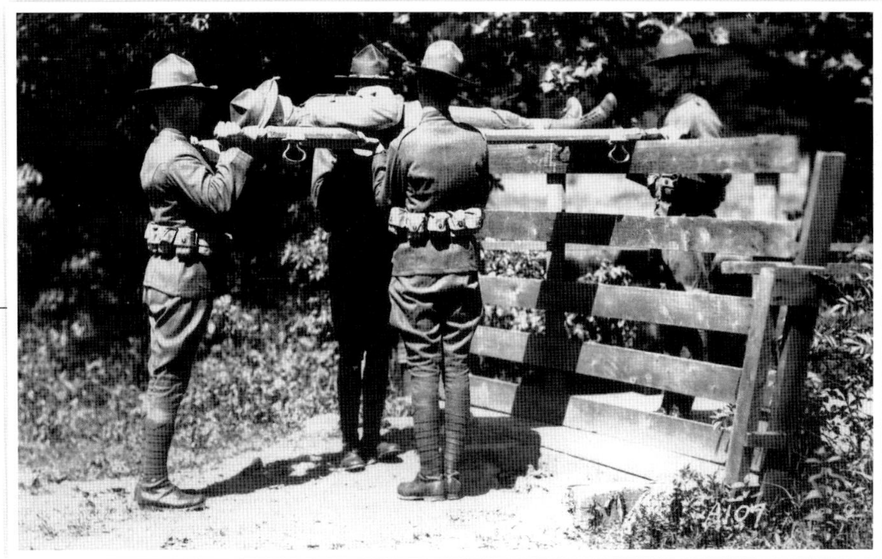

Litter Squad Clearing an Obstacle with a Loaded Litter
Soldiers at the front could be miles from motorized transport. Soldier - Litter drill, described in Training Regulation 405-50, was a vital part of the medical department curriculum.

(MSFF Illustrated Album, copy 7, 1930. Stimson Library Special Collections)

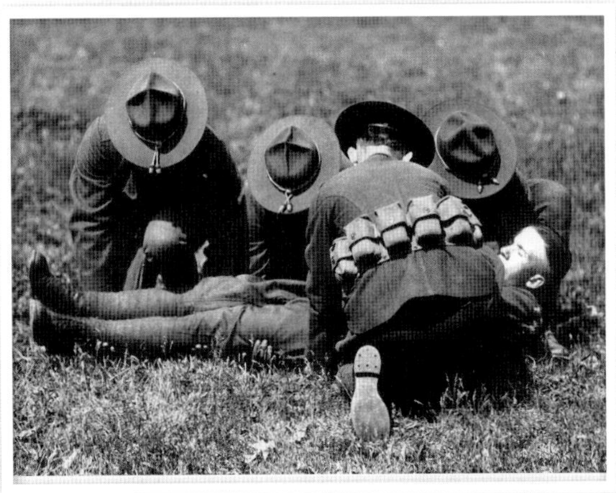

Litter Squad Picking Up Patient
The Litter Squad had to be thoroughly trained in this procedure as outlined in War Department Training Regulation 405-50.

(MSFF Illustrated Album, copy 7, 1930. Stimson Library Special Collections)

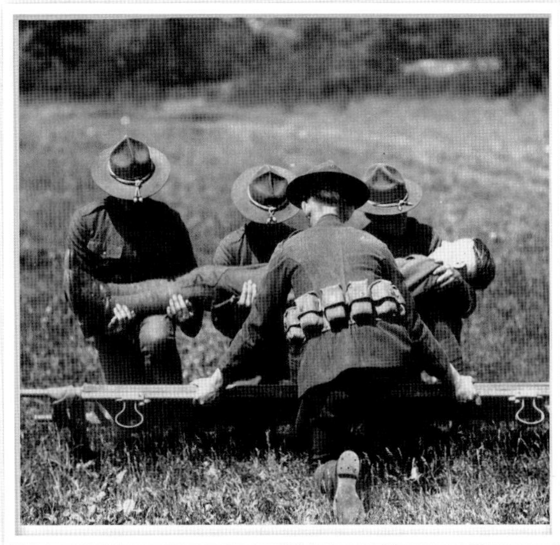

Patient Being Placed on Litter
The patient was held on bent knees while the litter was placed in position. The bearers always knelt on the knee toward the patient's feet.

(MSFF Illustrated Album, copy 7, 1930. Stimson Library Special Collections)

The scale of wartime training had revealed one great challenge that the Medical Field Service School (MFSS) could not address: its limited physical size. The post itself could not host field exercises by units larger than a battalion. The postwar AMEDD needed more room than could be acquired in the Carlisle area. The sun-baked and brush-dotted expanse of Fort Sam Houston, Texas, was accordingly chosen as the new home of the MFSS. On 8 February 1946, the first unit from the school, the 32nd Medical Battalion, entrained for Texas and arrived at the post three days later. Other elements of the school quickly followed, most of them taking up new quarters in the old 9th Infantry Regiment Quadrangle. No one could have guessed it at the time, but the MFSS would continue to serve at its new home at Fort Sam Houston until it entered its second century of duty to the Army and the nation.

(A History of the Medical Field Service School at Carlisle Barracks, 1920-1946, by 1st Lt France F Jordan, 24 April 1961, Stimson Library Special Collections)

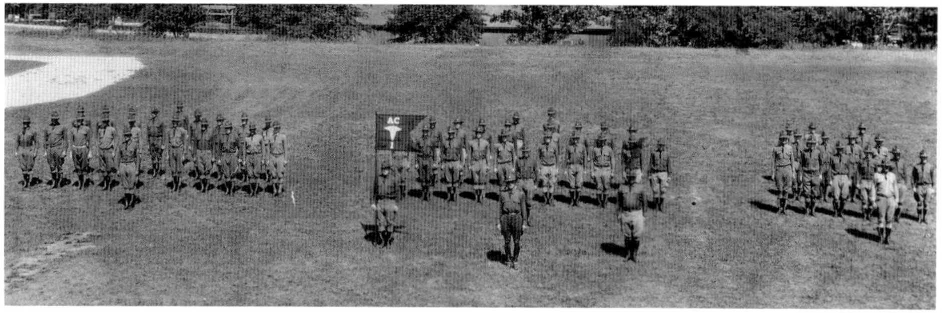

The Motor Ambulance Company
Each Medical Regiment had one ambulance battalion which consisted of two motor and one animal drawn company. This company was also divided into a Company Headquarters and two platoons.

(MSFF Illustrated Album, copy 7, 1930. Stimson Library Special Collections)

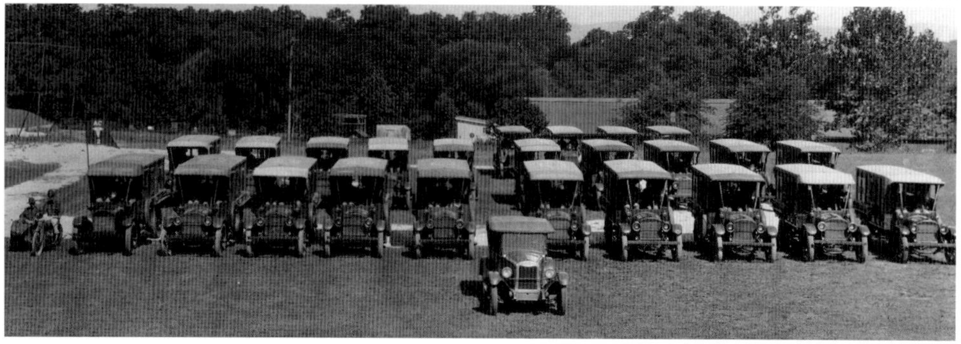

The Motor Ambulance Company
This company also had ten ambulances in each of the two platoons. Four ¾ ton trucks, one motor car and one motorcycle were included in the transportation.

(MSFF Illustrated Album, copy 7, 1930. Stimson Library Special Collections)

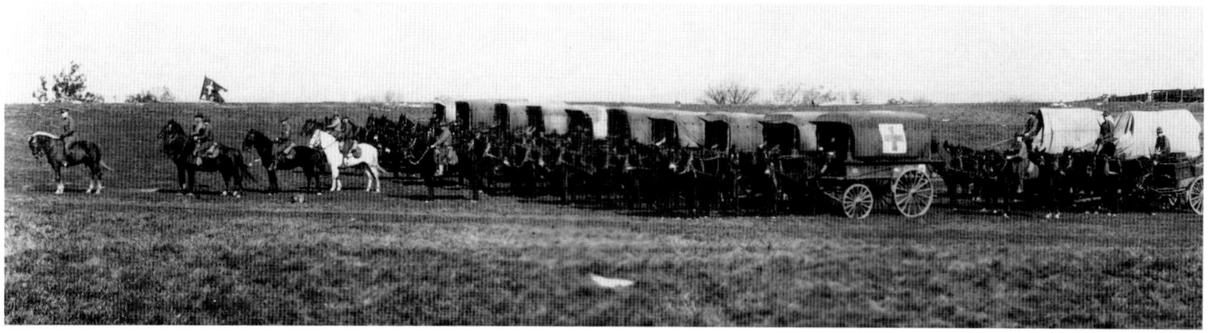

The Animal Drawn Ambulance Company of the Medical Regiment
This company was divided into a Company Headquarters and two platoons. It was principally used where roads were not suitable for motor ambulances.

(MSFF Illustrated Album, copy 7, 1930. Stimson Library Special Collections)

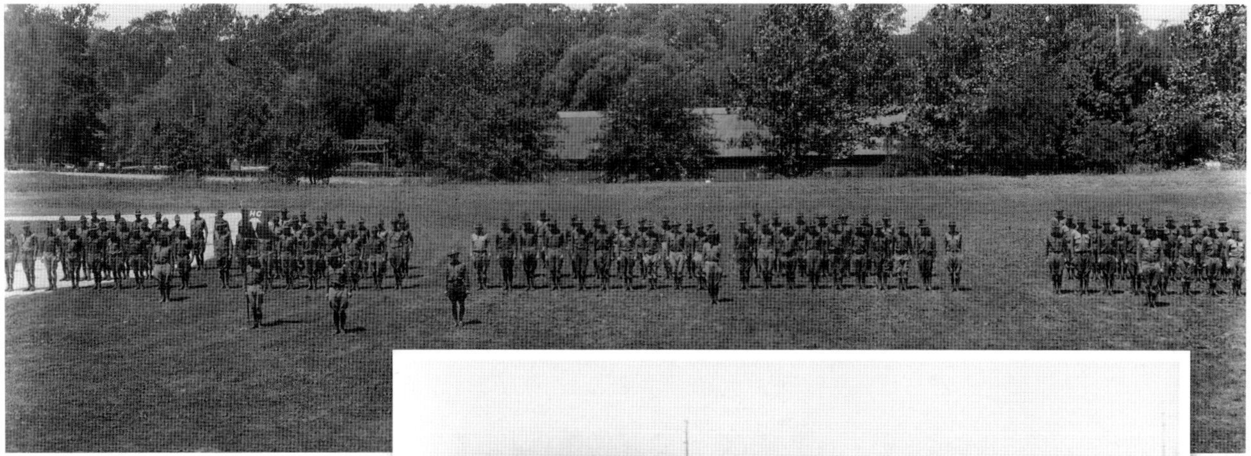

The Hospital Company
Each medical regiment had one Hospital Battalion which consisted of three such Hospital Companies. This company was divided into a Company Headquarters and two platoons. It established a Hospital Station for the sorting and necessary treatment of the sick and wounded of the Division to prepare them for transportation to the rear.

(MSFF Illustrated Album, copy 7, 1930. Stimson Library Special Collections.)

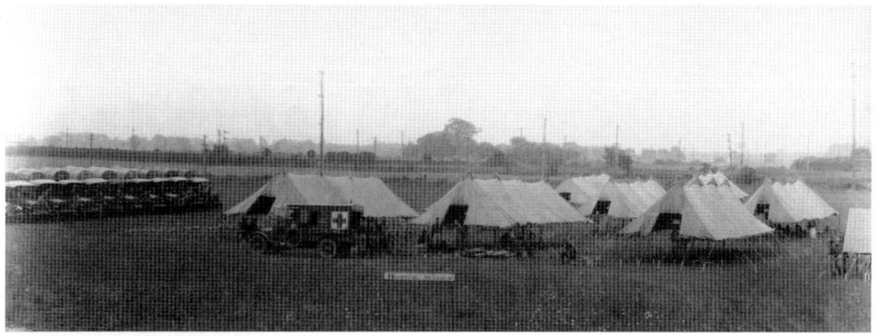

The Hospital Station
During combat, the sick and wounded were transported by ambulance companies from collecting stations to the Hospital Station. This illustrates the only Basic Unit which included the admission, property, gas, bathing, surgical, shock, evacuation and company headquarters tents. Ward tents were added when expansion was necessary.

(MSFF Illustrated Album, copy 7, 1930. Stimson Library Special Collections)

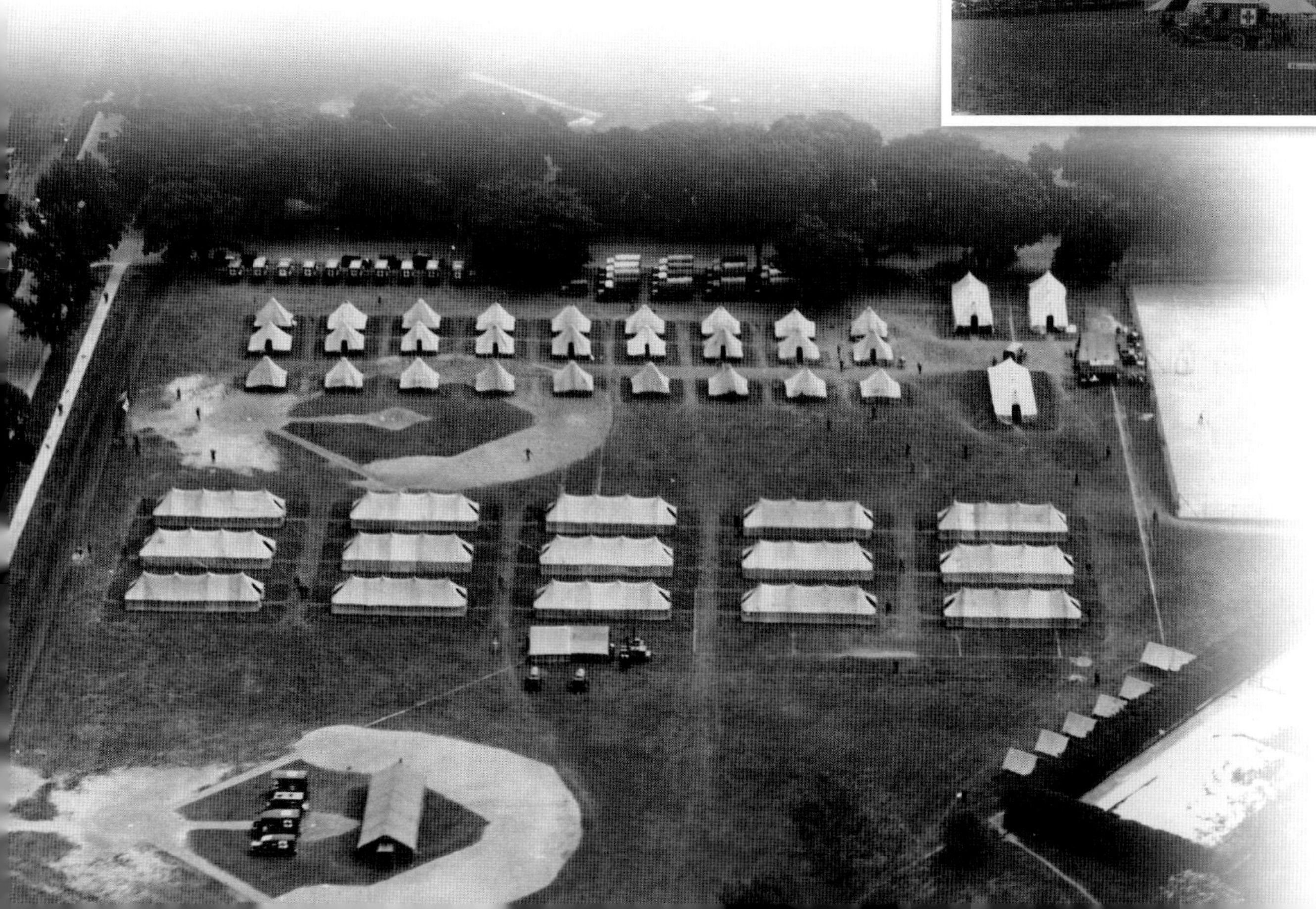

Aerial View of a Hospital Station
Established on the Washington Monument grounds by the First Medical Regiment.

(MSFF Illustrated Album, copy 7, 1930. Stimson Library Special Collections)

The Veterinary Lead Line
Veterinary Aid Stations were evacuated by means of the lead line. Four of these lines were provided for the company.

(MSFF Illustrated Album, copy 7, 1930. Stimson Library Special Collections)

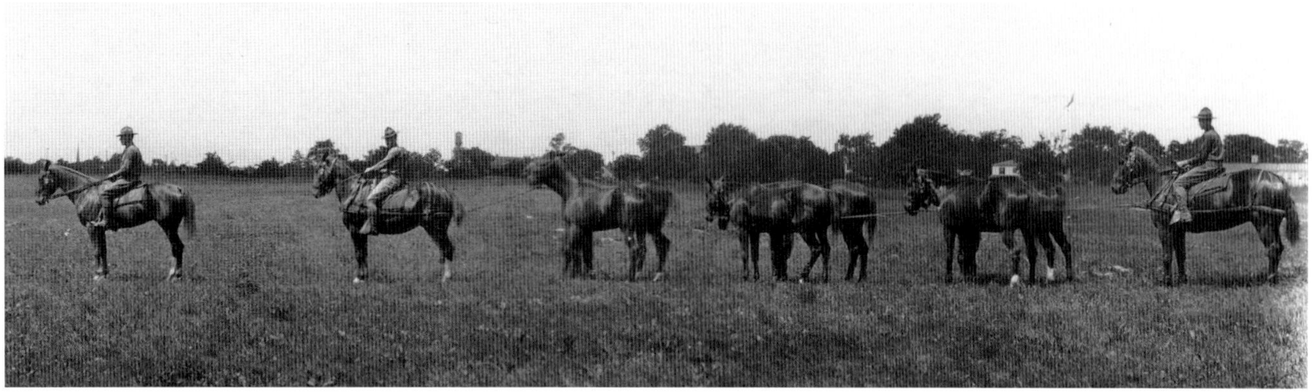

The Veterinary Collecting Station
This station was established for the treatment of sick and wounded animals which were collected from the Regimental Veterinary Aid Stations. They were examined at this station, sorted for further evacuation or destruction or returned to the unit from which they came.

(MSFF Illustrated Album, copy 7, 1930. Stimson Library Special Collections)

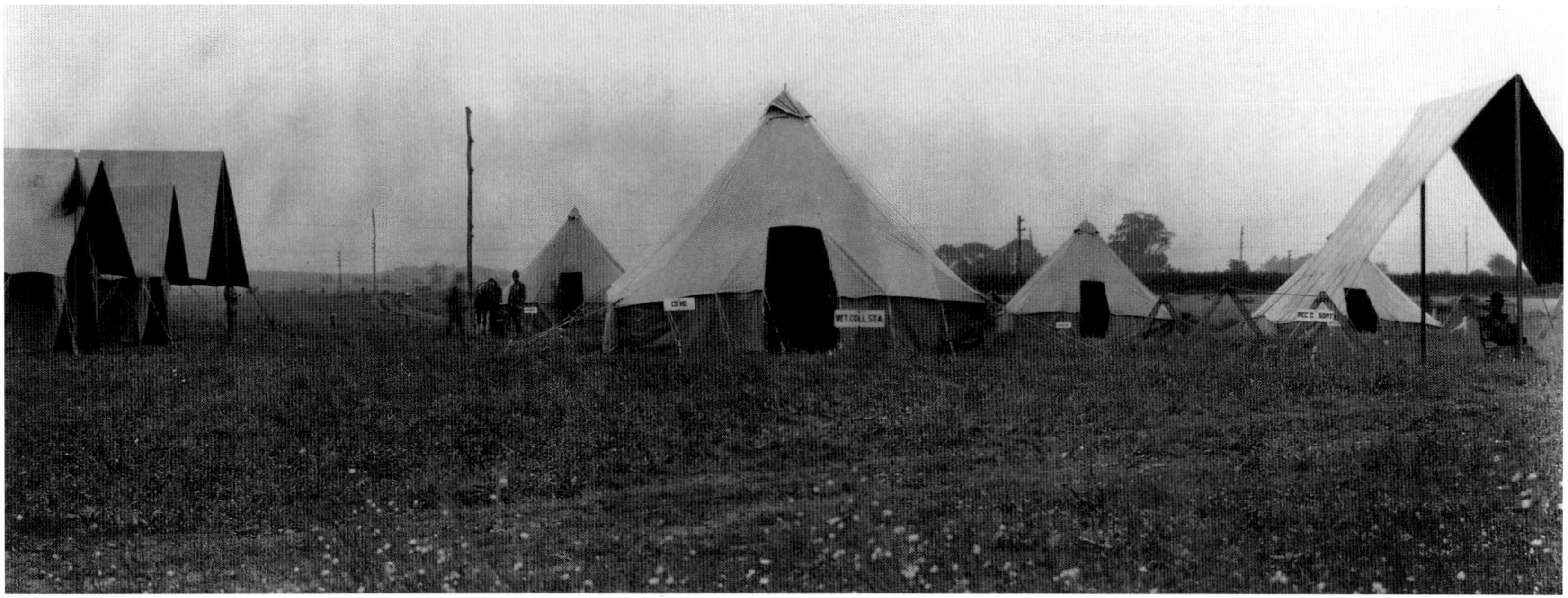

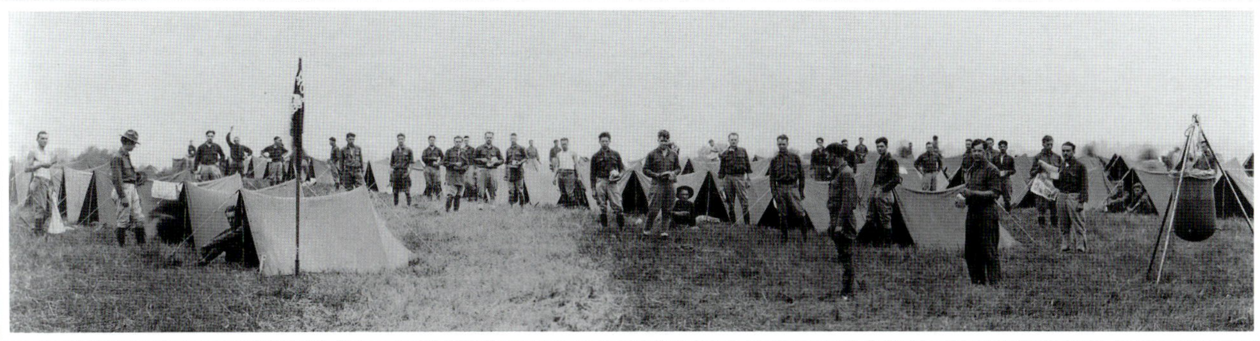

The Reserve Officers' Training Corps (ROTC) Battalion in "Pup Tent" Encampment

The shelter tent was established at the end of the day's practice march. This was an interesting part of the practical training of the ROTC students in Field Services.

(MSFF Illustrated Album, copy 7, 1930. Stimson Library Special Collections)

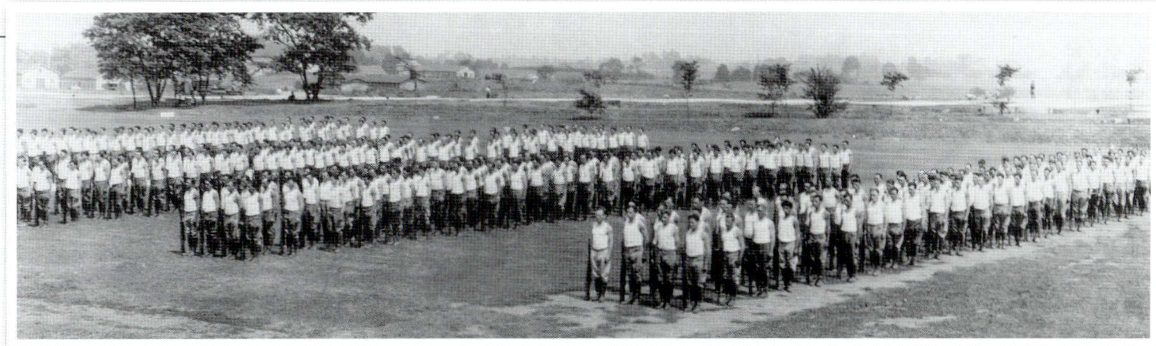

ROTC Battalion Formed for Physical Exercise with Rifles

This exercise was performed as a silent drill and trained the students in proper posture, coordination and precision of movement.

(MSFF Illustrated Album, copy 7, 1930. Stimson Library Special Collections)

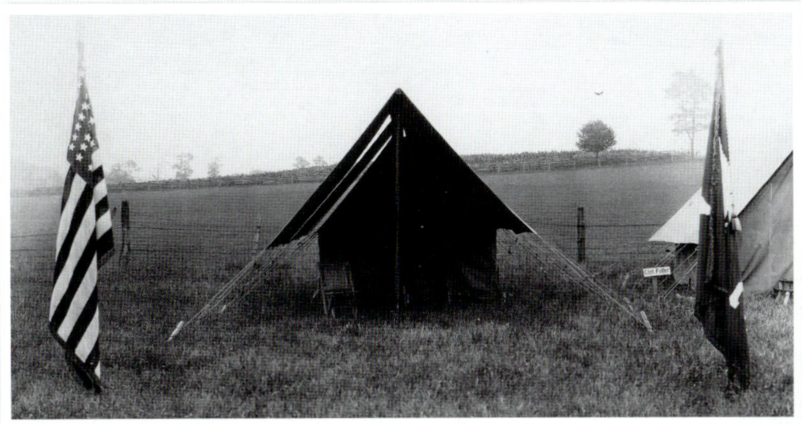

The Commanding Officers Tent

The National Colors were always saluted when passed.

(MSFF Illustrated Album, copy 7, 1930. Stimson Library Special Collections)

Evening Parade of the ROTC Battalion at Carlisle Barracks

This battlefield consisted of four companies. Each company was in command of ROTC students under the direction of regular officers.

(MSFF Illustrated Album, copy 7, 1930. Stimson Library Special Collections)

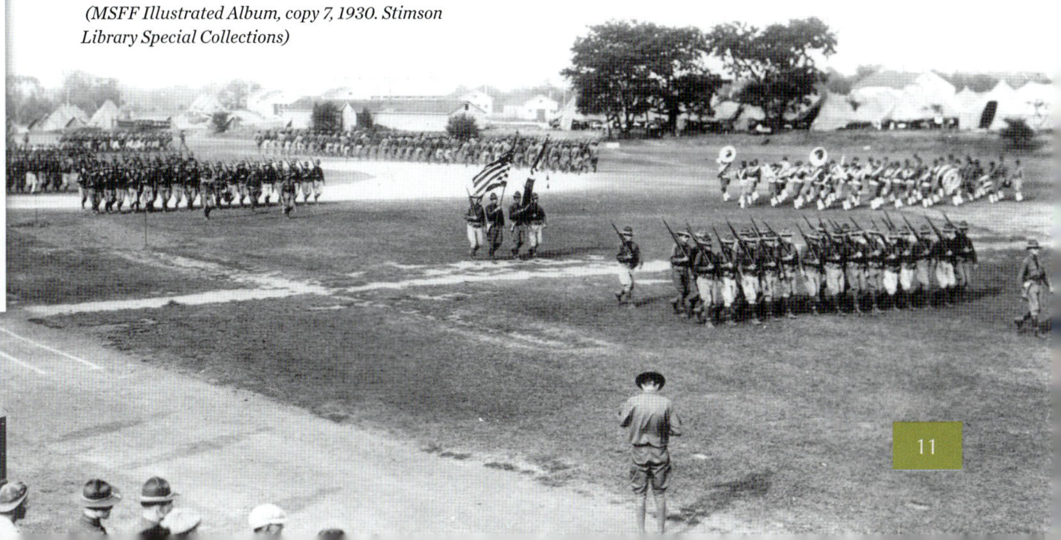

1946 - 1949

In November 1945, the War Department converted Fort Sam Houston into the Army's principal medical training installation. It started with the transfer of the MFSS from Carlisle Barracks to Fort Sam Houston at the beginning of 1946. The MFSS arrived with the 32nd Medical Battalion, the 141st Medical Training Battalion, the 142nd Medical Training Battalion, the 323rd Army Band, and the schools of Neuropsychiatry and Roentgenology. On August 1946, the Army Forces Training Center (Infantry) at Fort Sam Houston was redesignated as the Army Service Forces Training Center (Medical). Training cadres were provided from the Medical Training Group, Army Service Forces Training Center at Camp Crowder, and the Medical Training Section, Fort Lewis.

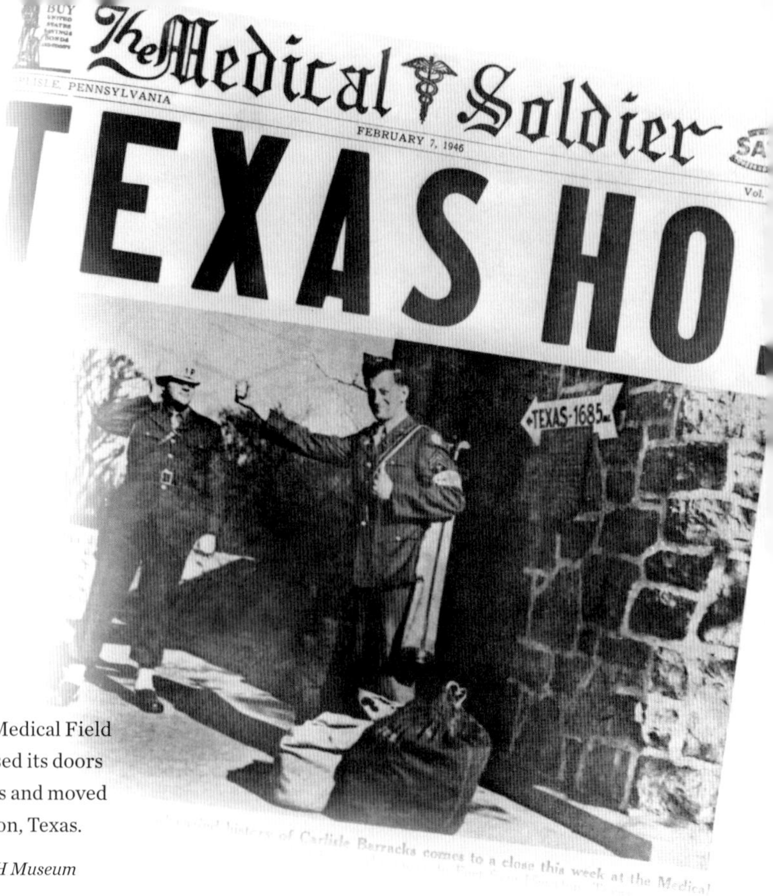

In early 1946, the Medical Field Service School closed its doors at Carlisle Barracks and moved to Fort Sam Houston, Texas.

(U.S. Army Photo, FSH Museum Photo Collection)

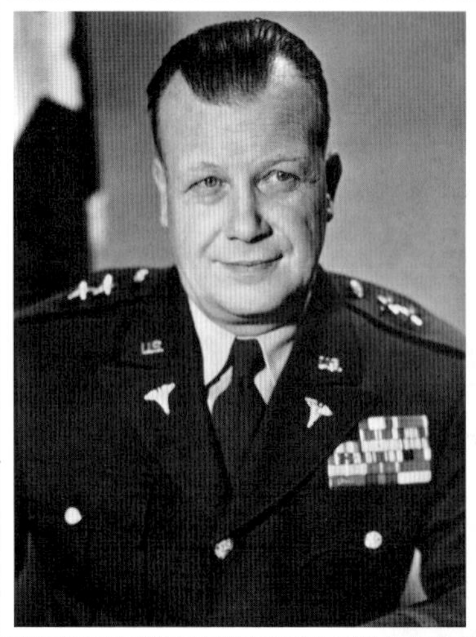

MG William E. Shambora
As a colonel, MG Shambora was the first commandant of the AMSS and responsible for the transition from Carlisle Barracks to Fort Sam Houston.

(U.S. Army Photo, FSH Museum Photo Collection)

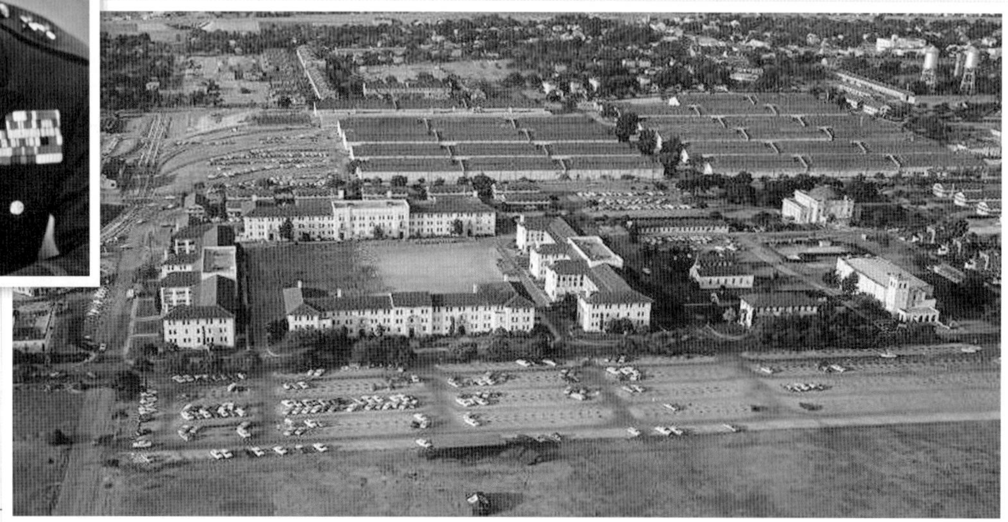

A New Home for MFSS
A pre-1949 aerial view of the 9th Infantry barracks quadrangle with field hospital tents set up on the parade ground.

(U.S. Army Photo, FSH Museum Photo Collection)

Brooke Army Medical Center (BAMC) was activated on 1 February 1946 to command various medical activities at Fort Sam Houston. Under BAMC's command was the Medical Field Service School (MFSS), the Army Service Forces Training Center Medical (ASFTC Medical), Medical Department Enlisted Technician School and Brooke Army Hospital. ASFTC Medical was inactivated in December 1946.

(Fort Sam Houston during the Korean War, 1950-1953, FSH Museum Publication, 2000, pp 5-6)

The MFSS designation was changed to the Army Medical Service School (AMSS), and it took up residence in the former 9th Infantry barracks quadrangle and World War II temporary mobilization barracks at Fort Sam Houston.

The first MFSS instructional film produced by the Training Doctrine Branch debuted at the end of 1946. Titled "Therapeutic Exercise," it featured an Army surgeon talking to his staff about pertinent problems in the use of therapeutic exercise and illustrated the appropriate exercises to be used with patients with nerve, spinal cord, brain, and chest injuries. Equipment shown in the film included a Hubbard tank, whirlpool, and goniometer.

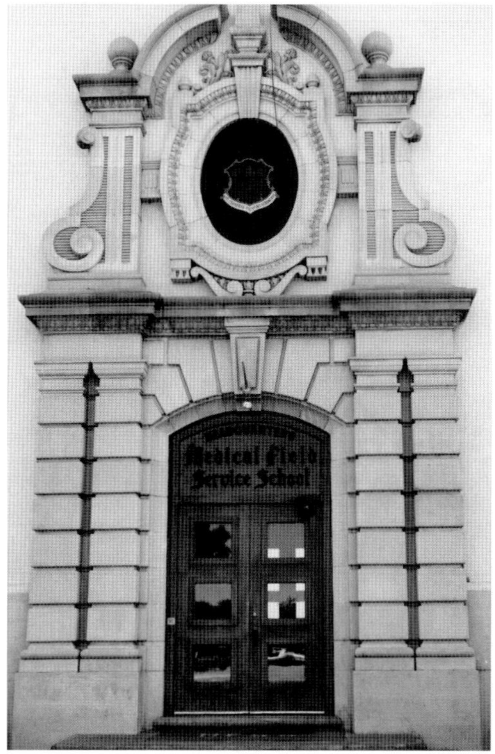

Entrance to the headquarters of the MFSS

(U.S. Army Photo, FSH Museum Photo Collection)

The first Officers' Basic Course commenced on 15 April 1946.

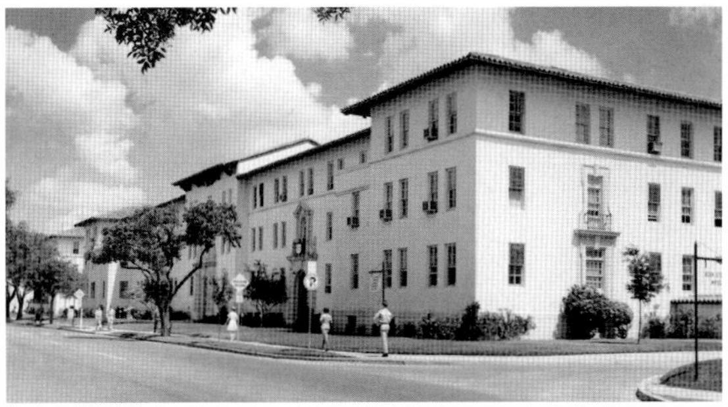

A view of the MFSS HQ from Stanley Road
The MFSS book store was across the street from headquarters.

(U.S. Army Photo, FSH Museum Collection)

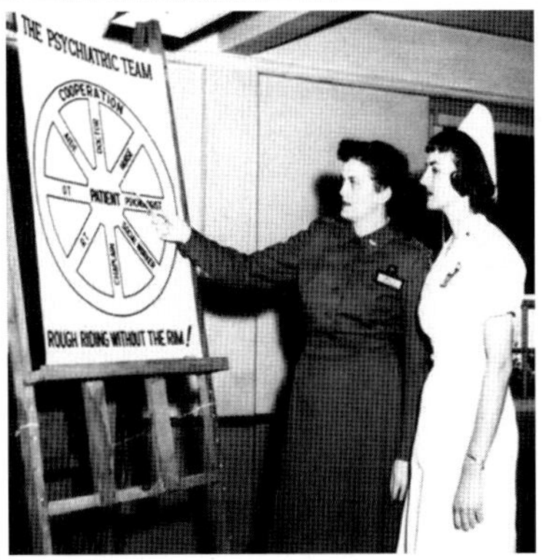

Personnel with the Neuropsychiatric School

(U.S. Army Photo, www.amedd.history.army.mil.)

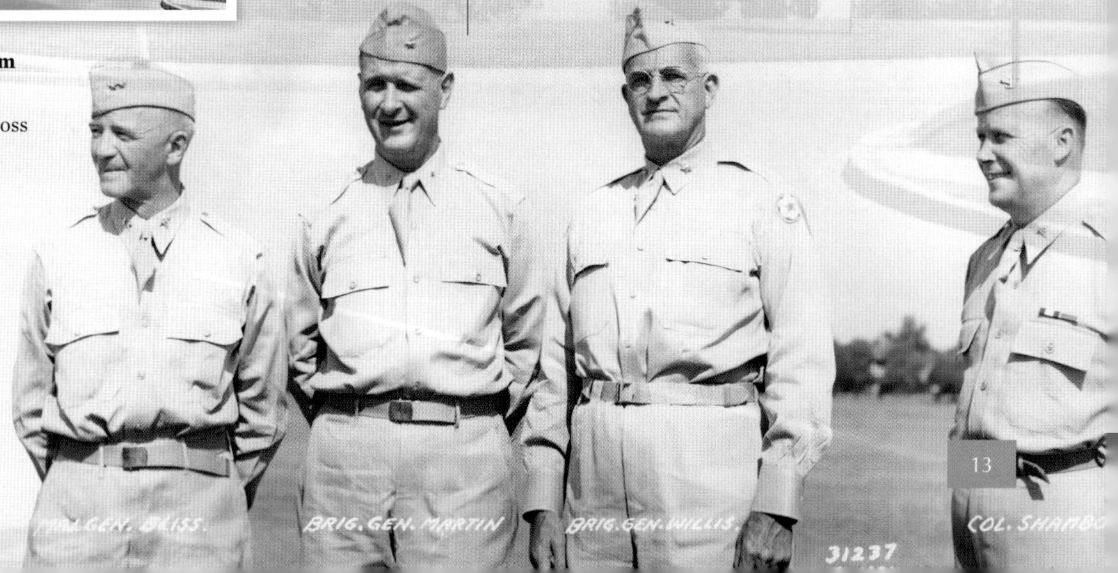

Medical Leadership at Ft. Sam Houston, 1946-1947
Major General Bliss,
Brigadier General Martin,
Brigadier General Willis,
Colonel Shambora

(U.S. Army Photo, FSH Museum Collection)

1947

On 15 January 1947, all independent schools operating under Brooke Army Medical Center (BAMC) were consolidated and absorbed by the AMSS, which was redesignated as the Medical Field Service School due to confusion between the Army School of Medicine at Walter Reed and the AMSS.

Field training at Camp Bullis was put on hold while a commission from the United States Department of Agriculture surveyed the area for a method to control a heavy infestation of Lone Star ticks, *Amblyomma Americanum* (L.), which carry Rocky Mountain spotted fever, tularemia (rabbit fever) and Bullis fever, a disease transmitted by ticks peculiar to the Bullis terrain.

(AMSS Annual Report, 1947, p 3)

The Mission Statement came out of the 1947 SOP for the MFSS. A whopping 41 pages long, the SOP covered everything from organization and structure to the nitty-gritty of syllabi formats.

Mission of the Medical Field Service School (1947)

The Medical Field Service School is a designated special service school of the Department of the Army's school system. Although it operates directly under the supervision of The Surgeon General, it conforms to the policies and requirements for all Army Service Schools.

Its mission is to provide systematic and progressive training in medical field services for Medical Department personnel to qualify them for duty with medical units of The Surgeon General, Army Field Forces, and Air Forces; specifically, to instruct and train Medical Department personnel of the Regular Army, National Guard, Reserve Corps, and Reserve Officers' Training Corps in professional and technical subjects that pertain to the Medical Department and that relate to the Medical, Dental, and Veterinary Services thereof. Emphasis is placed on medical support of tactical units in combat. Also, to act as an agency of The Surgeon General in the development of doctrine and progressive training methods for the medical service.

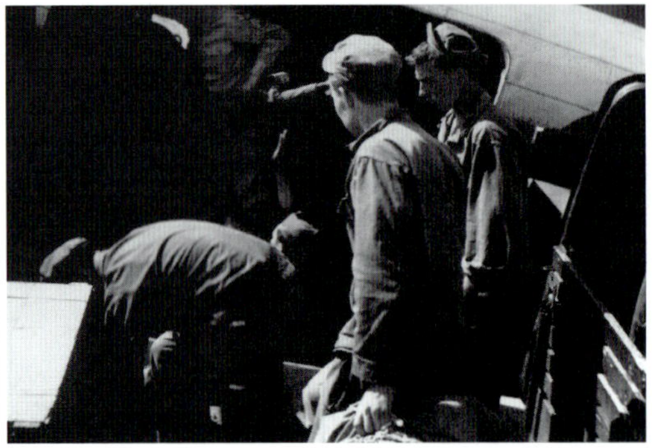

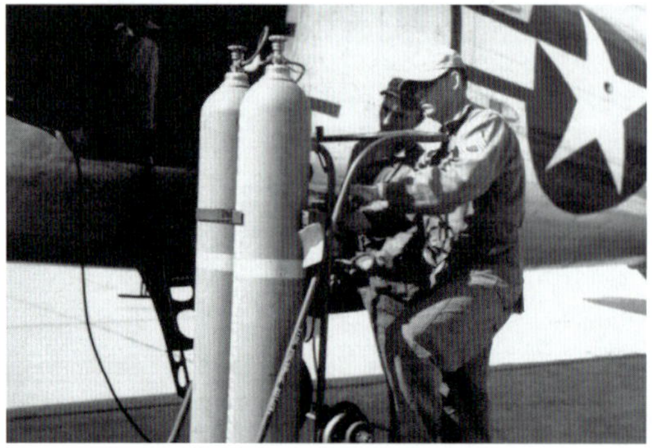

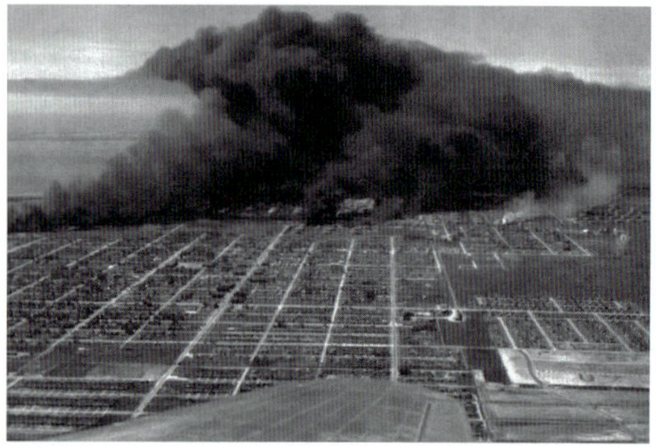

The Texas City Disaster

MFSS personnel and supplies deployed to assist with patient evacuation from the historic Texas City Disaster. Smoke billowed from the Texas City fires, caused by the explosion of 2,300 tons of ammonium nitrate.

(AMSS Annual Report, 1947)

Texas City Disaster

MFSS doctors, nurses, and medical transportation personnel, as part of the Fourth Army Disaster Team, responded, along with the Navy, Coast Guard, Marine Reserve and Texas National Guard medical personnel, to the April 16-17 Texas City Disaster, the largest industrial accident in U.S. history. The disaster began on board the SS *Grandchamp,* a cargo vessel docked at the port of Texas City. The vessel, laden with 2,300 tons of ammonium nitrate (fertilizer), exploded, and the resulting chain of fires and explosions flattened most of Texas City and killed at least 581 people. Much of MFSS participation in the disaster relief was involved in the reactivation of the hospital at Fort Crockett Station, providing staff, supplies and transportation of the injured to Fort Crockett and supporting hospitals in Galveston; and providing first aid, food, water, and comfort to the remaining city residents until the Red Cross disaster operations could take over.

(AMSS Annual Report, 1947, Inclusion 9, p 4)

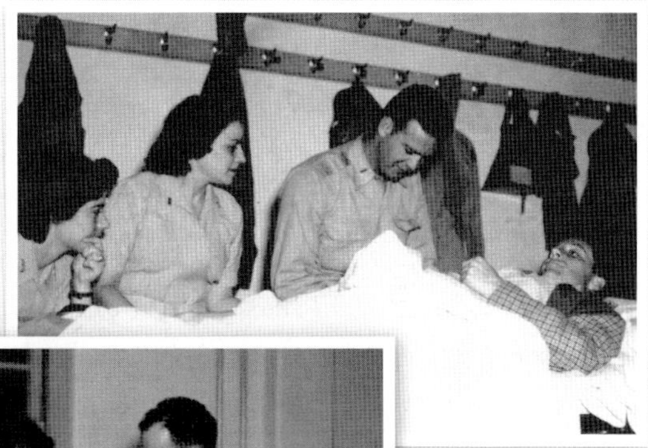

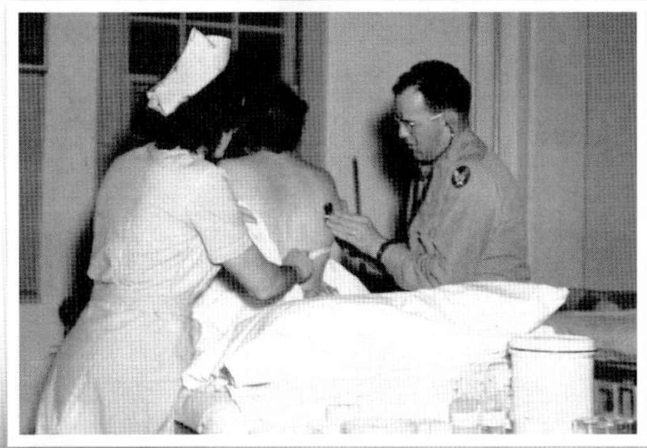

Army Medical personnel examined and transported disaster victims.

(Photos from AMSS Annual Historical Report, 1947)

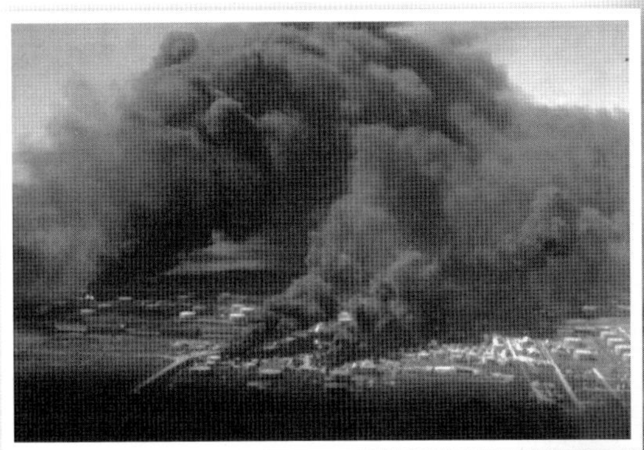

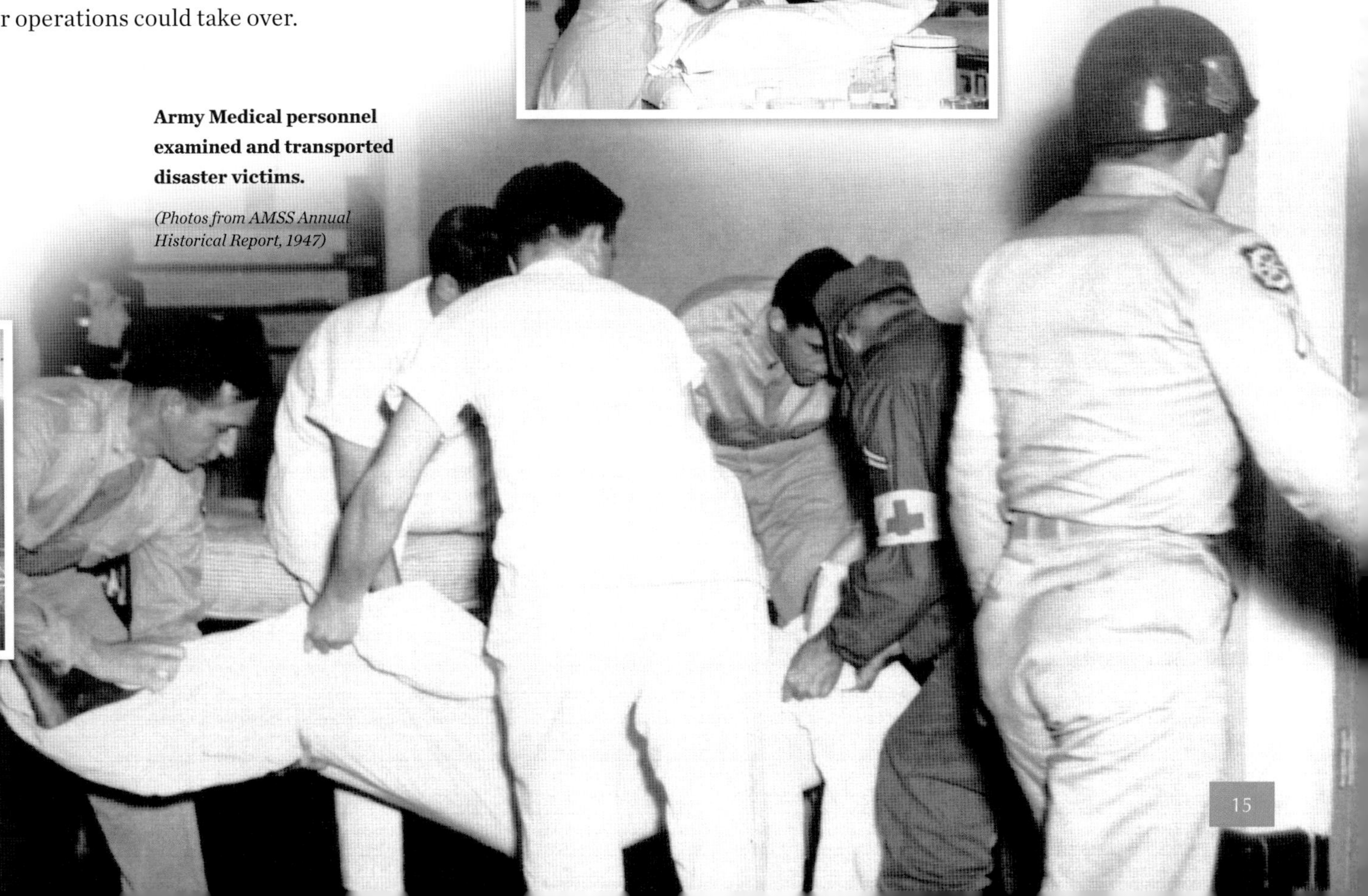

1947

The MFSS was housed in 285 buildings of all types, grouped in several locations around Fort Sam Houston.

"...in view of the present shortage of trained personnel throughout the Army, and the school in particular, it follows, ipso facto, that the school faculty and cadre are put to the unhappy task of maintaining liaison, training, police, and security of large and dispersed areas, a situation that would not be current were the school housed more compactly and adequately than at present."

(AMSS Annual Report, 1947, p 4)

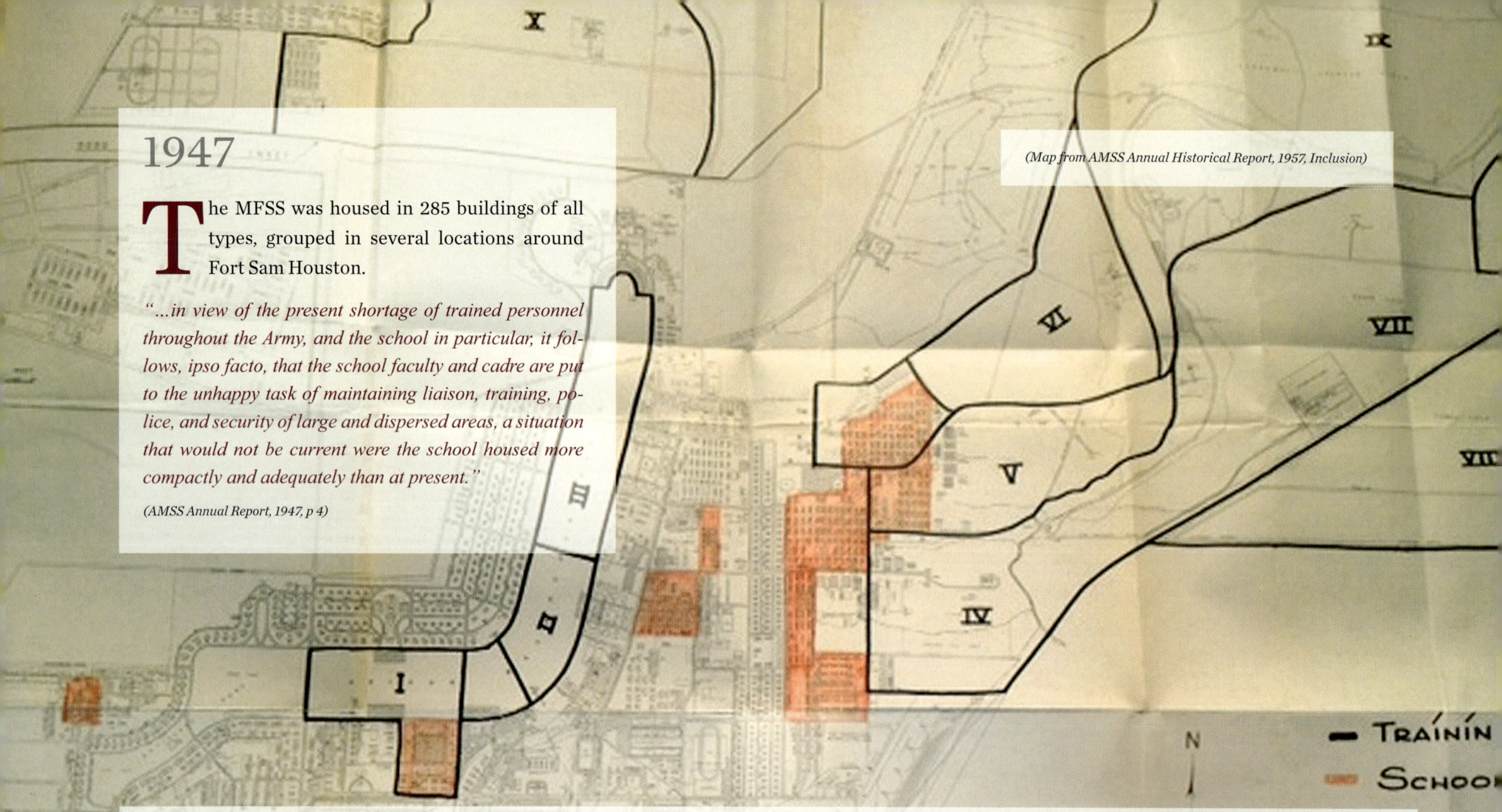

(Map from AMSS Annual Historical Report, 1957, Inclusion)

MFSS mission coverage was extended to endeavors far different from its original purpose. By the end of 1947, it offered 15 training courses for commissioned officers and 17 technical courses for enlisted personnel. The Medical Department Officers' Basic Course, a 40-week training program, opened to eligible members of the Army, Navy, and Air Force. Its scope of instruction was in leadership; Army and medical administration; Army dental service; field medicine and surgery; military neuropsychiatry; nursing service; preventive medicine; tactics, techniques and logistics; and the Army veterinary service. The Medical Department Officers' Associate Basic Course, an eight-week training program, explained the duties and functions of the Medical Department to officers of the regular Army, Reserve Corps, National Guard and other U.S. military branches.

One of the most notable courses founded in 1947 was the Hospital Administration Course. In 1951, it became the Army-Baylor University Program in Hospital Administration. The concept for the course stemmed from BG Martin's experience as a surgeon serving the Fifth Army in Italy. In that post, BG Martin saw the necessity of better trained ancillary personnel so that physicians could focus on patient care and not resource management.

A sanitary demonstration area was constructed along the Salado Creek to represent a basic set-up to teach the rudiments of field sanitation from the standpoints of expediency and improvisation. Special emphasis was placed on basic construction, location and minimizing special materials and equipment.

(AMSS Annual Report, 1947, Inclusion 3)

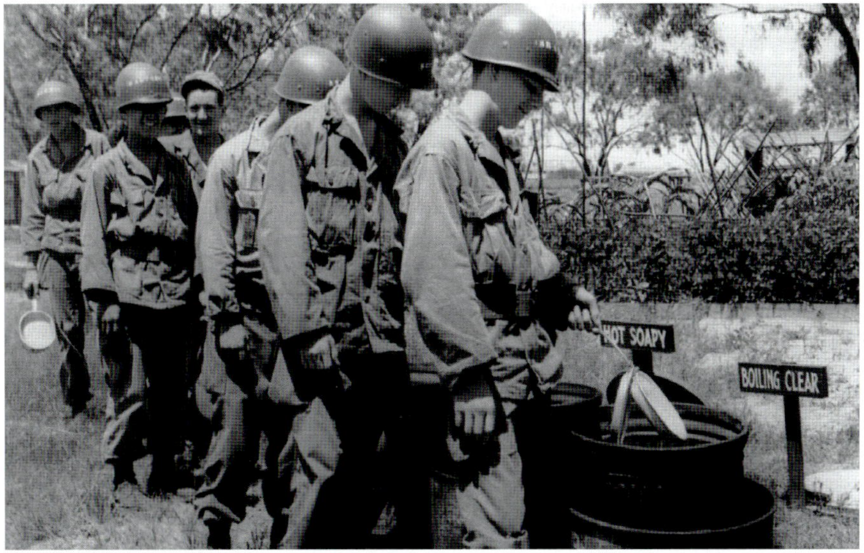

Mess kit cleaning demonstration

(Photos from AMSS Annual Historical Report, 1947, Inclusion 3)

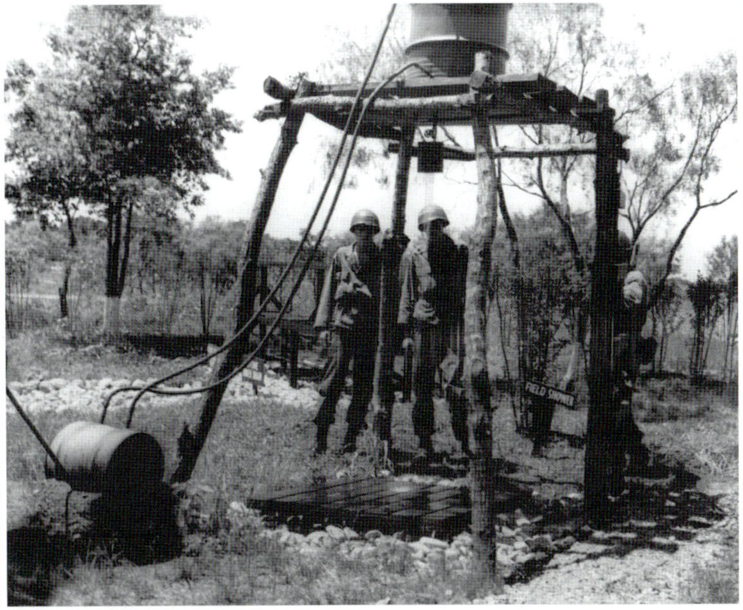

A field shower constructed from fuel drums

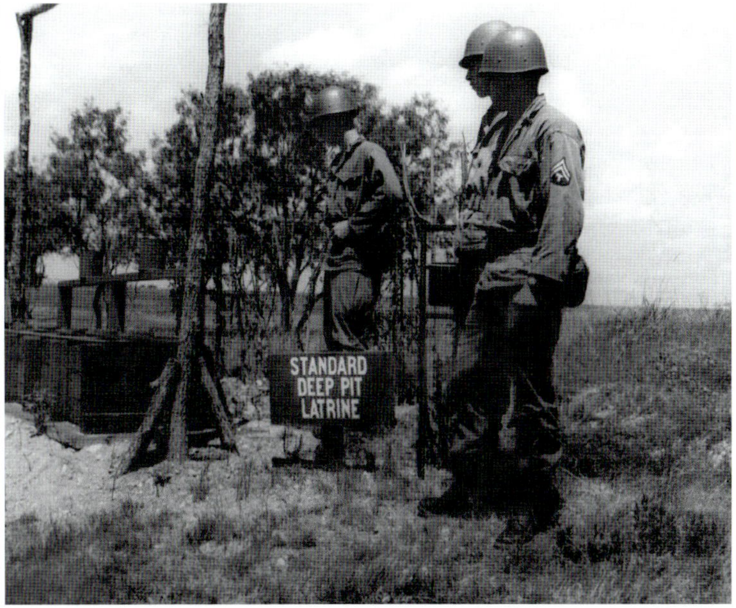

A basic four-hole-deep pit latrine

1947

The four art departments on Post were combined in November 1946 to create the Visual Aids Section of the MFSS. Staffed with one officer, three enlisted personnel and five civilian artists, the Visual Aids Section created all artwork required throughout BAMC. The section's most important job of 1947 was the Army Week Exhibit and drawings for training manuals compiled by the Department of Training Doctrine.

(AMSS Annual Report, 1947, Inclusion 5)

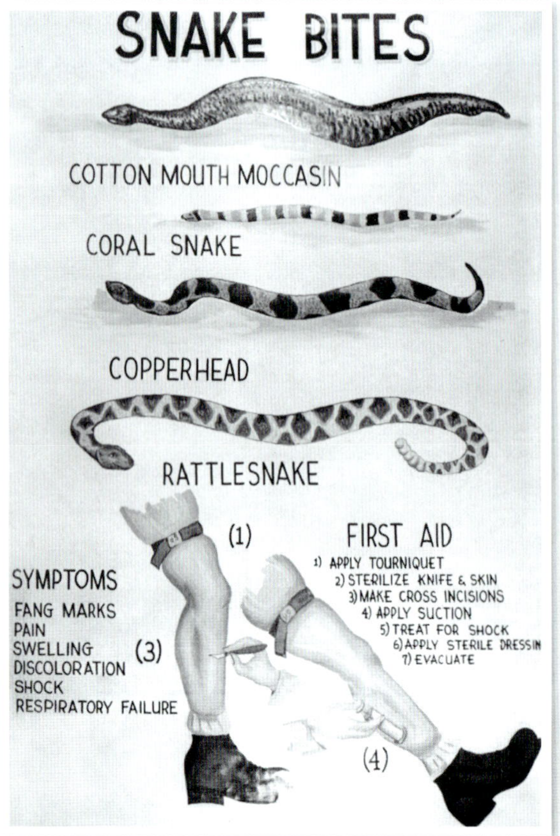

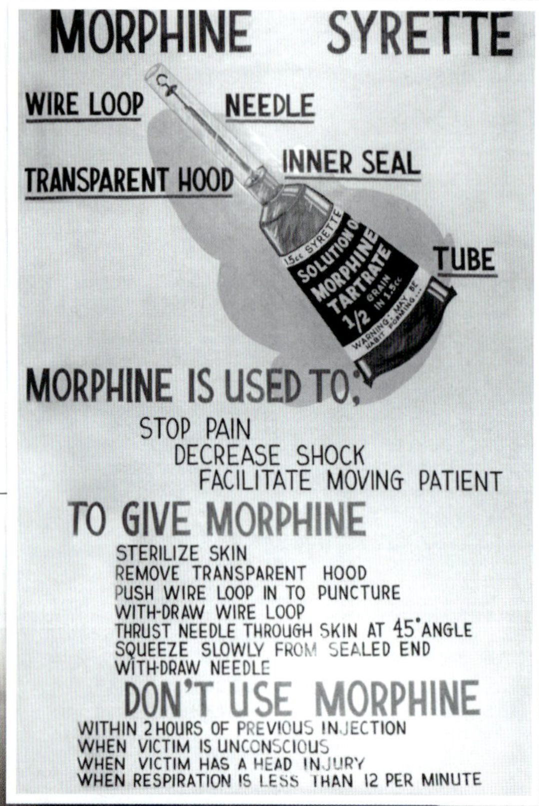

Instructional boards created by the Visual Aids Section in 1947

(AMSS Annual Historical Report, 1947, Inclusion 5)

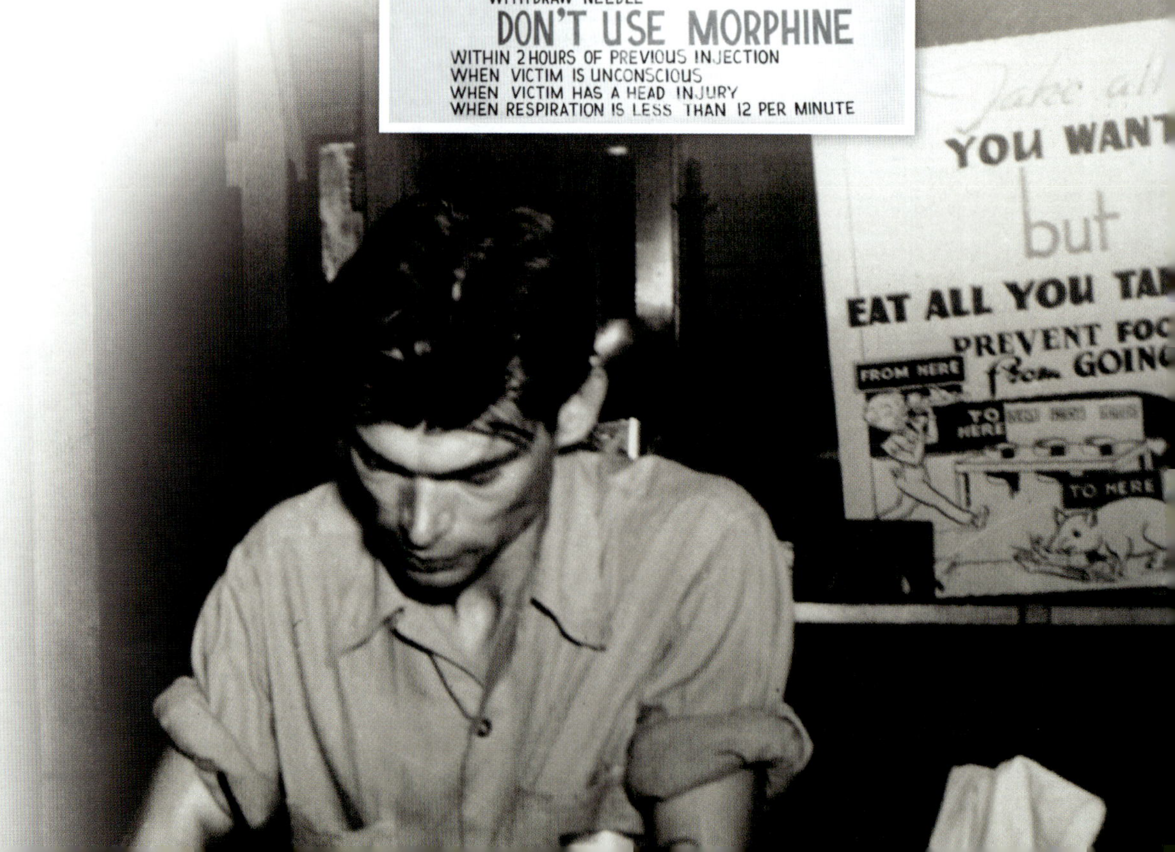

A civilian employee of the Visual Aids Section

(AMSS Annual Historical Report, 1947, Inclusion 5)

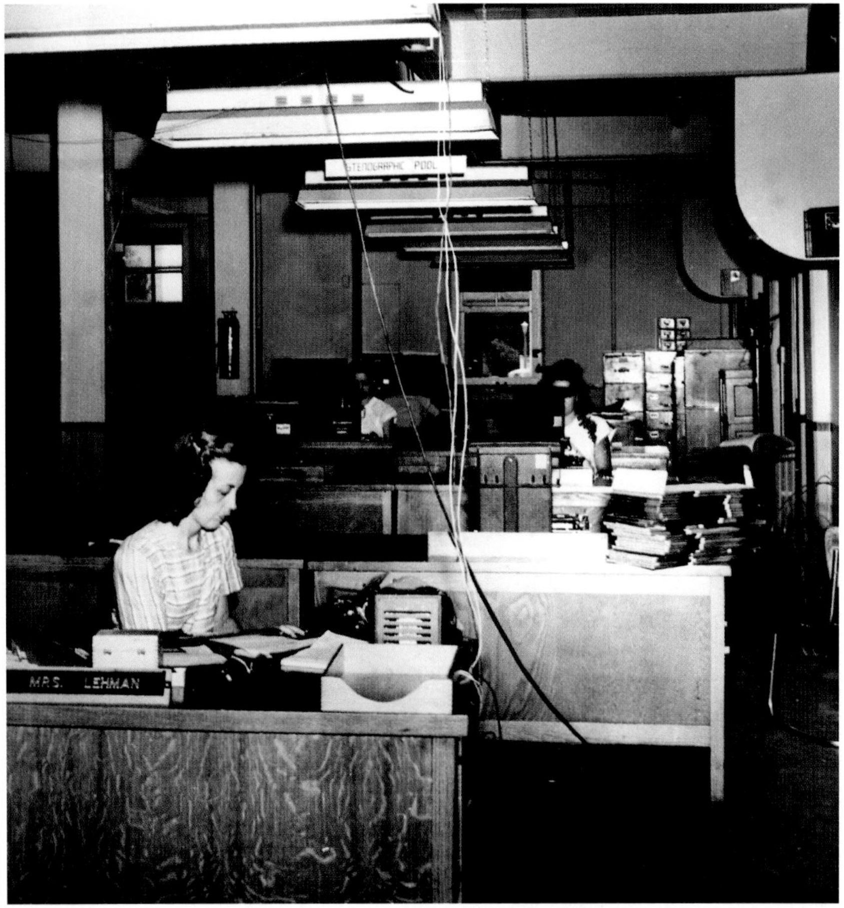

The Stenographic Pool of the Department of Training Doctrine

(AMSS Annual Historical Report, 1947, Inclusion 5)

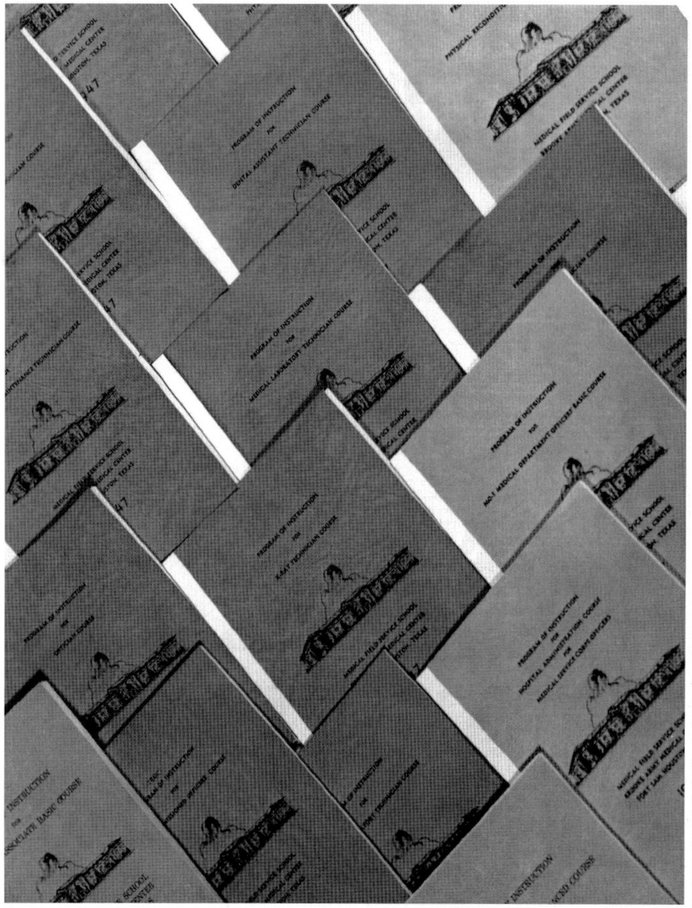

A sampling of Programs of Instruction manuals published by the MFSS in 1947

(AMSS Annual Historical Report, 1947, Inclusion 5)

1947

Army Week, celebrated 6-12 April 1947, was a public affairs event, when the mess halls, library, classrooms, and other facilities, as well as a large display of vehicles and equipment, were open to the general public. Parades, ceremonies, the Jodie Team's expert drill, exhibits and a realistic "amputation" operation were demonstrated twice daily.

(AMSS Annual Report, 1947, Inclusion 10)

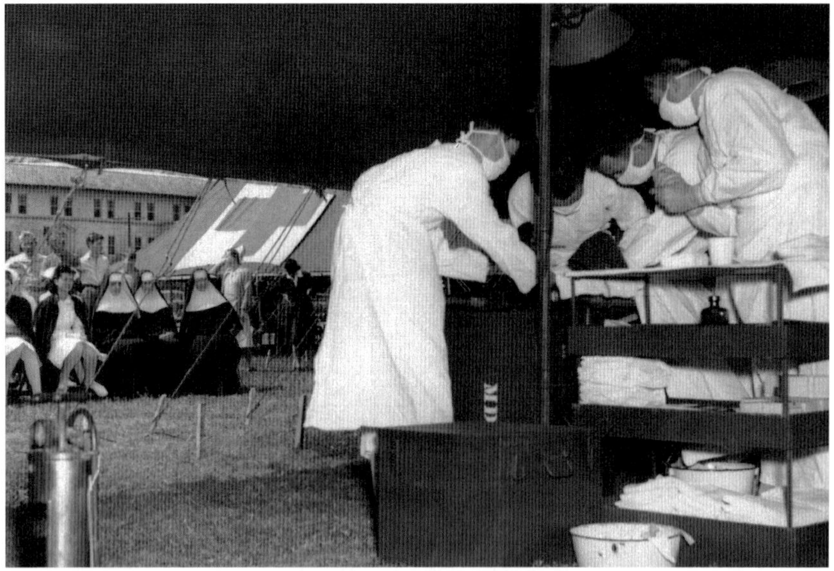

Army Surgeons conduct a realistic amputation twice daily during Army Week

(AMSS Annual Report, 1947, Inclusion 10)

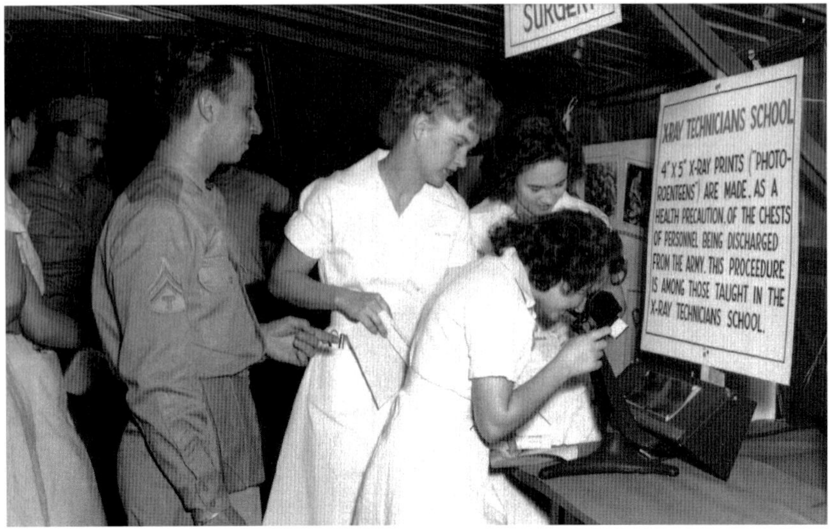

The X-Ray Technician School's exhibit during Army Week

(AMSS Annual Report, 1947, Inclusion 10)

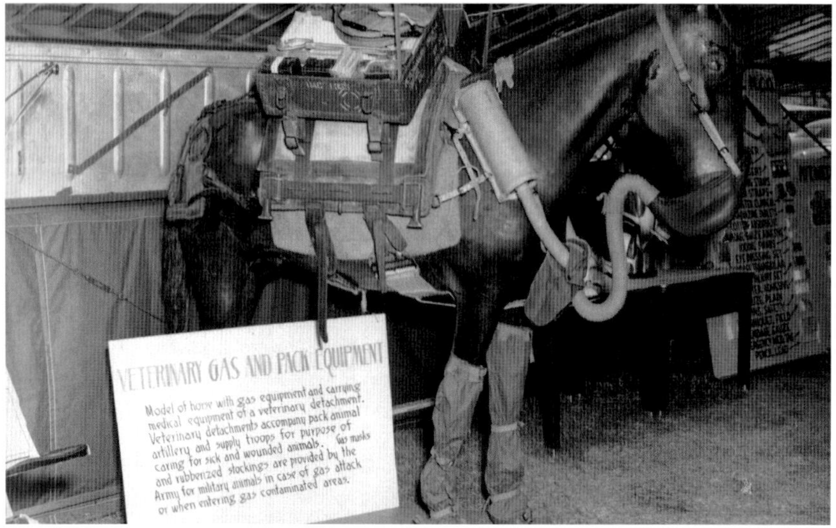
VETERINARY GAS AND PACK EQUIPMENT
Model of horse with gas equipment and carrying medical equipment of a veterinary detachment. Veterinary detachments accompany pack animal artillery and supply troops for purpose of caring for sick and wounded animals. Gas masks and rubberized stockings are provided by the Army for military animals in case of gas attack or when entering gas contaminated areas.

Veterinary Gas and Pack Equipment
Gas masks and rubberized boots were provided to Army animals when entering a gas contaminated area.

(AMSS Annual Report, 1947, Inclusion 10)

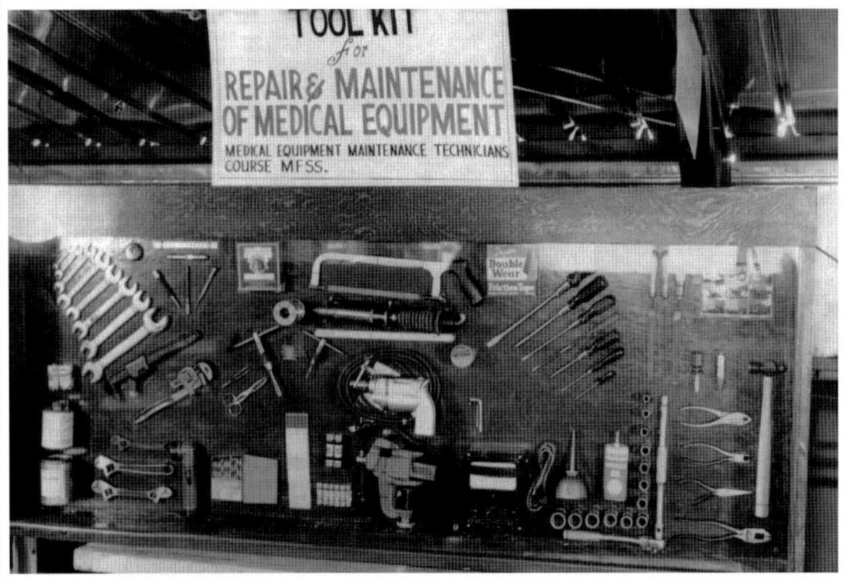

Medical Equipment Repair
Repair and maintenance training extended from medical equipment to include instruction on the proper maintenance of MFSS medical facilities.

(AMSS Annual Report, 1947, Inclusion 10)

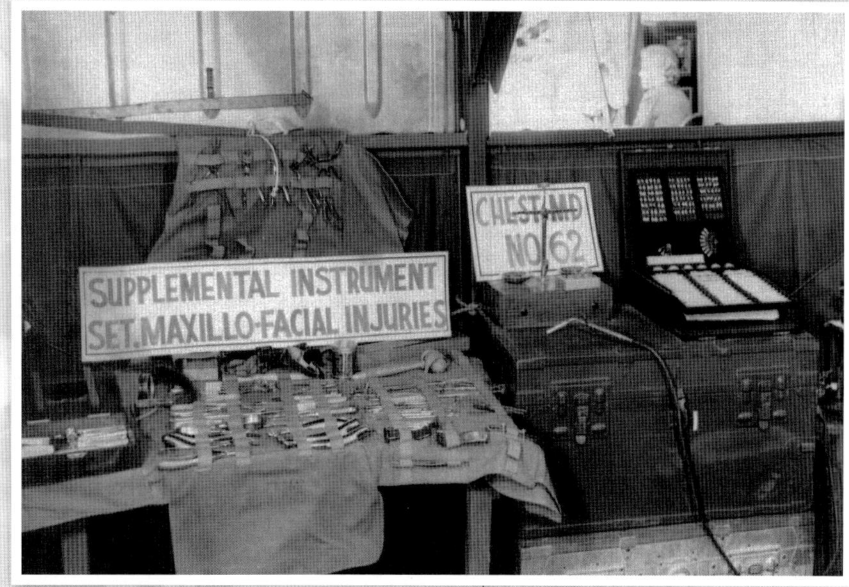

Officer, NCO and Private medical kit displays

(AMSS Annual Report, 1947, Inclusion 10)

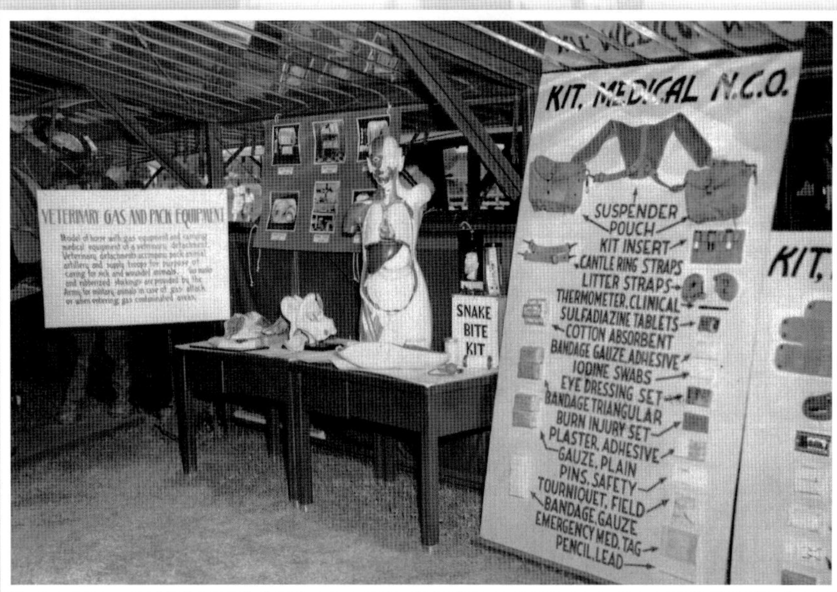
VETERINARY GAS AND PACK EQUIPMENT
SNAKE BITE KIT
KIT, MEDICAL N.C.O.
SUSPENDER
POUCH
KIT INSERT
CANTLE RING STRAPS
LITTER STRAPS
THERMOMETER, CLINICAL
SULFADIAZINE TABLETS
COTTON ABSORBENT
BANDAGE GAUZE ADHESIVE
IODINE SWABS
EYE DRESSING SET
BANDAGE TRIANGULAR
BURN INJURY SET
PLASTER, ADHESIVE
GAUZE, PLAIN
PINS, SAFETY
TOURNIQUET, FIELD
BANDAGE, GAUZE
EMERGENCY MED. TAG
PENCIL, LEAD

Officer, NCO and Private medical kit displays

(AMSS Annual Report, 1947, Inclusion 10)

1947

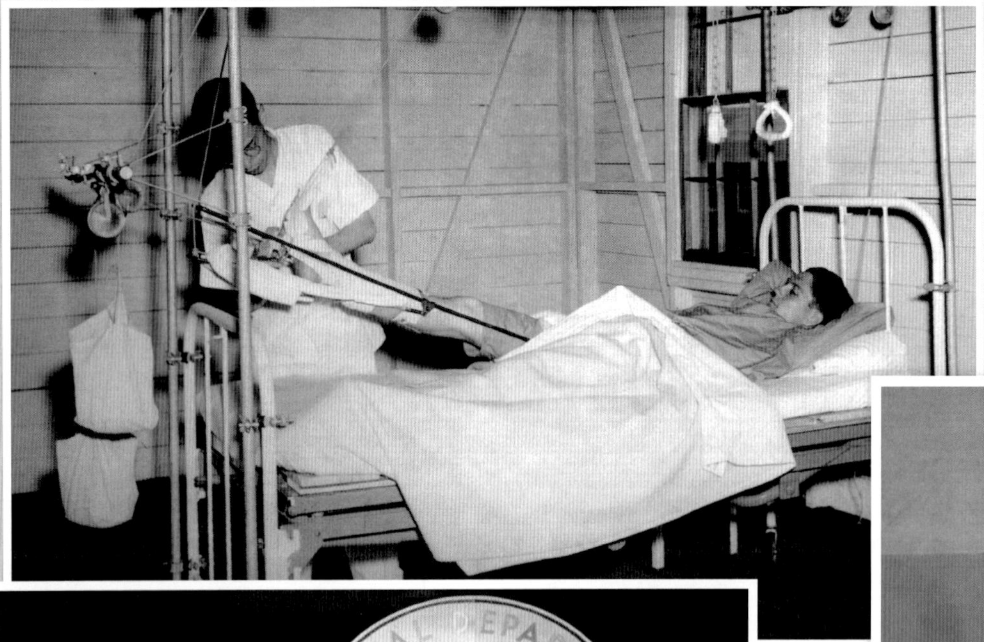

Medical Technicians Course
The Medical Technicians Course trained students in the use of weighted traction.

(AMSS Annual Report, 1947)

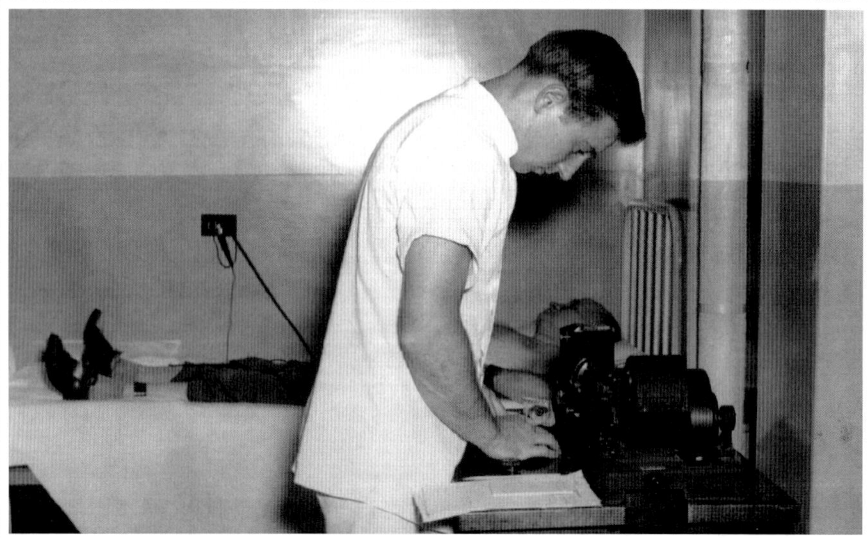

Electroencephalography Technicians Course
The Electroencephalography (EEG) Technicians Course taught soldiers the first line method for the diagnosis of tumors, stroke and epilepsy.

(AMSS Annual Report, 1947)

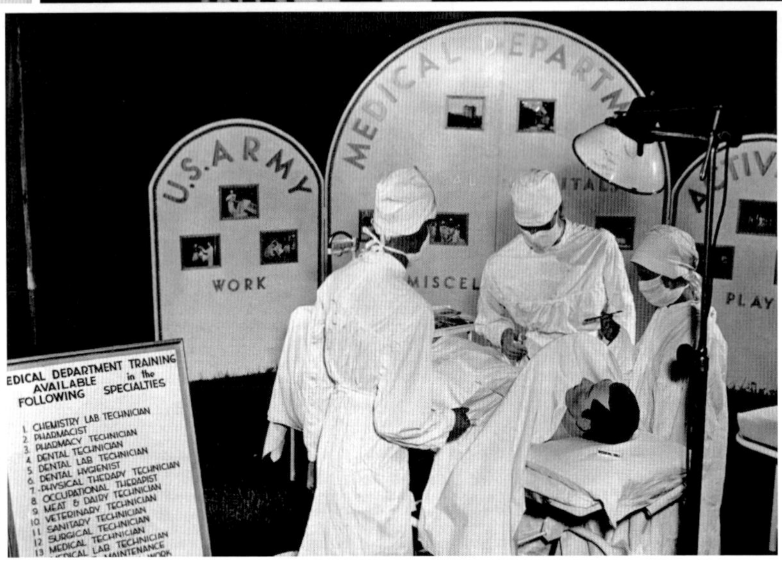

Surgical Technicians Course
Surgical Technicians Course students demonstrate their training with mannequins during Army Week.

(AMSS Annual Report, 1947)

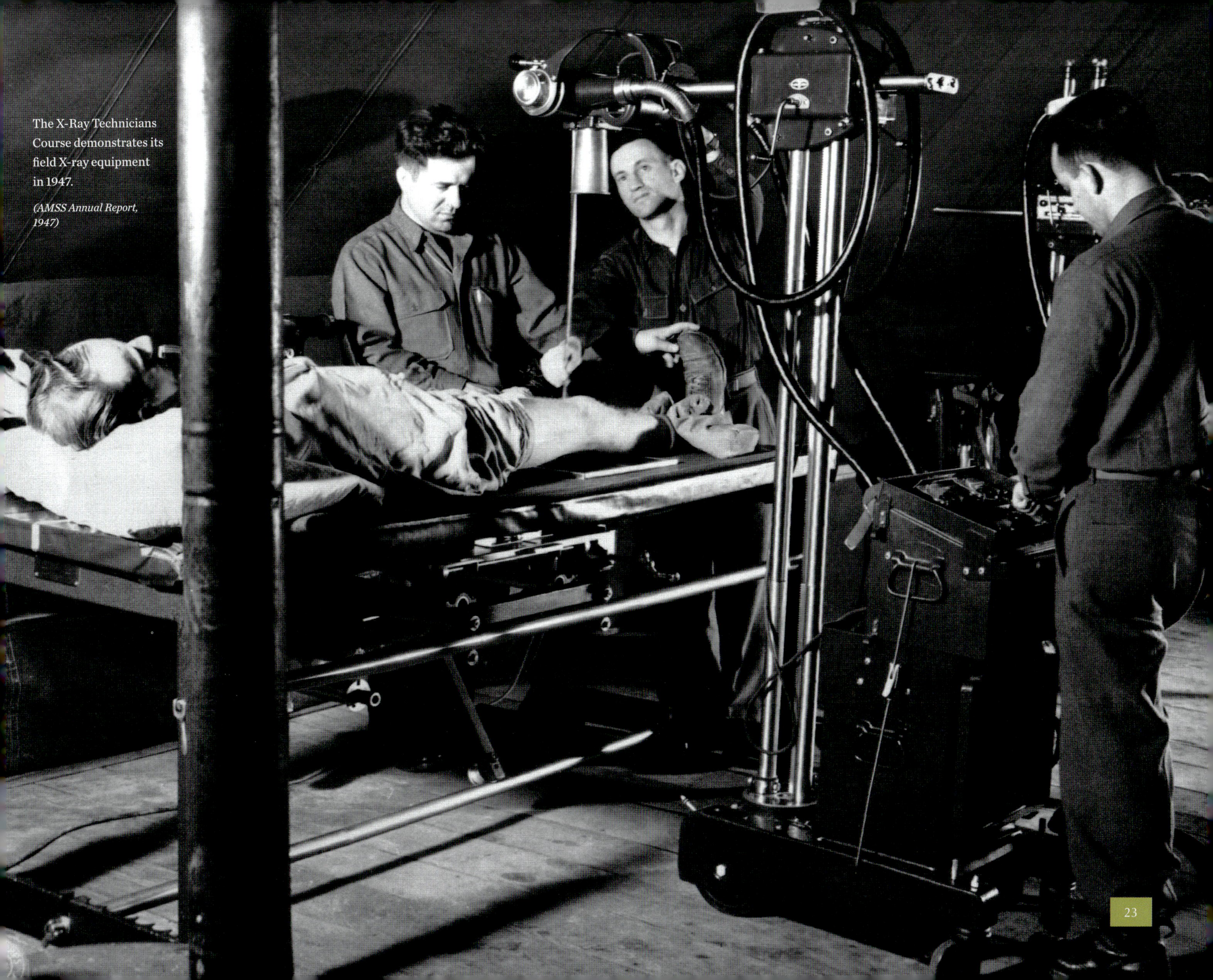

The X-Ray Technicians Course demonstrates its field X-ray equipment in 1947.

(AMSS Annual Report, 1947)

1947

The library, operated under the direct supervision of the School Secretary, was considered one of the most valuable adjuncts to the MFSS and was the source of daily information, reference material, and collateral reading.

(AMSS Annual Report, 1947, Inclusion 7)

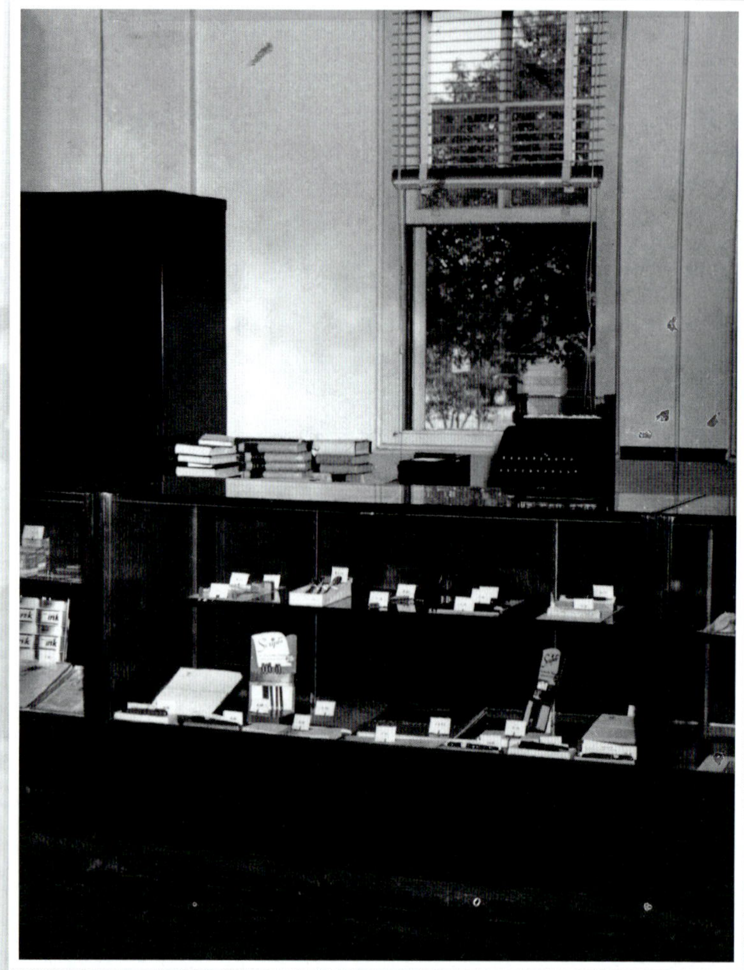

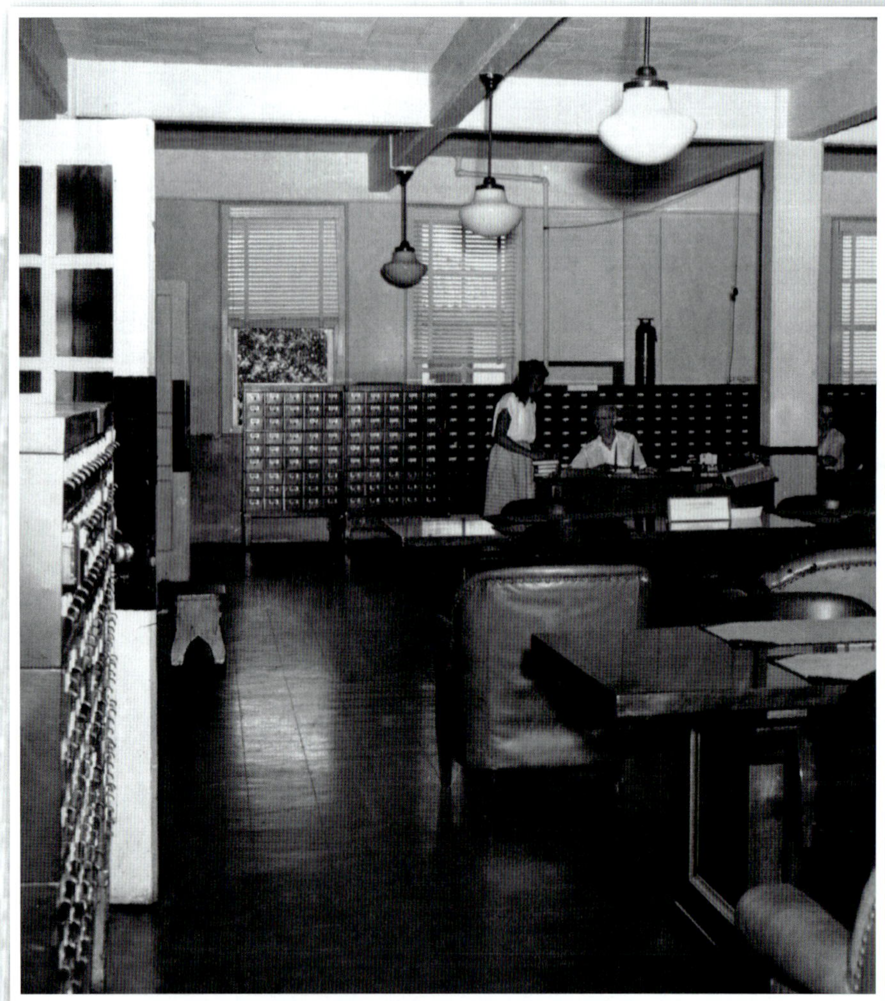

School Supplies
The library had a small counter that sold school supplies.

(AMSS Annual Historical Report, Inclusion 7)

Library
The MFSS Library, 1947.

(AMSS Annual Historical Report, Inclusion 7)

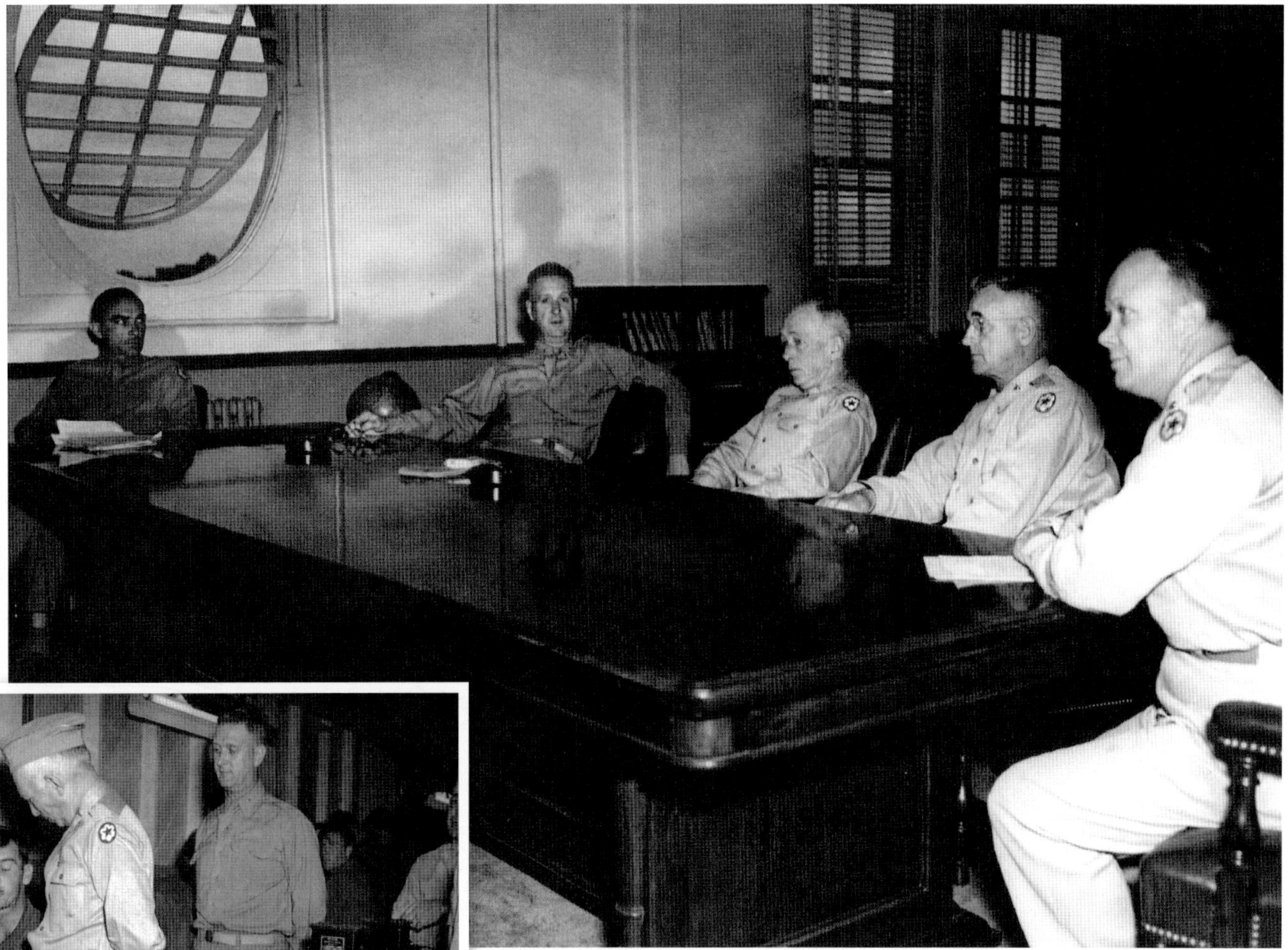

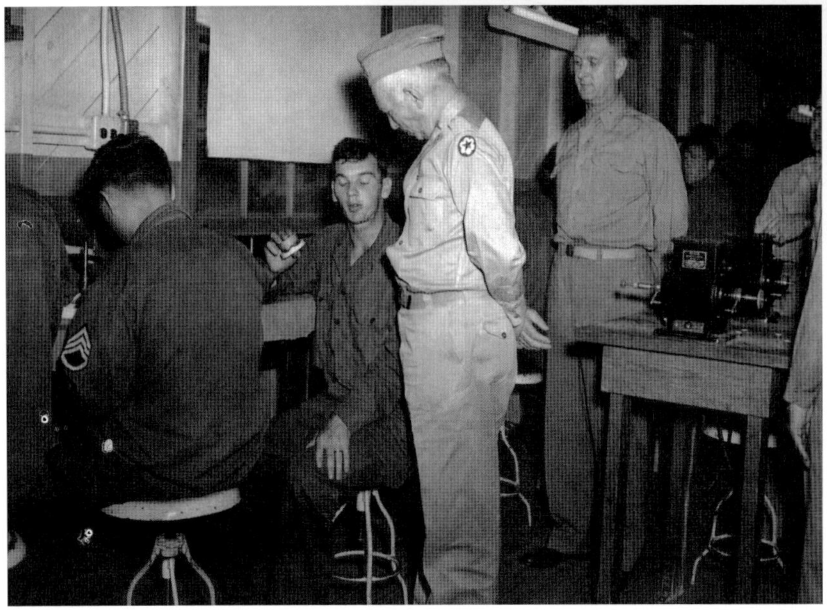

Visit from the Surgeon General

MG Norman T. Kirk (center), Surgeon General of the Army, discusses the merits of MFSS training with a soldier during his April 1947 visit.

(AMSS Annual Report, 1947)

1947

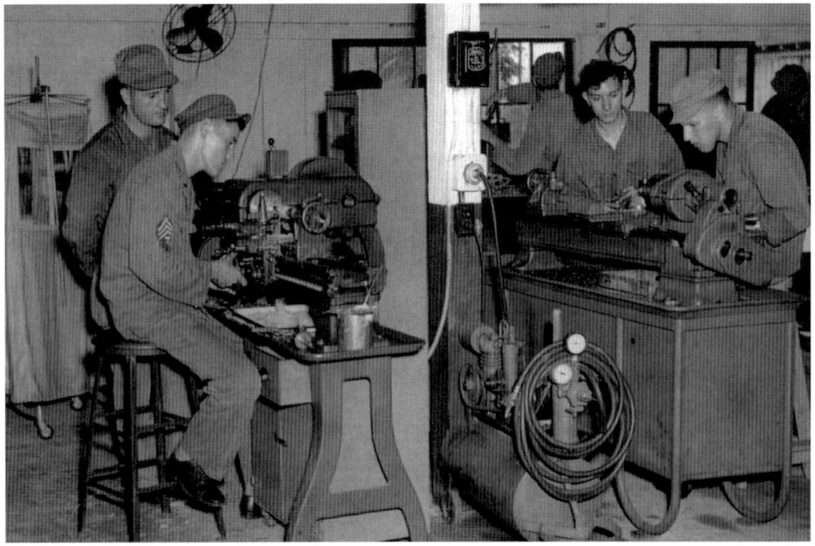

The Medical Equipment Maintenance Technicians Course

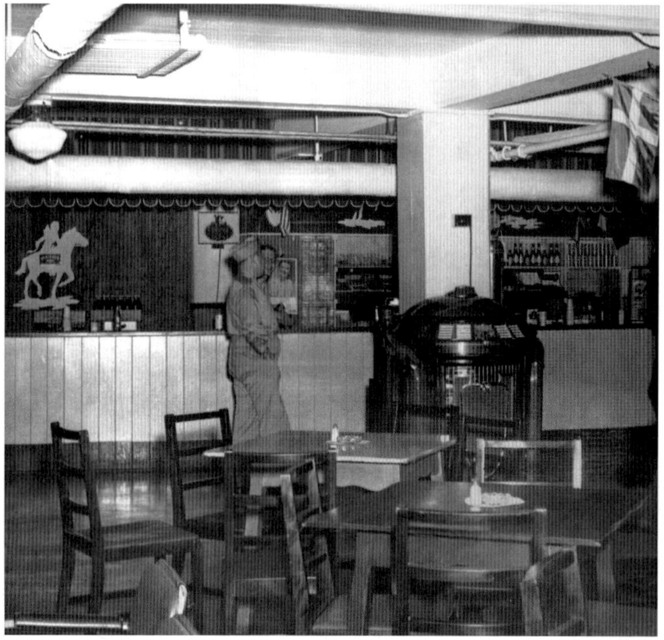

The Student Officers' Club contained a lounge, game room, tap room, bowling alley, billiards and ping-pong tables, check-cashing service, and refreshment counter.

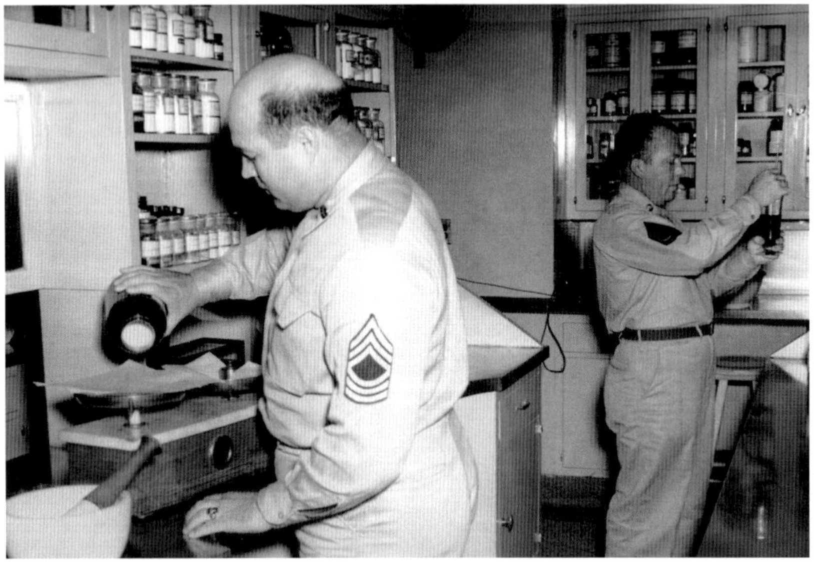

(Photos from AMSS Annual Report, 1947, Inclusion 13)

The Pharmacy Technicians Course

In January 1947, MAJ Stanley J. Weidenkopf, Sanitary Corps, Department of Preventive Medicine, MFSS, observed operations during Task Force FRIGID and Task Force WILLIWAW in and near Fairbanks, Alaska. His observations, included in the 1947 Annual Historical Report, highlighted the medical-related effects of cold weather on personnel, motor vehicles, armament and equipment involved in medical operations.

(AMSS Annual Report, 1947, Inclusion 14)

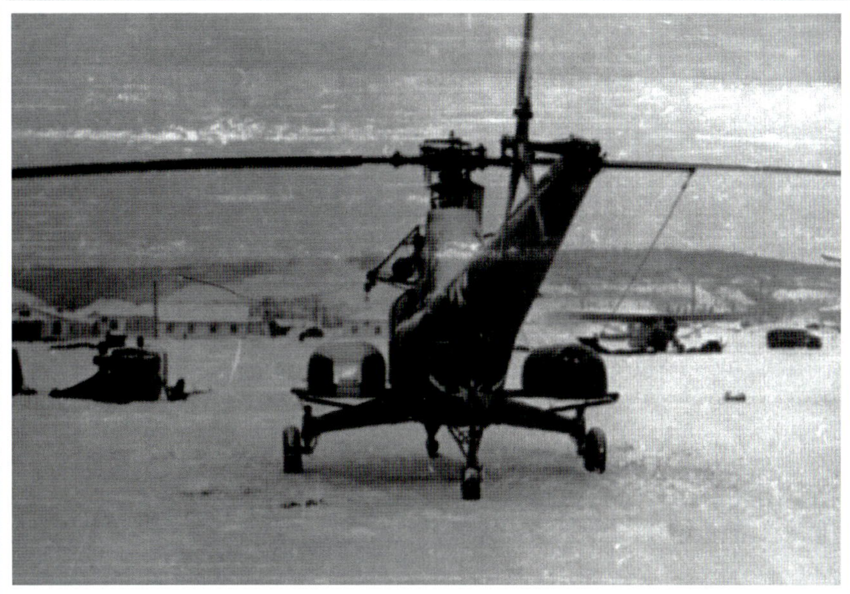

"Specially equipped helicopters were employed for air evacuation of wounded... a standard machine equipped with a coffin-like capsule on either side of the fuselage, each carrying one litter case. Greatest disadvantage: planes are not flown at temperatures below minus 40 degrees F...short daylight hours low visibility due to frozen fog, etc."

(AMSS Annual Report, 1947, Inclusion 14)

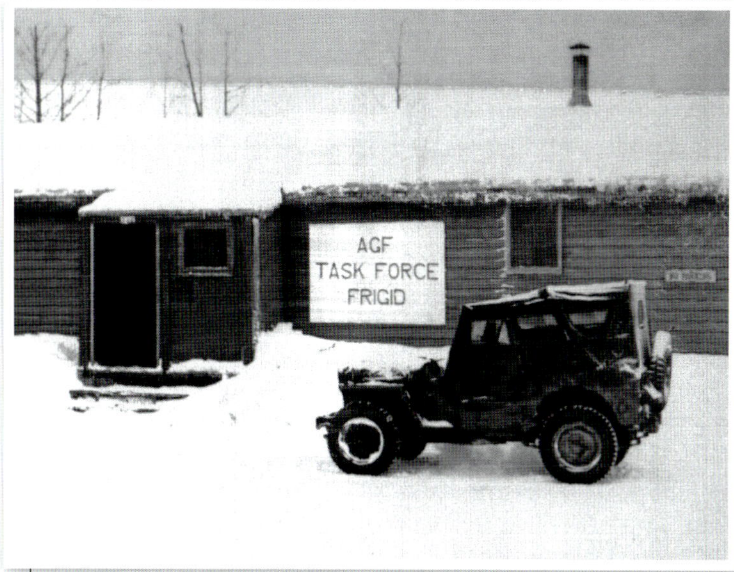

Headquarters Building for Army Ground Forces Task Force FRIGID

(Photos from AMSS Annual Historical Report, 1947, Inclusion 14)

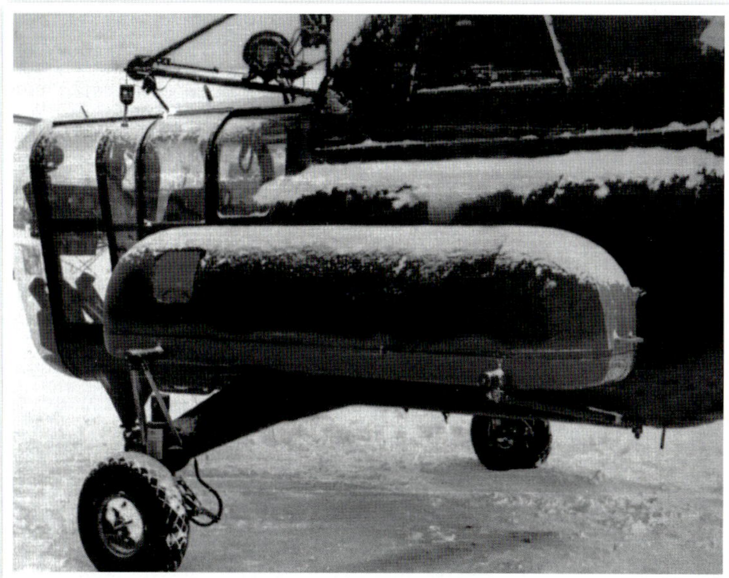

1948

The gradual expansion of training activities during the year saw a huge increase in administrative work handled by the Adjunct's Office. It logged approximately 11,000 pieces of incoming correspondence and 15,000 pieces of outgoing mail, in addition to numerous routine boards, special orders, and memoranda in 1948. The school was unable to hire competent clerk-typists because compensation was not sufficient to entice or retain qualified personnel. This shortcoming was mentioned not once, but five times within the 1948 Annual Report.

(AMSS Annual Report, 1948, p 4)

"The construction of a centralized modern school building, as recommended in the Technical Report for Fiscal Year 1947, would not only eliminate these training obstacles, but also provide optimum training conditions for instructors and students alike."

(AMSS Annual Report, 1948, p 2)

While there were an adequate number of vehicles in the motor pool, the school suffered from a shortage of trained drivers to transport students from Post to Randolph Field, Camp Bullis, and Salado Creek.

(AMSS Annual Report, 1948, p 3)

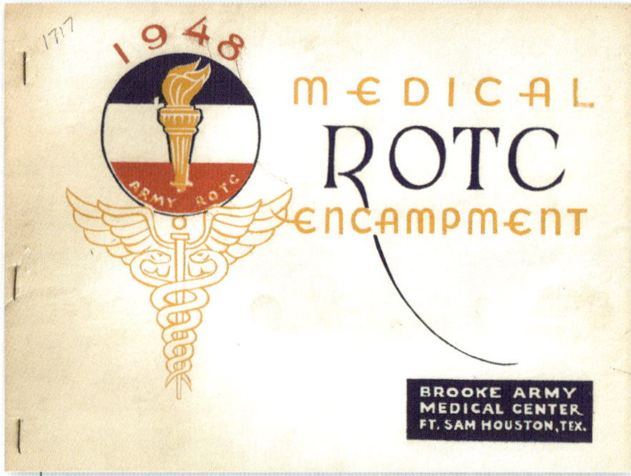

The 1948 Medical ROTC encampment at BAMC was the largest single service summer camp ever held in the nation at that point in time. The training was held under the guidance of the MFSS who trained some 585 cadet personnel that summer.

(Stimson Library Special Collections)

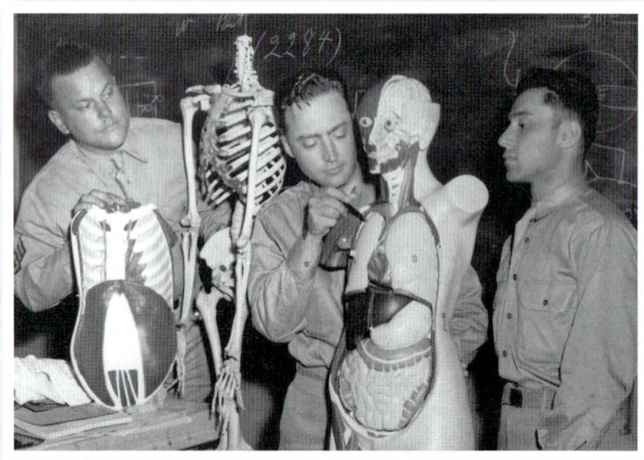

Student soldiers learned on "Matilda the Model."

(Stimson Library Special Collections)

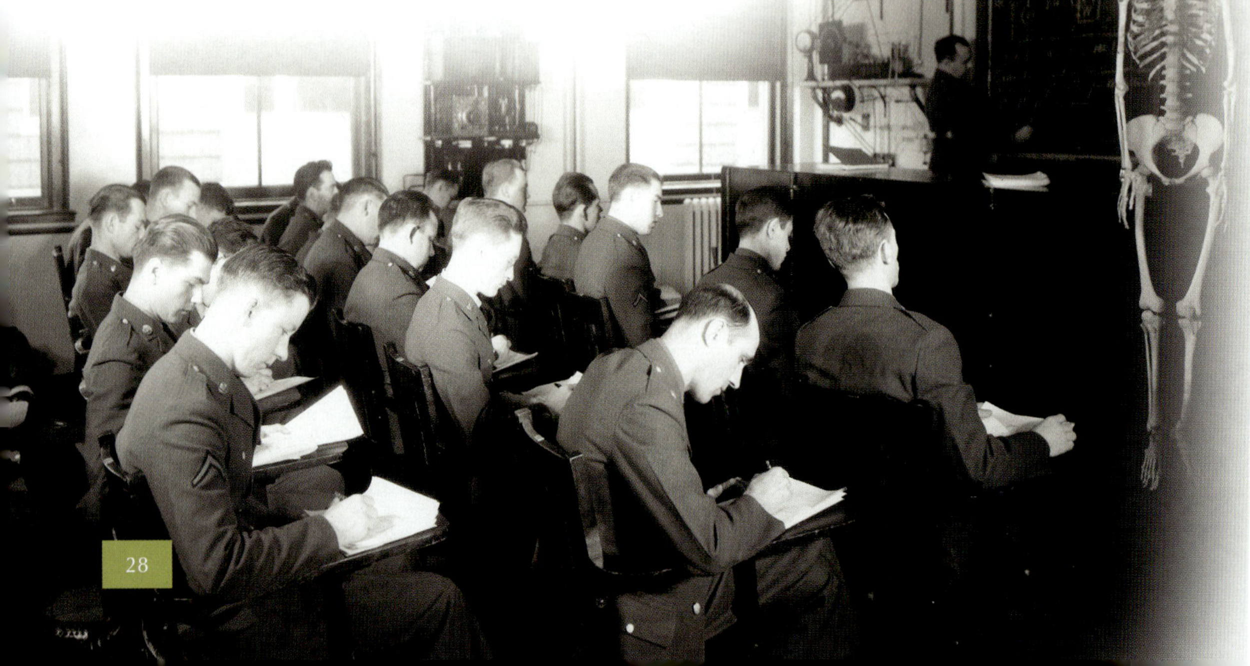

Anatomy and Physiology class, circa 1948

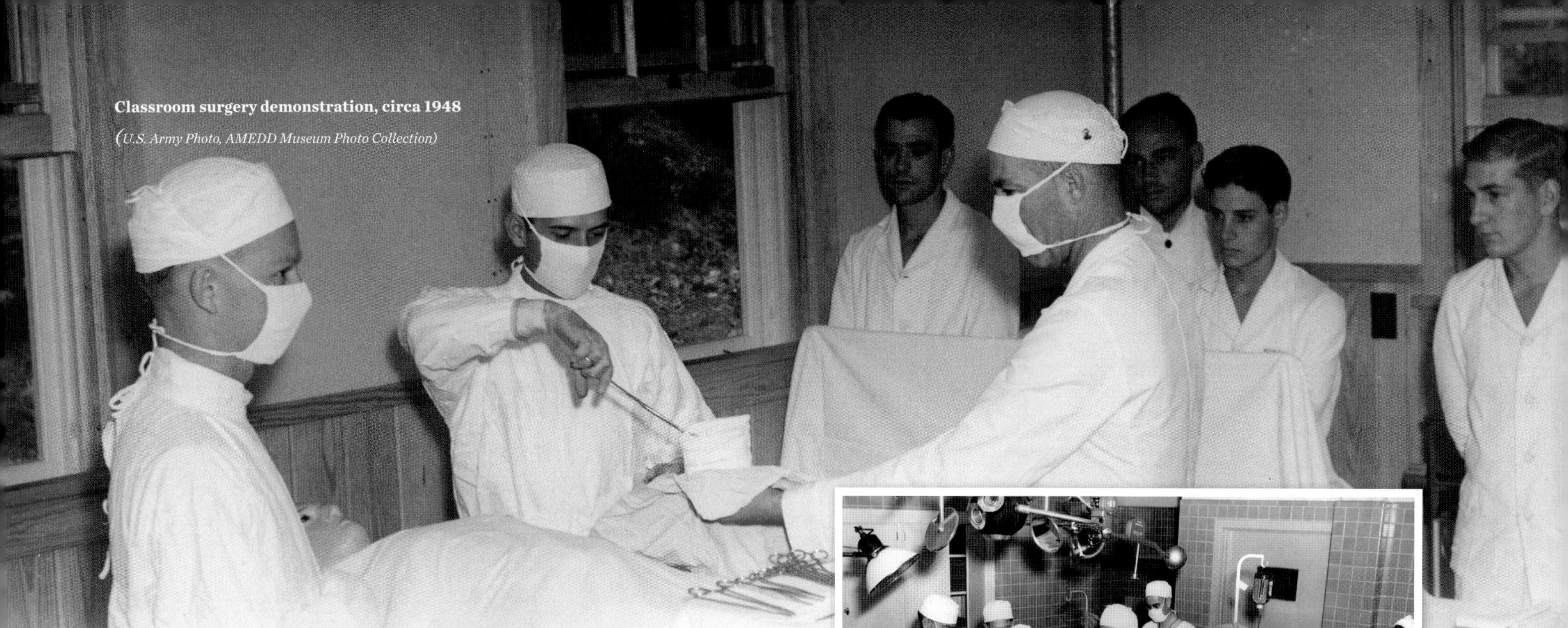

Classroom surgery demonstration, circa 1948

(U.S. Army Photo, AMEDD Museum Photo Collection)

The MFSS encountered an issue of unqualified instructor personnel in 1948. The final recommendation of MG Martin, MFSS Commandant, in the 1948 Annual Report was that "...whenever possible personnel assigned to the Medical Field Service School for duty as instructors should be experienced, qualified, and desirous of performing duty as instructors. It is further recommended that these instructors be assured, insofar as is consistent with current personnel policies, of a tour of duty of at least two years."

(AMSS Annual Report, 1948, p 41)

The 323rd Army Band, 187th Malaria Control Detachment, 188th Malaria Control Detachment, and 212th Malaria Survey Detachment assisted the MFSS with its general mission.

(AMSS Annual Report, 1948, p 4)

The Personnel Branch focused its efforts on properly designating primary occupational specialties for military personnel and implementing the Army Career Guidance Plan for warrant officers and enlisted personnel in 1948.

(AMSS Annual Report, 1948, p 6)

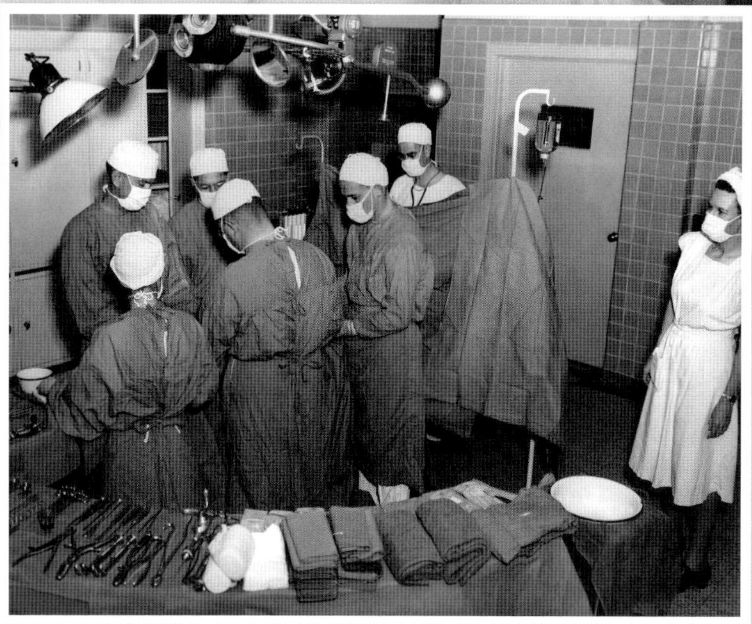

General instructs students

MG John M. Willis (fourth from left) and a surgical team demonstrate operation techniques for MFSS students on 8 Jan 1948. MG Willis was the eighth Commandant of the Army Medical Field Service School, and first Commander of BAMC.

(U.S. Army Photo, AMEDD Museum Photo Collection)

1948

In November 1948, the position of civilian coordinator for the school was abolished, and an Employee Utilization Section at Headquarters, Brooke Army Medical Center, was organized to administer civilian affairs.

(AMSS Annual Report, 1948, p 8)

The Food Service Section operated between three and five messes, serving almost a million meals during the calendar year. It received a superior rating when inspected by Major MacDonald of the Food Service Section, Office of the Quartermaster General, Washington, D.C.

(AMSS Annual Report, 1948, pp 8-9)

An eight-week course of instruction in physical reconditioning was conducted at the Medical Field Service School, Fort Sam Houston, Texas, beginning 26 April 1948. The purpose of the course was to qualify officers to activate, organize, and administer programs of physical reconditioning.

(Bulletin, March 1948, p 185)

In response to the Randolph Act, enacted by Congress in 1946 to provide a preventive medicine program to Federal employees, the Army began to train a cadre of preventive medicine specialists through civilian schools of public health. A practical course in field aspects of preventive medicine was offered by the MFSS in 1948, and by May of that year, the Army Medical Department Research and Graduate School announced plans to introduce a course in preventive medicine comparable to a master's degree in public health.

(Bulletin, May 1948, p 346)

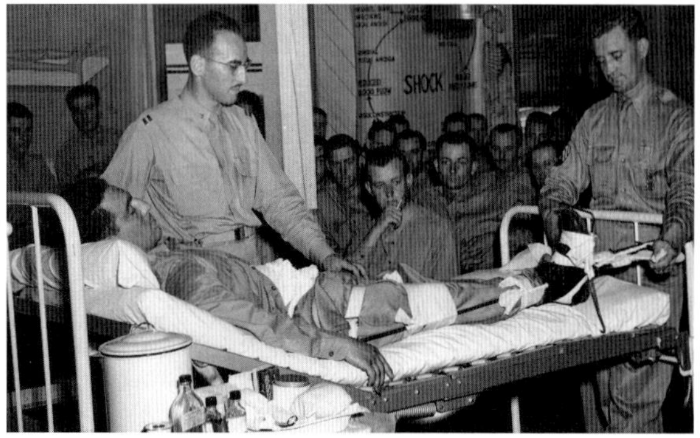

Classroom casting instruction, circa 1948

(U.S. Army Photo, AMEDD Museum Photo Collection)

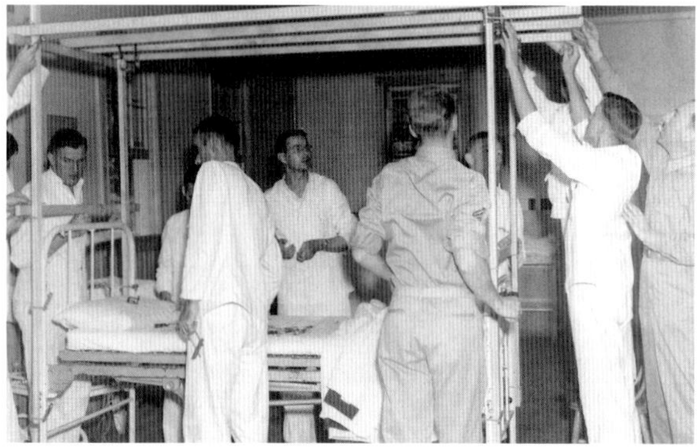

Learning to assemble a hospital bed, circa 1948

(U.S. Army Photo, AMEDD Museum Photo Collection)

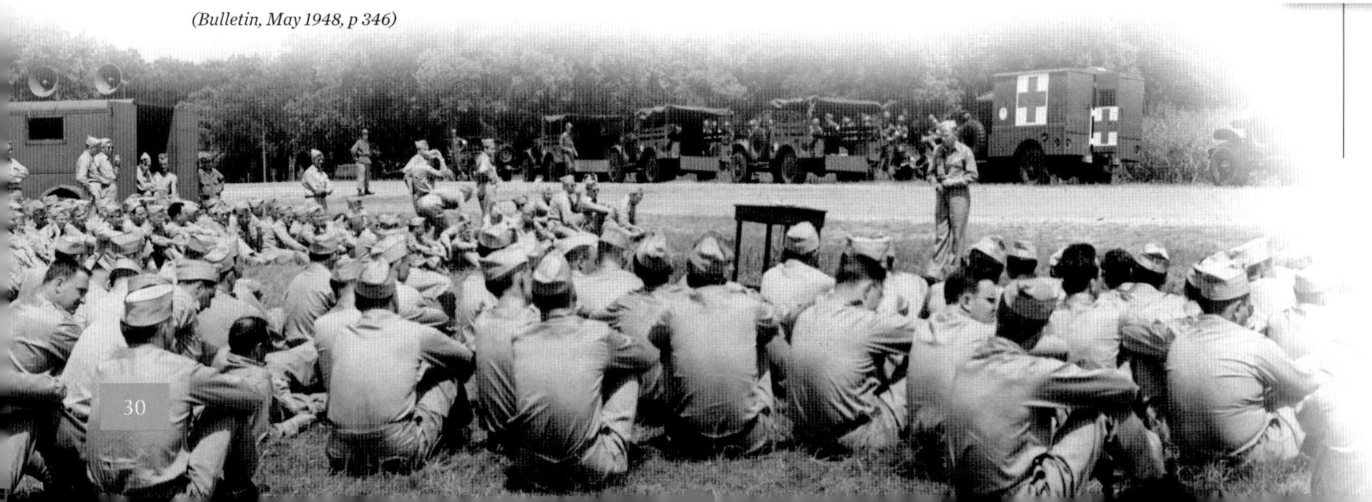

Drivers and convoy training course, circa 1948

(U.S. Army Photo, AMEDD Museum Photo Collection)

In September 1948, the MFSS began the two-month Basic Medical Department Female Officers Course, a prerequisite for acceptance into a twelve-month physical therapy training program. The course consisted of a well-integrated program of six months of didactic instruction at BAMC and then a six-month applicatory phase at select general hospitals. Women accepted into the program had to apply for and accept a commission in the Women's Medical Specialist Corps section of the Officers' Reserve Corps and request an active duty extension of two years. The criteria for applicants was very narrow—applicants had to be between 21 and 26 years of age; a U.S. citizen; single, widowed, or divorced; without dependents under 14 years of age; possess high moral character and personal qualifications; and meet physical qualifications as set forth in Army regulations, as well as have a degree in physical education from an accredited school or university.

(Bulletin, August 1948, p 595)

Six complete extension course series were available to Reserve nurses through the MFSS in October 1948. The courses counted toward eligibility for promotion and retirement and applied to all Reserve nurses.

(Bulletin, Oct 1948, p 821)

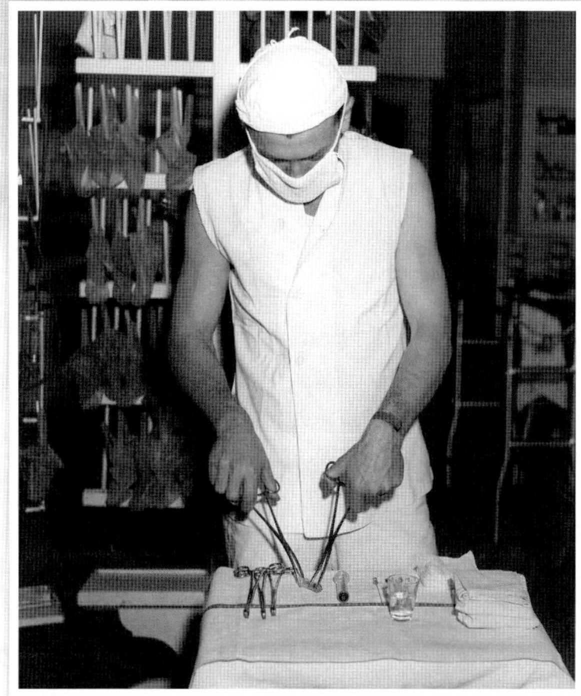

Demonstration of proper instrument sterilization technique, 1948

(U.S. Army Photo, AMEDD Museum Photo Collection)

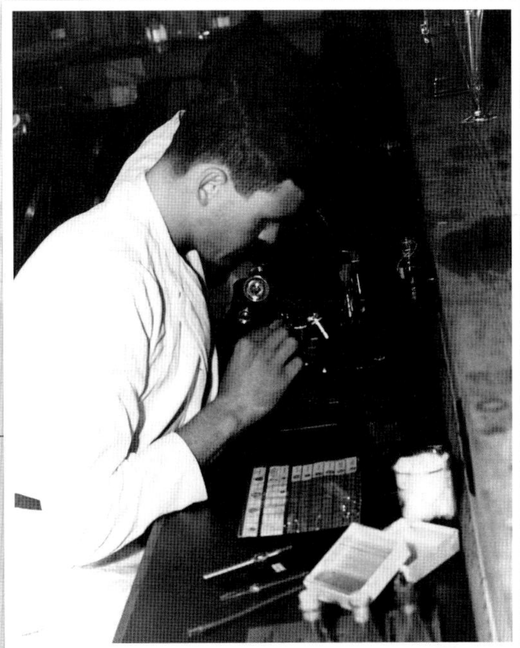

Learning to read lab slides, circa 1948

(U.S. Army Photo, AMEDD Museum Photo Collection)

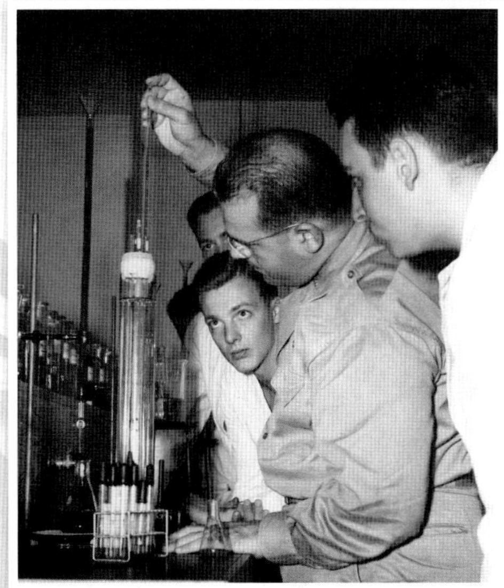

Removing specimen from a test tube holder, circa 1948

(U.S. Army Photo, AMEDD Museum Photo Collection)

1949

No major changes were made in the grounds and facilities available to the MFSS in 1949. The barracks continued to be converted into classrooms, but were found inadequate as instructional facilities, even after extensive remodeling.

AMSS Annual Report, 1949, p 2)

The Department of Nursing was established as the number of women increased in the Female Officer Basic Course, Medical Department Officer Advance Course, and Hospital Administration. The increase also required additional supervision for the technical aspect of the Enlisted Hospital Course.

(AMSS Annual Report, 1949, p 2)

The Women's Auxiliary Corps (WAC) Student Detachment was organized 23 March 1949 to provide administrative care and supervision for WAC students attending the Enlisted Technician Course. A cadre of two officers and six enlisted personnel, housing, a day room, lounge, and office facilities in Building 2266 were assigned to the detachment.

(AMSS Annual Report, 1949, p 10)

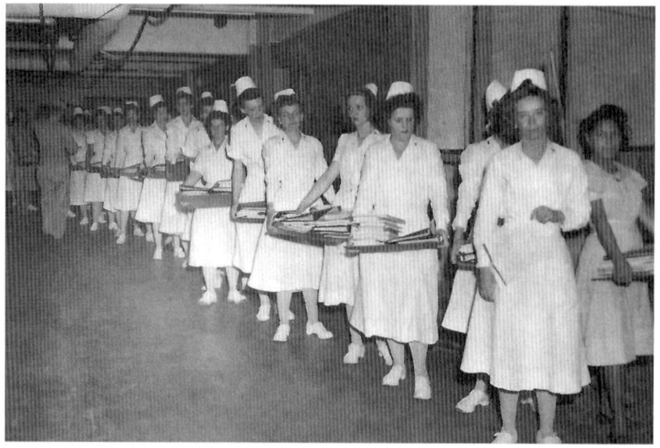

New students processing for Female Officer Basic Course

(AMSS Annual Report, 1949, fig 2)

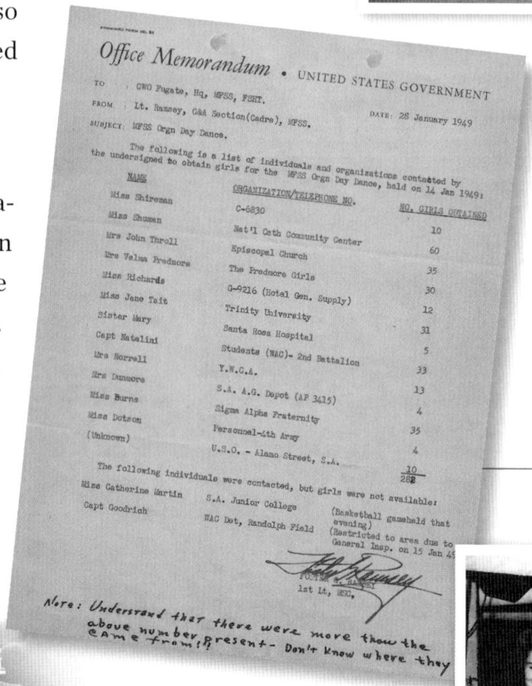

Office Memorandum • UNITED STATES GOVERNMENT

TO : CWO Fugate, Hq, MFSS, FSHT.

FROM : Lt. Ramsey, G&A Section(Cadre), MFSS. DATE: 28 January 1949

SUBJECT: MFSS Orgn Day Dance.

The following is a list of individuals and organizations contacted by the undersigned to obtain girls for the MFSS Orgn Day Dance, held on 14 Jan 1949:

NAME	ORGANIZATION/TELEPHONE NO.	NO. GIRLS OBTAINED
Miss Shireman	C-6830	10
Miss Shuman	Nat'l Cath Community Center	60
Mrs John Throll	Episcopal Church	35
Mrs Velma Predmore	The Predmore Girls	30
Miss Richards	G-9216 (Hotel Gen. Supply)	12
Miss Jane Tait	Trinity University	31
Sister Mary	Santa Rosa Hospital	5
Capt Natalini	Students (WAC)- 2nd Battalion	33
Mrs Norrell	Y.W.C.A.	13
Mrs Dunmore	S.A. A.G. Depot (AP 3415)	4
Miss Burns	Sigma Alpha Fraternity	35
Miss Dotson	Personnel-4th Army	4
(Unknown)	U.S.O. - Alamo Street, S.A.	10
		282

The following individuals were contacted, but girls were not available:

Miss Catherine Martin	S.A. Junior College	(Basketball gameheld that evening)
Capt Goodrich	WAC Det, Randolph Field	(Restricted to area due to General Insp. on 15 Jan 49

FOSTER S. RAMSEY
1st Lt, MSC,

Note: Understand that there were more than the above number present- Don't know where they came from!?

Local San Antonio organizations received open invitations for female members to attend the Organization Day Dance. The handwritten post script on the bottom suggests that there was no shortage of young women in San Antonio interested in meeting eligible young men training at the MFSS.

(AMSS Organization Day File, 1949)

The WAC Student Detachment in formation

(AMSS Annual Report, 1949, fig 3)

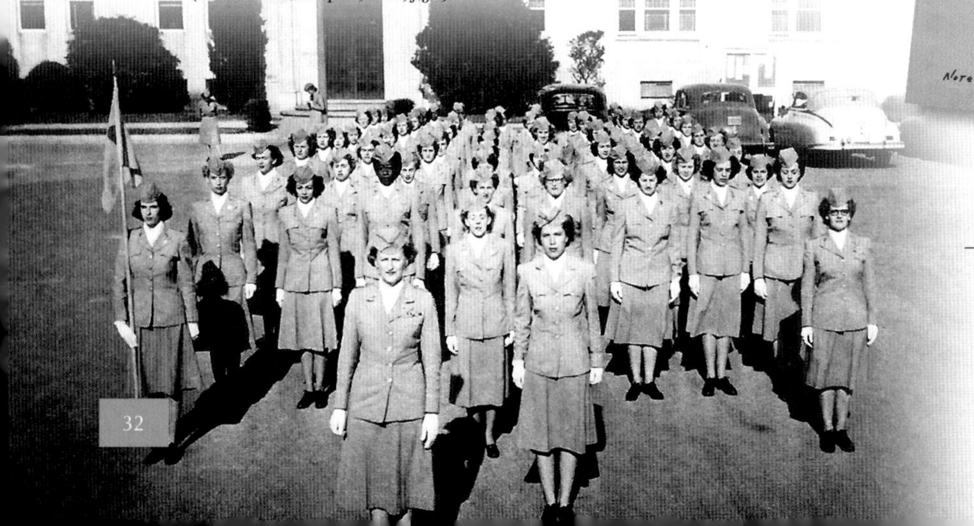

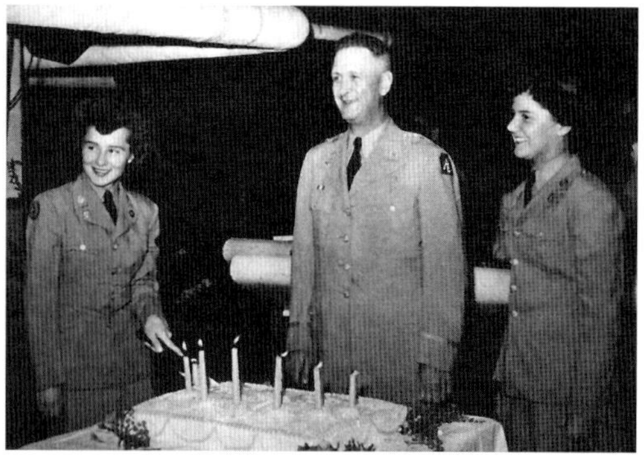

MG Joseph I. Martin at WAC Student Detachment Reception

(AMSS Annual Report, 1949, fig 4)

Fort Sam Houston was considered "exceptionally well provided with diversified recreational and athletic facilities." The swimming pools, located in the training battalion and Salado Creek (Officers' Club), were great favorites with students and staff alike; more than 10,000 people visited them per month during the summer. Other activities included ping-pong, bowling, volleyball, basketball, baseball, horseshoe, and golf tournaments. Supervised tours were arranged through the Special Services Officer and the United Service Organizations (USO) Director. The USO conducted tours to Monterrey, Mexico, on long holiday weekends.

(AMSS Annual Report, 1949, p 12)

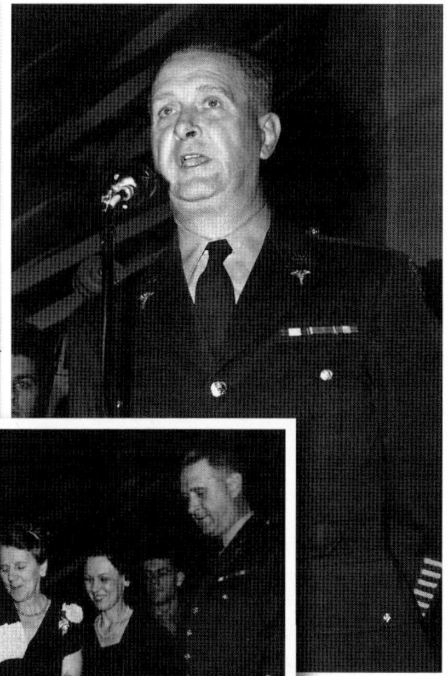

Dance!
MG Martin called the opening dance for the Organizational Day Dinner 14 January 1949.

(AMSS Organization Day File, 1949)

The Third Enlisted Training Battalion was inactivated and consolidated with the First Training Battalion. This move streamlined administrative coordination and functions and proved to provide substantial savings in overhead and personnel. Transfer of property and personnel was provided by General Order No. 19, 9 September 1949, Headquarters, MFSS.

(AMSS Annual Report, 1949, p 3)

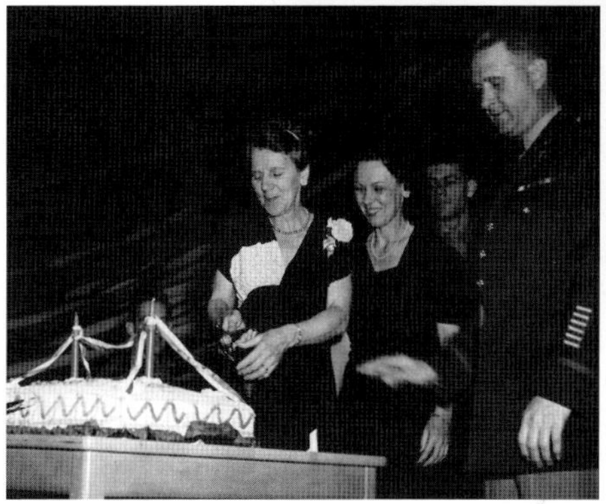

Organization Day
MG Martin and Mrs. Martin cut the Organization Day Cake.

(AMSS Organization Day File, 1949)

Students enjoyed a competitive round of Bingo as part of Organization Day. Prizes ranged from television sets to beauty salon services.

(AMSS Organization Day File, 1949)

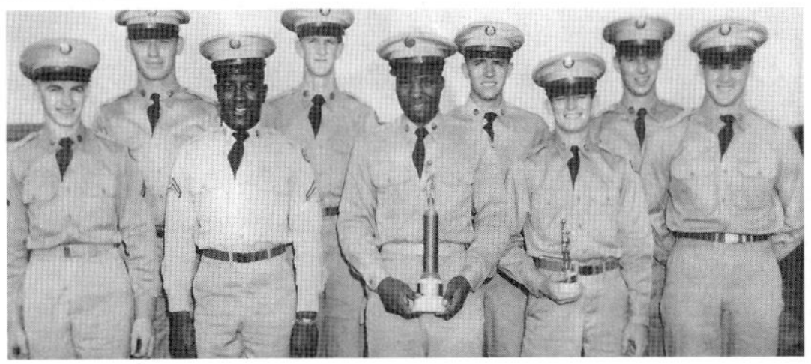

Army-wide Champs
The AMSS wins the Army-wide Basketball Championship.

(AMSS Annual Report, 1949, fig 5)

1949

As the MFSS became increasingly responsible for development of civilian training materials, a Civilian Component Section was created in the Secretary's Office in April 1949. It provided a focal point for the editing, proof reading, printing, binding, and distribution of Civilian Component Headquarters subject schedules, lesson plans, and lectures.

(AMSS Annual Report, 1949, p 3)

The Liaison Section was given the status of a faculty department and redesignated the Department of Combined Arms as a greater emphasis was placed on unification and coordination between all armed forces services in both training and combat. In June 1949, an Air Force officer was assigned to the school as the official Air Force representative and subject matter instructor on Air Force affairs.

(AMSS Annual Report, 1949, p 3)

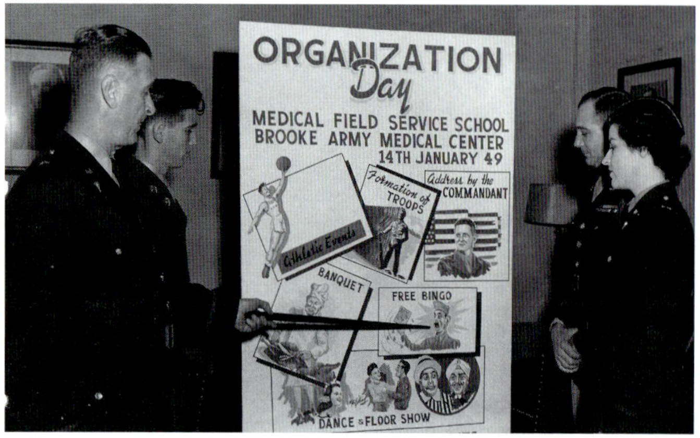

Organization Day was one of the largest events of the year with invitations, flyers and posters posted throughout the Post and the city.

(AMSS Organization Day File, 1949)

Information training in geopolitics

(AMSS Annual Report, 1949, Fig 11)

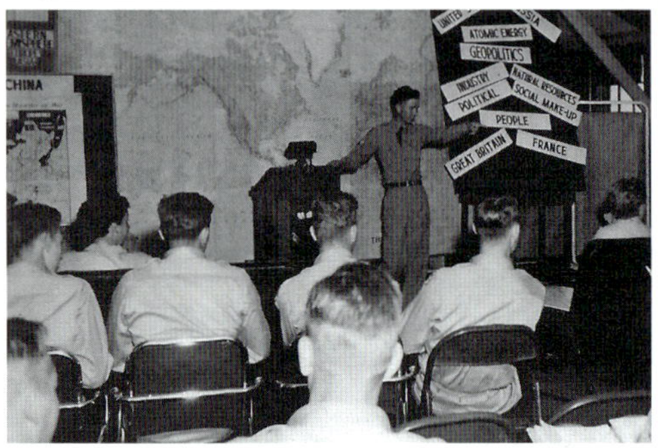
CHINA
ATOMIC ENERGY
GEOPOLITICS
INDUSTRY
POLITICAL
NATURAL RESOURCES
SOCIAL MAKE-UP
PEOPLE
FRANCE
GREAT BRITAIN

Hand drawn flyer for the 1949 Organization Day

(AMSS Organization Day File, 1949)

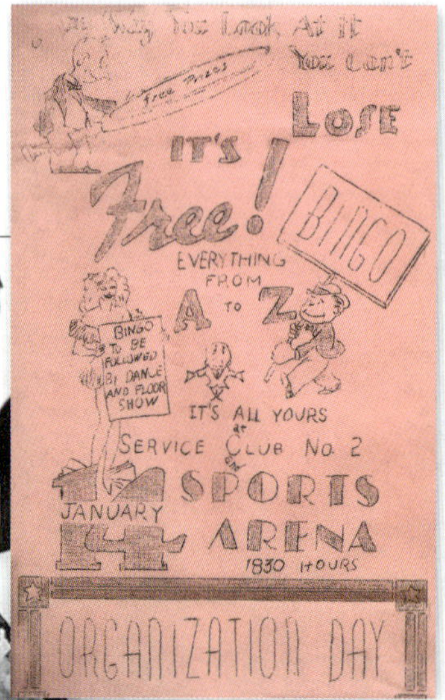
You Can't
Lose
IT'S
Free!
BINGO
EVERYTHING FROM A TO Z
BINGO TO BE FOLLOWED BY DANCE AND FLOOR SHOW
IT'S ALL YOURS
SERVICE CLUB No 2
JANUARY 14
SPORTS ARENA
1930 HOURS
ORGANIZATION DAY

The Commandant, Faculty and Staff Holiday Greeting Card

(AMSS Annual Report, 1949, insert)

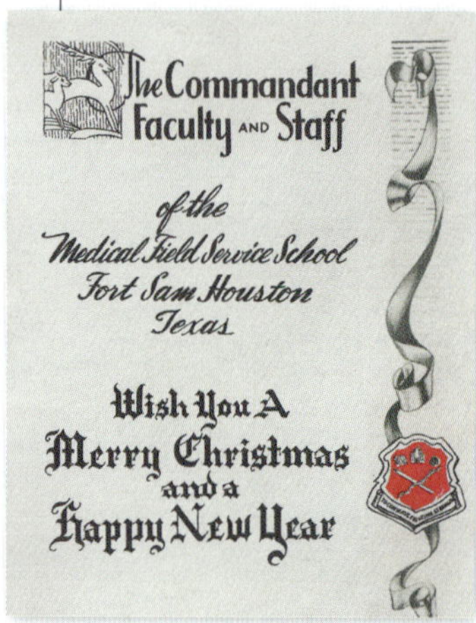
The Commandant
Faculty and Staff
of the
Medical Field Service School
Fort Sam Houston
Texas
Wish You A
Merry Christmas
and a
Happy New Year

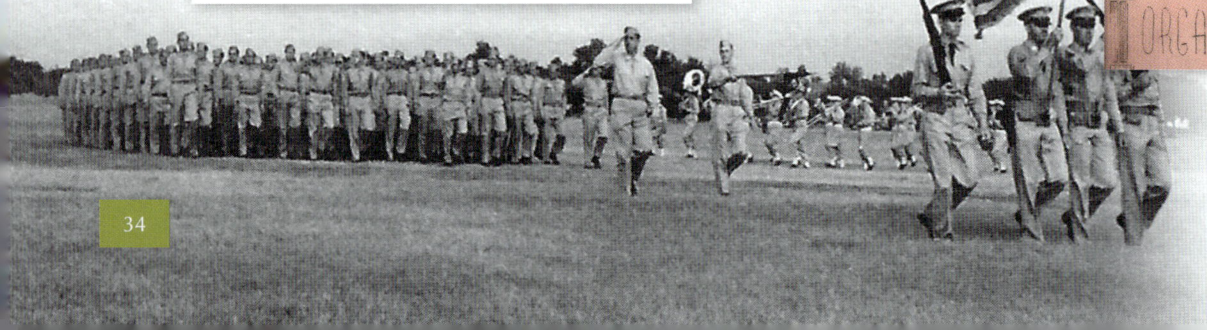

ROTC Graduation Parade

(AMSS Annual Report, 1949, Fig 33)

1949 saw the movement of 124 enlisted men to the Medical Department of the Air Force. While the Technical Service Unit of the MFSS strength dropped, there was no loss in manpower as those who transferred were assigned to Section A of the 2206th Hospital Squadron at BAMC. While this prevented overnight depletion of key specialists, it caused problems in the oversight of pay, discipline, and promotions.

(AMSS Annual Report, 1949, p 5)

On 13 May 1949, the students in the Physical Therapy Training Course at the MFSS completed their first phase of training. The ten Reserve officers in the Women's Medical Specialist Corps were assigned to hospitals to receive the second six-month phase of training.

There continued to be issues with obtaining qualified instructors. The importance of maintaining adequate and competent teaching staff was reiterated in the Annual Report.

(AMSS Annual Report, 1949, p 6)

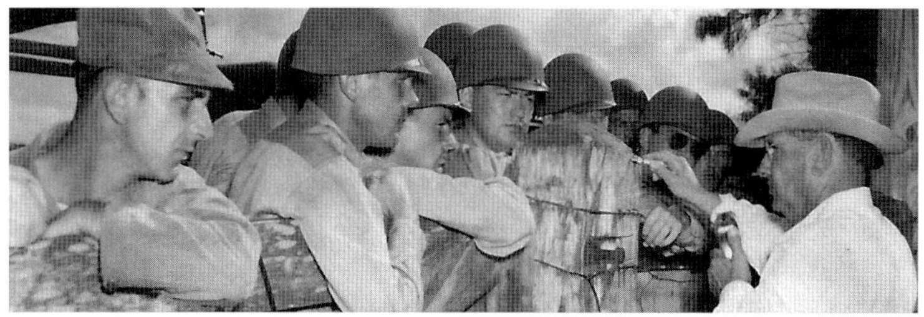

King Ranch

Students in the ROTC Veterinary Course received instruction on the genetics of Santa Gertrudis cattle and observed cattle under range conditions at the King Ranch.

(AMSS Annual Report, 1949, fig 35)

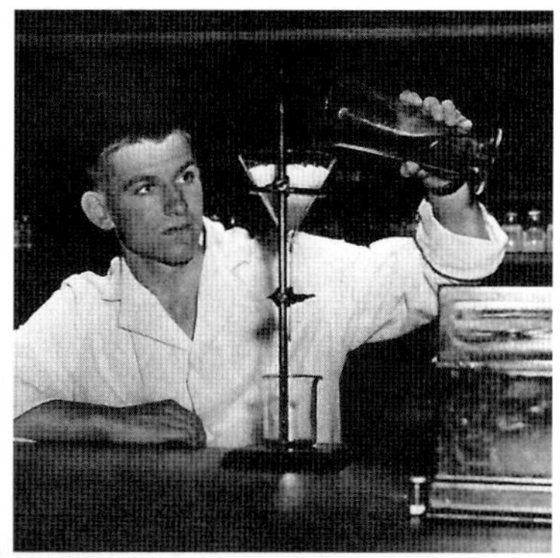

Laboratory equipment for pharmacy course

(AMSS Annual Report, 1949, fig 26)

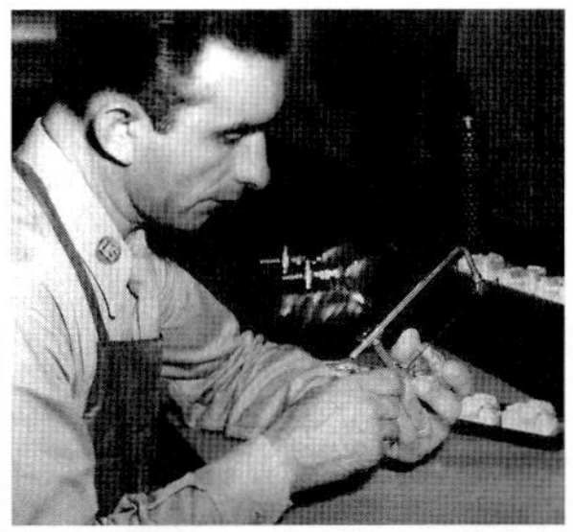

Practical exercises in dental mechanics

(AMSS Annual Report, 1949, fig 28)

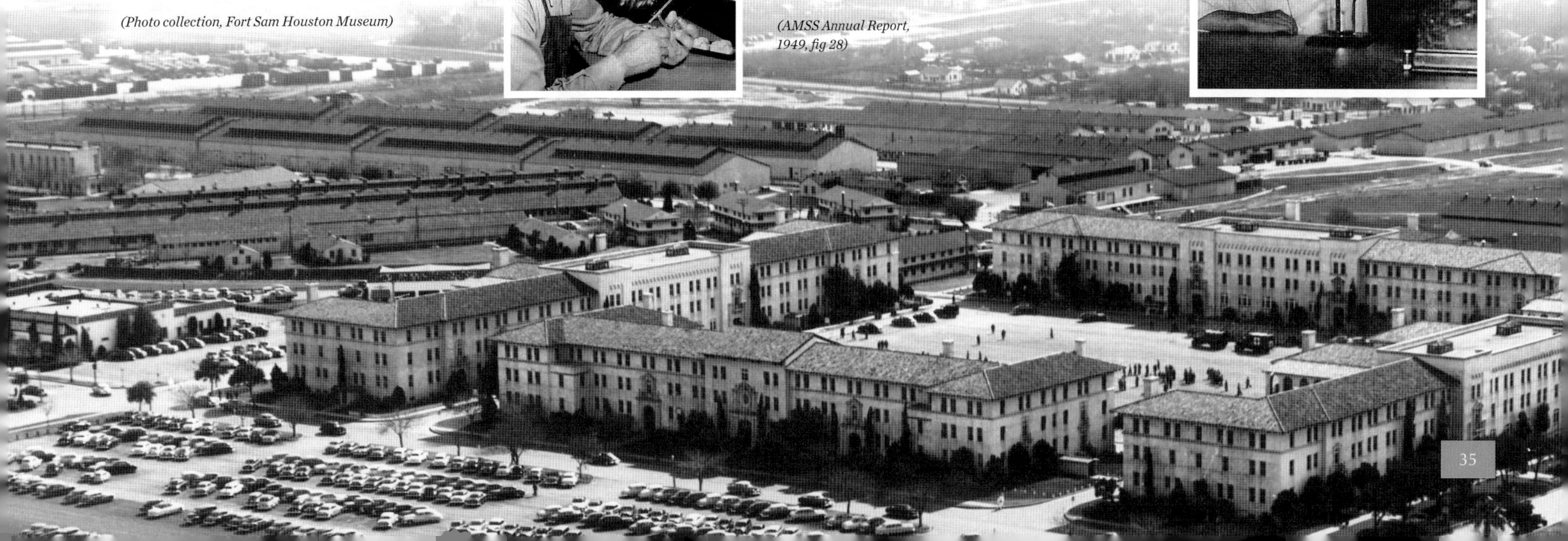

The MFSS Headquarters Building circa 1949

(Photo collection, Fort Sam Houston Museum)

1949

The chief source of enlisted instructors was the unassigned student body. An over-authorized allotment of enlisted personnel in the last quarter of 1949 made it difficult to properly assign personnel to duties related to their primary MOS. This created serious morale problems for both the soldiers and administrators attempting to place them in meaningful assignments.

(AMSS Annual Report, 1949, p 7)

A four-hour course, "Techniques in Instruction," was conducted periodically for officers and enlisted personnel by the Department of Training, but was found inadequate. It was expanded to an eight-week course for officers only.

(AMSS Annual Report, 1949, p 26)

The first Army child guidance clinic to preserve and prevent mental health problems among young dependents of military personal was set up at the Brooke General Hospital. Enlisted and officer students enrolled in the School of Neuropsychiatry at the MFSS used the clinic for observation and training purposes. Therapeutic techniques such as group therapy, play therapy, and classic office interviews were tested.

(Bulletin, June 1949, pp 449-457)

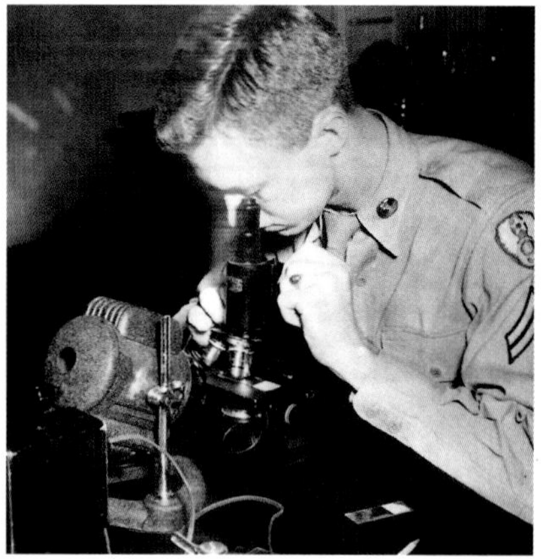

Practical application of medical laboratory procedures

(AMSS Annual Report, 1949, fig 22 & 23)

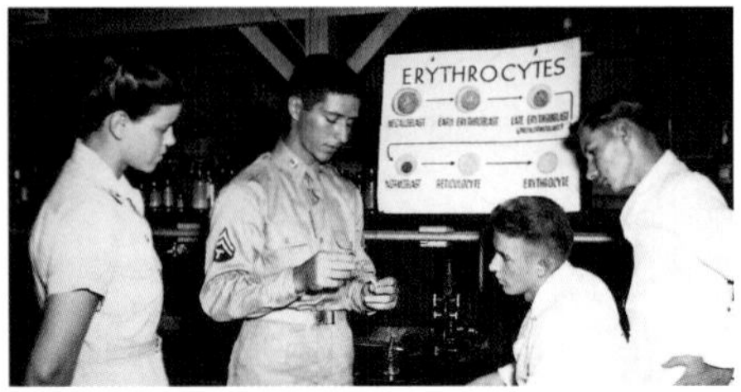

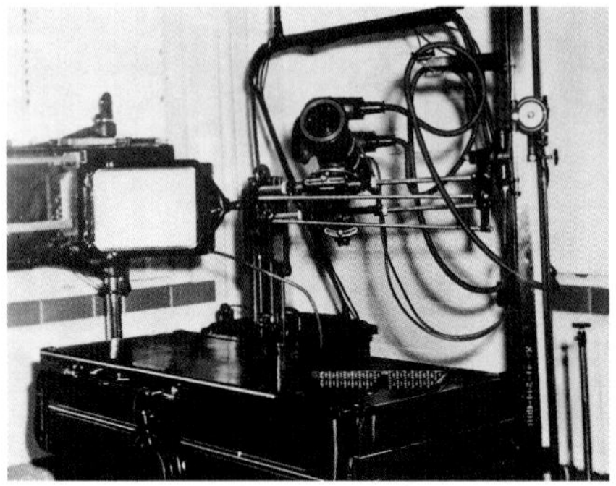

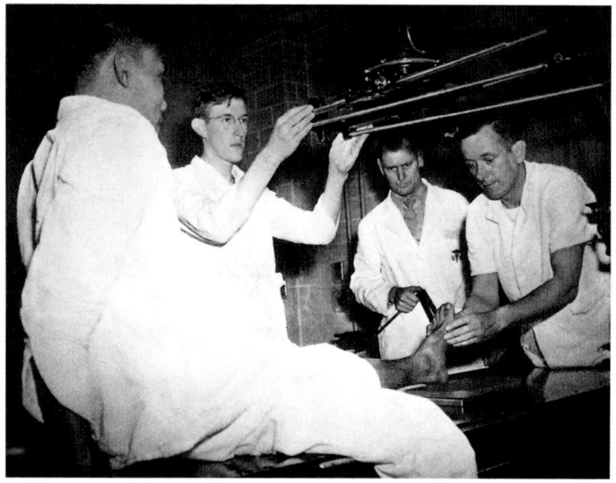

X-ray procedure demonstration and equipment

(AMSS Annual Report, 1949, figs 24 & 25)

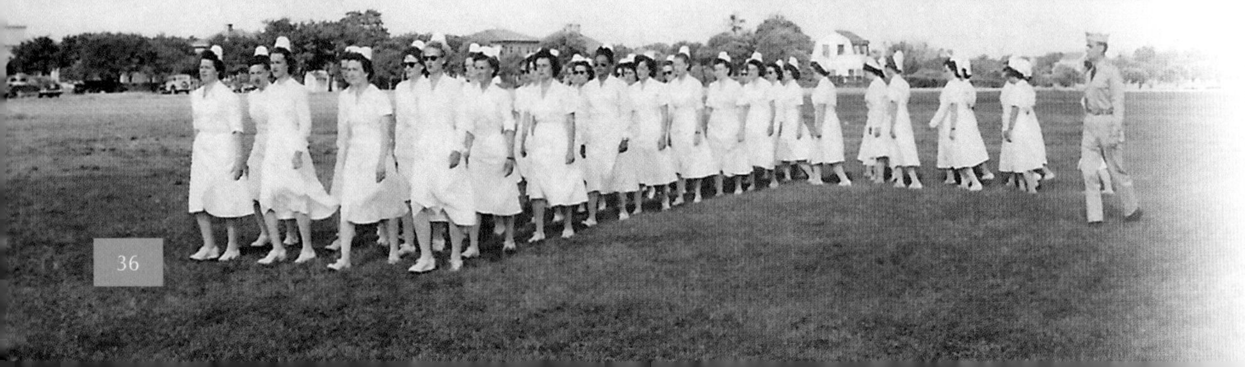

Student nurses executing drill formations

(AMSS Annual Report, 1949, fig 21)

The Extension Department was tasked with preparing and revising 78 correspondence subcourses. It graded a total of 64,047 exams during the 1949 reporting period.

(AMSS Annual Report, 1949, p 18)

The entire second class of the Advance Medical Department Officer's Course and faculty members were transported by air to Ft. Benning, Georgia, to witness a realistic ground troop demonstration, and then to Eglin Field, Florida, for OPERATION COMBINE, an air evacuation exercise.

(AMSS Annual Report, 1949, p 26)

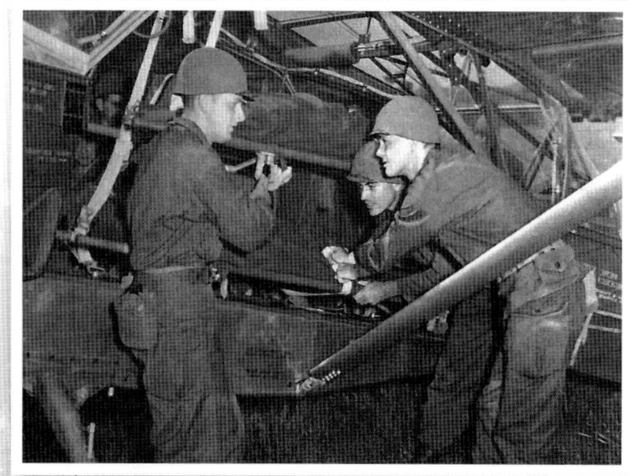

ROTC students demonstrating air evacuation techniques

(AMSS Annual Report, 1949, fig 32)

Students receiving instruction in remedial reading techniques

(AMSS Annual Report, 1949, figs 36, 37 & 38)

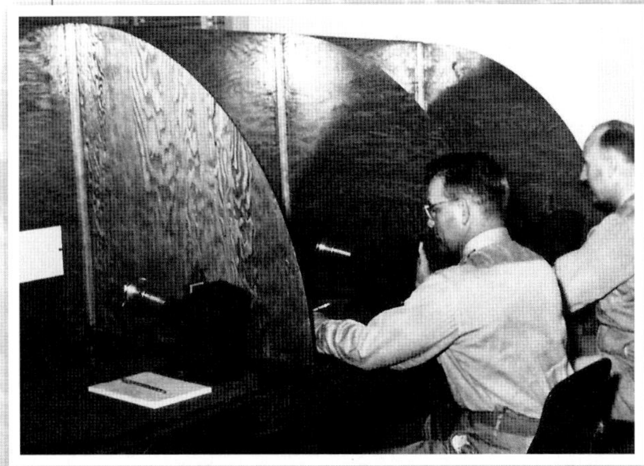

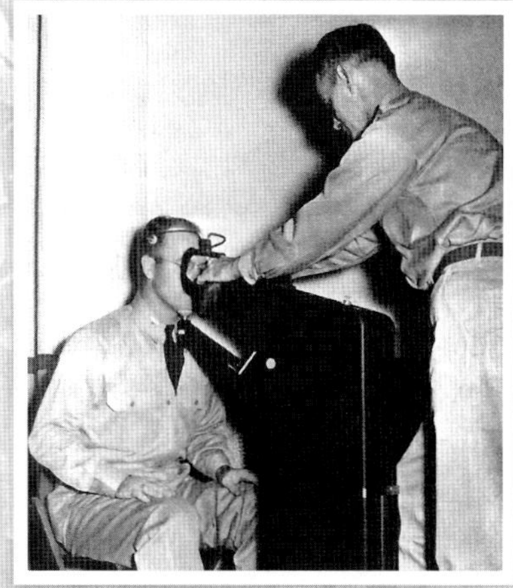

A, B, and C Companies, 1st Battalion, MFSS, Armistice Day Parade, downtown San Antonio

(AMSS Annual Report, 1949, fig 17)

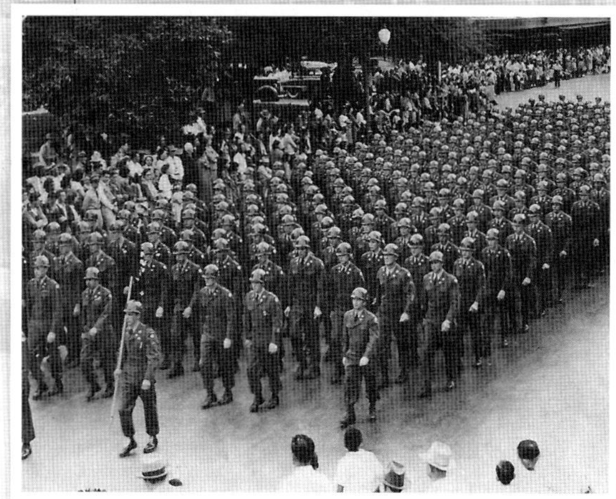

Headquarters of the Medical Field Service School

(AMSS Annual Report, 1949, fig 1)

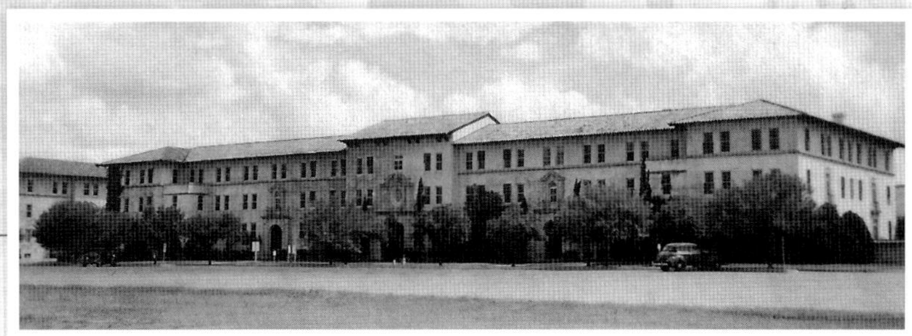

1950 - 1959

The Bulletin of the U.S. Army Medical Department and the Naval Medical Bulletin consolidated and published its first issue in January 1950 as *The United States Armed Forces Medical Journal.*

(Officers' Reserve Corps [ORC] Training Bulletin, Medical Department U.S. Army, published by the Medical Field Service School [MFSS], FSH, TX, October 1950, p 3)

MSG Edward Austin shows clippings of MFSS activities to a young newcomer, PVT Donald Sedlaw, of Detroit, MI, age 17. MSG Austin served at the MFSS most of his 32 years in the Army, first at Carlisle Barracks, then at BAMC.

(AMSS Annual Report, 1950)

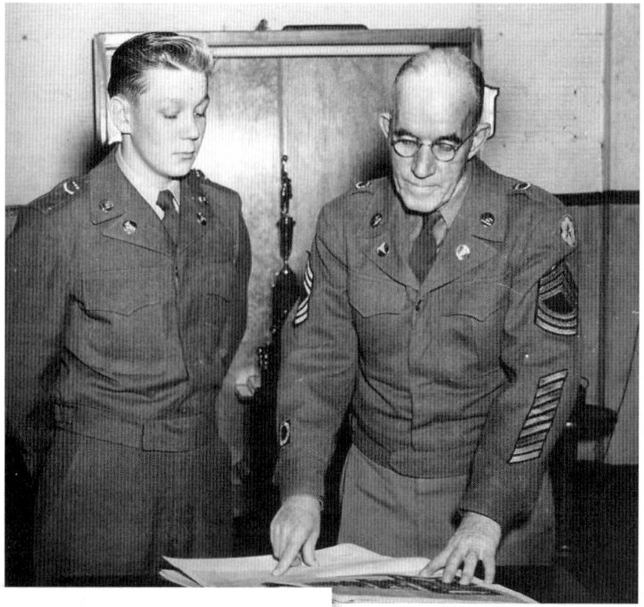

WAC Uniform
On 6 April 1950, members of the Women's Army Corps (WAC) student detachment were given an opportunity to view the WAC uniform which was contemplated for future issues.

(AMSS Annual Report, 1950, p 16)

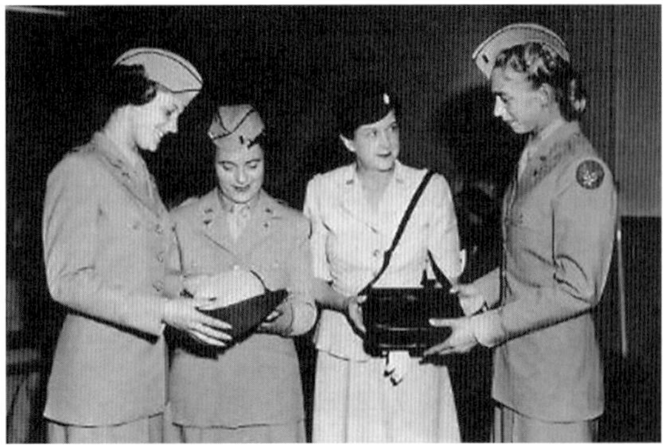

During a two-week active duty training at the MFSS, 103 members of the Officers' Reserve Corps saw demonstrations of an ambulance shuttle system. The training covered manual carries of patients, improvised litters, and conversions of standard Army vehicles to patient carriers. A variety of vehicles were involved, including the 2 ½, 1 ½, and ¾-ton trucks; a ¼-ton jeep with trailer; a half-track armored vehicle; a scout car, and the M29C, commonly called the "Weasel."

(ORC Training Bulletin, Medical Department U.S. Army, published by the MFSS, FSH, TX, 1 September 1950, p 1)

A large influx of wounded from Korea in the fall of 1950 increased the need for Red Cross housing on post, forcing female officers who served as instructors to obtain off-post quarters.

(AMSS Annual Report, 1950, p 19)

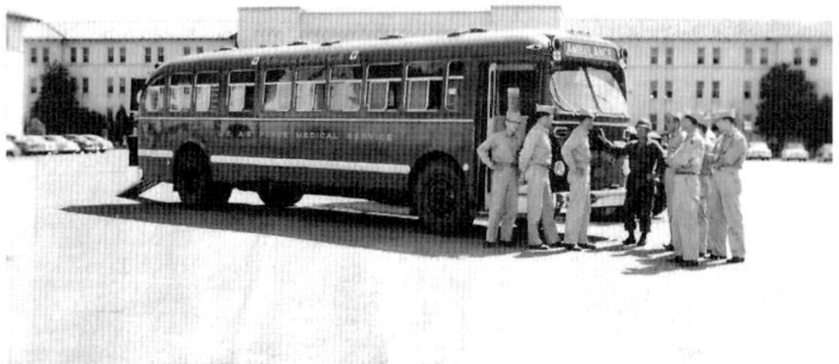

Ambulance, circa 1952

(AMSS Annual Historical Report, 1951)

The Graphic Arts Section was key to education and training at the MFSS during the 1950s. It created displays and exhibits for Armed Forces Day, the San Antonio International Trade Fair, and exhibits throughout the school. It designed and built numerous training aids for the newly activated Medical Replacement Training Center and developed a three-dimensional aids shop that produced models, mock-ups and three dimensional training aids that illustrated effects of atomic explosions and anatomical models. It also prepared a Training Aids Catalog which contained training charts and diagrams readily available through their department.

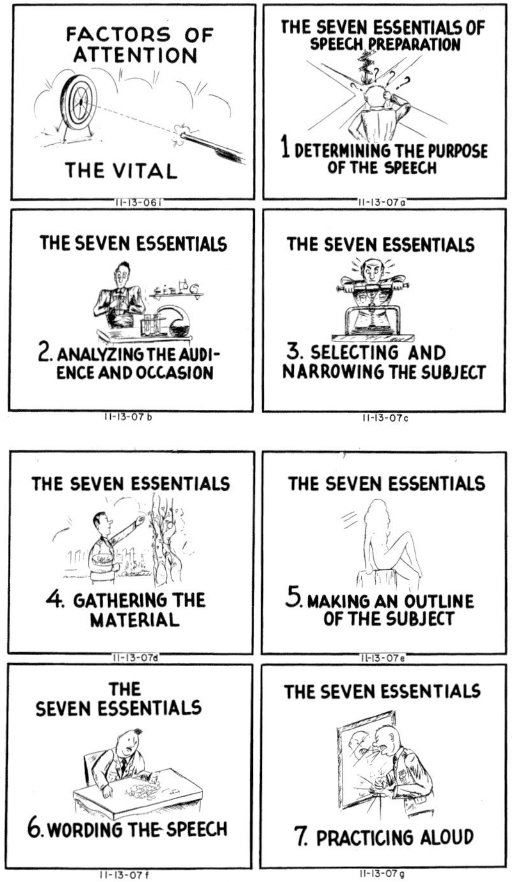

The Seven Essentials
A training aid for speech preparation from the 1950 Training Aids Catalog.

(AMSS Annual Report, 1950, p 16)

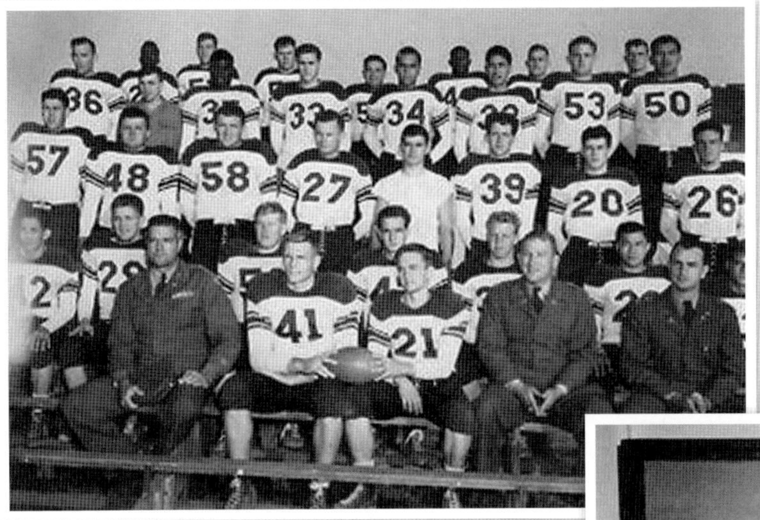

The MFSS 1950 football team, the "Comets"

(AMSS Annual Report, 1950)

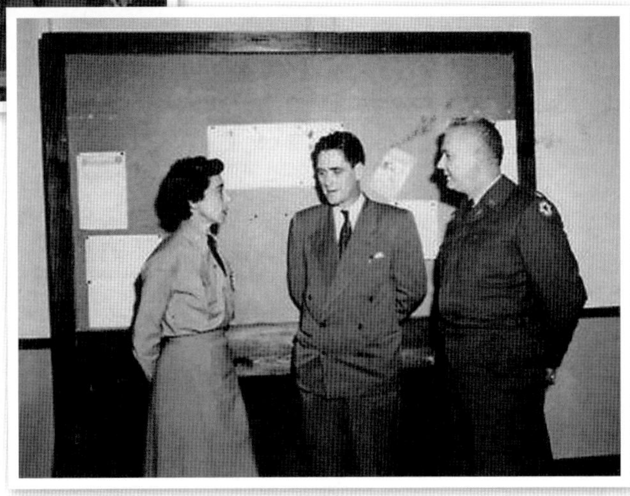

Guest Speaker, Dr. Earl Elkins, Director of Physical Therapy Department at Mayo Clinic, with MAJ Snyder and LTC Tate

(AMSS Annual Report, 1950)

1950

The Vu-Graph overhead projector was adopted by the MFSS as a training device, opening a whole new field of graphic training aids.

(AMSS Annual Report, 1950, pg 21)

The MFSS implemented a Civilian Components Section in compliance with Army-wide policy. The primary mission of the section was to coordinate the preparation and distribution of instructional material to civilian components — Officer Reserve Corps (ORC), Reserve Officer Training Corps (ROTC), and National Guard (NG).

(ORC Training Bulletin, Medical Department U.S. Army, published by the MFSS, FSH, TX, 1 August 1950)

Women Officers Basic Class on the steps of the School of Aviation Medicine

(AMSS Annual Report, 1950)

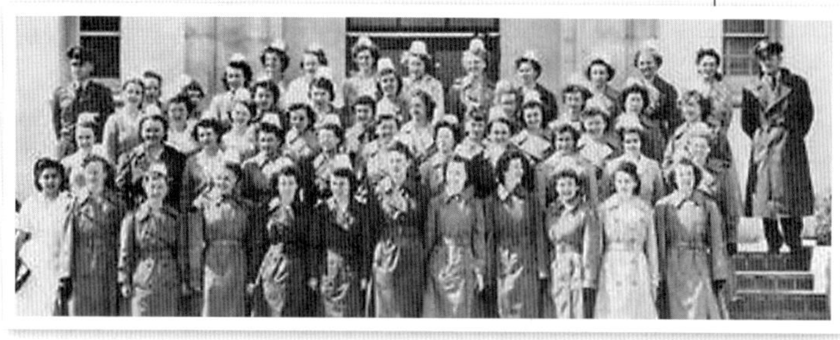

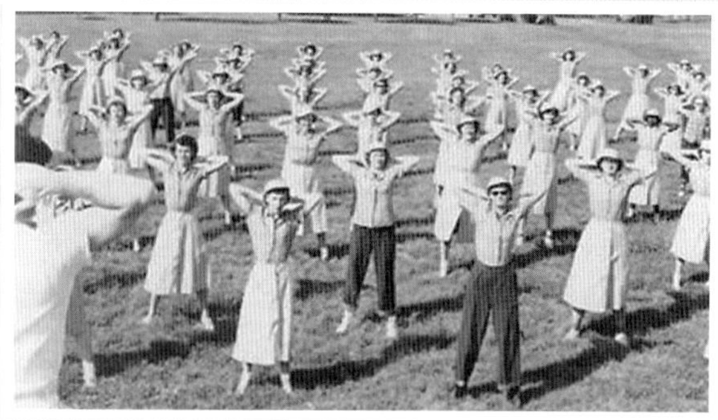

Women Officers Basic Class at calisthenics

(AMSS Annual Historical Report, 1950)

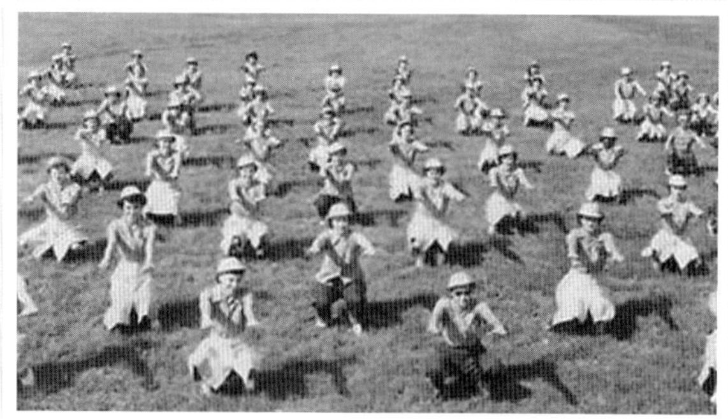

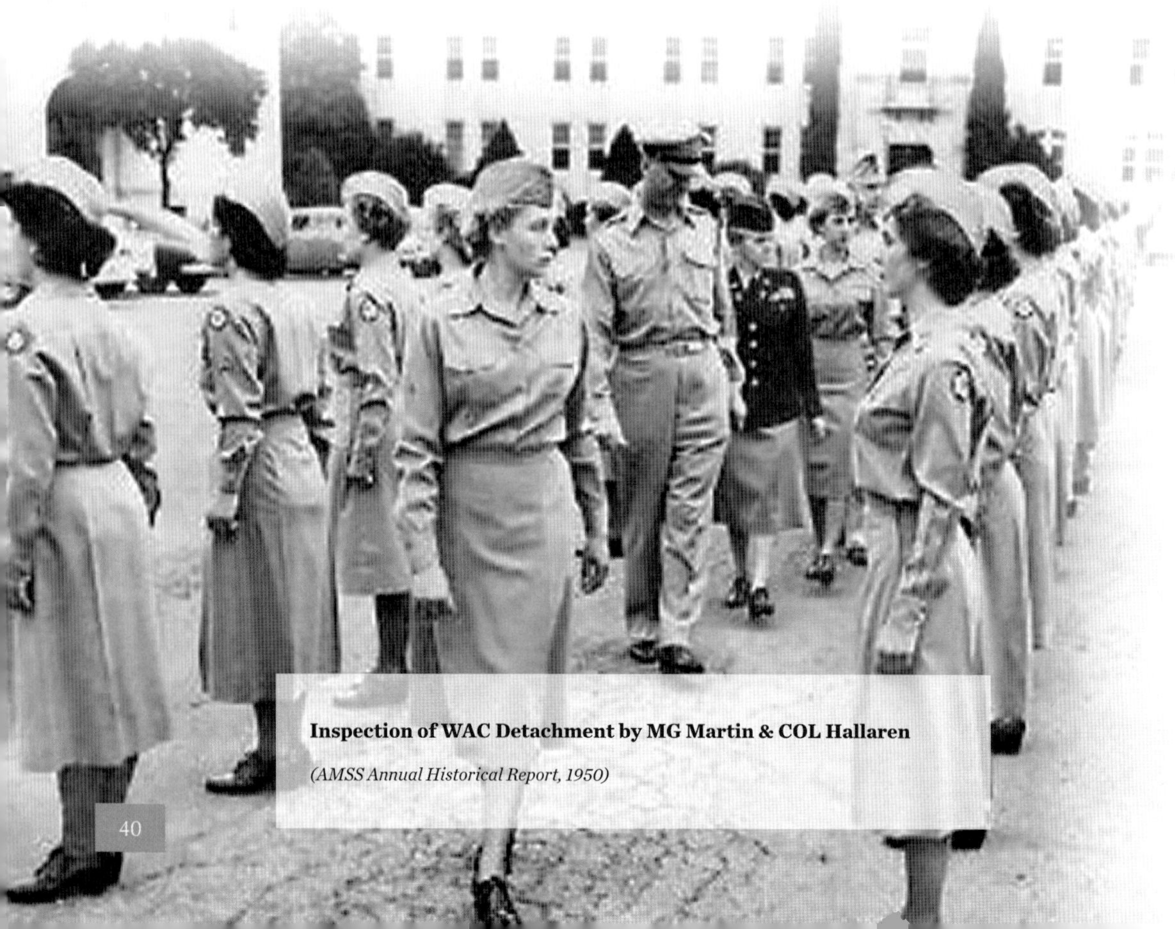

Inspection of WAC Detachment by MG Martin & COL Hallaren

(AMSS Annual Historical Report, 1950)

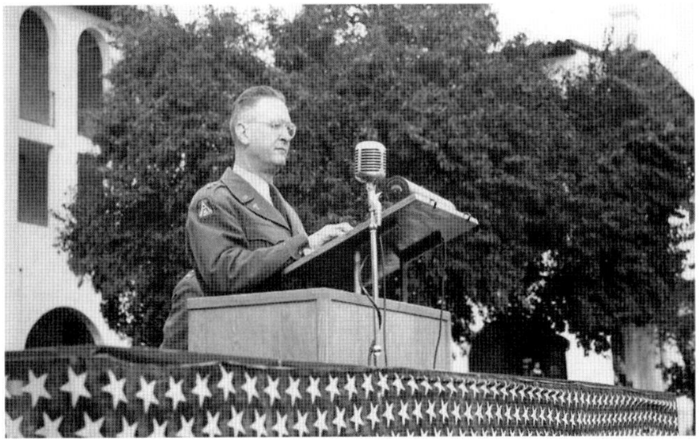

Organization Day
MG Martin addresses the troops during Organization Day.

(AMSS Annual Report, 1950)

Muster
Troops of the MFSS muster in formation in the Quadrangle to hear MG Martin deliver School Commandant's Organization Day Speech.

(AMSS Annual Report, 1950)

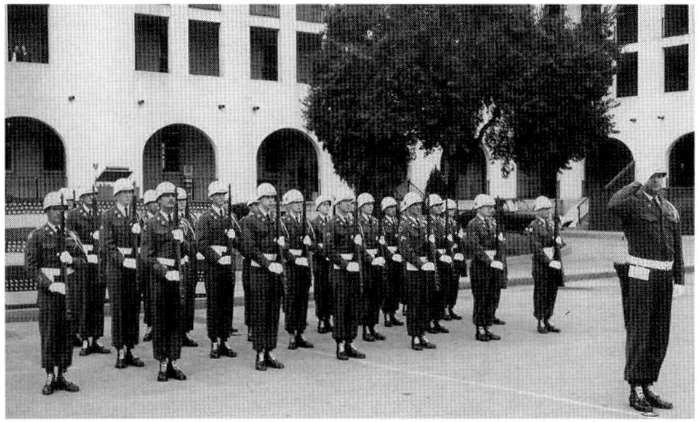

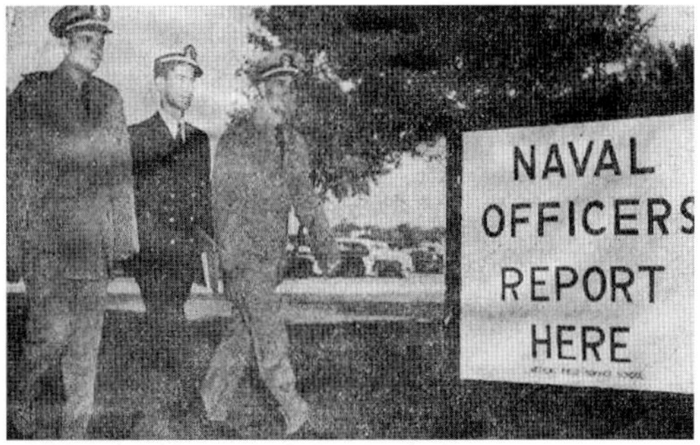
NAVAL
OFFICERS
REPORT
HERE

U.S. Navy
The Navy assigned more than 600 Naval Reserve doctors to Army posts nationwide to ease a shortage of physicians. Several of the doctors-on-loan served at the MFSS.

(U.S. Army Photo, 1950)

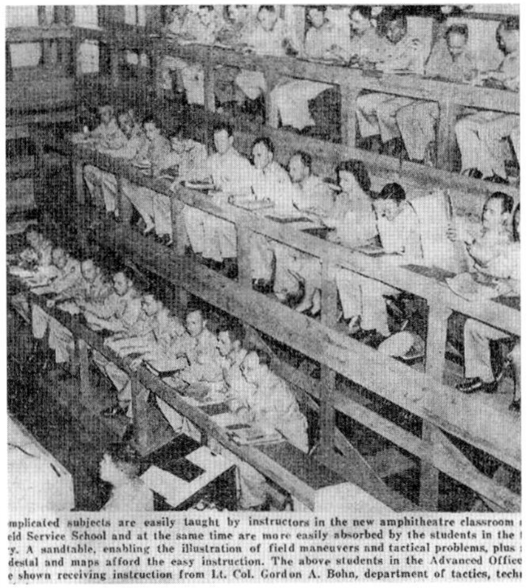
mplicated subjects are easily taught by instructors in the new amphitheatre classroom
eld Service School and at the same time are more easily absorbed by the students in the
y. A sandtable, enabling the illustration of field maneuvers and tactical problems, plus
destal and maps afford the easy instruction. The above students in the Advanced Office
e shown receiving instruction from Lt. Col. Gordon A. Bohn, department of tactics, tech

Ampitheater
Students attend tactical maneuver training in the "new" amphitheater classroom at the MFSS.

(AMSS Annual Report, 1950)

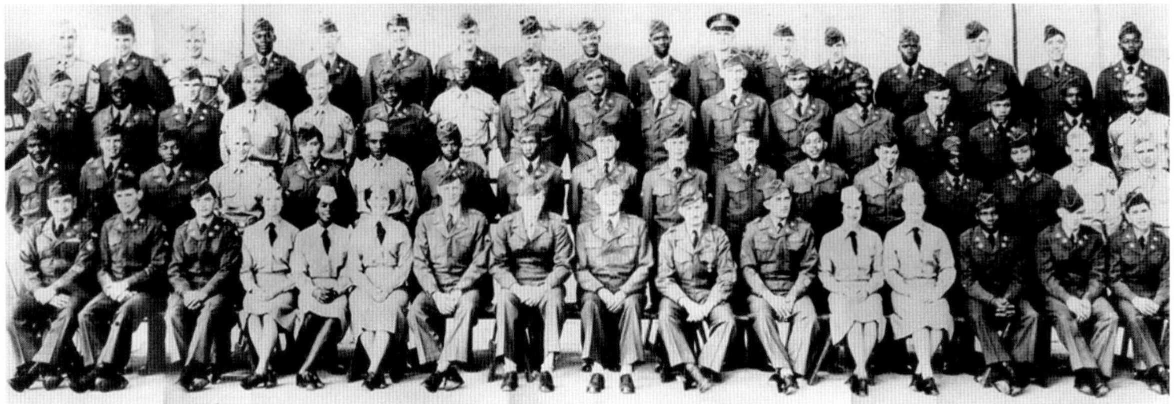

Class 168, Company A, 3rd Battalion, MFSS Surgical Technician Course
This image from October 1950 includes a number of Air Force troops (male individuals in khaki uniforms are Air Force personnel).

(U.S. Army Photo, Fort Sam Houston Museum Collection)

1950

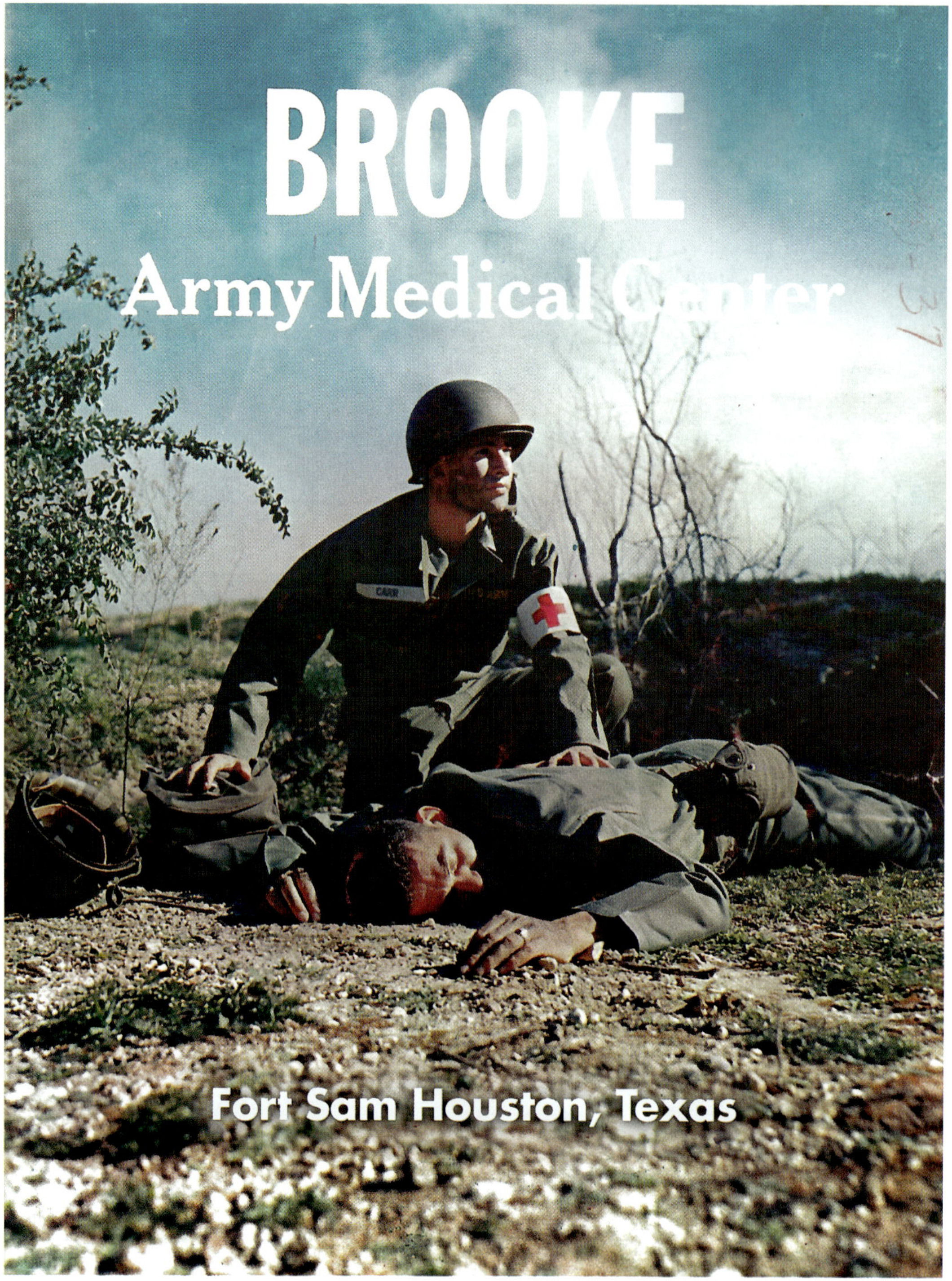

In 1950, BAMC produced a view book documenting research, training, and technology at the MFSS and BAMC.

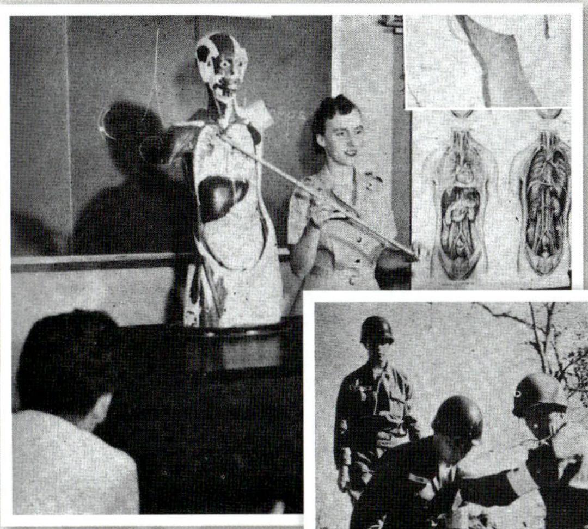

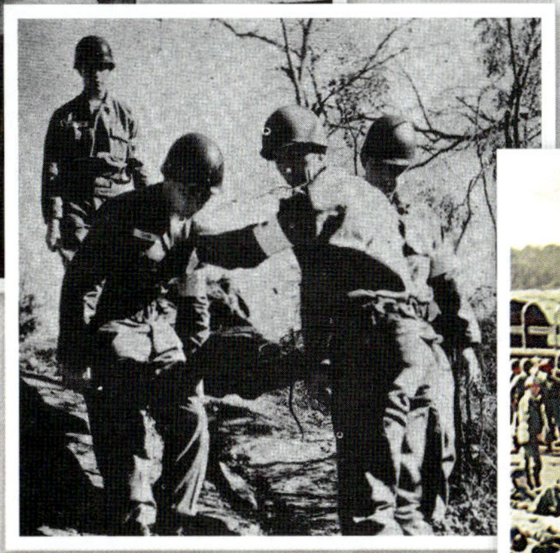

1950 Viewbook

A collage of images from the 1950 Viewbook highlighting MFSS training.

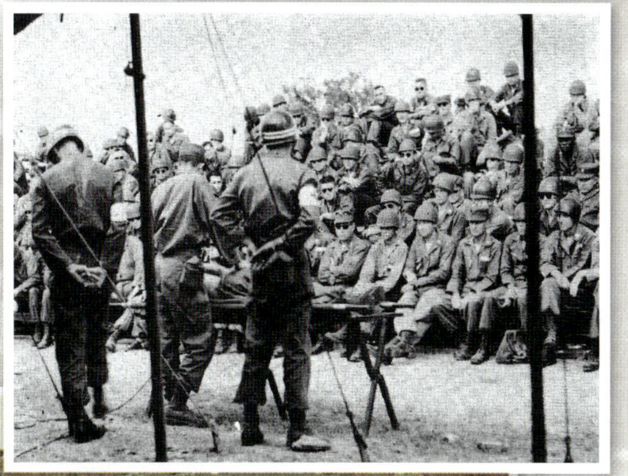

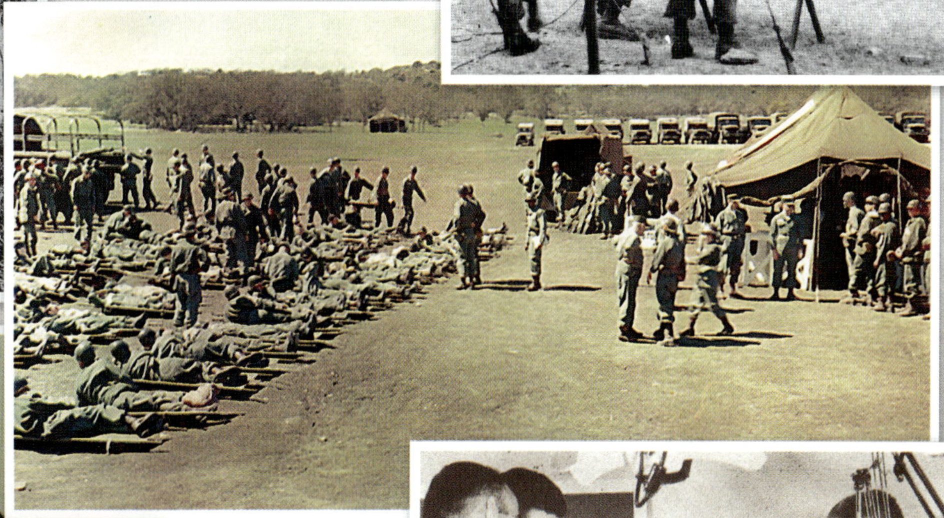

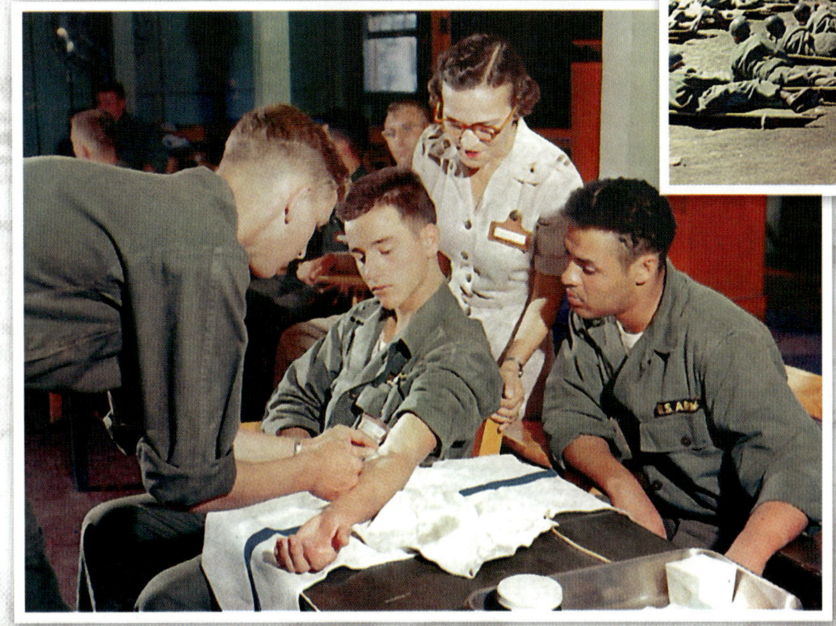

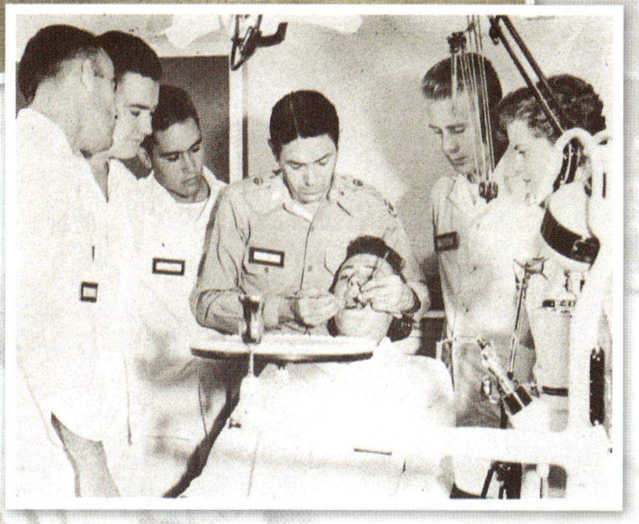

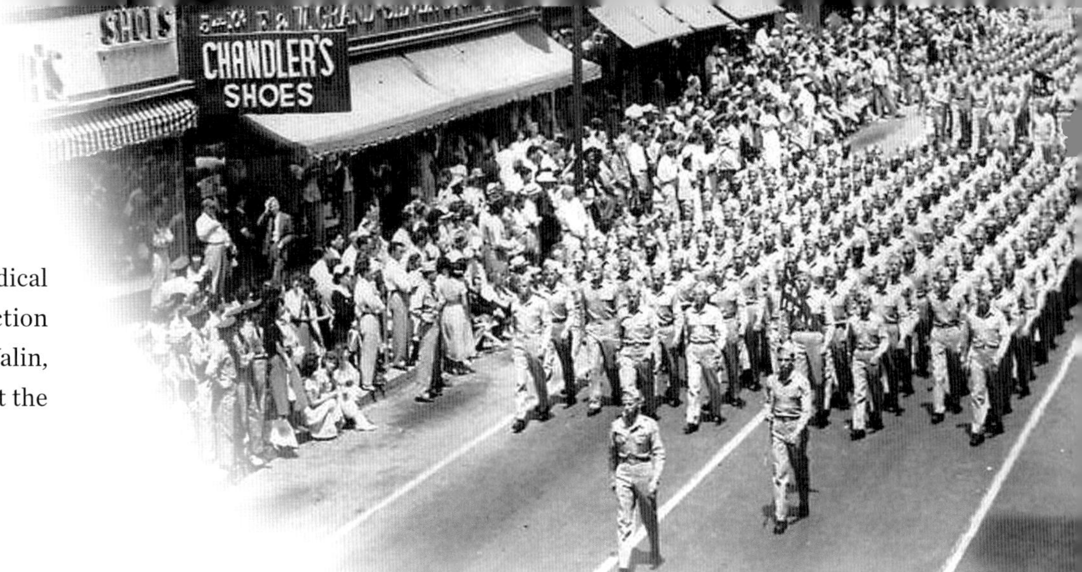

1951

The U.S. Army Medical Service and Royal Canadian Army Medical Corps formed a cooperative to standardize medical instruction and equipment between the two armies. COL J.C. Van Valin, Director of the Department of Tactics, Techniques, and Logistics at the MFSS was appointed to head up the U.S. Army's liaison team.

("Brooke Colonel to Head Team," San Antonio Evening News, 4 January 1951)

The first two women doctors to report for duty to the Army Medical Corps since WWII MAJ Theresa T. Woo and MAJ Ruth E. Church attend a four-week orientation course at the MFSS in February of 1951. MG Martin at center.

("First Two," San Antonio Express, 8 February 1951)

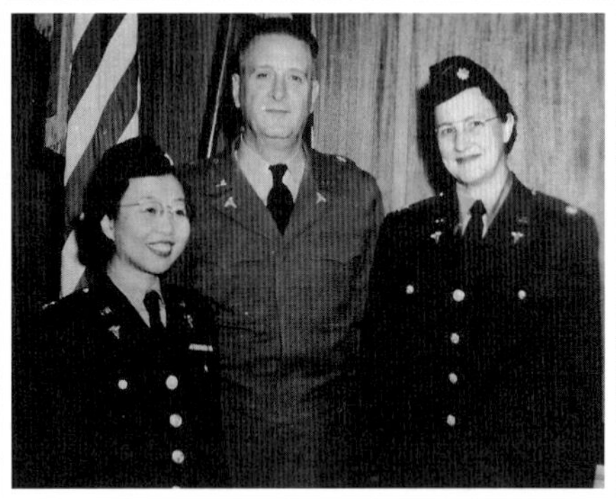

During the first quarter of 1951, more than 500 officers arrived at the MFSS for their basic military training, including 165 women officers. Shortly after their arrival, 1,000 new enlisted medical soldiers arrived for training. Both groups were the largest to report to the MFSS at that time.

("500 Due for Medic Course," San Antonio Evening News, date unknown, 1951; "1,000 Arrive at Ft. Sam," San Antonio Evening News, date unknown, 1951)

LTC Theodore J. Dalton was named commanding officer of the newly organized Fourth Battalion created to accommodate the increase in student population.

("MFSS Activates New Battalion," Army Post Times, 11 May 1951)

In honor of Armed Forces Day, part of Armed Forces Week, traditionally held the third weekend of May, the MFSS paraded in downtown San Antonio, placed window displays in storefront windows, and held demonstrations on MacArthur Field highlighting the research, technology, and training taking place at Fort Sam Houston.

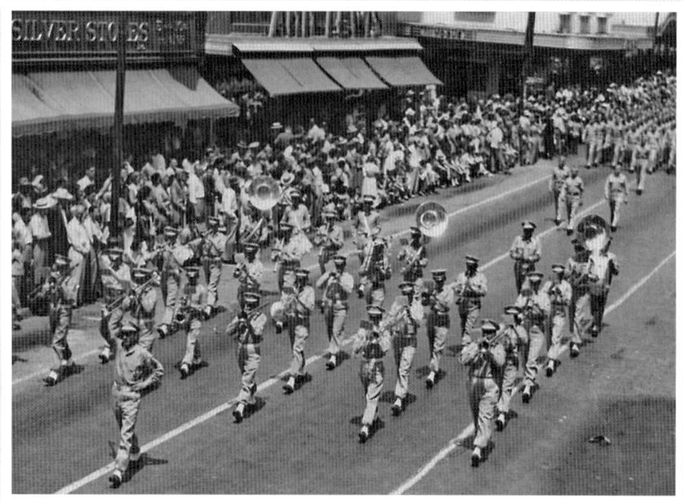

The 323rd Army Band and troops march in the 1951 Armed Forces Day Parade in downtown San Antonio.

(Armed Forces Day Report, May 19-20, 1951, Stimson Library Special Collections)

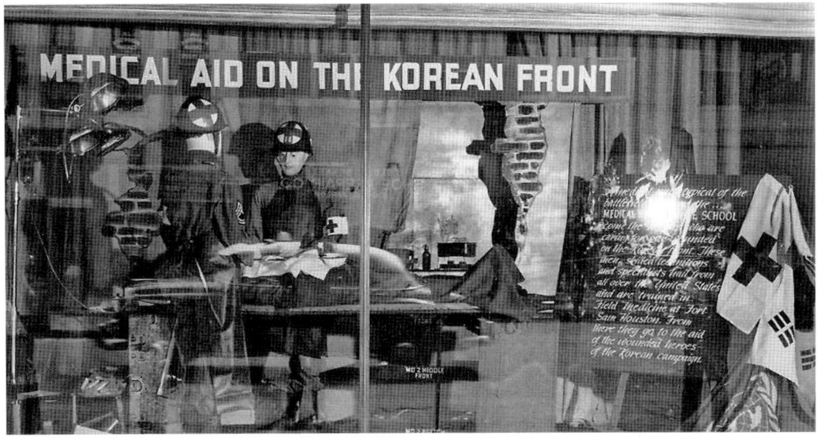

Store-front displays of surgical instruments and a battalion aid station were placed in the windows of the Wolff & Marx Company on Soledad Street and Joskes of Texas, then San Antonio's largest department store on Alamo Plaza.

(Armed Forces Day Report, May 19-20, 1951, Stimson Library Special Collections)

Static exhibits about field service, effects of radiation, and supply movement were set up at Fort Sam Houston to instruct the general public on the MFSS mission and history.

(Armed Forces Day Report, May 19-20, 1951, Stimson Library Special Collections)

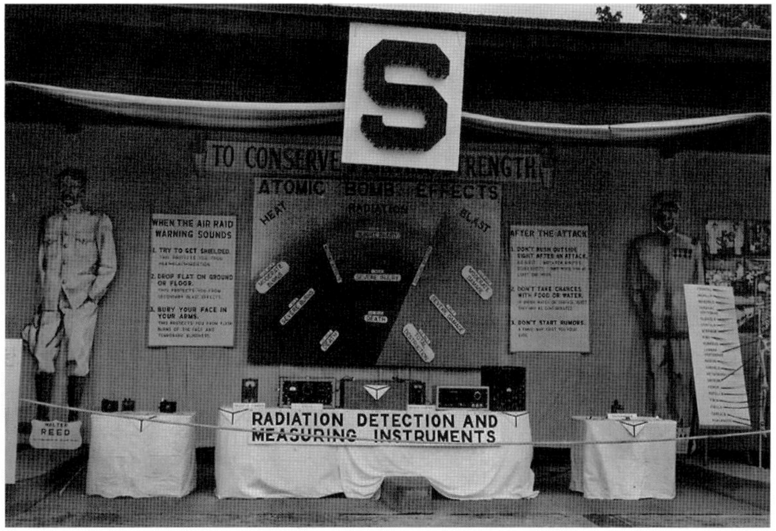

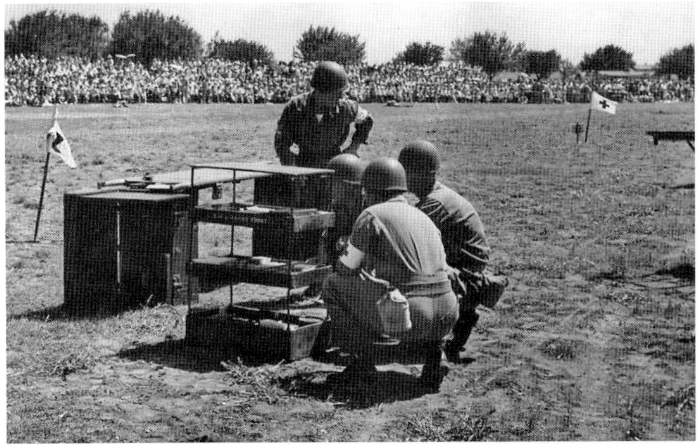

Patient care at point of injury and MEDEVAC operations were recreated at MacArthur Field.

(Armed Forces Day Report, May 19-20, 1951, Stimson Library Special Collections)

Medical troops load a patient into ambulance during exercises.

(Armed Forces Day Report, May 19-20, 1951, Stimson Library Special Collections)

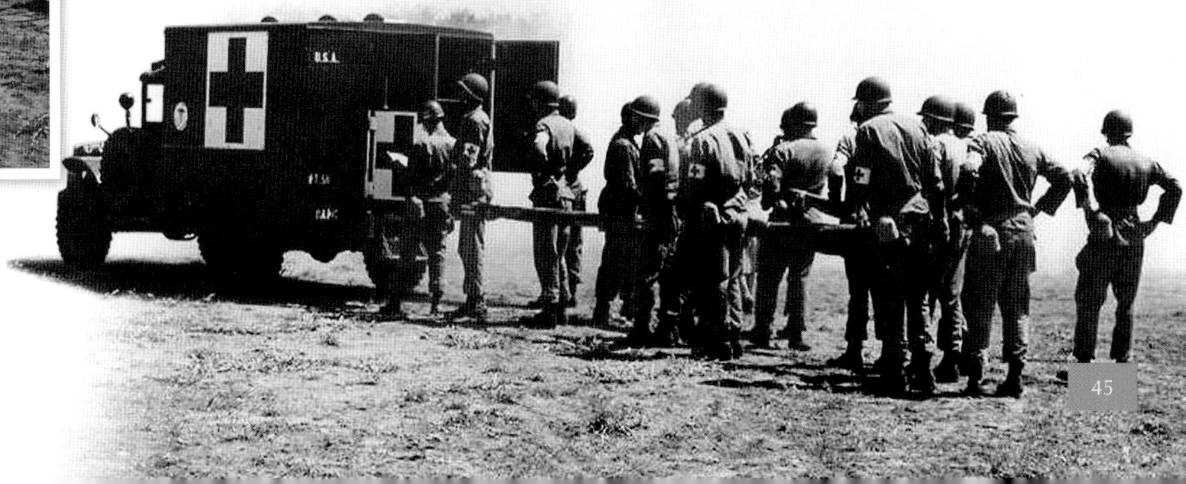

1951

The first woman officer of the Medical Service Corps, CPT Dorothy V. Parker, reported to duty at the MFSS in June of 1951.

("Woman Officer to Train Here," San Antonio News Express, June 1951)

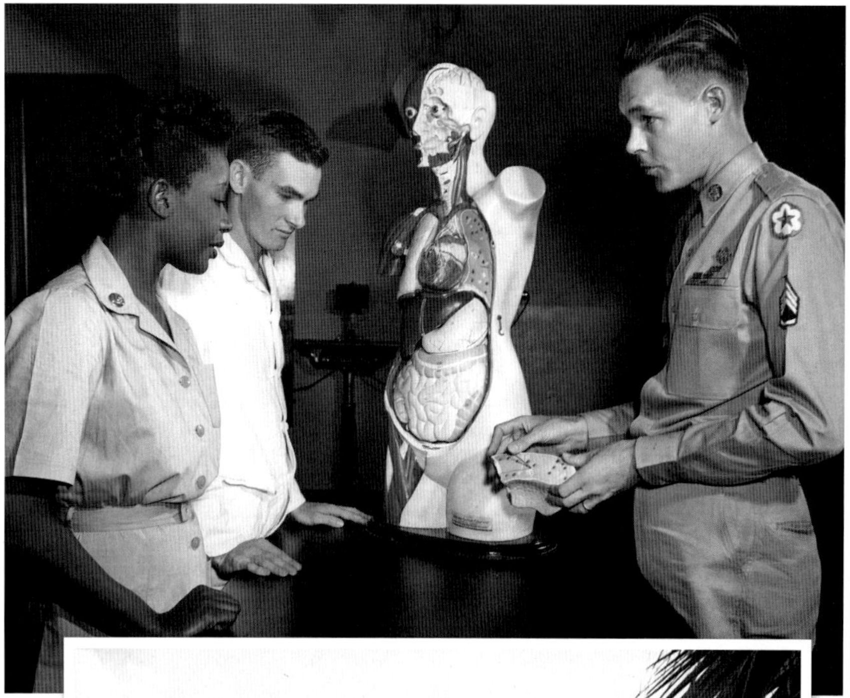

The sectional torso nicknamed "Matilda" assisted SGT Fowler as he instructed PVT Bertia Lewis and PVT Claude Blackburnon on the finer points of lung structure.

(U.S. Army Photo, AMEDD Museum Photo Collection)

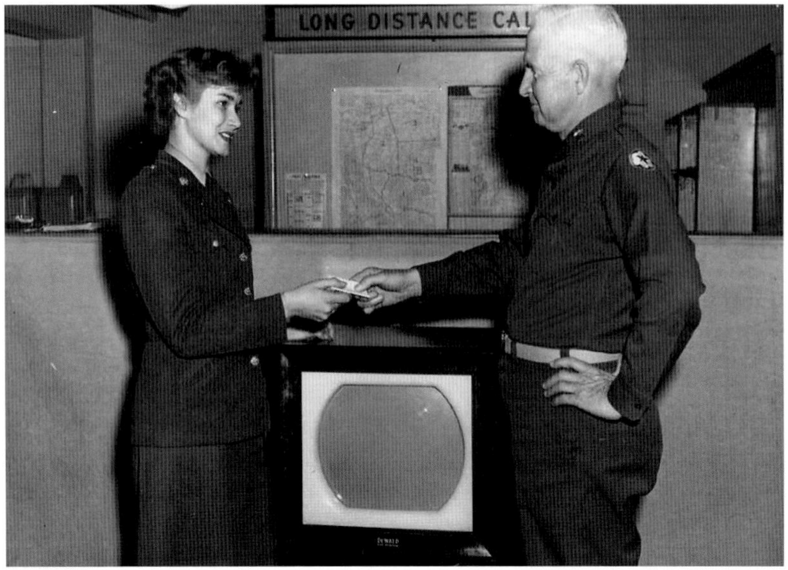

LTC Harvey Wilson, MFSS Acting Chief of Troops Division (right), awards PVT Helen Daniels, Nurse Practitioner Technician student, a television set given as the grand door prize on Organization Day.

(Organization Day file, 1951, Stimson Library Special Collections)

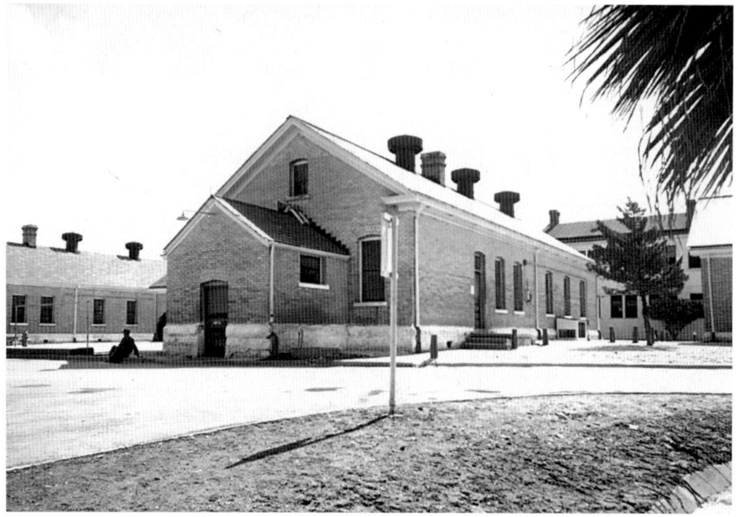

Company A area in Reception Center, Infantry Post

(U.S. Army Photo, Fort Sam Houston Museum Photo Collection)

The "Doctor Commando," BG Crawford F. Sams, became Assistant Commandant of the MFSS. BG Sams acquired his nickname from a Collier's magazine article detailing his heroic mission behind enemy lines to obtain proof of the nonexistence of bubonic plague among Communist Koreans.

("Brooke General's Exploits Behind Lines Told," San Antonio Light, 23 September 1951, p 11-A)

On 2 November 1951, PVT Roland Forte became the 100,000th student to graduate from the MFSS. The output of total students had doubled since the arrival of the MFSS at Fort Sam Houston in 1946. 20,000 alone had graduated since the beginning of the Korean War.

("100,000th Medical Grad," San Antonio Light, 2 Nov 1951)

Members of the 498th Preventive Medicine Company began an ectoparasitic survey of malaria-diseased bats at local caves.

("Army Trying to Determine If Bats Transmit Malaria," San Antonio Express, 18 November 1951)

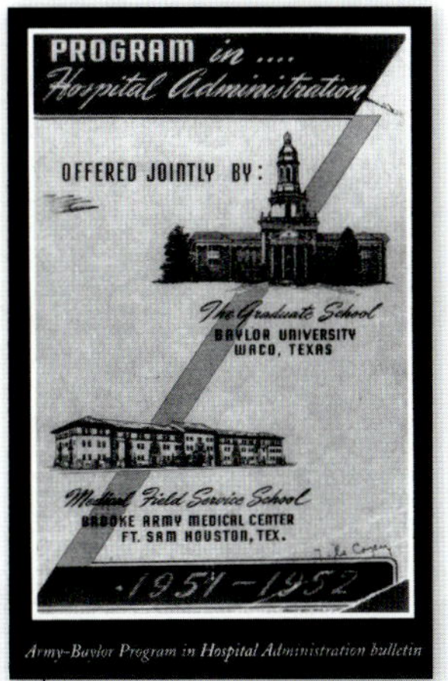
PROGRAM in ....
Hospital Administration
OFFERED JOINTLY BY:
The Graduate School
BAYLOR UNIVERSITY
WACO, TEXAS
Medical Field Service School
BROOKE ARMY MEDICAL CENTER
FT. SAM HOUSTON, TEX.
1951 - 1952
Army-Baylor Program in Hospital Administration bulletin

The "Doctor Commando"
BG Crawford F. Sams

(U.S. Army Photo, Fort Sam Houston Museum Photo Collection)

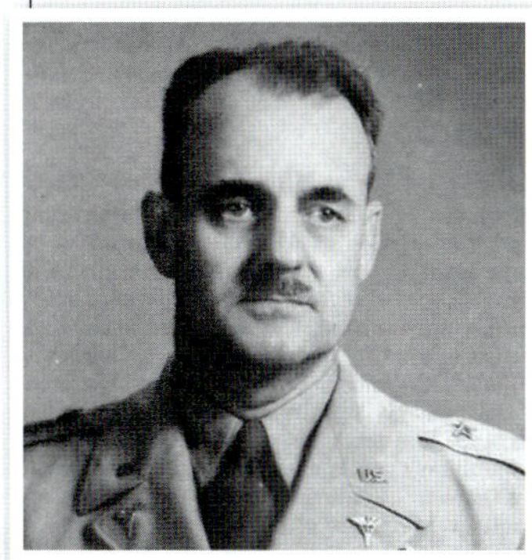

MG Martin and Mrs. Martin cut the birthday cake commemorating the fourth anniversary of the MFSS during Organization Day at NCO Club No. 2.

(Organization Day file 1951, Stimson Library Special Collections)

The Army-Baylor Program offered its first program in Hospital Administration in 1951.

(Army-Baylor Bulletin 1951, Stimson Library Special Collections)

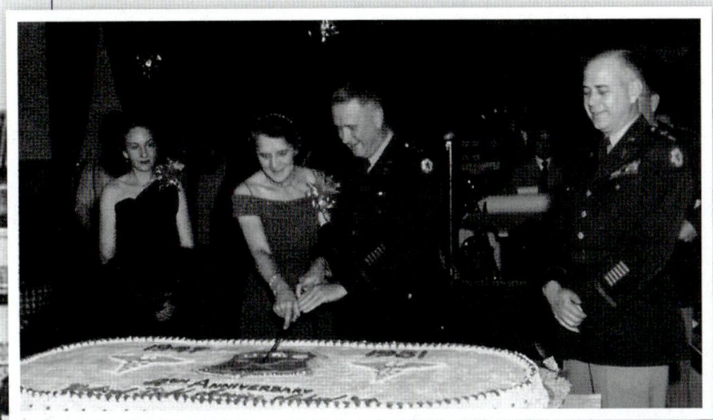

Formation in the 9th Infantry Quadrangle prior to MG Martin's Organization Day speech.

(Organization Day file 1951, Stimson Library Special Collections)

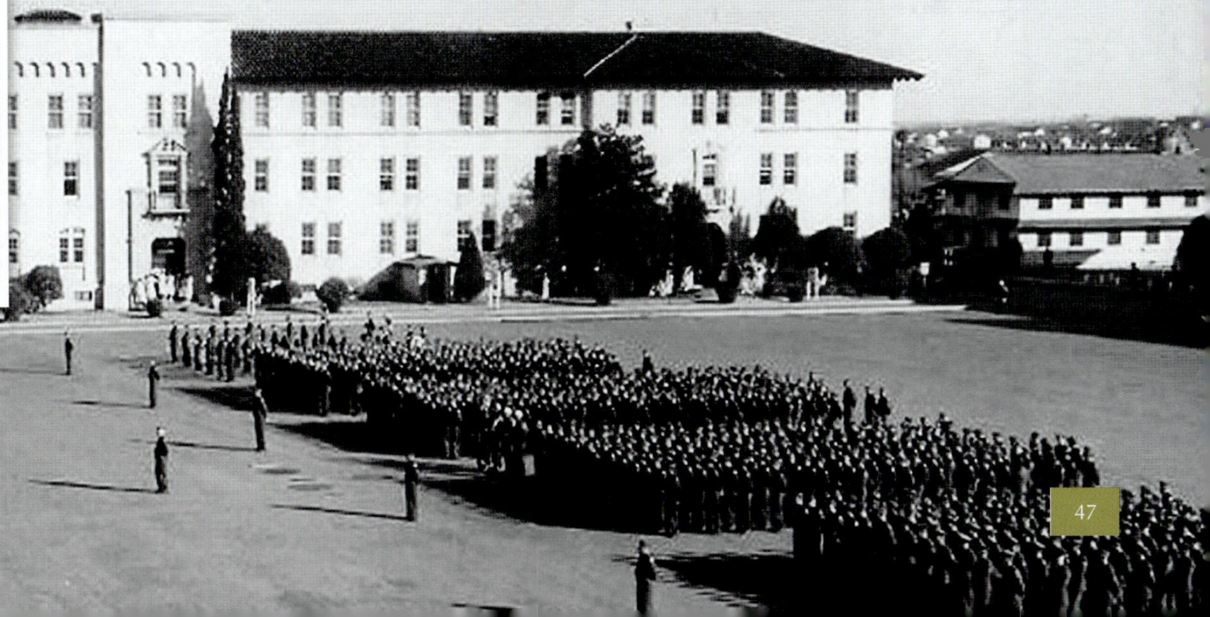

1952

In July 1952, the MFSS became the first Army medical installation to add helicopters to its training facilities. LT Joseph L. Bowler was appointed head of the MFSS aviation section. At the time, LT Bowler held the record for the most casualty evacuations during the Korean War.

("Two 'Flying Windmills' Added As MFSS Shapes Aviation Section," Army Post Times, 11 July 1952)

The MFSS held its first "Think Fast and Then Act Deliberately" course. An all male officer course, it involved both day and night field exercises designed to teach students tactics against guerilla techniques.

("Think Fast! Act Deliberately!," ORC: the Army Medical Service Training Bulletin, Vol III, No. 1, BAMC, FSH, TX, April 1952, p 2)

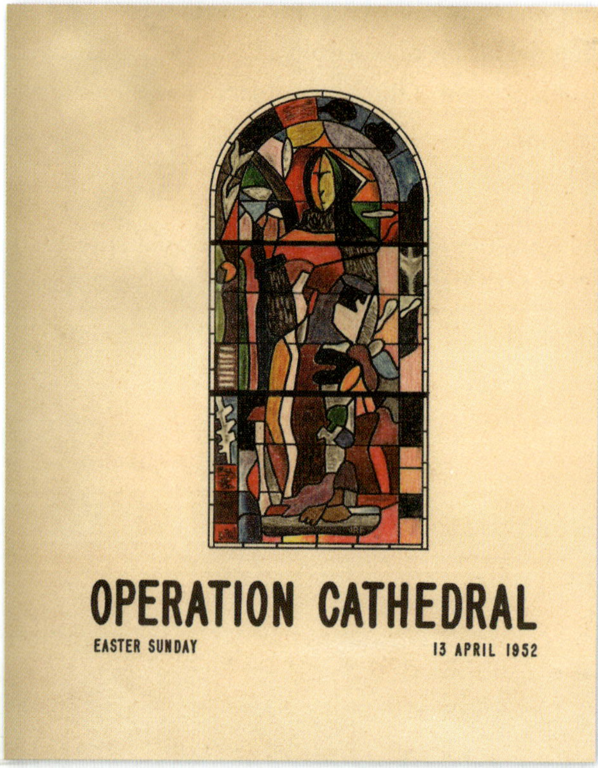

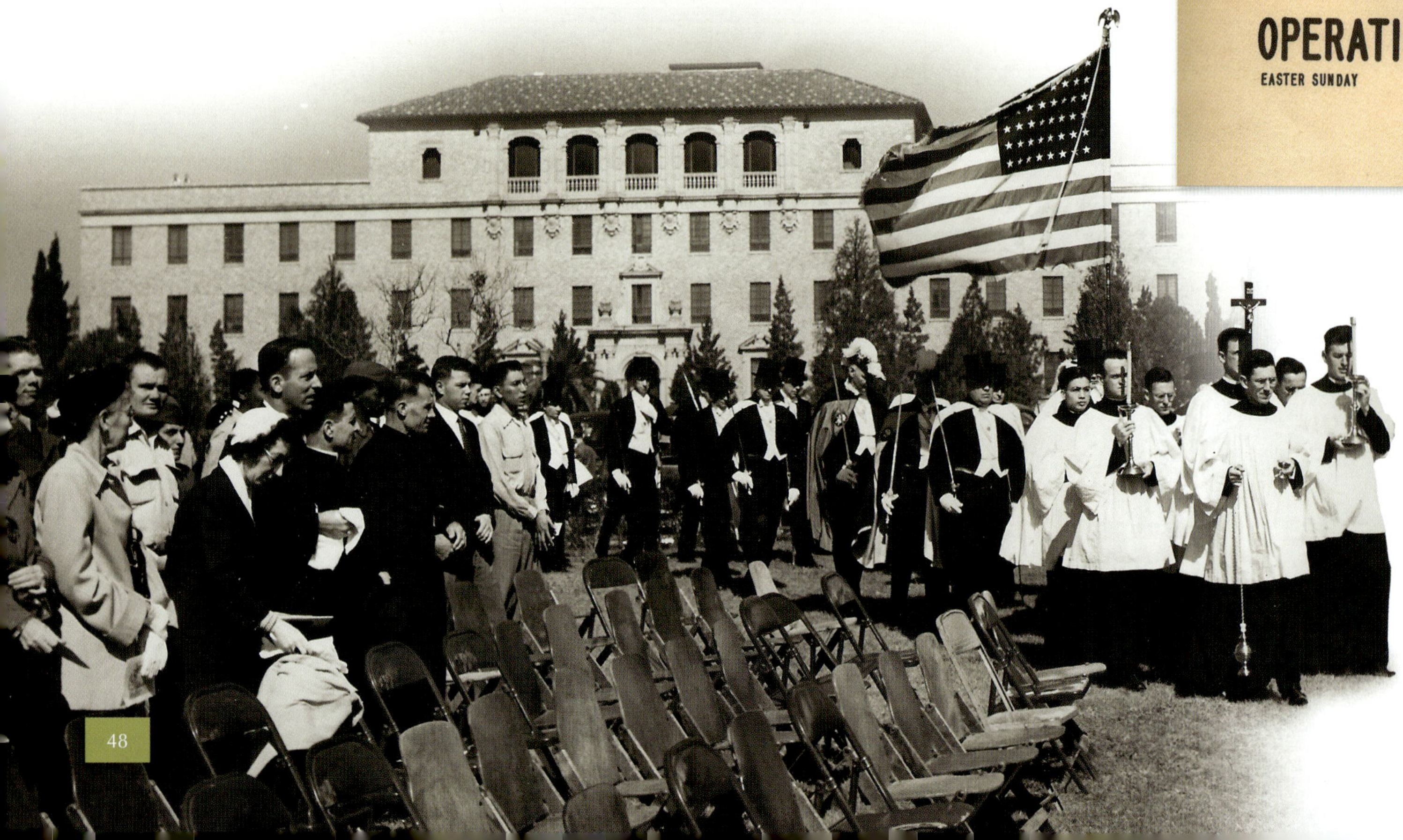

Seminarians from the De Mazenod Seminary and members of the San Antonio Fourth Degree Knights of Columbus participated in the Easter Sunday pontifical field mass on MacArthur Field. The mass was part of an overall Easter weekend program named "Operation Cathedral."

(Operation Cathedral OPORD, 1952, Stimson Library Special Collections)

A portable weight rack was devised and put into use at BAMC by MFSS students with the Physical Therapy Program as a time and labor-saving device.

("Portable Weight Rack," ORC: the Army Medical Service Training Bulletin, Vol. III, No. 2, BAMC, FSH, TX, July 1952)

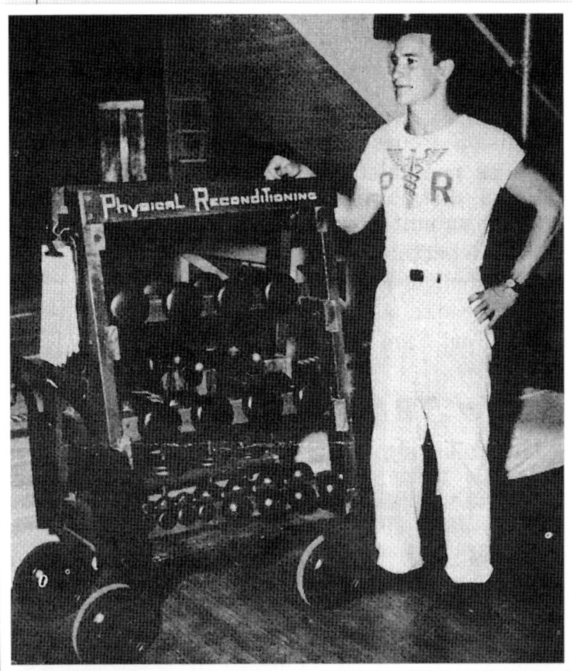

"Medical aid men" begin their training on the new ambulance truck M43, designed to accommodate five litter or eight ambulatory patients.

("New Ambulance Type Truck," ORC: the Army Medical Service Training Bulletin, Vol. III, No. 4, October 1952, p 3)

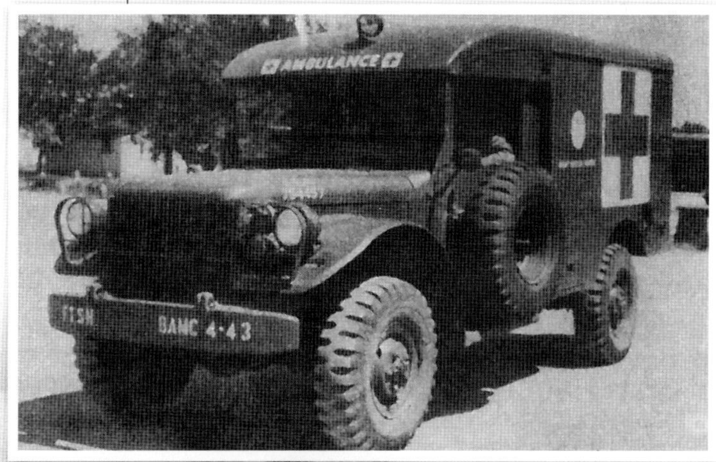

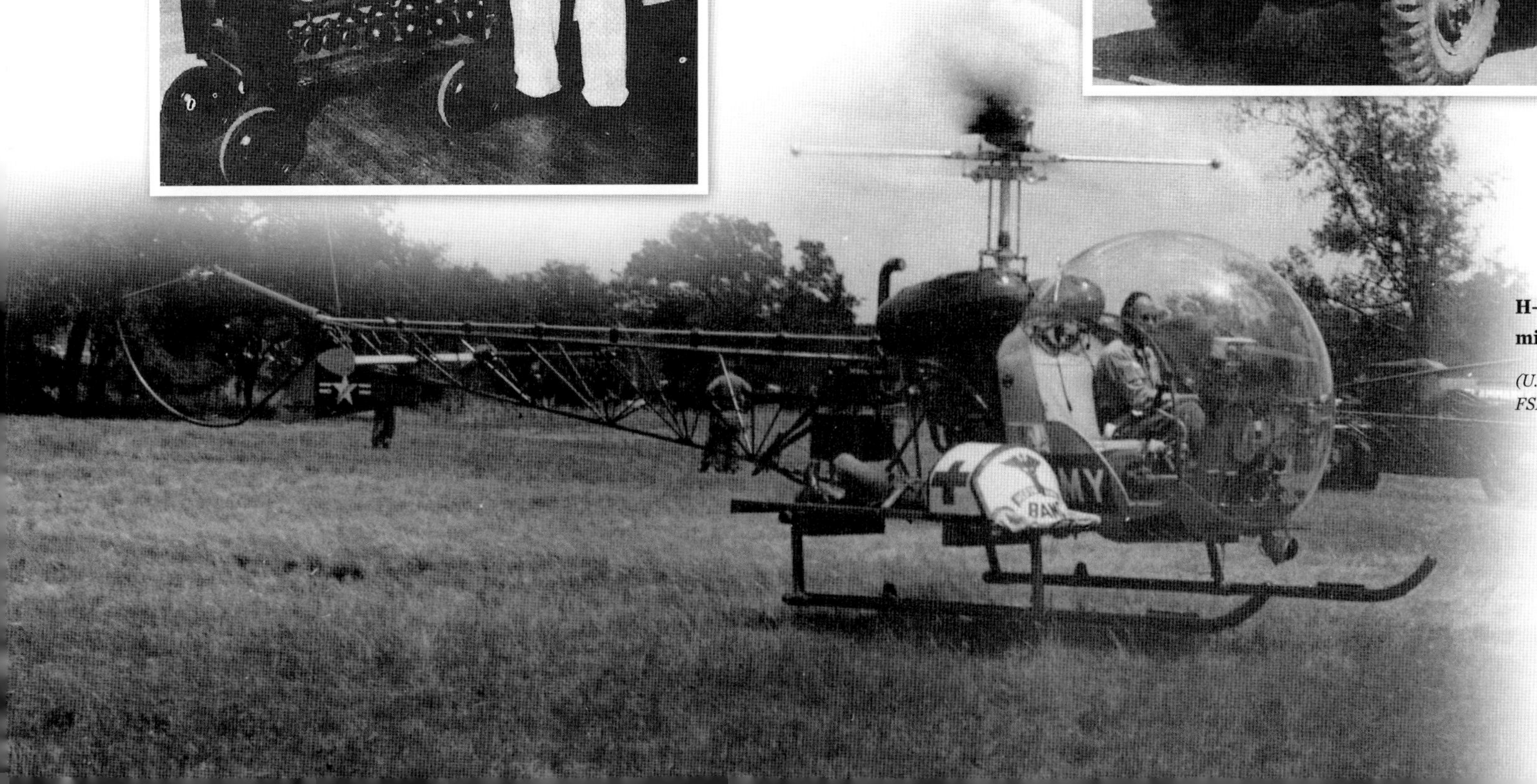

H-13 helicopters land on a mission to BAMC, circa 1952

(U.S. Army Photo, FSH Museum Photo Collection)

1952

Two hundred and forty-eight pharmacy and veterinary ROTC Cadets completed a six-week training camp at the MFSS in August of 1952. They attended courses on Military Courtesy, Organization of the Army, Chemical Warfare, Dismounted Drill, and Map Reading. The veterinary students completed their training with a three-day exercise at the King Ranch in Kingsville, Texas.

("ROTC Summer Camp," ORC: the Army Medical Service Training Bulletin, Vol. III, No. 2, BAMC, FSH, TX, July 1952)

A scrapbook page shows the difference between what the Army wanted the MFSS student barracks to look like and what they really looked like in 1952.

(FSH Museum Photo Collection)

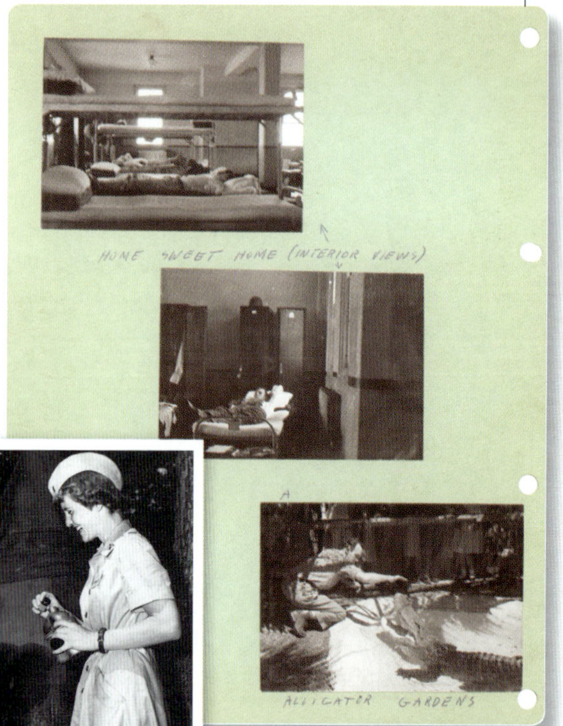

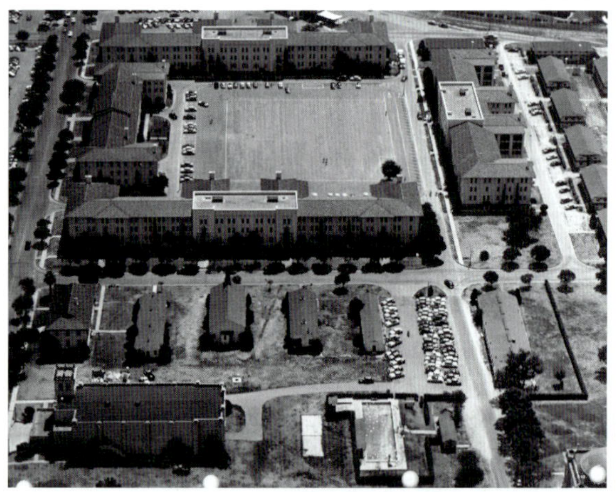

Aerial view of the 9th Infantry Quadrangle, 1952

(U.S. Army Photo, FSH Museum Photo Collection)

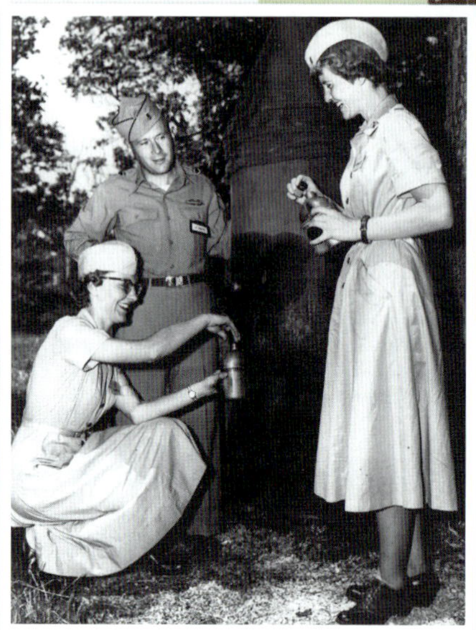

Army Nurses in the Women's Officer Basic Course receive instruction on water purification, 6 May 1952.

(U.S. Army Photo, AMEDD Museum Photo Collection)

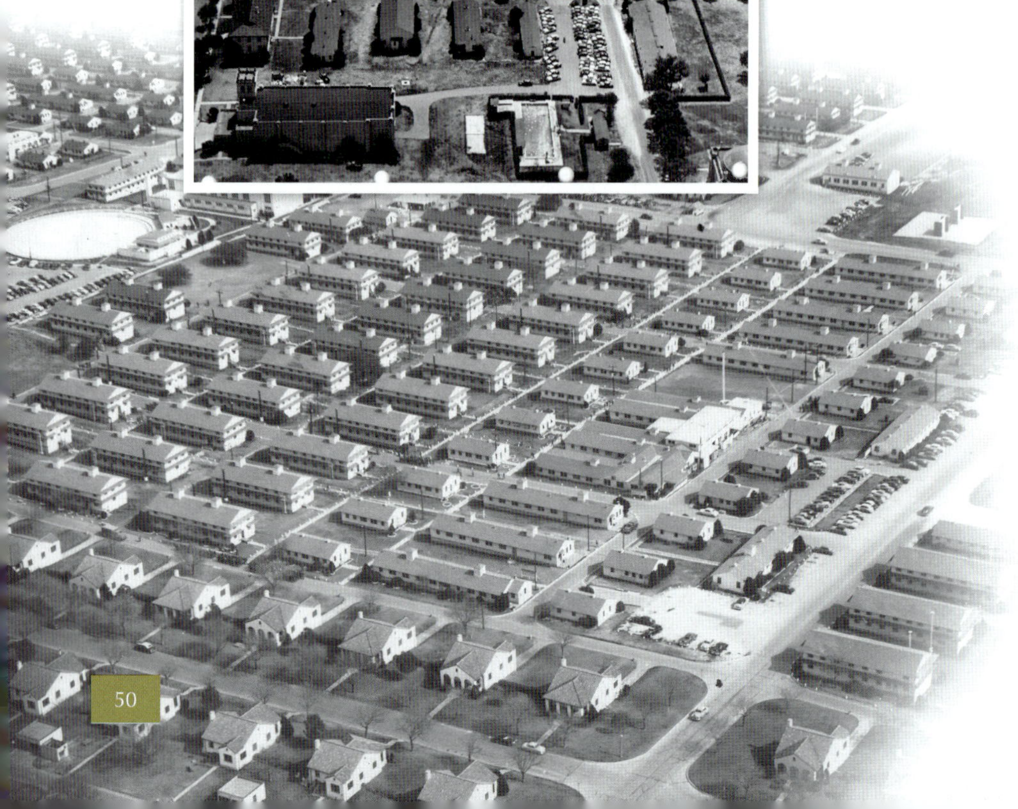

Medical Replacement Training Center, 1952, in mobilization barracks area along Garden Street between Schofield and Hardee Roads

(U.S. Army Photo, FSH Museum Photo Collection)

A logistical command post exercise and map maneuver designated as LOGEX 52 ½ was conducted at Camp Bullis by the MFSS from 2-13 September 1952. LOGEX 52 ½ was a scaled-down version of previous training exercises and allowed more observation of students by proctors. Two hundred total personnel participated, in comparison to the 1,500 participants of the LOGEX 52 carried out earlier in the year.

("LOGEX 52 ½," ORC: the Army Medical Service Training Bulletin, Vol. III, No. 4, BAMC, FSH, TX, October 1952)

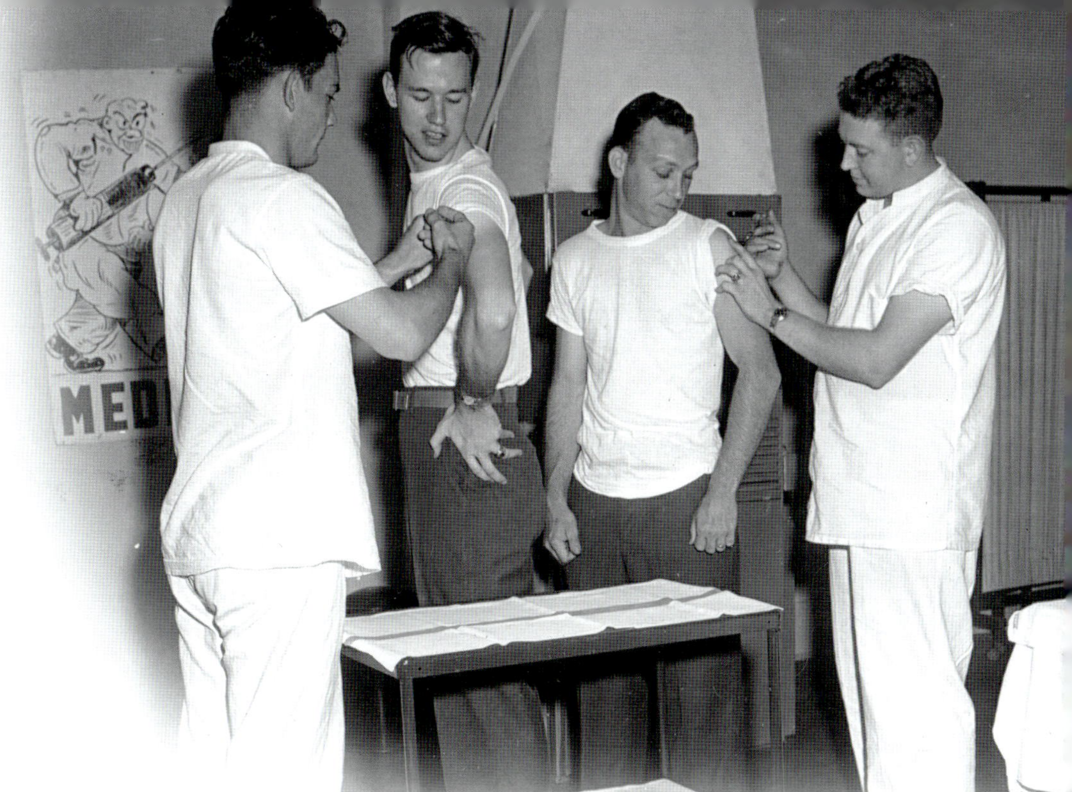

Shots

(U.S. Army Photo, FSH Museum Photo Collection, 1952)

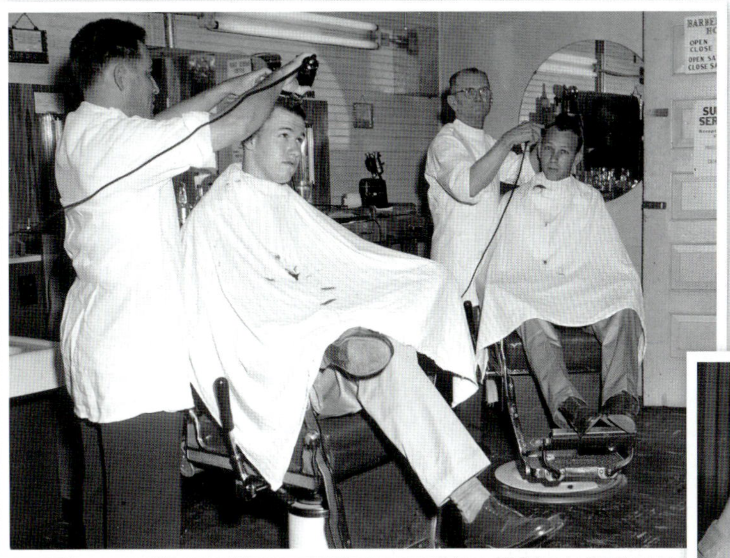

The barber shop was located in building 615

(U.S. Army Photo, FSH Museum Photo Collection, 1952)

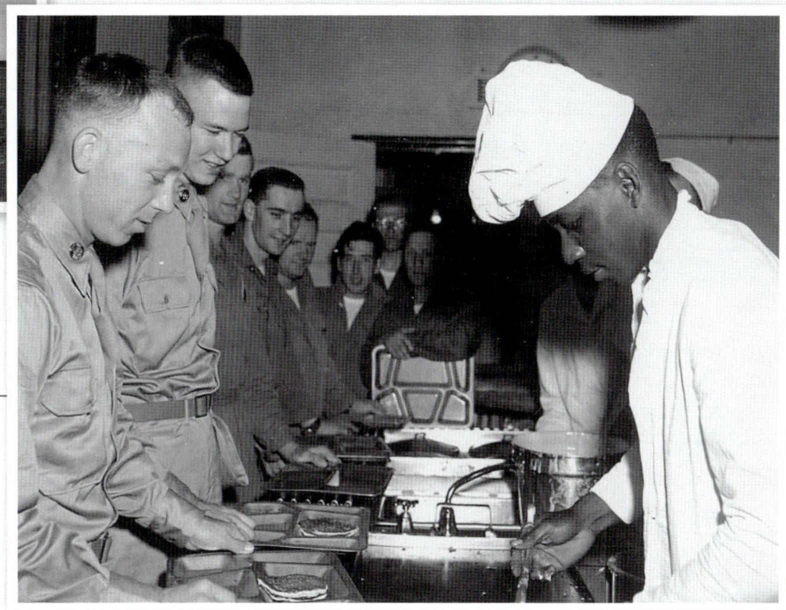

The chow line at one of the many mess halls

(U.S. Army Photo, FSH Museum Photo Collection, 1952)

1952

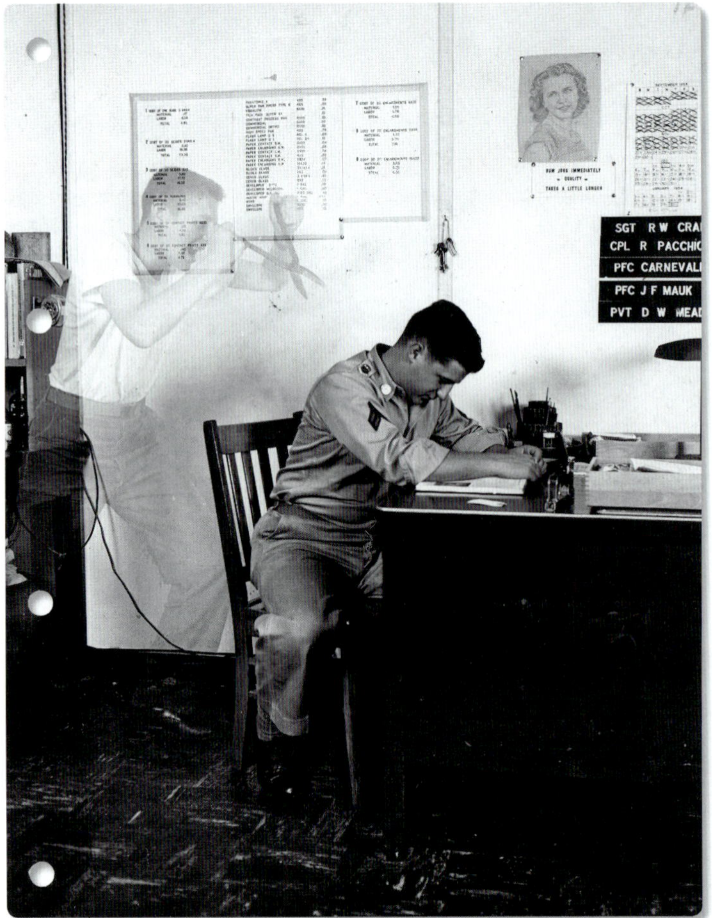

Student Pranks

Soldiers working the photo lab of the Training Aids Department playing around with a "ghost" image.

(FSH Museum Photo Collection, 1952)

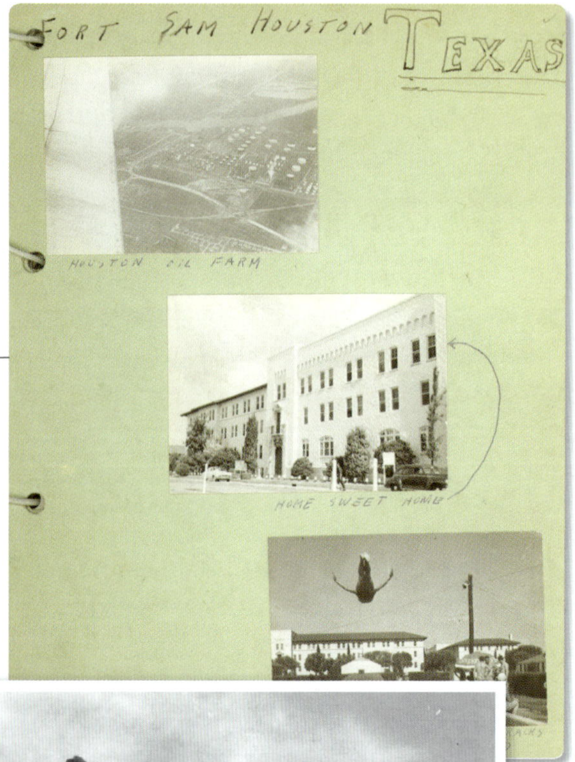

Student Photo Memoirs

A former student's photo album reveals fond memories of the pool and MFSS carnival.

(FSH Museum Photo Collection, 1952)

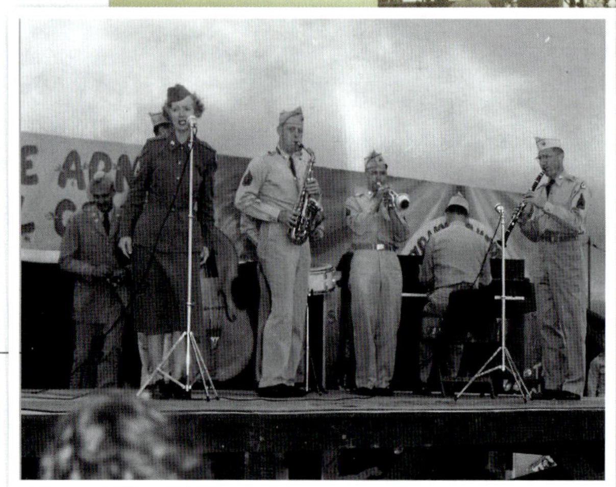

Swing

The 323rd Band performs at Organization Day 19 May 1952.

(Organization Day File, 1952, Stimson Library Special Collections)

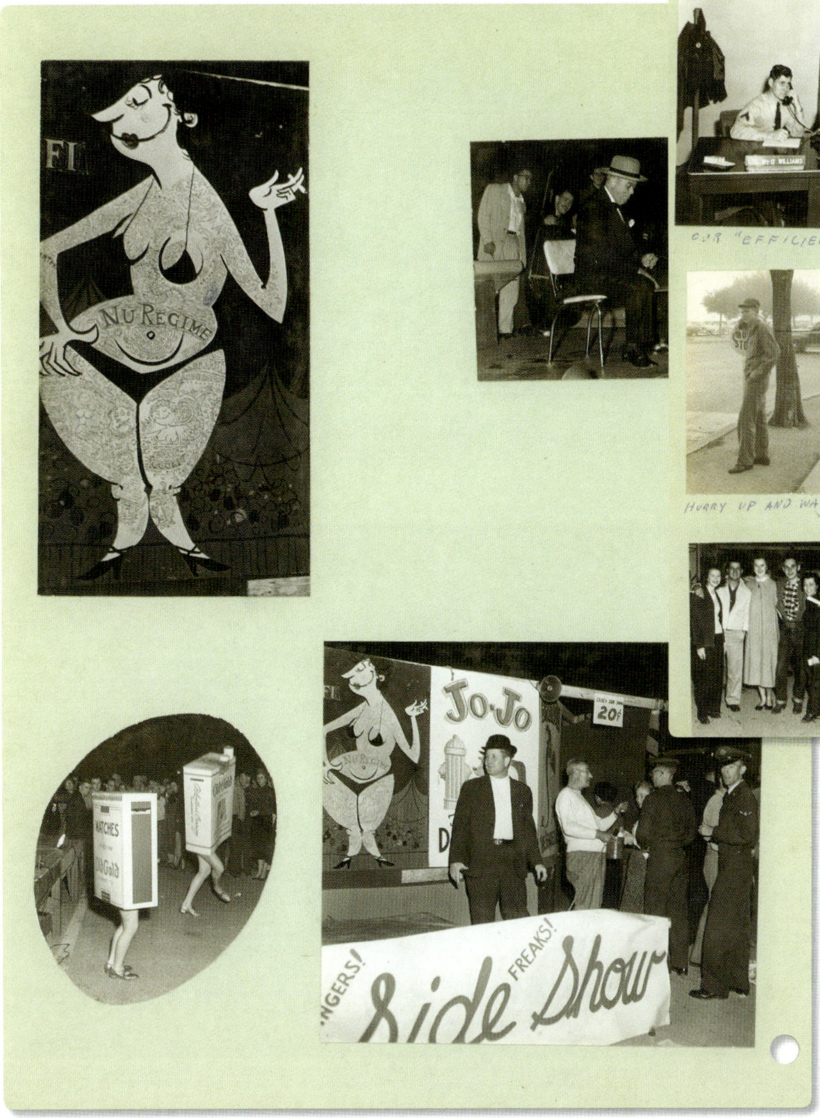
FIFI
NU REGIME
Jo-Jo
20¢
FREAKS!
Side Show

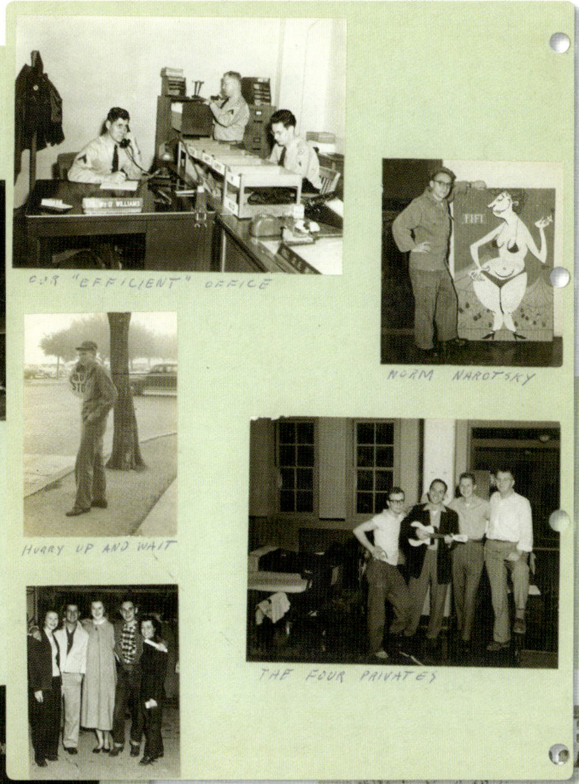
OUR "EFFICIENT" OFFICE
NORM NAROTSKY
HURRY UP AND WAIT
THE FOUR PRIVATES

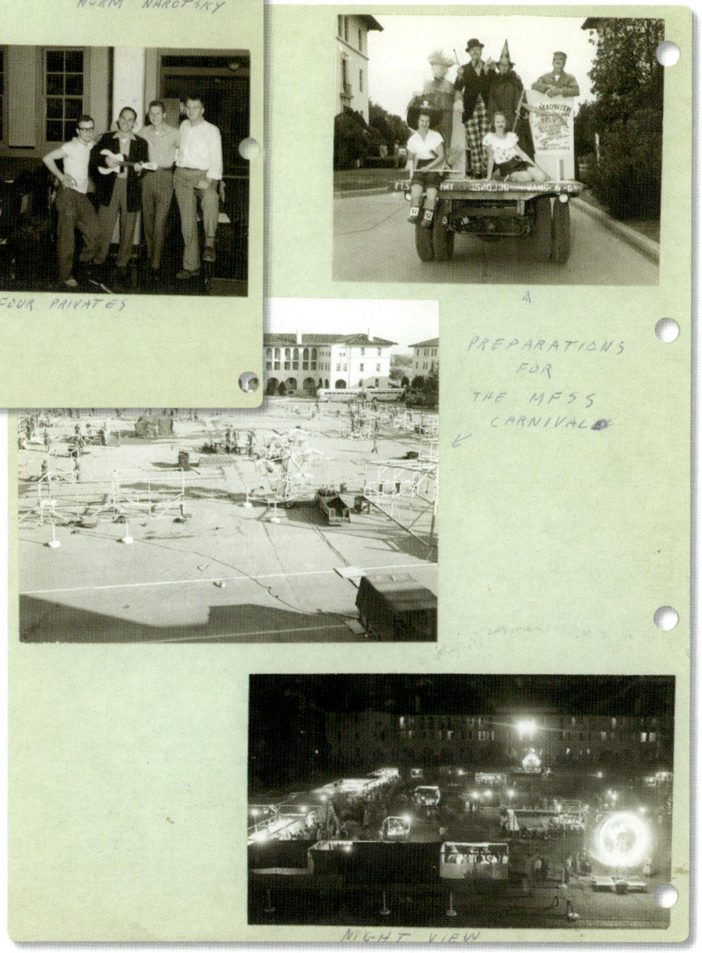
PREPARATIONS FOR THE MFSS CARNIVAL
NIGHT VIEW

Student Life

The MFSS sponsored a carnival that involved students, cadre, and civilians alike.

(FSH Museum Photo Collection, 1952)

1953

The Stimson Library obtained a medical exhibit on loan from the Armed Forces Medical Library detailing President Grover Cleveland's secret operation for jaw cancer aboard the yacht Oneida. It was the first time the documents had been seen outside of Washington, D.C.

("Medical Journal Being Displayed at MFSS Library," Army Post Times, 10 April 1953)

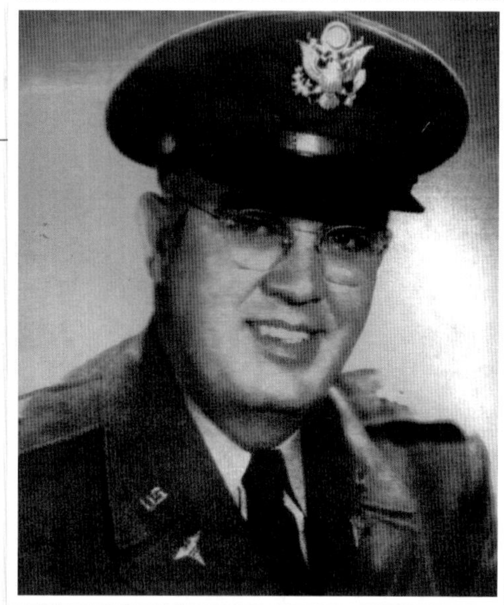

BG James P. Cooney
MG Joseph I. Martin, Commandant of the MFSS and Deputy Commanding General of BAMC, assumed command of BAMC in April of 1953. He was succeeded at the MFSS by BG James P. Cooney.

The Majestic
The latest methods and equipment used by the Medical Field Service School were staged at a four-day display in front of and within the Majestic Theater in downtown San Antonio in conjunction with the premiere of the Humphrey Bogart and June Allyson movie "Battle Circus."

("4-Day Display Staged by MFSS at Majestic," Army Post Times, 3 April 1953)

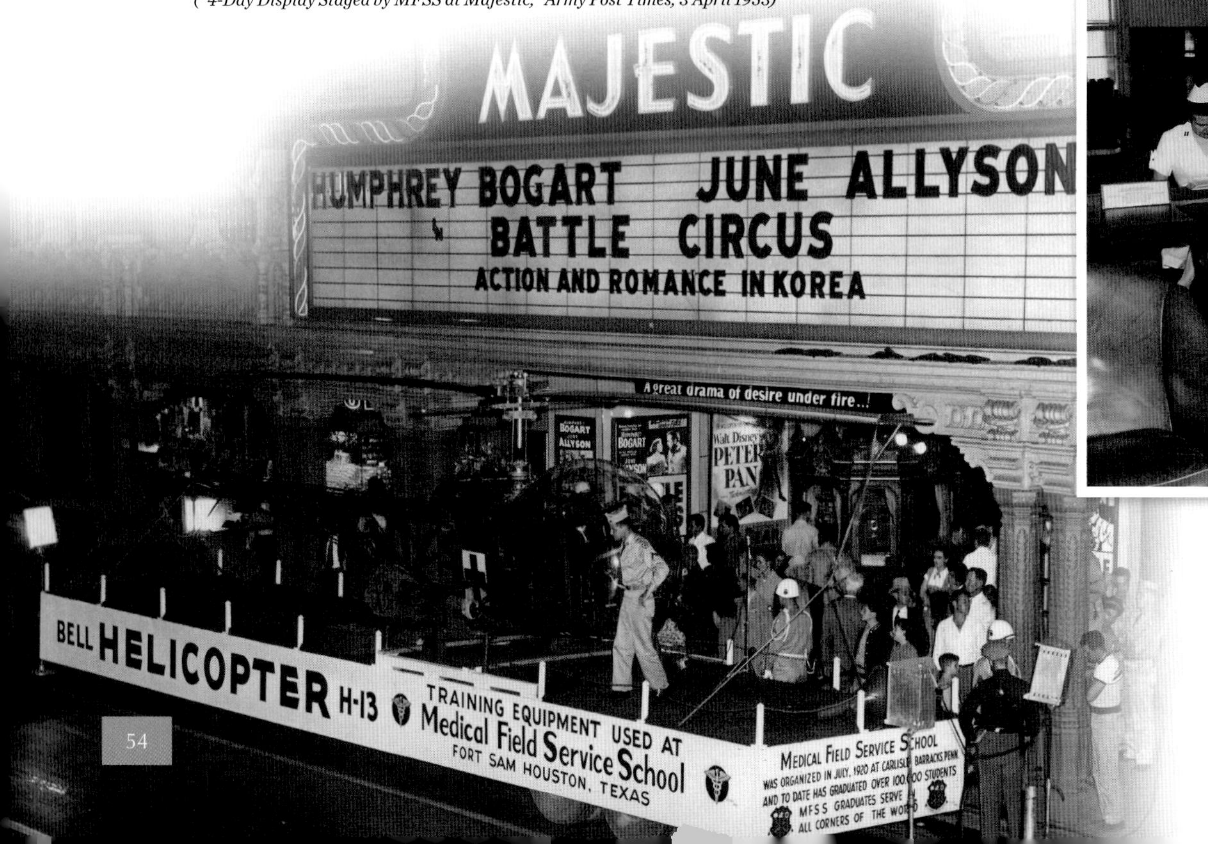

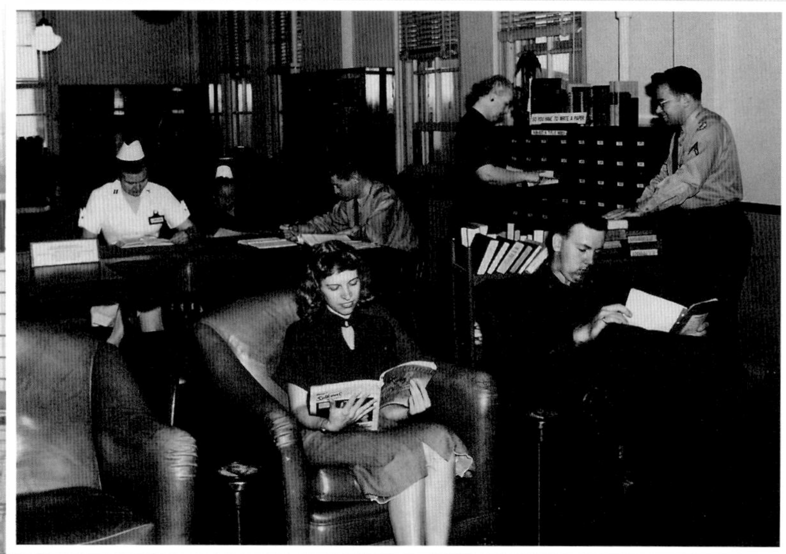

Stimson Library
Long-time civilian librarian, Mrs. Beth Simpson (third from right), is seen searching the card catalog in the Stimson Library, January 1953.

(MFSS Scrapbook 1950-1953, Stimson Library Special Collections)

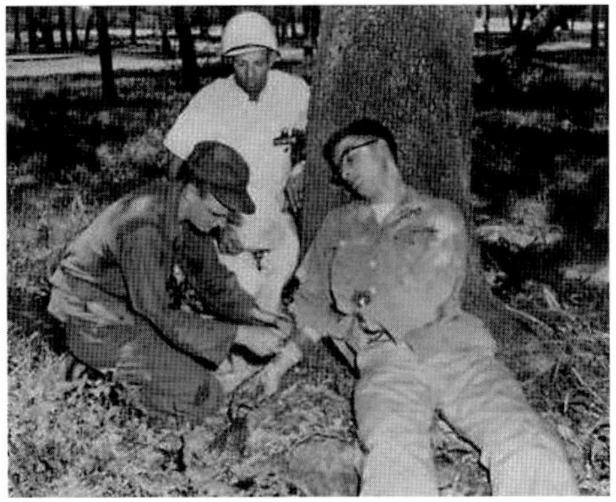

An exercise in the practical application of emergency medical treatment

(U.S. Army Medical Service School Annual Report of Army Medical Service Activities, Fort Sam Houston, 1953, p 70)

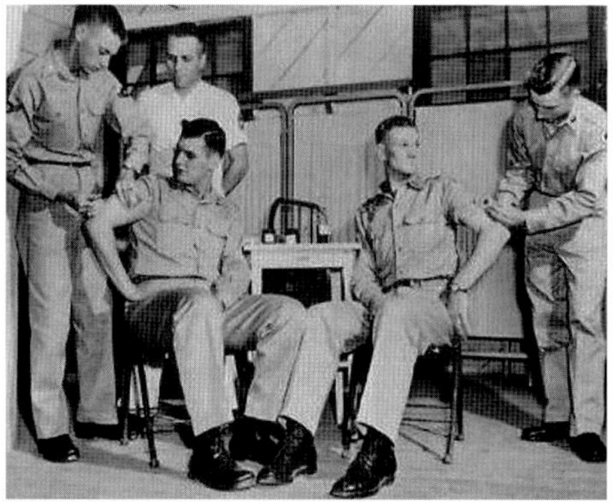

Medical Intermediate Course immunization practical application

(U.S. Army Medical Service School Annual Report of Army Medical Service Activities, Fort Sam Houston, 1953, p 71)

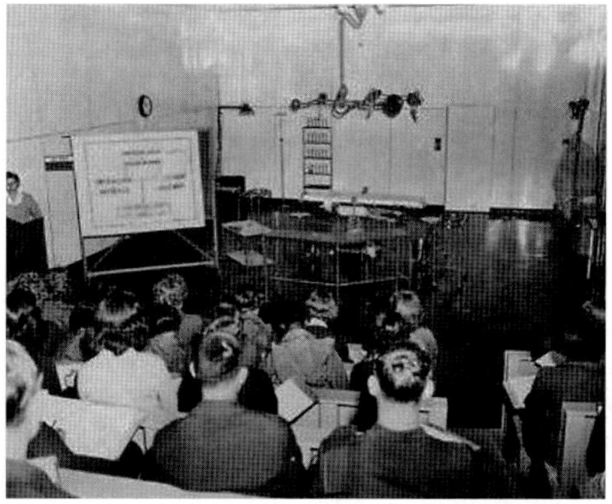

Practical demonstrations of operating room techniques during enlisted hospital procedures training

(U.S. Army Medical Service School Annual Report of Army Medical Service Activities, Fort Sam Houston, 1953, p 70)

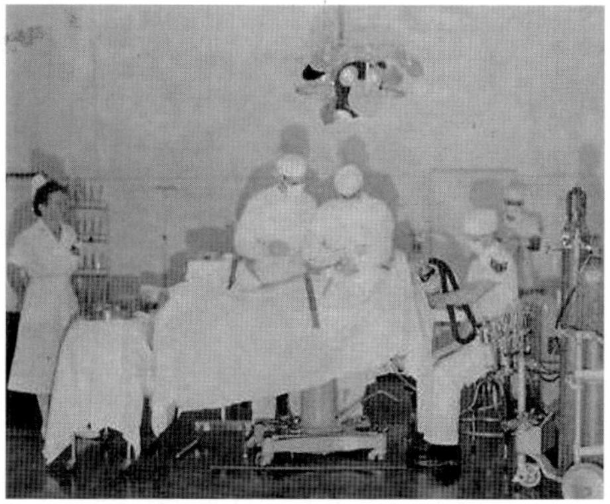

Medical Intermediate Course mock appendectomy

(U.S. Army Medical Service School Annual Report of Army Medical Service Activities, Fort Sam Houston, 1953, p 71)

In June 1953, the MFSS added a Piasecki H-25, "Army Mule," to its fleet of H-13 helicopters. The H-25 was the Army's latest means of transporting the sick and wounded. A demonstration of the aircraft was conducted by the Medical Service Branch, Department of Tactics, Techniques and Logistics, at Camp Bullis. Camp Bullis provided a perfect setting for such training because the rough terrain resembled much of Korea. The H-25 joined the "big three" of front line casualty evacuation: the litter, the litter jeep, and the ambulance. The H-25 was a critical addition because it could provide speed, which was essential in battlefront pick-up.

("MFSS Hosts Tandemeer Editor," Army Post Times, 5 June 1953; "Army Medics Demonstrate Use of H-25," Tandemeer, July-August 1953)

1953

The addition of the H-25 coincided with the initiation of a helicopter pilot program for Medical Service Corps officers. Announced in the Standard Garrison Organization (SGO) Circular, No. 82, 2 July 1953, the program consisted of 22 weeks of pilot training at the Army Aviation School, Fort Sill, Oklahoma. Successful completion of the program qualified the officer as an Army aviator and awarded him MOS 1066, Helicopter Pilot. Follow-on assignments were to units at Brooke Army Medical Center, overseas commands, and a few to the staff and faculty of the MFSS and the Army Aviation School at Fort Sill.

(The Army Medical Service Reserve Training Bulletin, Vol IV, No. 3, BAMC, FSH, TX, July-Sept 1953, p 2)

That summer the utility of helicopters for air evacuation was demonstrated by three H-13 helicopters from the MFSS 53rd Medical Detachment, which participated in the week-long 6th Annual International Aviation Exposition in Detroit.

("MFSS Sends Helicopters to Perform in Exposition," Army Post Times, July 30)

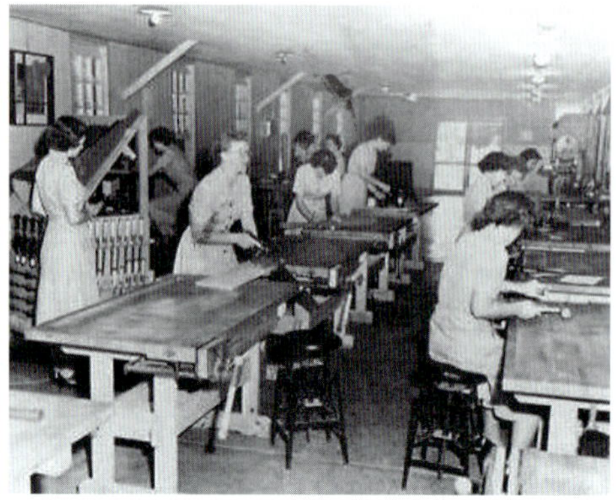

Occupational therapy workshop

(U.S. Army Medical Service School Annual Report of Army Medical Service Activities, Fort Sam Houston, 1953, p 73)

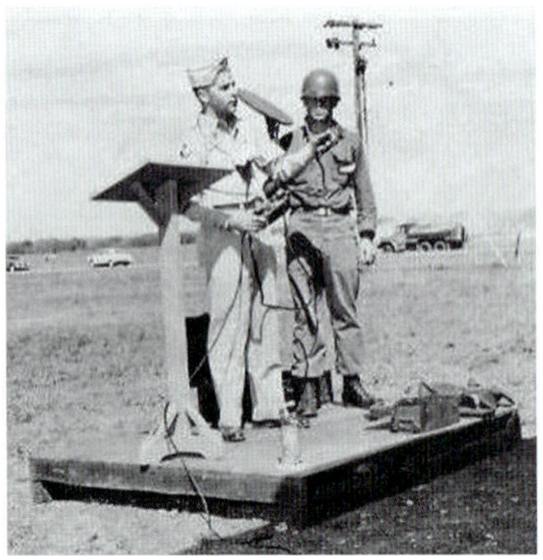

Instruction in mine warfare

(U.S. Army Medical Service School Annual Report of Army Medical Service Activities, Fort Sam Houston, 1953, p 73)

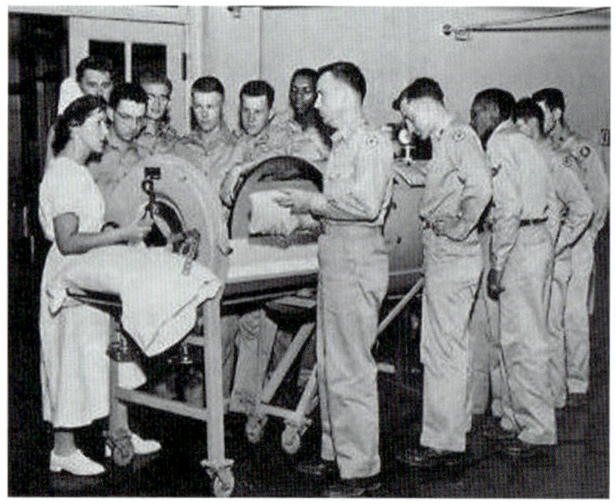

Explanation in the operation of a respirator for operating room technicians

(U.S. Army Medical Service School Annual Report of Army Medical Service Activities, Fort Sam Houston, 1953, p 72)

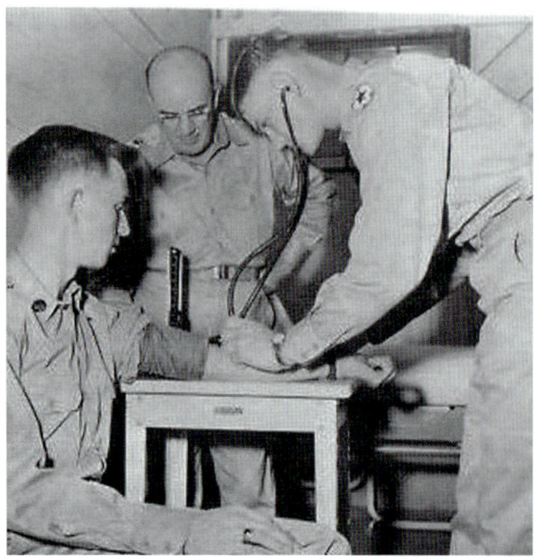

Medical Intermediate Course use of sphygmomanometer practical application

(U.S. Army Medical Service School Annual Report of Army Medical Service Activities, Fort Sam Houston, 1953, p 72)

Medical Service officer personnel entering active duty received eight hours of training in weapons familiarization and battle indoctrination as part of the Basic Course at the MFSS. The weapons instruction covered the nomenclature, characteristics, capabilities, disassembly and assembly, care and cleaning, operations, function, safety factors, and safety precautions of the U.S. Carbine, Caliber .30.

(The Army Medical Service Reserve Training Bulletin, Vol IV, No. 3, BAMC, FSH, TX, July-Sept. 1953, p 3)

MG William E. Shambora, MC, Assistant Commandant of the Medical Field Service School in 1946, returned to Fort Sam Houston to serve as Commander of Brooke Army Medical Center.

(The Army Medical Service Reserve Training Bulletin, Vol. IV, No. 4, BAMC, FSH, TX, Oct-Dec 1953, p 1)

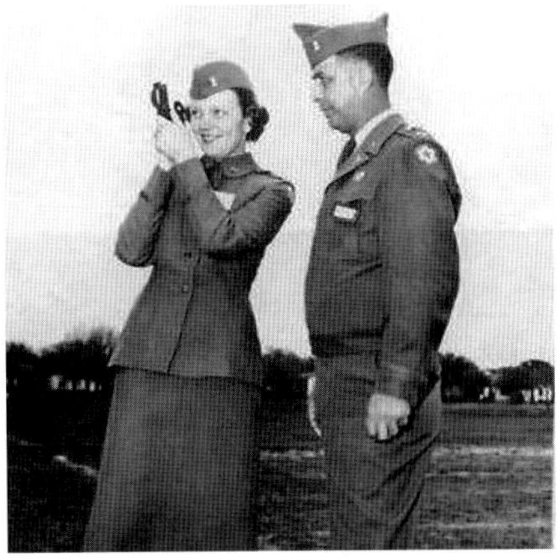

Instruction in map reading

(U.S. Army Medical Service School Annual Report of Army Medical Service Activities, Fort Sam Houston, 1953, p 74)

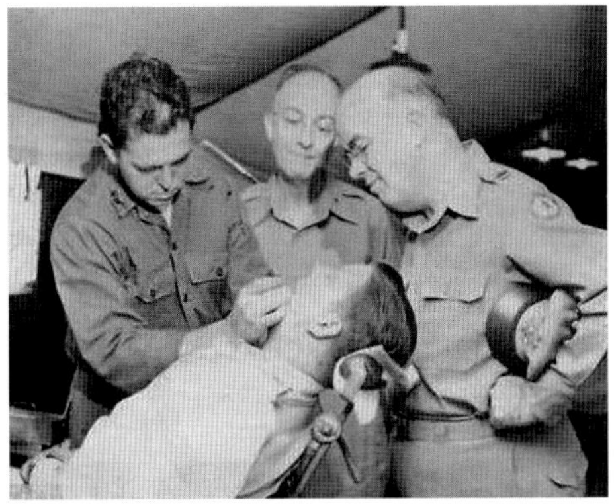

Medical Field Service School's second annual field dental clinic exercise in minor dental operation

(U.S. Army Medical Service School Annual Report of Army Medical Service Activities, Fort Sam Houston, 1953, p 75)

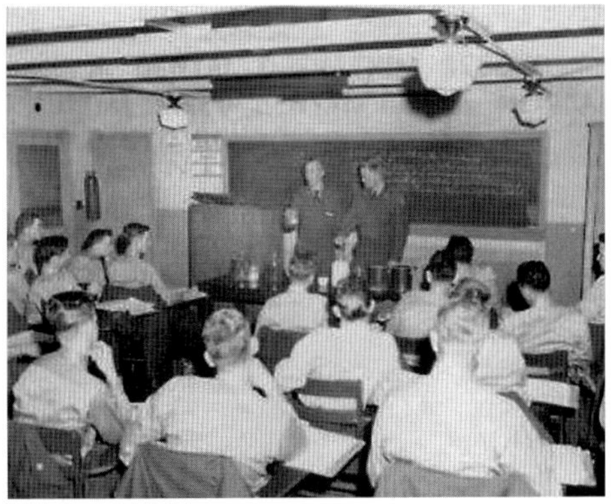

Preventive Medicine Course demonstration

(U.S. Army Medical Service School Annual Report of Army Medical Service Activities, Fort Sam Houston, 1953, p 74)

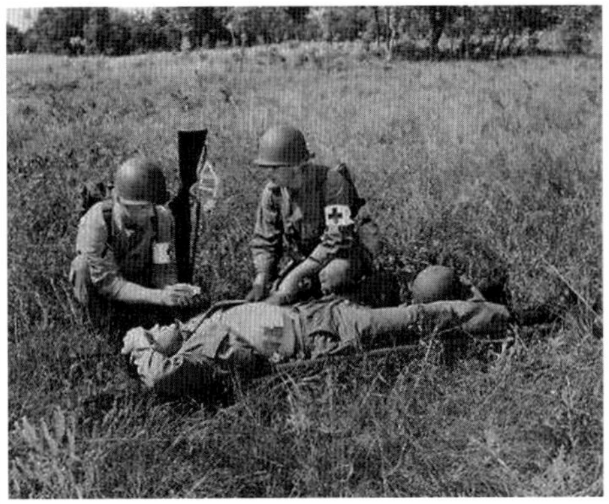

Exercise in treatment to a battle casualty by company aid man

(U.S. Army Medical Service School Annual Report of Army Medical Service Activities, Fort Sam Houston, 1953, p 76)

1953

Civilian consultants were noted as having an increasingly important role in the Army Medical Service since the civilian consultant program was established just prior to WWII. Their numbers had risen to 1,553 consultants (approved by the Surgeon General) in 1953. Many of these served at the MFSS. The important benefits of civilian consultants were listed as:

1. Promoting better integration of civilian and Army surgeons during a national emergency.
2. Introducing improved methods of diagnosis and treatment of the sick and wounded and advances in the field of preventive medicine.
3. Playing a prime role in Army residency training programs and care of patients at the hospital level.
4. Augmenting Army medical research.
5. As an advisory body on medical personnel and administrative matters, consultants were considered to be of inestimable value to the Surgeon General and other levels of Army Medical Service commands.

(The Army Medical Service Reserve Training Bulletin, Vol IV, No. 3, BAMC, FSH, TX, Oct-Dec. 1953, p 3)

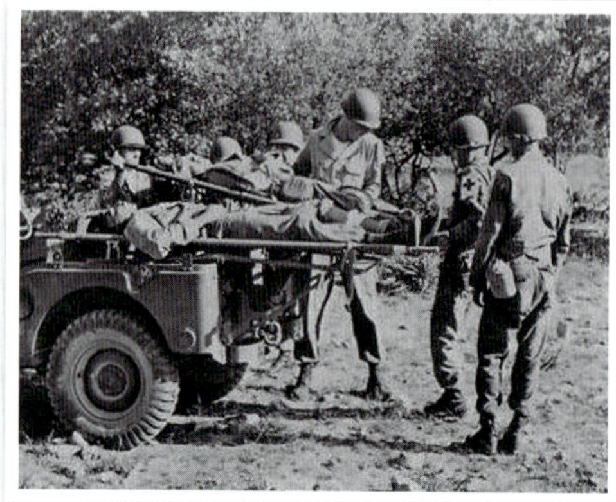

How to execute the evacuation of a patient by litter jeep from the Battalion Aid Station to the Collecting Station

(U.S. Army Medical Service School Annual Report of Army Medical Service Activities, Fort Sam Houston, 1953, p 78)

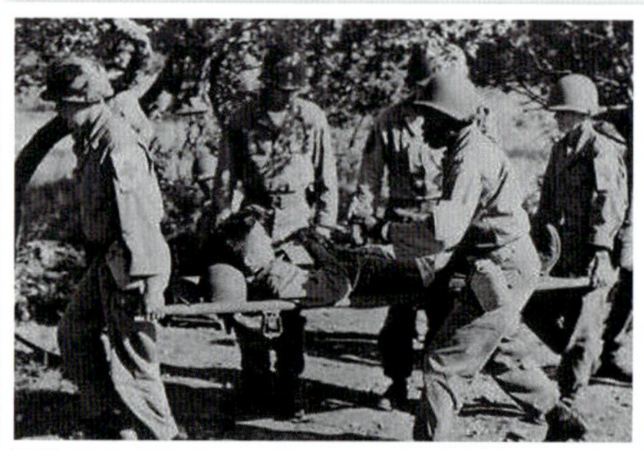

Entering the Battalion Aid Station for treatment

(U.S. Army Medical Service School Annual Report of Army Medical Service Activities, Fort Sam Houston, 1953, p 77)

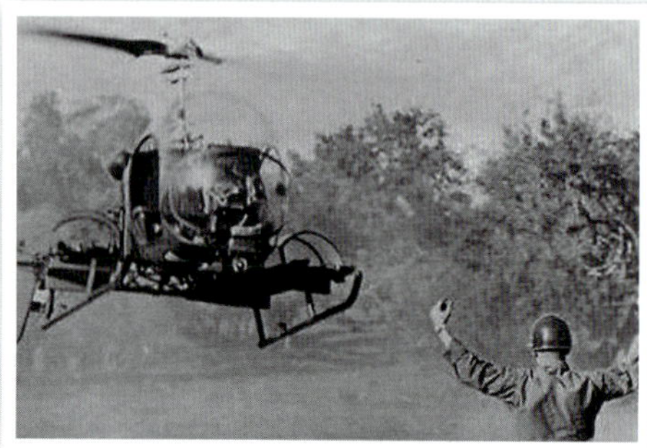

A demonstration in the arrival of a helicopter at the Battalion Aid Station for seriously wounded casualties

(U.S. Army Medical Service School Annual Report of Army Medical Service Activities, Fort Sam Houston, 1953, p 78)

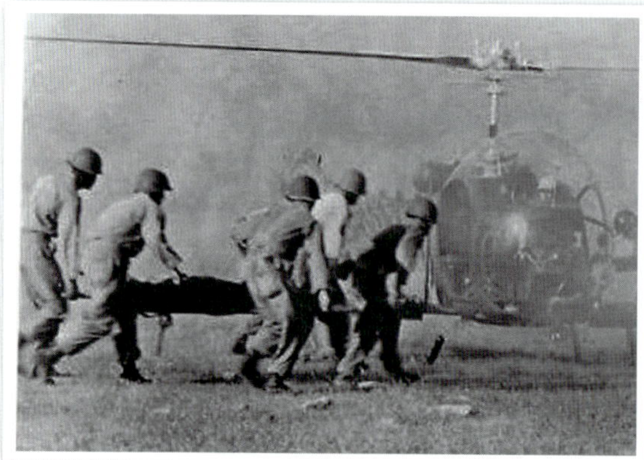

Loading of a seriously wounded casualty at the Battalion Aid Station

(U.S. Army Medical Service School Annual Report of Army Medical Service Activities, Fort Sam Houston, 1953, p 79)

"Realistic" is the only word that was used to describe the MFSS field demonstration that showed the work of the medical service of an infantry battalion under fire at Camp Bullis. Members of the 37th Medical Battalion participated in the exercise, providing aid station, litters, jeep ambulances, and air evacuation.

("True to Life Training," San Antonio Express Magazine, Dec. 11)

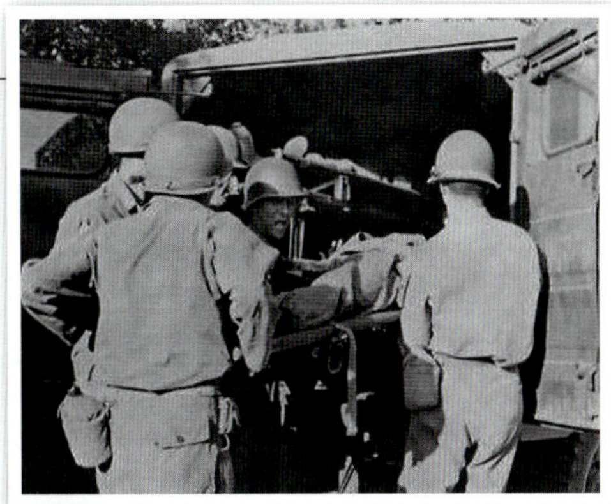

Training in the evacuation of a seriously wounded casualty from the collecting station

(U.S. Army Medical Service School Annual Report of Army Medical Service Activities, Fort Sam Houston, 1953, p 79)

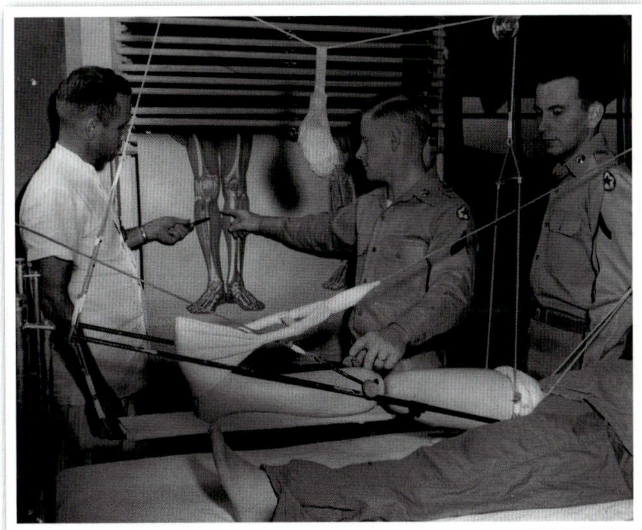

MSG Piederdella points out on the chart the best point to place a skeletal tracian pin on a model, 5 July 1953.

(U.S. Army Photo, AMEDD Museum Photo Collection)

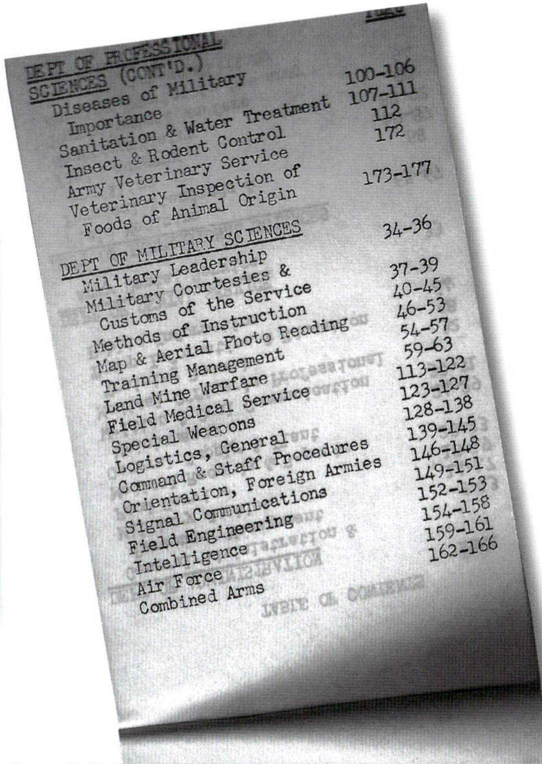

DEPT OF PROFESSIONAL SCIENCES (CONT'D.)

Diseases of Military Importance	100-106
Sanitation & Water Treatment	107-111
Insect & Rodent Control	112
Army Veterinary Service	172
Veterinary Inspection of Foods of Animal Origin	173-177

DEPT OF MILITARY SCIENCES

Military Leadership	34-36
Military Courtesies & Customs of the Service	37-39
Methods of Instruction	40-45
Map & Aerial Photo Reading	46-53
Training Management	54-57
Land Mine Warfare	59-63
Field Medical Service	113-122
Special Weapons	123-127
Logistics, General	128-138
Command & Staff Procedures	139-145
Orientation, Foreign Armies	146-148
Signal Communications	149-151
Field Engineering	152-153
Intelligence	154-158
Air Force	159-161
Combined Arms	162-166

Page

167
168
169-171
178-184
185-191
192-194

Military Justice	195
Unit Supply	196
Medical Records & Reports	

DEPT OF DENTAL SERVICE

Operation of the Dental Service	197-210

DEPT OF PROFESSIONAL SCIENCES

Emergency Medical & Surgical Procedures	211-216
Veterinary Food Inspection Service	217-220
Veterinary Animal Service	221-228
Veterinary Laboratory Service	229-230

3

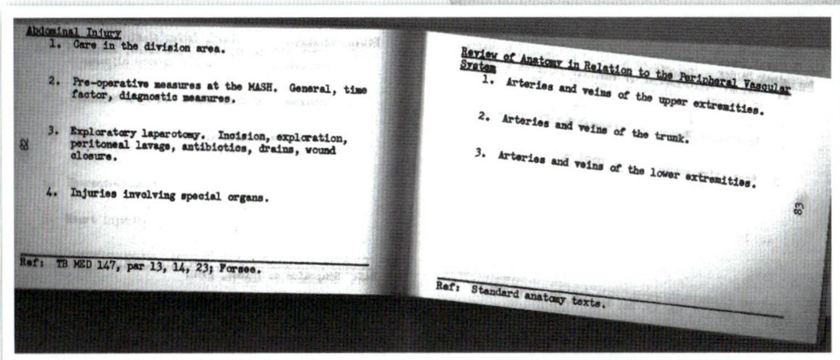

Abdominal Injury

1. Care in the division area.
2. Pre-operative measures at the MASH. General, time factor, diagnostic measures.
3. Exploratory laparotomy. Incision, exploration, peritoneal lavage, antibiotics, drains, wound closure.
4. Injuries involving special organs.

Ref: TB MED 147, par 13, 14, 23; Forsee.

Review of Anatomy in Relation to the Peripheral Vascular System

1. Arteries and veins of the upper extremities.
2. Arteries and veins of the trunk.
3. Arteries and veins of the lower extremities.

Ref: Standard anatomy texts.

Syllubs 1,2,3

Hip-pocket syllabi were a common teaching tool in the 1950s.

(Stimson Library Special Collections)

1954

"6,100 theater size tickets arranged in kaleidoscope pattern of colors on a huge plywood panel control the activities of 2,500 MFSS students every week. These ticketed boards give students an 'at-one-glance' picture of sequence of instruction among other things. "

("6,100 Tickets Control All Brooke Center Student Work," San Antonio Express, 13 Jan 1954)

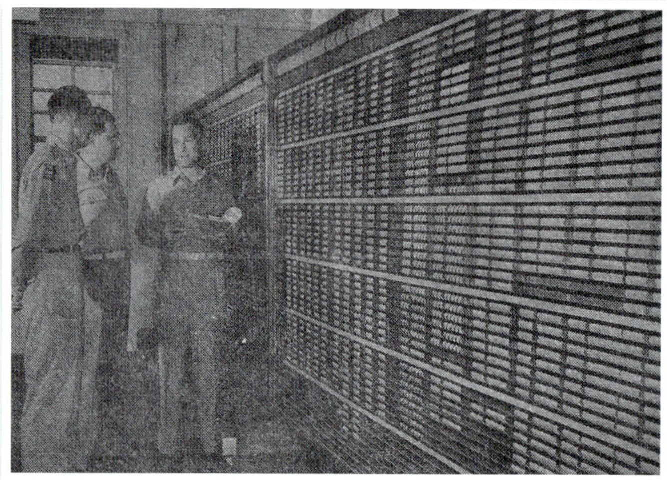

Witte Memorial Museum exhibited John Groth's sketches and watercolors of Army nurses, at work and play. The pictures were part of a permanent collection of the MFSS and loaned to the museum in honor of the 53rd Anniversary of the Army Nurse Corps.

("Witte Exhibit Tells Story of Army Nurses in Korea ," San Antonio Express, 27 Jan 1954)

SGT Theodore Greenwald points to a Thompson splint as SFC Lawrence Stewart considers a picture of a U.S. Army Nurse in Korea, as portrayed by John Groth. The men, members of the 307th Airborne Medical Battalion, 82 Airborne division, know the rigors of combat medics – both were aidmen in Korea. They visited the Witte Museum while at the Medical Field Service School on a demonstration parachute drop, 27 January 1954.

(U.S. Army Photo, "Museum Tour," 1954 MFSS Scrapbook, Stimson Library Special Collections)

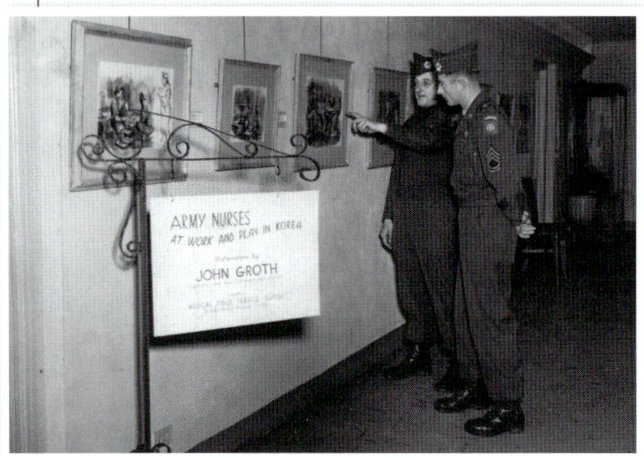

Watercolors and sketches of Army nurses

("Witte exhibit tells story of Army Nurses in Korea," San Antonio Express, Jan 1954) (Digital images downloaded from http://history.amedd.army.mil/art/korea.html)

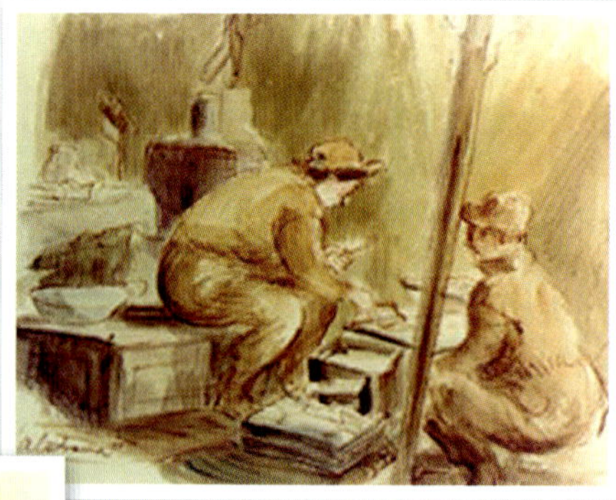

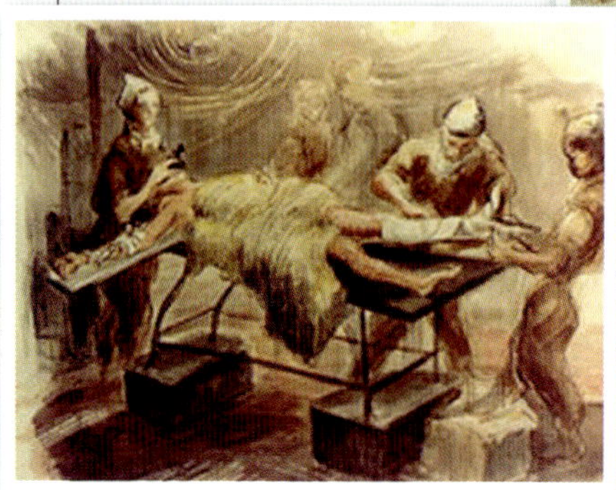

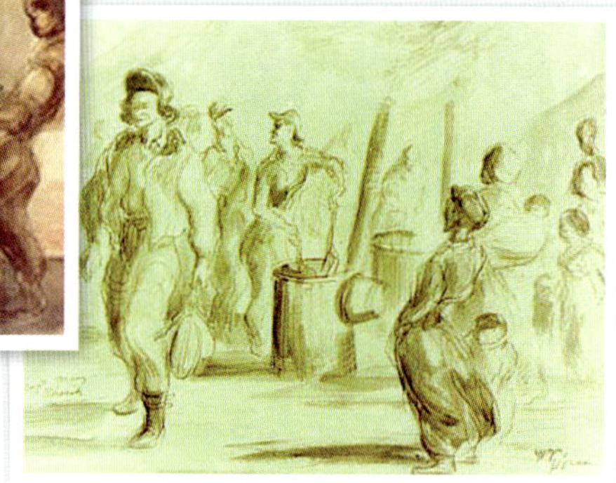

The MFSS conducted a demonstration of the transportation of the sick and wounded at the 12-21 February San Antonio Livestock Exposition. The aim of the exhibit was to educate the public in the transporting of patients from the most forward combat zone through medical channels to the main general hospital.

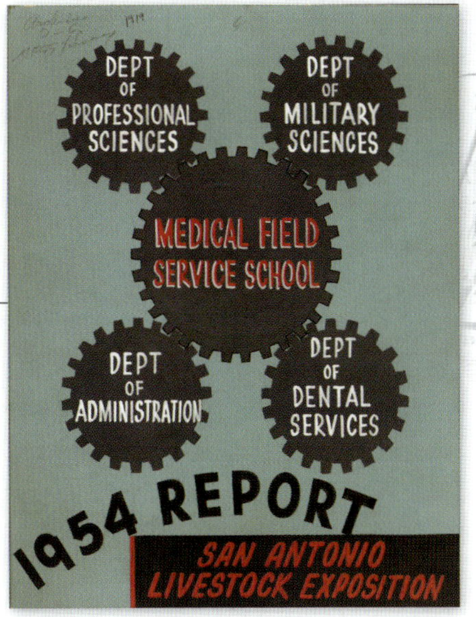

San Antonio Livestock Exposition Report cover

(San Antonio Livestock Report 1954, Stimson Library Special Collections)

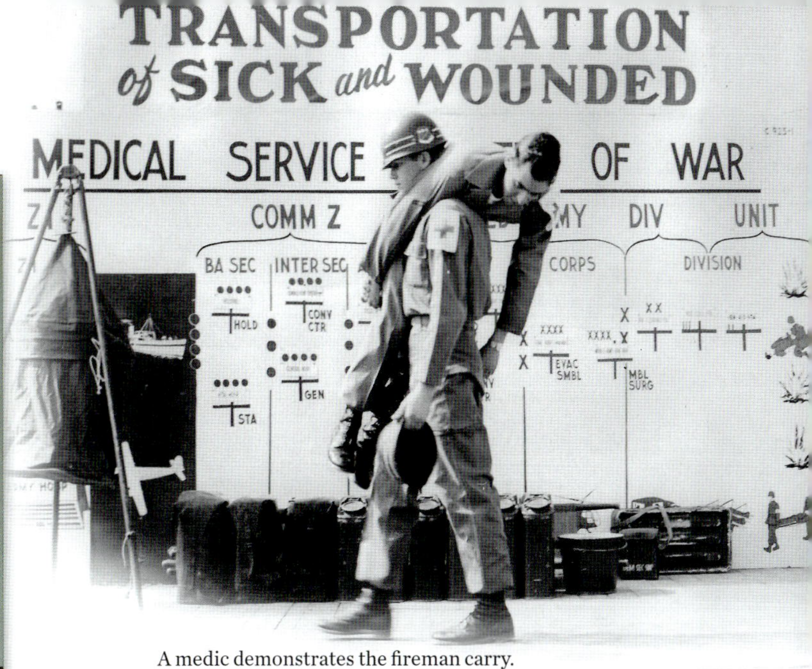

A medic demonstrates the fireman carry.

(San Antonio Livestock Report 1954, Stimson Library Special Collections)

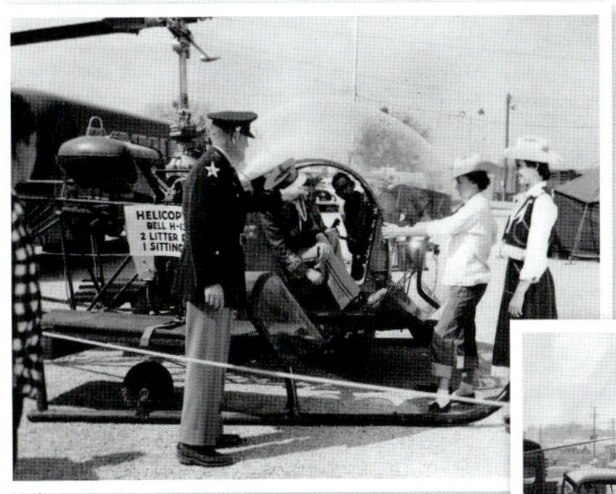

The H-13 air evacuation exhibit captivated a couple of young livestock go-ers.

(San Antonio Livestock Report 1954, Stimson Library Special Collections)

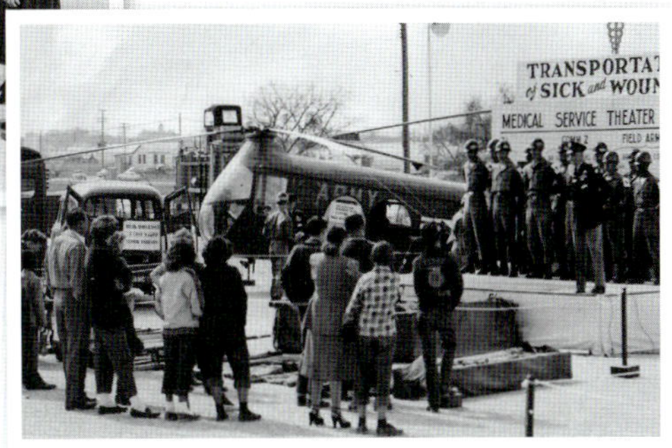

The ¾ ton ambulance, ½ ton ambulance and H-25 Piasecki Helicopter can be seen in the background of the exhibit.

(San Antonio Livestock Report 1954, Stimson Library Special Collections)

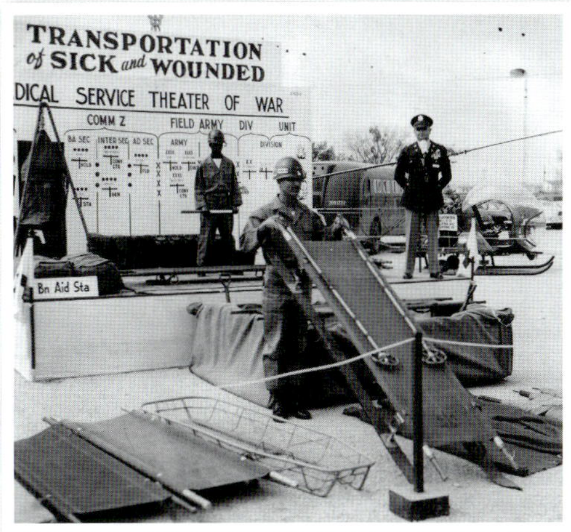

The litter demonstration included exhibits of 12 different kinds of litters: straight wood pole, aluminum, steel pole, stokes, litter mounted on skis, blanket, blanket with poles, field jacket with poles, sandbag with poles, door, rafts with poles, and a 7-litter raft.

(San Antonio Livestock Report 1954, Stimson Library Special Collections)

1954

Mrs. Lucille Leone, Assistant Surgeon General and Chief Nurse Officer of the U.S. Public Health Service, Department of Health, Education & Welfare (HEW), visited Brooke Army Medical Service School to address students at the MFSS on nursing education in the U.S.

("Chief Nurse Officer of U.S. Public Health Service Visits," Army Post Times, Feb 1954)

In March 1954, MG William E. Shambora, BAMC Commander, activated the Medical Training Center, the Army's only basic training unit for combat aidmen and hospital corpsmen. The Medical Training Center was made a component of BAMC and was placed under the command of Brigadier General L. Holmes Ginn, Jr. MG Shambora also activated a unit within the Medical Training Center for training conscientious objectors for Army duty. The unit was the only one of its kind within the Army. Men in the unit were given eight weeks of basic military training with the exception that they were not required to train with weapons. Three hundred and ninety-seven conscientious Soldiers were trained by October 1954.

("MFSS Has Only Unit of Kind For Training Conscientious Objectors For Army Duty," Military Service Review, 8 October 1954)

Approximately 338 ROTC students attended the Army Medical Service Summer ROTC Camp. The ROTC cadets received training in the professional and technical procedures of military medicine. The primary purpose of the summer camp training was to familiarize the cadets with their responsibilities and duties as prospective officers in the armed services.

("ROTC Camp Opens Here for Medics," Army Post Times, June 1954)

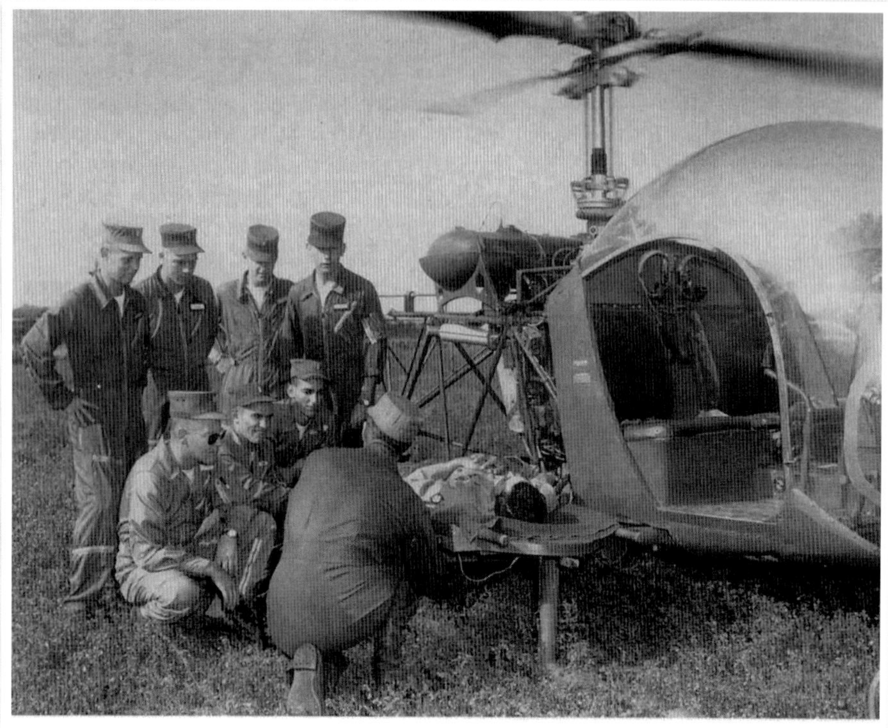

Buckle up

A class of Medical Service Corps officers learns how properly to strap a patient and litter on an H-13 helicopter, October 1954.

(U.S. Army Photo. Digital image downloaded from www.history.amedd.mil)

In June 1954, 11 helicopters from BAMC's 274th and 57th Helicopter Detachment, as well as the Aviation Section of the MFSS, evacuated 85 passengers, hundreds of pounds of baggage, and U.S. mail stranded on a train from the flood-hit Del Rio, Texas, area. For two weeks, the BAMC and MFSS helicopters (H-25s and H-13s) continued disaster relief efforts to areas stricken on both sides of the Rio Grande of Nuevo Laredo and Ciudad Acuña. The smaller of the helicopters, the H-13, was able to make rooftop landings to deliver supplies. Rescued people sang the praises of the entire operation, particularly the helicopter pilots.

("Operation Copter Follows Flood Crest Down Rio Grande," San Antonio News, June 1954; "Brooke Helicopters Join in Flood Rescue," Army Post Times, 1 July 1954; "Brooke AMC 'Chopper' Continues Mercy Flights," Army Post Times, 8 July 1954)

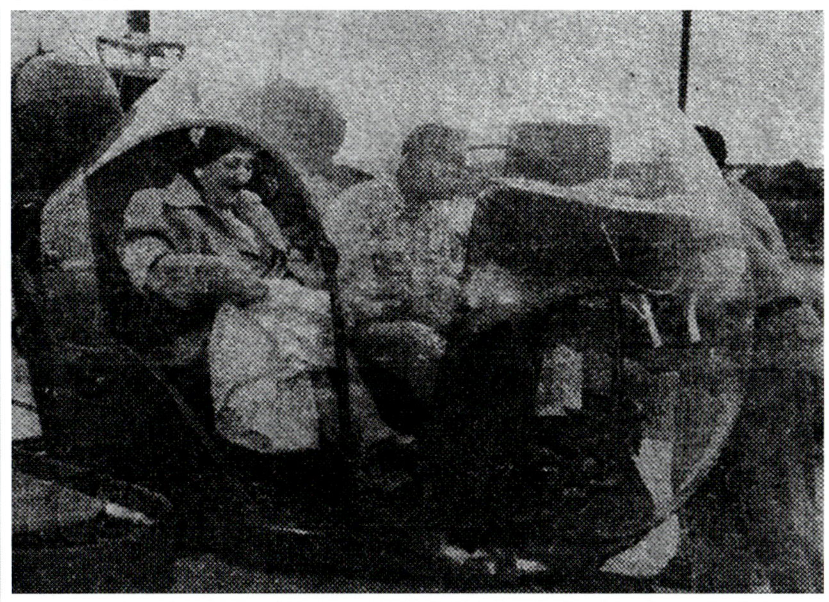

Passenger rescued

An MFSS pilot flies a passenger stranded on a train during the floods caused by Hurricane Irene to safety.

(U.S. Army Photo)

The new enlisted "Medical Records" class began at the MFSS the second week of July 1954. Specifically designed to train administrative personnel for supervisory positions, the course included instruction in medical records, office statistics, admission, disposition, and the hospital command operations.

("New 'Medical Records' Class Begun this Week," Army Post Times, 8 July 1954)

The first Turkish dental officer, MAJ Enver Plumer, began studies at the MFSS in September 1954.

("First Turkish Dentist Starts MFSS Course," Army Post Times, 2 September 1954)

COL Irene Galloway made her first visit to Ft. Sam Houston as the WAC Director. She conferred with commanders and was the guest of honor at a meeting for all enlisted WAC personnel.

("WAC Director Makes First Official Visit," Army Post Times, 21 April 1954)

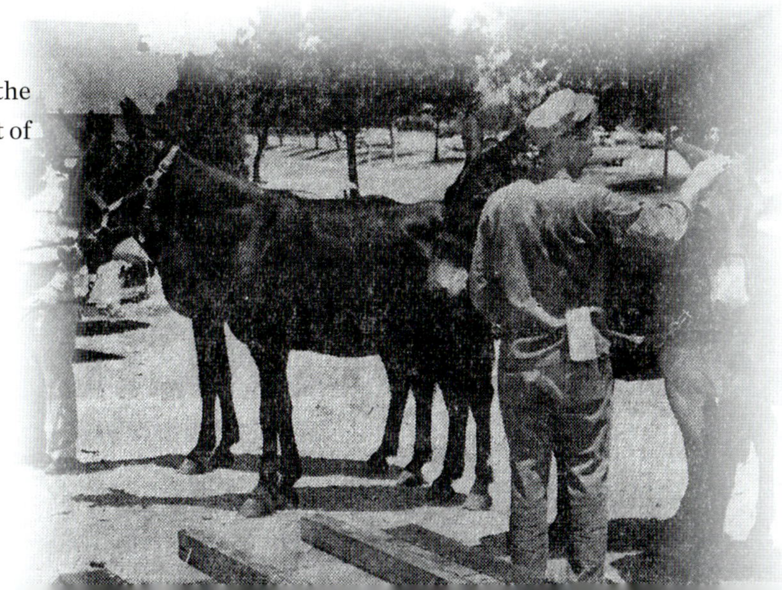

A six-mule train team was temporarily assigned to Fort Sam Houston from Camp Carson, Colorado, for use in the ROTC Veterinary Training Program.

("Sounds of Mules Braying at Fort Sam Thrills Vet," San Antonio Express, 12 Aug 1954)

1954

The first enlisted course in Meat and Dairy Hygiene began in the Fall of 1954. Graduates of the eight-week course became Food Inspection Technicians and were eligible for assignments throughout Army installations worldwide.

("Meat, Dairy Course to Start Here," 9 Sep 1954)

The first three Japanese officers to train at the MFSS arrived in September of 1954.

(Army Post Times, 8 Sep 1954)

A litter obstacle course was designed and installed at Camp Bullis in October 1954. Developed to train and remind the medical community that despite the advancement of helicopter ambulances and motor vehicles that "go anywhere," the first transportation of a wounded soldier consists of aidmen and litter bearers.

("Serving the Troops, Military Service Review," 8 Oct 1954)

The Brooke Nursing School becomes the first accredited vocational nursing school in the San Antonio area in October of 1954.

("Brooke Nursing School First Accredited in SA," Army Post Times, 28 Oct 1954)

In early October, the Turkish Surgeon General, MG HawzaVahit Gogen, began a 14-day visit to observe basic medical training at the Medical Training Center, advanced instruction at the MFSS, treatment of burn patients at the Surgical Research Unit's ward, and operations of the centralized medical laboratories at Fourth Army. The Turkish general's visit was the first of a series of consultations between medical officers of the United States and members of the North Atlantic Treaty Organization (NATO). Later in the year, BG Hak-Shin, the first Surgeon General of Korea, and BG Jesus Lozoya-Solis of Mexico conducted similar visits.

("BAMC Host To Turkish General," Army Post Times, 7 October 1954; "Brig Gen. Hak-Shin at BAMC," Army Post Times, 9 Dec 1954; "Top Mexican Medical Head to Visit S.A.," San Antonio Express, 12 Jan 1955)

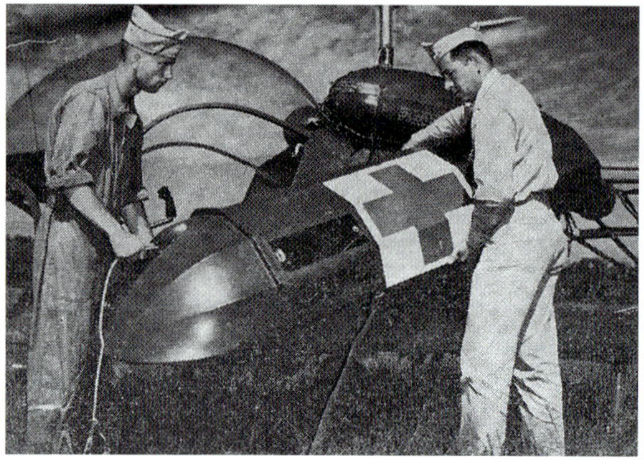

The Bell Helicopter Corporation debuted its new H-13 ambulance helicopter at the MFSS on 18 August 1954. The new ambulance helicopter was designed to convert between carrying cargo and patients.

("New Ambulance 'Copter' Shown," San Antonio Express, 18 Aug 1954)

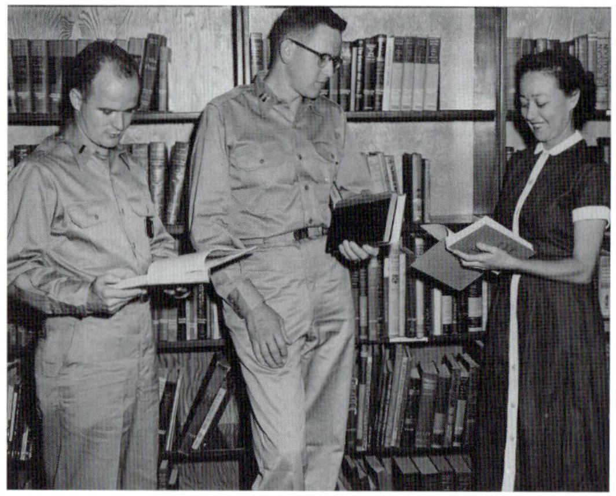

Miss Stortz of the MFSS Library, CPT Edward Crane, and LT Frank O'Toole peruse the stacks.

(MFSS Scrapbook 1954, Stimson Library Special Collections)

On 9 December, student officers at the MFSS watched airborne medics of the 11th Airborne Medical Battalion, part of the 11th Airborne (Angels) Division stationed at Fort Campbell, Kentucky, drop over 15,000 pounds of equipment from six C-119 Flying Boxcars at Brooks Air Force Base.

("Student Officers Watch Airborne Medics Perform," Army Post Times, 10 December 1954)

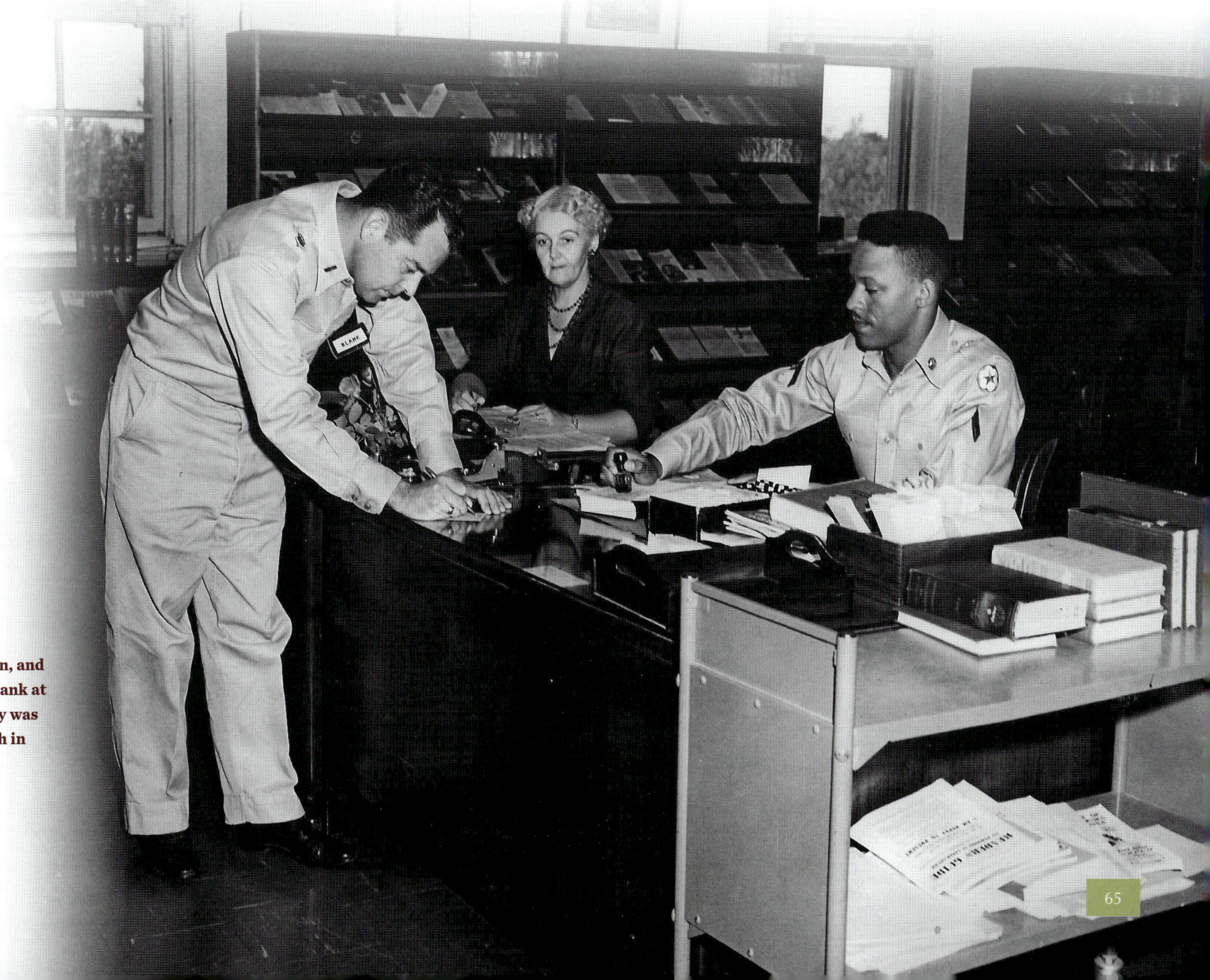

Mrs. Simpson, Chief Librarian, and PFC Johnson assist LT Jay Blank at the MFSS Library. The library was named "Section" of the month in October of 1954.

(MFSS Scrapbook 1954, Stimson Library Special Collections)

1955

In February 1955, the MFSS began maintaining the U.S. Army Medical Museum.

Full military honors were accorded to BG Jesus Lazoya-Solis, director of the Central Military Hospital of Mexico City, when he visited BAMC for a general tour and briefing on hospital operations.

("Top Mexican Medical Head Visits BAMC," San Antonio Express, 12 Jan 1955)

"Nurses from the MFSS show their appreciation for the apartments by the care and concern with which they furnish them. Originally designed as minimally furnished barracks, most of the girls prefer to augment the apartments with their own trimmings and basic items of their own choice."

("Army Nurses Preserve Gracious Living Niceties," San Antonio Express, 30 Jan 1955)

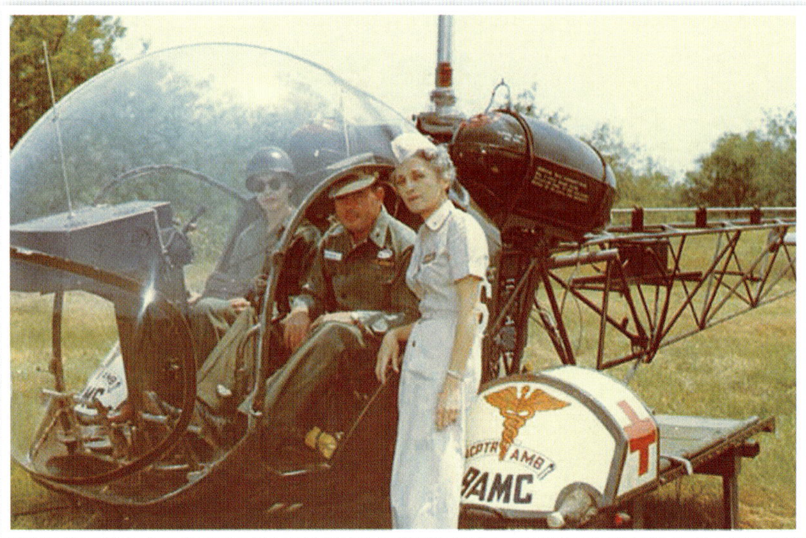

Brooke Army Medical Center in early 1950's, Korean War era. Army nurse with helicopter crews. COL Agnes Maley, ANC, meets a medical transport helicopter at BAMC.

(U.S. Army Photo. Digital image downloaded from http://history.amedd.army.mil/art/korea.html)

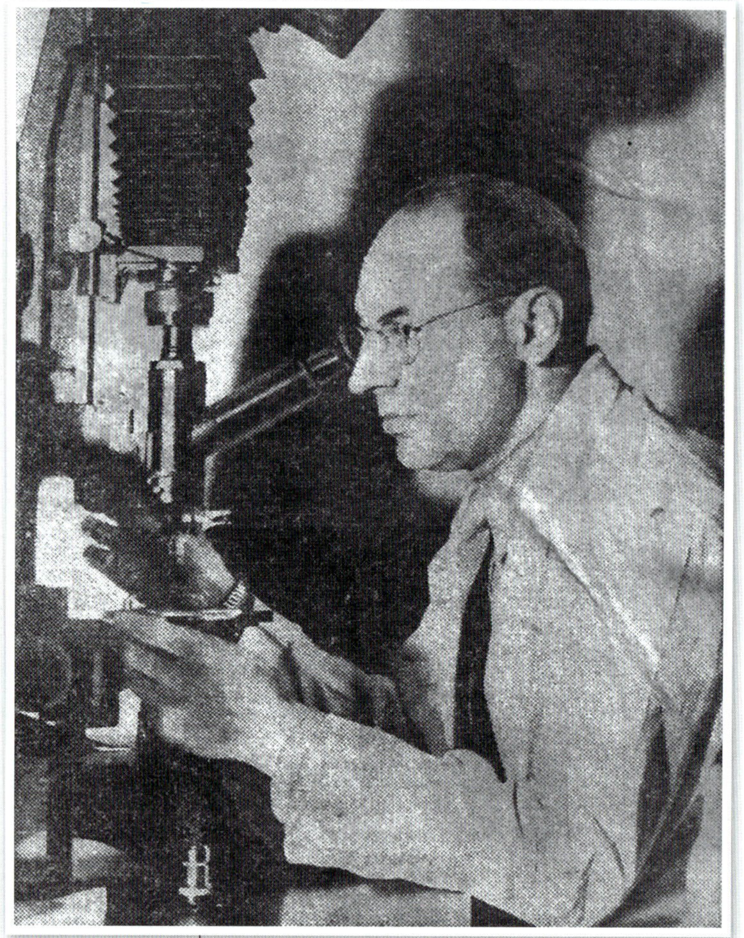

BG Elbert DeCoursey, the new commanding general of the MFSS, peers into a microscope. "I like a microscope. They teach us a lot and that's just it, we get right back to teaching. What good is research if you don't learn from it? MFSS is the best assignment of my career and is the ultimate opportunity to teach military medicine."

("MFSS Commander Likes Microscope Best," San Antonio Light, 2 Aug 1955)

The Army adjusted its enlisted personnel management system to separate Non-Commissioned Officers (NCOs) from "Specialists" in upper enlisted grades. The system adjustment reinforces the NCO's authority, responsibility and respect by making a distinction between leadership responsibilities and positions of technical expertise.

("New MOS System to Begin Soon," Army Post Times, 5 May 1955)

In October 1955, the MFSS's name was changed to Army Medical Service School (AMSS) again.

("Medical Field Service School Has New Name," San Antonio News, 2 Nov 1955)

Breaking the ice

The Army's first commissioned male nurse, reports to Brooke. 2LT Edward Lyon's arrival was no surprise as he had been the subject of news stories, radio interviews and television appearances. "Someone had to break the ice," Lyon said of his unique role.

("First Army Male Nurse Now Training at Brooke," San Antonio Express, 20 October 1955)

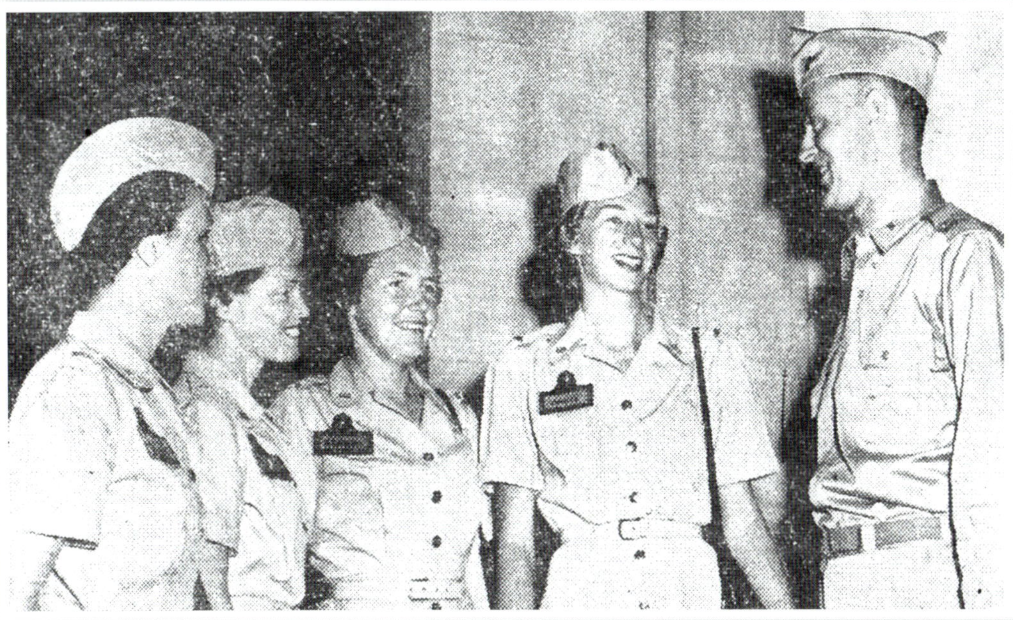

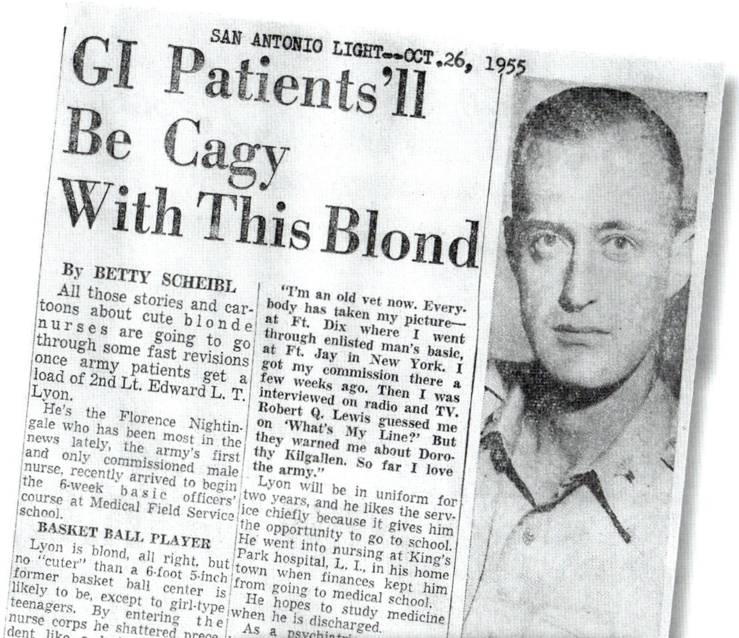

SAN ANTONIO LIGHT--OCT.26, 1955

GI Patients'll Be Cagy With This Blond

By BETTY SCHEIBL

All those stories and cartoons about cute blonde nurses are going to go through some fast revisions once army patients get a load of 2nd Lt. Edward L. T. Lyon.

He's the Florence Nightingale who has been most in the news lately, the army's first and only commissioned male nurse, recently arrived to begin the 6-week basic officers' course at Medical Field Service school.

BASKET BALL PLAYER

Lyon is blond, all right, but no "cuter" than a 6-foot 5-inch former basket ball center is likely to be, except to girl-type teenagers. By entering the nurse corps he shattered precedent like a lockjawed lobster chomping down on an old thermometer.

Lyon, interviewed at MFSS, is enjoying his fame while it asts, knowing that another offi-er and gentleman will be in he corps in a few weeks. (He's ue to arrive at Brooke Army Iedical center Nov. 9.)

OTHER NURSES

Then there are the 75 non-mmissioned male nurses al-ady in the army, many of hom are expected to win the utenancies they are encour-ed to apply for.

These will add up to a hoard manly pulse takers who rt gold bars and "flashbulb tans."

ut now there's only one— n, an ebullient young t whose picture has been n oftener recently than the ibs of some amateur ographers.

nments the 25-year-old hetist:

"I'm an old vet now. Everybody has taken my picture— at Ft. Dix where I went through enlisted man's basic, at Ft. Jay in New York. I got my commission there a few weeks ago. Then I was interviewed on radio and TV. Robert Q. Lewis guessed me on 'What's My Line?' But they warned me about Dorothy Kilgallen. So far I love the army."

Lyon will be in uniform for two years, and he likes the service chiefly because it gives him the opportunity to go to school. He went into nursing at King's Park hospital, L. I., in his home town when finances kept him from going to medical school.

He hopes to study medicine when he is discharged.

As a psychiatri-

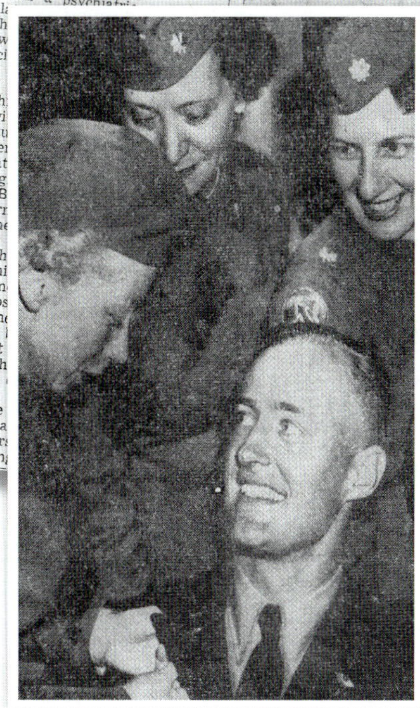

1956

A platoon of the 520th Medical Ambulance Company was sent to Ft. Greeley, Alaska, to take part in a maneuver exercise involving evacuation of battle casualties. The purpose was to experience real world training in sub-zero weather.

("49 BAMC Soldiers Take Part in Exercise Moose Horn in Alaska," San Antonio News, 1 February 1956)

38 paramedics from the 307th Airborne Medical Battalion, Ft. Bragg, N.C., set up a medical clearing station in 16 ½ minutes after both men and equipment were parachuted from "flying boxcars" during a demonstration at Brooks Air Base for 500 student officers, including AMSS students.

("Para-Medics Make Jump for 500 Student Officers," Talon, 5 February 1956)

The 520th Medical Clearing Company, 566th Medical Ambulance Company and the 712th Preventive Medical Company (all from the 37th Med BN at the AMSS) received unit decorations for outstanding service during WWII. More than 3,000 soldiers marched in the parade following the awards.

("Three Medical Units Get Unit Decorations," Talon, 8 March 1956)

MAJ Edith Aynes, a nursing instructor at the AMSS, retired after 22 years of service. A popular class director and instructor, she concerned herself with the problems and challenges of the Army Nurse Corps. She is also widely known as the author of the Army Nurse's Pledge and the song, "The Nurse's Prayer."

("Famous Nurse Retires after 22 Years," Talon, 3 May 1956)

The Nurse's Prayer

Hear my prayer in silence before Thee as I ask for courage each day.

Grant that I may be worthy of the sacred pledge of my profession

And the lives of those entrusted to my care.

Help me to offer hope and cheer in the hearts of men and my country,

For their faith inspires me to give the world and nursing my best.

Instill in me the understanding and compassion of those who led the way,

For I am thankful to You for giving me this life to live.

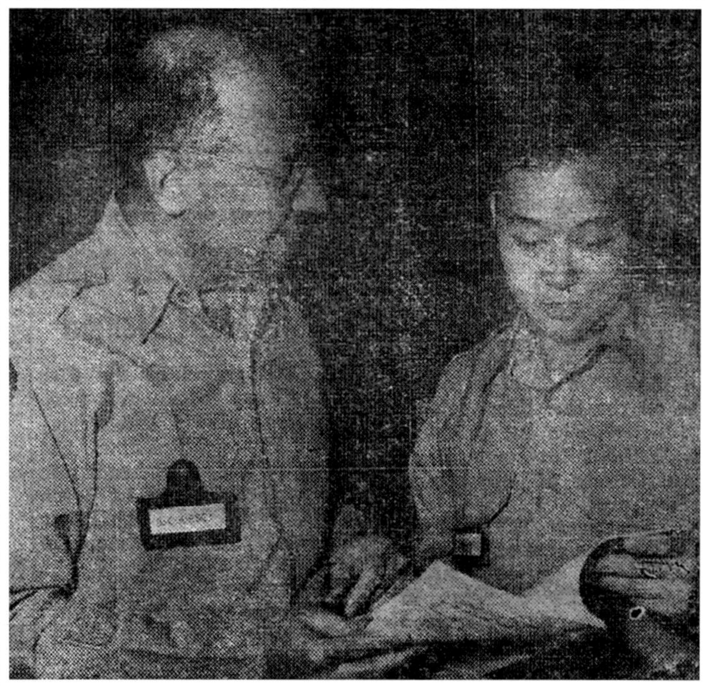

BG Elbert DeCoursey, left, Commandant of the AMSS, and MAJ Wu David Tachin, Republic of China, review training aids in preparation for arrival of non-English speaking Chinese students.

("Chinese Army Office...MAJ to Translate AMSS Course," Talon, 8 November 1956)

COL Egberto Bermudez, Chief Surgeon of the Nicaraguan Army and personal physician to the President of Nicaragua, spent 4 days touring BAMC. He was briefed on the mission and daily operations of BAMC and also observed basic and advanced medical training at the MTC.

("Nicaraguan Chief Surgeon Tours BAMC," Talon, 21 June 1956)

In 1956, the 3273rd Air Force Technical Training Squadron was a component of the Army Medical Service School. COL Jacob B. Martin, a former Medical Administrative Corps Army Officer, who transferred to the United States Air Force in 1950, was assigned command of the squadron.

("COL Martin is New CO of AMSS AF Squadron," Talon, Aug 1956)

MAJ Leo K. Nonn became the first medical officer in the Federal Army of Western Germany, officially organized 1 January 1956, to visit Brooke Army Medical Center. MAJ Nonn made the AMSS his headquarters during his three week stay.

("From New Army...German Officer Visits Here," Talon, 6 Sep 1956)

Five Chinese medical and dental officers arrived at BAMC to serve as translators for 25 top ranking Chinese students scheduled to attend classes at the AMSS in January of 1957. The group was preceded by their liaison officer, who was also a translator, MAJ Wu David Tachin. MAJ Tachin and the group worked in conjunction with instructors and other personnel to have reference materials, films, and training aids translated for student use before the students' arrival.

("5 Translators Arrive at BAMC," Talon, 21 Nov 1956)

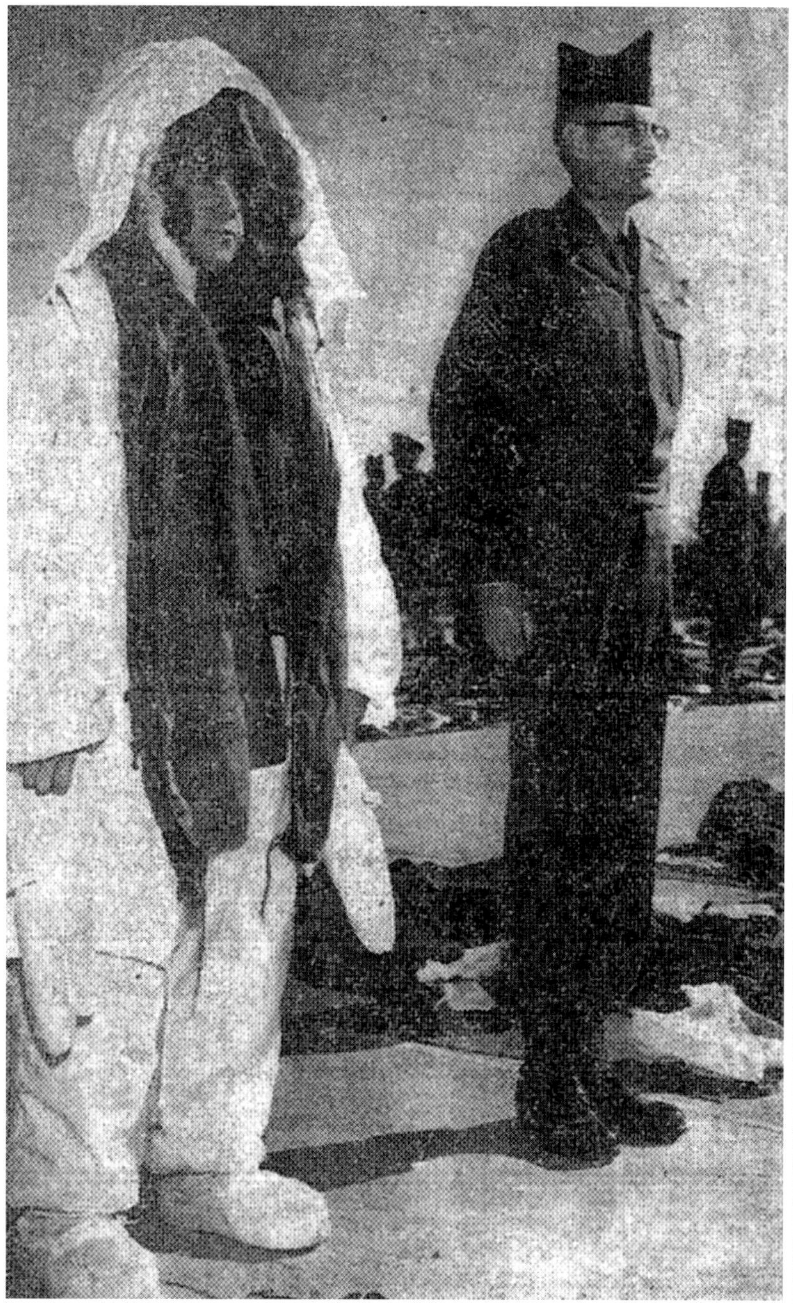

SGT Alfonso J. Steffanella models arctic clothing worn in Exercise Moose Horn as he awaits inspection by MG Shambora, BAMC Commander. Troops from the 520th Medical Clearing Company unload their gear in subzero weather as they arrive at Fort Greeley, Alaska.

(U.S. Army photo, MFSS Scrapbook 1955-56, Stimson Library Special Collections)

1956

Effective December 1956, the Department of Professional Sciences was reorganized into the Department of Medicine and Surgery, the Department of Neuropsychiatry, and the Department of Preventive Medicine.

(AMSS News Bulletin No. 2, 23 January 1957)

Trying to stay warm
37 soldiers from the 520th and 12 soldiers from the 57th Med Det (helicopter ambulance) provided medical support during the Arctic maneuver.

(U.S. Army photo, MFSS Scrapbook 1955-56, Stimson Library Special Collections)

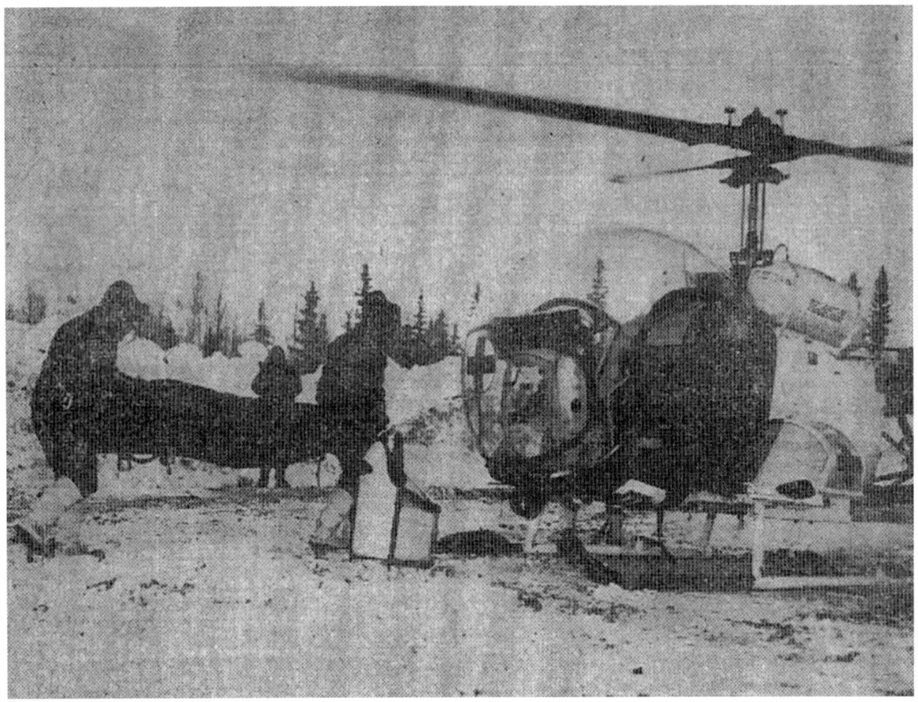

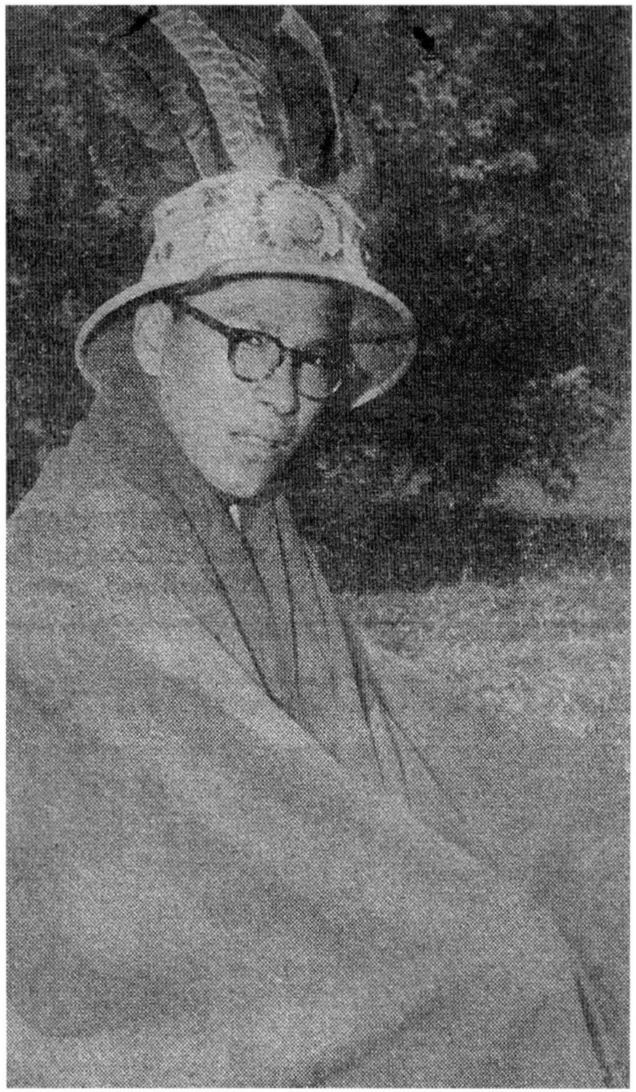

Cooling off
PVT Peter Mahmeah, a Kickapoo Indian from Shawnee, Oklahoma, demonstrates what he says is an old Indian system of keeping comfortable in the summer by covering up with a blanket to keep out the heat. He is a dental technician student at the AMSS, BAMC.

("Cooling Off," San Antonio Evening News, 7 August 1956)

The program for the Eighth Medical Instructors' Conference hosted at the AMSS

(Stimson Library Special Collections)

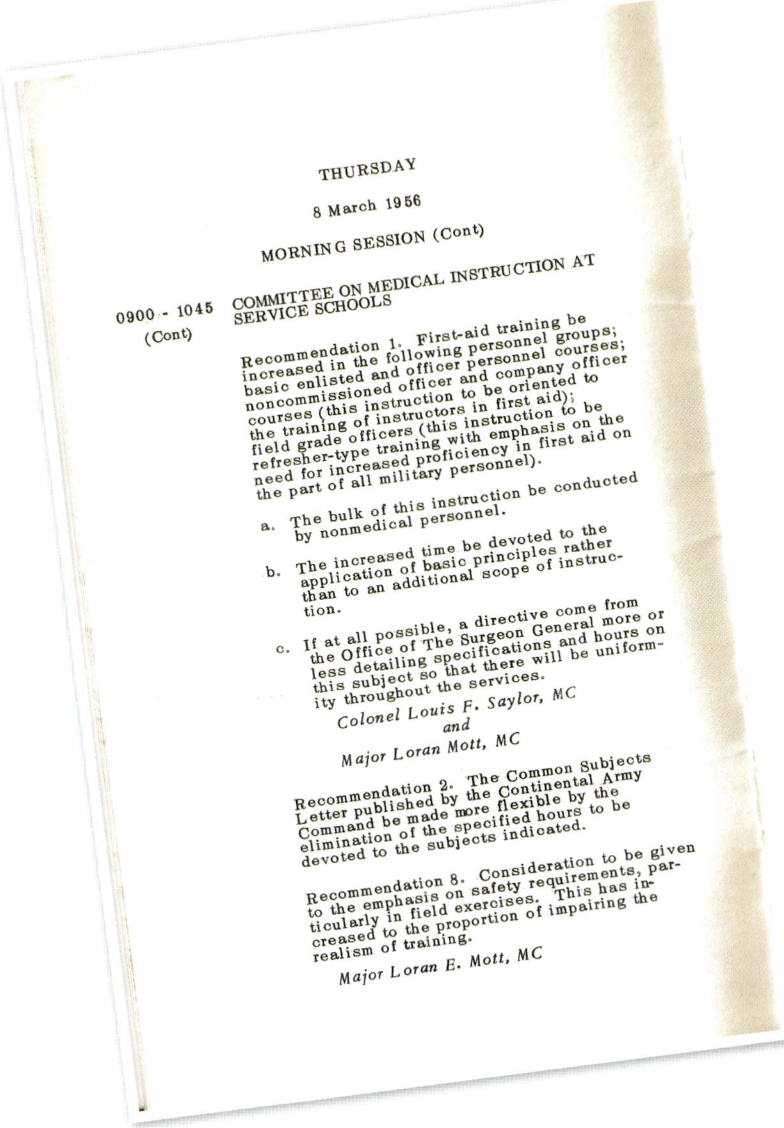

THURSDAY

8 March 1956

MORNING SESSION (Cont)

0900 - 1045 (Cont) COMMITTEE ON MEDICAL INSTRUCTION AT SERVICE SCHOOLS

Recommendation 1. First-aid training be increased in the following personnel groups; basic enlisted and officer personnel courses; noncommissioned officer and company officer courses (this instruction to be oriented to the training of instructors in first aid); field grade officers (this instruction to be refresher-type training with emphasis on the need for increased proficiency in first aid on the part of all military personnel).

a. The bulk of this instruction be conducted by nonmedical personnel.

b. The increased time be devoted to the application of basic principles rather than to an additional scope of instruction.

c. If at all possible, a directive come from the Office of The Surgeon General more or less detailing specifications and hours on this subject so that there will be uniformity throughout the services.

Colonel Louis F. Saylor, MC
and
Major Loran Mott, MC

Recommendation 2. The Common Subjects Letter published by the Continental Army Command be made more flexible by the elimination of the specified hours to be devoted to the subjects indicated.

Recommendation 8. Consideration to be given to the emphasis on safety requirements, particularly in field exercises. This has increased to the proportion of impairing the realism of training.

Major Loran E. Mott, MC

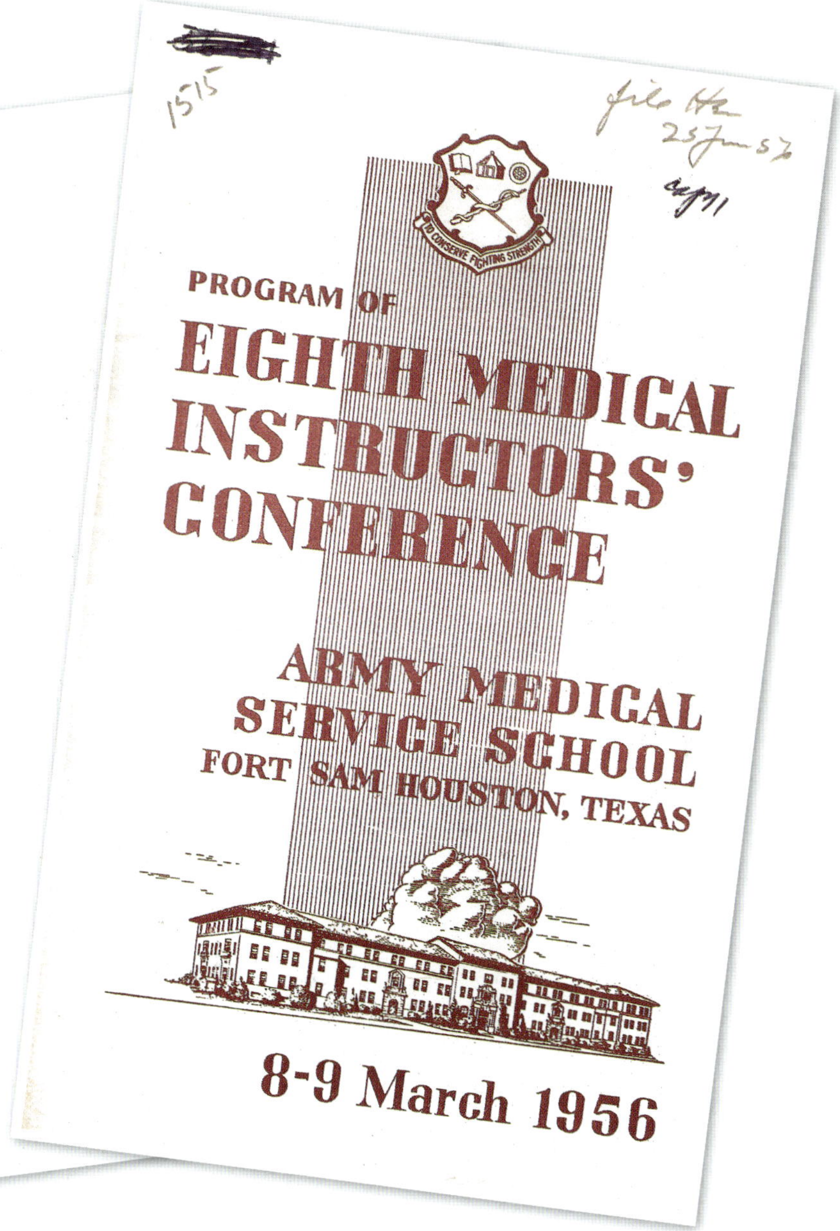

Sunday, Nov. 3, 1957 SAN ANTONIO LIGHT 5-D

Color May Alter Your Whole Personality

By MARGIE TAYLOR

Do you always reach for the bread in the red wrapper? Do you keep buying the cereal in the blue box, even though your family takes ages to eat it up?

Don't be surprised—there's a reason for these choices, according to Lt. Col. Vincent I. Hack, chief of the training aids and facilities branch at Brooke Army Medical center. Col. Hack conducts extensive research at Brooke in the psychology of color, a new field of personality analysis and adjustment.

Women will become more and more aware of the scientific use of color in coming years, Col. Hack believes. He predicts that by 1965 women will be coloring their hair and eyebrows shades of blue, green, orange—to either complement or change their personality characteristics. There will be personality analysts to assist women.

As a basis for his beliefs, Col. Hack must obtain a physical, psychological or physiological reaction to a color time after time, and obtain a significant result. He refuses to venture any ideas which he has not proved.

* * *

Color can be a powerful force, he contends; a force which can cause a complete personality change, or cause mental disturbance. As more people realize the results of color in their home, office and clothes, he expects many revolutions in industry.

For instance, professors giving a 45-minute lecture have been "beamed" repeatedly with colored lights. These invisible beams, faster than the eye, were blinked at the instructors throughout a lecture. When a red light was used—which has the longest wave length and causes increased physical and mental activity—the professor finished his lecture in about half an hour, and snapped at a student for little reason. Under a blue beam the same professor took an hour and 15 minutes for his lecture, lounged on the desk and leaned against the blackboard.

* * *

The color analyst has conducted tests with normal persons and blind persons, all placed in a room and asked to hold out their hands. Under a blue light the hands would gravitate toward each other; under yellow they would be straight ahead; under red light, increased mental activity caused the hands to swing outward.

* * *

Col. Hack believes a woman is going to "wear her personality" in future years. Women with quick tempers usually associated with red hair may be dying their hair red; or combating the trait with cooler, quieter colors. A woman can, even today, analyze herself by observing what color she has chosen for her car, and what color she selects to paint her living room walls.

Colors can be modified by personal aspirations, however, Col. Hack points out. A person may choose a color not because it suits his personality but because it appeals to the personality he would like to have!

* * *

What was referred to in the past as "good taste" now has a scientific background. Before experiments with color, people seemed to "have the feeling" for colors; hence red has become the sign of danger and means stop, green is soothing and, in traffic lights for instance, means "go ahead."

* * *

In color preference, women usually choose red; men prefer blue. Children of either sex choose red; older persons suffer from what Col. Hack calls a "blue starvation" and choose blue above all other colors. Only the center of the eye, made up of minute cones, are receptive to the wave lengths of the different colors. Chickens, for instance, have eyes completely made of cones, and this extra sensitivity is what makes them get up at daylight and retire when its dark. Bats, whose eyes are all rods, have reverse sensitivity and therefore reverse sleeping habits.

* * *

A red dress can do wonders for a woman! Tests with men at Brooke showed that, when they were shown a good looking woman in a white light, there was little or no change in brain response. The same woman under a red light, however, made their hearts beat faster, blood pressure rise, endocrine response shoot up, and their respiratory rate become a pant! Complexions look best under red-tinted lights; worst under blue.

* * *

Red objects appear closer, heavier, wider. Industries that have changed to blue-colored packaging find the back-ache rate of employees cut in half.

Tests have shown that people associate shape with color. Shown a circle, 80 per cent of all races and both sexes will say it is red. Squares are called blue; triangles are yellow. A "blue-type" person will most likely reach for a square box in preference to a cylinder.

Col. Hack's field is training aids; therefore his research does not reach further into this new and challenging field. Through his studies, the 400 instructors at Brooke have been rated and a color chart prepared to suit their personalities. Complementary colors are then used in assembling training aids for these professors. They are also shown how to use color during the day; a stimulating red after lunch when students tend to be drowsy; cooler, quieting blues and greens for classes which follow invigorating physical training exercises.

Col. Hack will enlarge on his theories on the psychology of color at a public lecture at 8 p. m. this Sunday at Bolivar hall, La Villita, under the auspices of the Coppini Academy of Fine Arts.

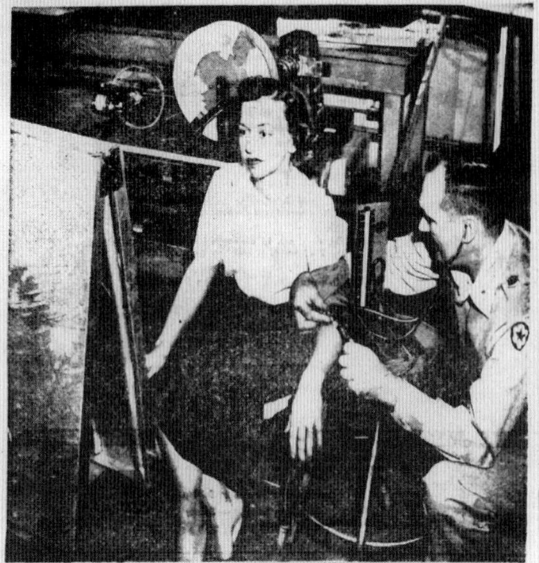

COLOR CHANGES PERSONALITY, ANALYST DEMONSTRATES
Mrs. Annabelle Ahrens' blood pressure checked by Lt. Col. V. I. Hack while color flashes.

LTC Vincent L. Hack, Director of the Training Aids Section and the world's leading authority on the psychology of color (on the right), checks Mrs. Annabelle Ahrens' blood pressure while colors flash on a screen.

("Color May Alter Your Whole Personality," by Margie Taylor, San Antonio Light, 2 November 1957, article location in collection of the AMEDD Museum, LTC Vincent Hack files)

1957

January 1957 marked the beginning of the expanded Allied Officer Program at AMSS. The school initiated a special course for non-English speaking students. Twenty-five Chinese nationals, supported by LTC Choa as their interpreter, were the first to attend the course.

(AMSS News Bulletin No. 1, 16 January 1957)

Dental facilities were updated and enlisted dental students were offered two highly specialized courses: advanced dental laboratory procedures and dental assistant.

("For AMSS Dental Courses: Modern Facilities Provided," Talon, 17 January 1957)

The Surgical Research Unit, added in 1947, became a separate unit in 1953 to conduct extensive research, especially in burn treatment.

The Army Field Medical Service Development Unit, added circa 1957, worked under the Office of the Surgeon General.

("BAMC Observes 11th Anniversary Friday," Talon, 31 January 1957)

BG Elbert Decoursey, MFSS Commandant, addressed the International Medical Assembly of Southwest Texas in January 1957 on the increased use of radioactivity. His presentation discussed the hazards and benefits of the use of radioisotopes for everything from industry to medical treatment.

("Radioactivity Use Increased," San Antonio News, 28 January 1957)

OPERATION BLOWUP: The mass casualty exercise of 1,000 simulated casualties from a thermonuclear bomb blast took place over a five day period the last week in February at Camp Bullis.

("Top Officers Talk on Nuclear Effects," Talon, 28 February 1957)

LTC Vincent Hack and the Training Aids Section's BAMC float win two trophies in the Battle of Flowers and Flambeau Parades in 1957. The floats were designed to represented Atlantis and underwater scenery based on the movie "Beneath the 12 Mile Reef."

("BAMC Float Takes Two Trophies in SA Fiesta," Talon, 2 May 1957)

"Pete," BAMC's famous bleeding dummy, was a feature of the Army's static displays at the Armed Forces Day Open House. At his last public appearance, over 25,000 watched him go through his routine of demonstrating many types of open wounds. He was used at the Medical Training Center for instruction of basic medical aidmen and corpsmen.

("Bleeding Dummy Part of Exhibit," San Antonio News, 17 May 1957)

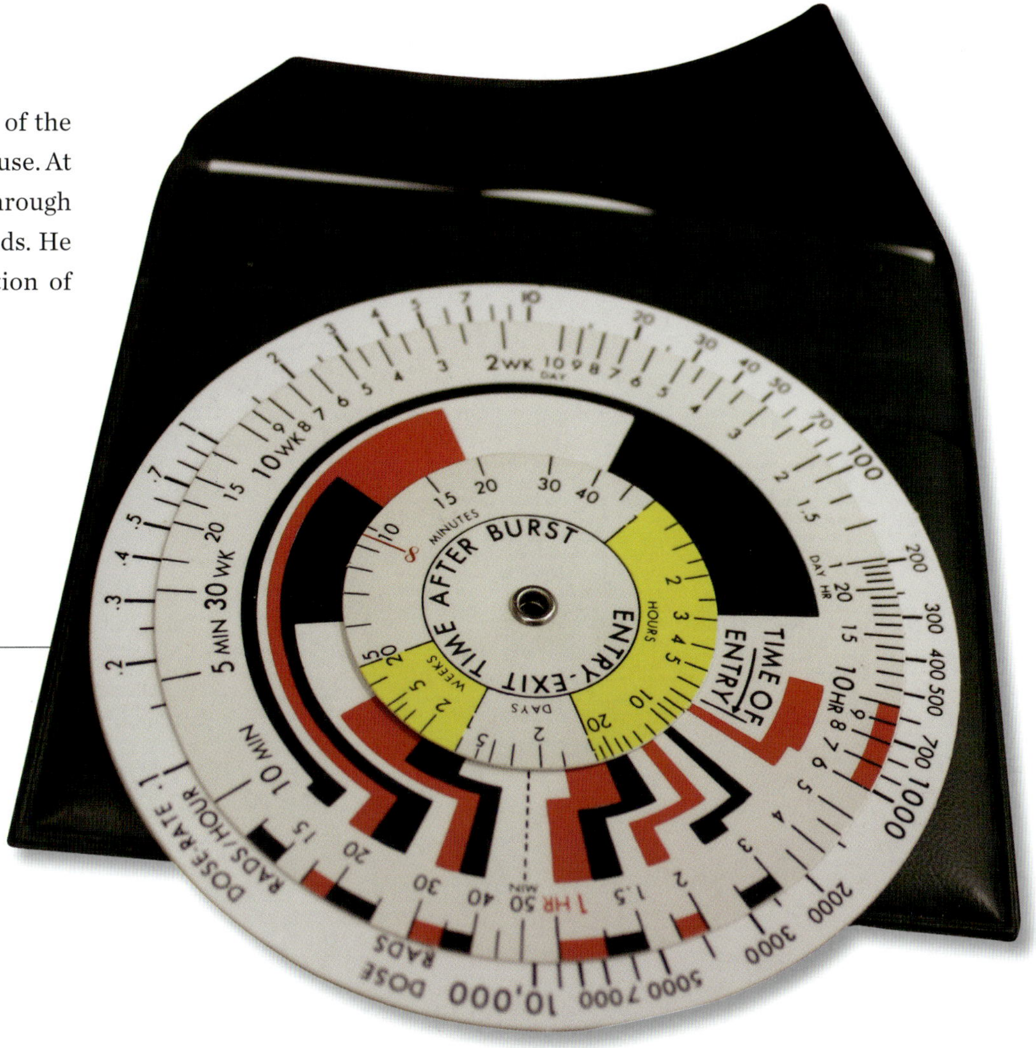

A RADIAC and Nuclear Yield Calculator Set (model: ABC-M28A1) used to calculate downwind hazard (predictor) for nuclear weapons detonation.

(Courtesy of Preventive Medicine Department, AMEDDC&S)

1958

1LT Ulka Sema Aran was the first woman to become an officer and a doctor in the Turkish Army. She was also the first allied woman physician to enroll in the 22-week course for company officers at the Army Medical School.

("Turkish Woman Doctor is the 'First,'" Talon, 31 July 1958)

BAMC was first in the San Antonio area to present an exhibit about some of the peaceful applications of atomic energy in the fields of industry, agriculture and medicine.

("AEC Exhibits 'Peaceful Atom' at Stimson Library," Talon, 14 August 1958)

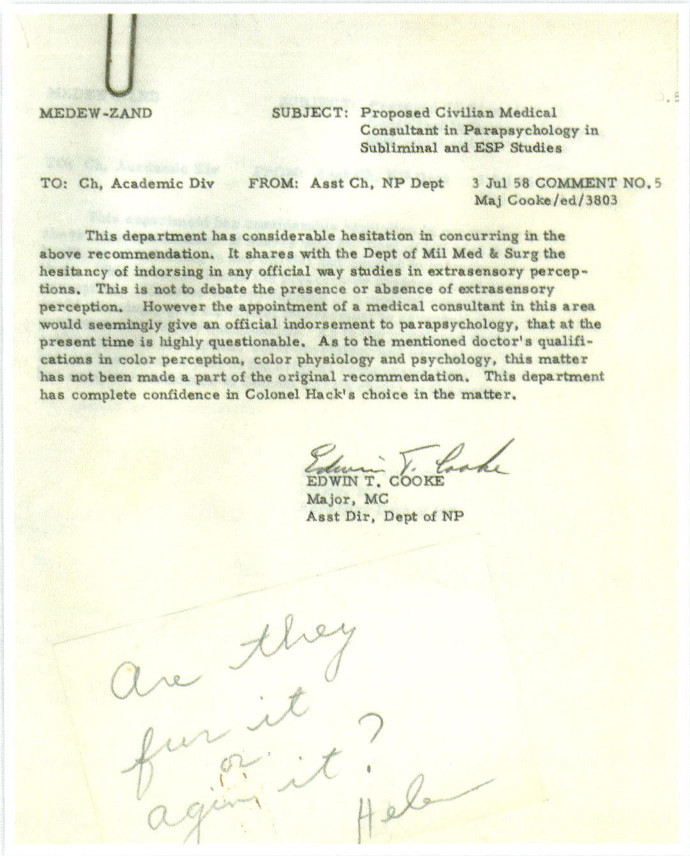

MEDEW-ZAND SUBJECT: Proposed Civilian Medical Consultant in Parapsychology in Subliminal and ESP Studies

TO: Ch, Academic Div FROM: Asst Ch, NP Dept 3 Jul 58 COMMENT NO. 5
Maj Cooke/ed/3803

This department has considerable hesitation in concurring in the above recommendation. It shares with the Dept of Mil Med & Surg the hesitancy of indorsing in any official way studies in extrasensory perceptions. This is not to debate the presence or absence of extrasensory perception. However the appointment of a medical consultant in this area would seemingly give an official indorsement to parapsychology, that at the present time is highly questionable. As to the mentioned doctor's qualifications in color perception, color physiology and psychology, this matter has not been made a part of the original recommendation. This department has complete confidence in Colonel Hack's choice in the matter.

EDWIN T. COOKE
Major, MC
Asst Dir, Dept of NP

Are they for it or agin it? Hel

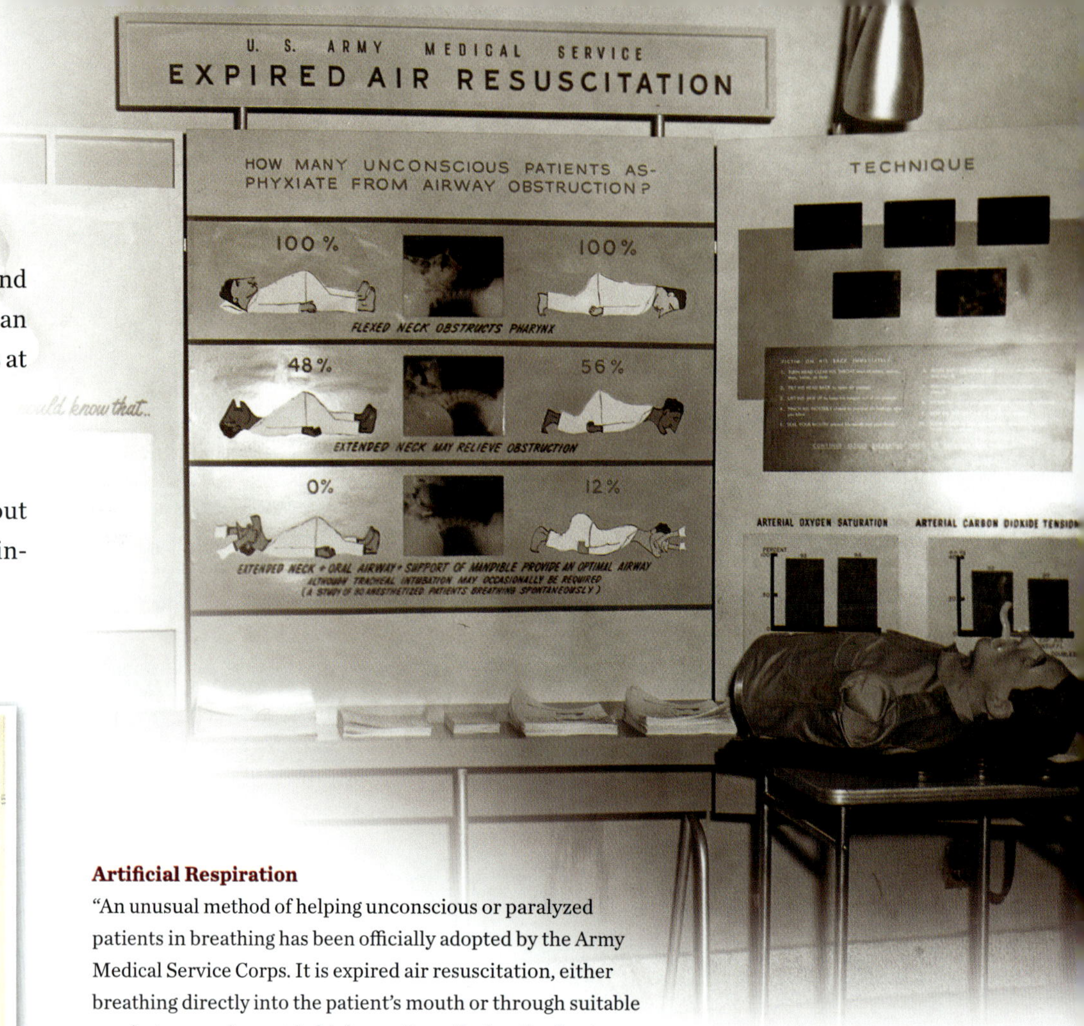

Artificial Respiration

"An unusual method of helping unconscious or paralyzed patients in breathing has been officially adopted by the Army Medical Service Corps. It is expired air resuscitation, either breathing directly into the patient's mouth or through suitable respiratory equipment in his lungs. Described as the 'best system available,' the procedure has been adopted at a time when new weapons could cause a greater number of casualties than ever before. The process is new only in recognition, for medical history has recorded resuscitation by mouth-to-mouth as much as 200 years ago."

("Army Adopts a Better Way of Artificial Respiration," Talon, 17 July 1958) (Image from the 1959 AMSS Livestock Show AAR, Stimson Library Special Collections)

In June 1958, LTC Vincent Hack, one of the AMSS innovators during the 1950s and 1960s, sought to hire a civilian medical consultant to conduct a study on extra sensory perception and subliminal color perception. The accompanying note suggests he met with an indeterminate response.

"SP4 Loren Henley, an instructor of basic medical lab procedures at the AMSS, was the first enlisted man at BAMC to be accepted for the Army's new college training program for enlisted personnel. Upon completion of the program, he will owe two years of service for each year of college training."

("AMSS Instructor First to Attend College," Talon, 11 Sept 1958)

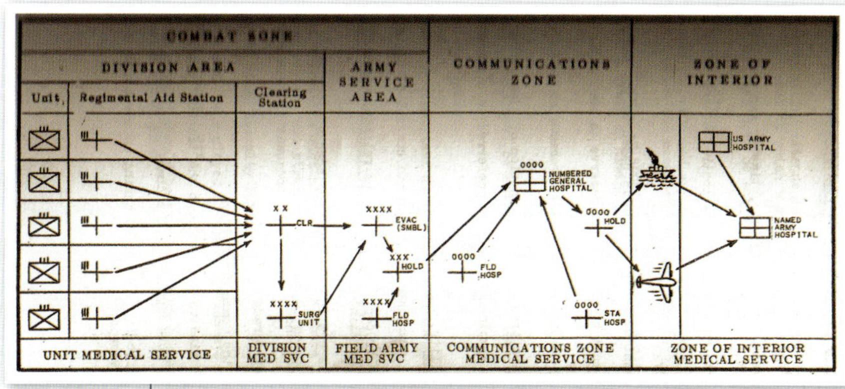

Levels of Medical Service

(Field Medical Service Handbook, Army Medical Service School, Brooke Army Medical Center, Fort Sam Houston, Texas, M925 Jun 58 (Rev), p 9, Stimson Library Special Collections)

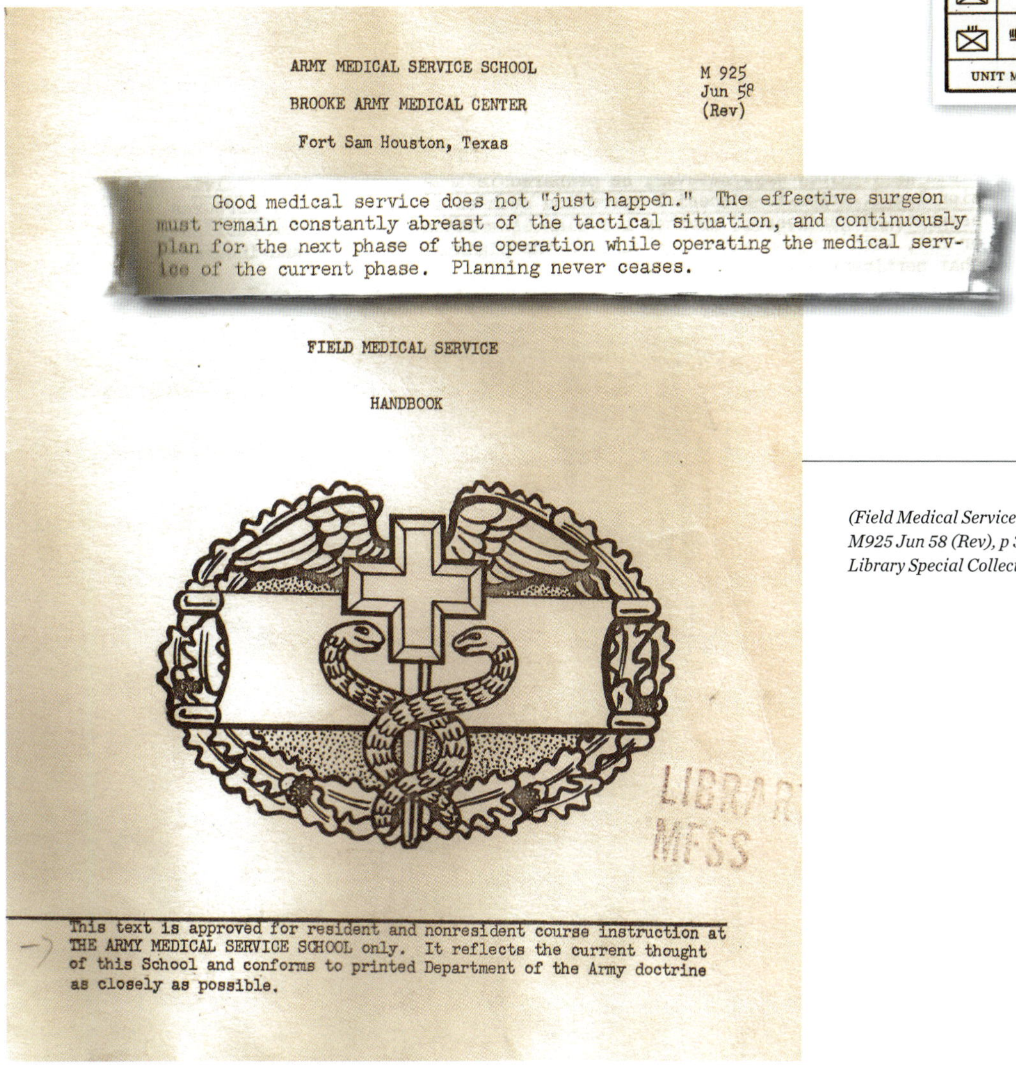

ARMY MEDICAL SERVICE SCHOOL

BROOKE ARMY MEDICAL CENTER

Fort Sam Houston, Texas

M 925
Jun 58
(Rev)

Good medical service does not "just happen." The effective surgeon must remain constantly abreast of the tactical situation, and continuously plan for the next phase of the operation while operating the medical service of the current phase. Planning never ceases.

FIELD MEDICAL SERVICE

HANDBOOK

This text is approved for resident and nonresident course instruction at THE ARMY MEDICAL SERVICE SCHOOL only. It reflects the current thought of this School and conforms to printed Department of the Army doctrine as closely as possible.

(Field Medical Service Handbook, M925 Jun 58 (Rev), p 37. Stimson Library Special Collections)

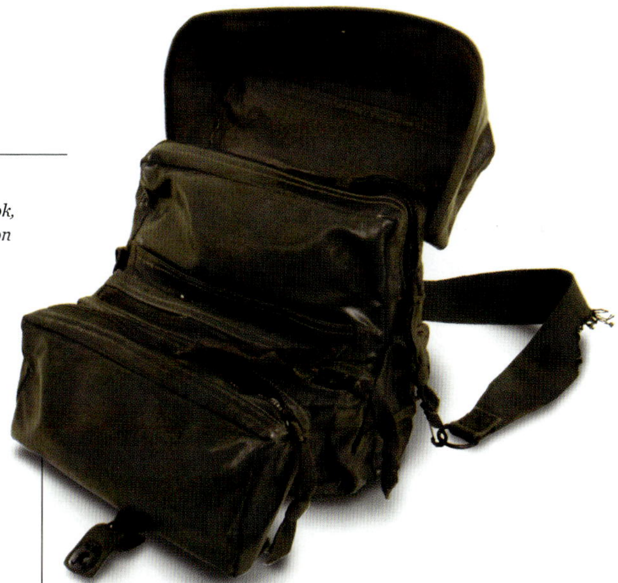

M3 Bag, circa 1958

The canvas M3 Combat Medic Bag made its first appearance about 1948. It was replaced by the rubberized M3 in June 1958. The Nylon Duck M3 arrived 13 years later in November 1971.

(AMEDD Museum Collection. Dates obtained from QM change memos)

1959

Designed for emergency care of nuclear and other casualties, the armed services designed a first aid medical packet to meet conditions immediately following a military disaster when no direct medical aid could be expected.

("Armed Services Devise First Aid Medical Packet for Use by Wounded," Talon, 16 Jan 1959)

AMSS claimed to have the best instructors possible due in part to the Academic Training Unit (ATU). The ATU training program lasted a minimum of three weeks during which time it prepared and perfected potential AMSS instructors' teaching techniques.

("Instructor Training / Instruction Pays Off," Talon, 29 Jan 1959)

CPT Manuel Santa Ursula of the Spanish Army and a student of the C4 AMSS program wished to pay tribute to San Antonio and rendered a colorful interpretation of his feelings as a temporary native. "I read, several days ago, that San Antonio is feminine. All right. She is shamefully sentimental. Delightfully flirtatious. Outrageously seductive. Dangerously engaging and at all times, charming. She is half a saint and half hussy, and I love her madly. So will you if you are not careful." Even though his intent was sincere in the best of ways, he acknowledged that he "was not careful" (in his choice of words).

("San Antonio, Flirtatious, Half Saint...Half Hussy," Talon, 26 March 1959)

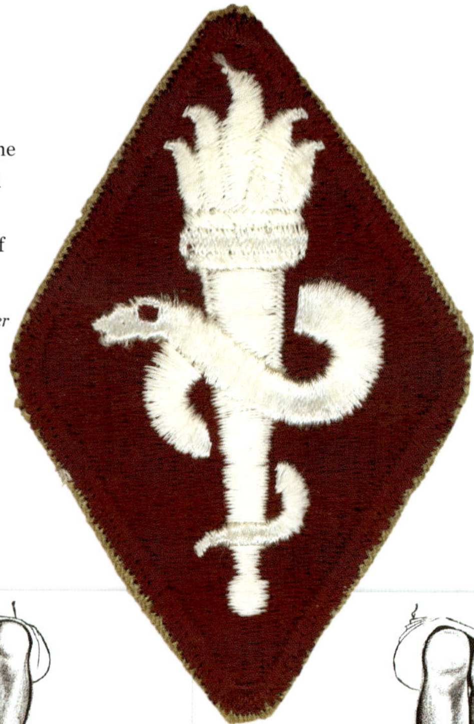

Medical Training Center Patch
Soldiers assigned to the Area Support Medical Company received a new patch in March of 1959 (ASMC).

("Medical Training Center gets Patch," Talon, 19 March 1959) (Patch from the AMEDD Museum Collection)

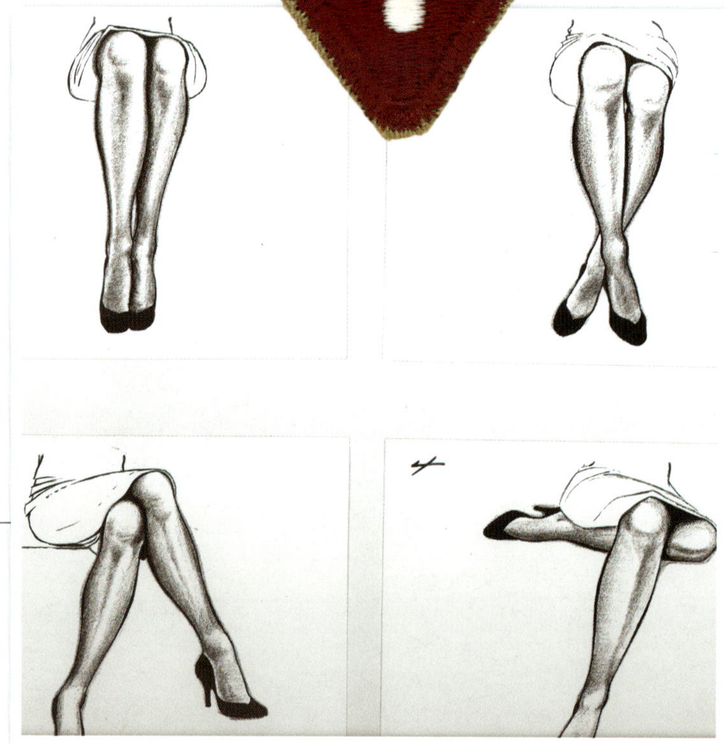

Body Language Studies
COL Vincent Hack, Chief of Training Aids at the AMSS, conducted a study that correlated the way women cross their legs with basic personality types. The study received the nickname "Learn through Leerin'" in the San Antonio Light.

("Learn Through Leerin': Gals Legs Reveal Personality," by Ann Gaddis, San Antonio Light, 11 Oct 1959; original leg images from LTC Vincent Hack files, AMEDD Museum)

1LT Johnson and 2LT Larsen were the first male candidates to be selected for and attend AMSS training for their future assignments as Army dieticians, an MOS previously restricted to women.

("Army's First Male Dieticians," Talon, 20 April 1959)

"Potential use of paper-based clothing items is being studied by the Quartermaster Corps during an extensive user test at BAMC. Medical personnel will wear-test during normal operations and the test data is expected to form the basis for consideration of further material development requirements."

("Disposable Paper-Based Clothing Tested at BAMC," Talon, 11 June 1959)

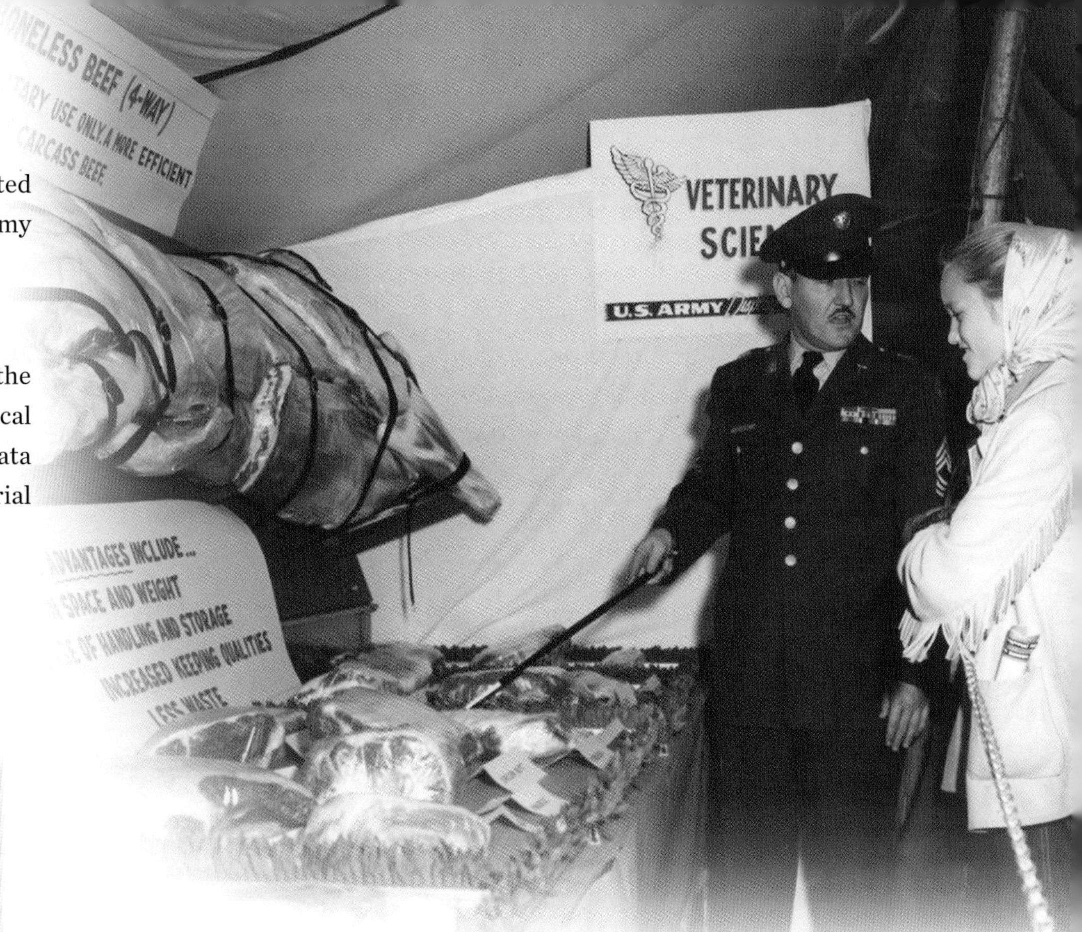

A Vet Corps master sergeant discusses the merits of a boneless beef carcass to a viewer at the 1959 San Antonio Livestock Show.

(U.S. Army Photo, AMEDD Museum Photo Collection)

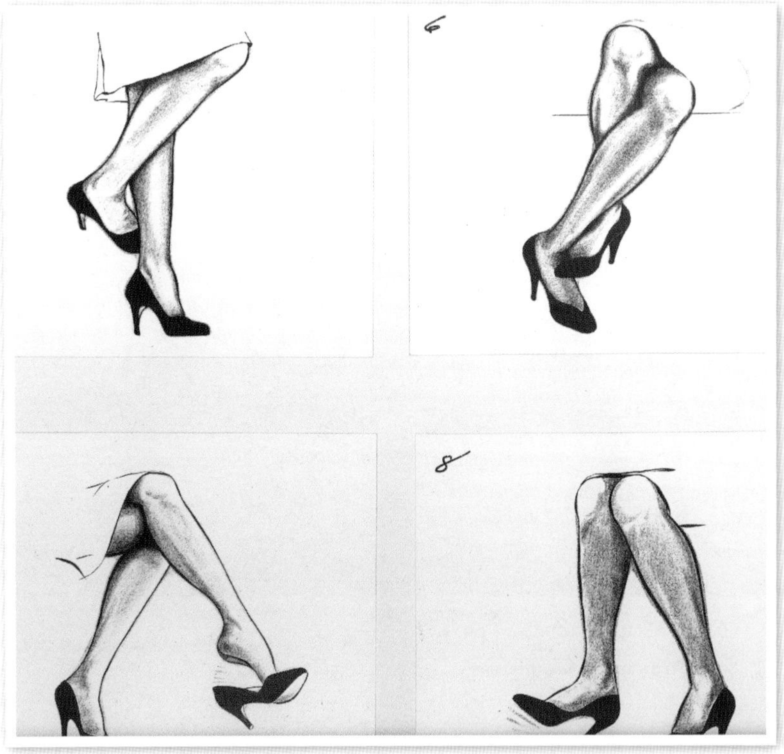

Dr. Monohan of the Royal Canadian Army Medical Corps and Filipina nurse Alderita Peregrino were both promoted at a ceremony at BAMC. Of the thousands of allied officers who attended the AMSS over the decades, CPT Monohan and 1LT Peregrino were the first to be promoted here.

("Two Allied Officers First to be Promoted at BAMC," Talon, 22 Oct 1959)

The Faculty Development Course was established in 1959 to educate instructors in teaching methods for the staff and faculty of the Army Medical Service School.

("FDU Teaches the Teachers," San Antonio Light, 10 Dec 1972, p 5-l)

1959

Annual Active Duty for Training of the 807th Hospital Center was held at the AMSS, BAMC, 31 May through 13 June 1959. This was the third consecutive year that the unit trained at the AMSS. It was the first time the 807th Hospital Center annual active duty training included a field exercise at Camp Bullis.

(807th Hospital Center: Annual Active Duty for Training 1959 After Action Report, Stimson Library Special Collections)

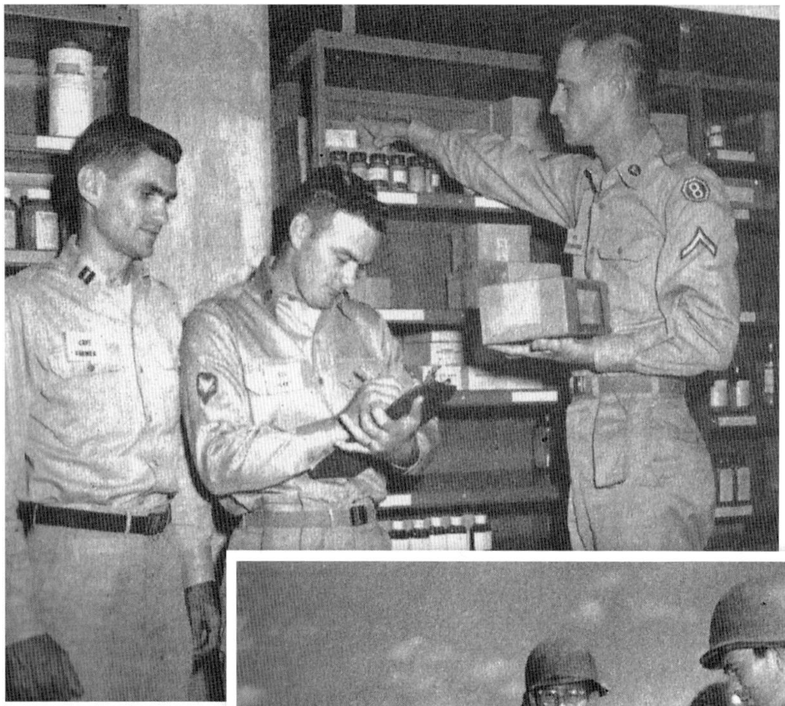

Checking pharmacy stores

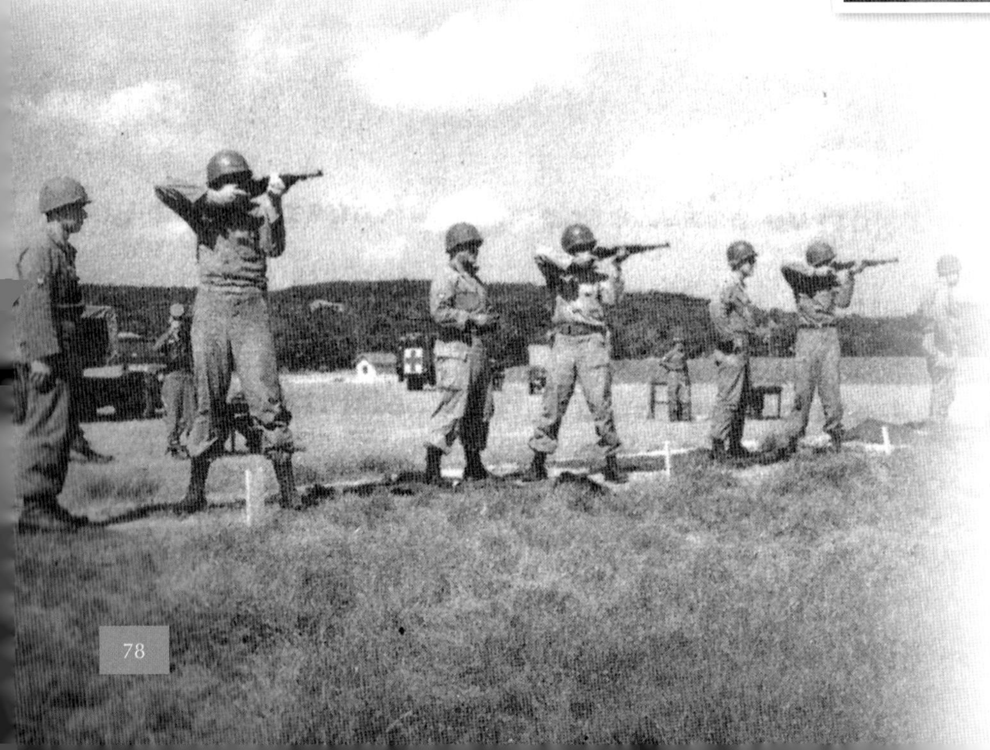

Weapons training at Camp Bullis

(Photos from: 807th Hospital Center: Annual Active Duty for Training 1959, After Action Report, Stimson Library, Special Collections)

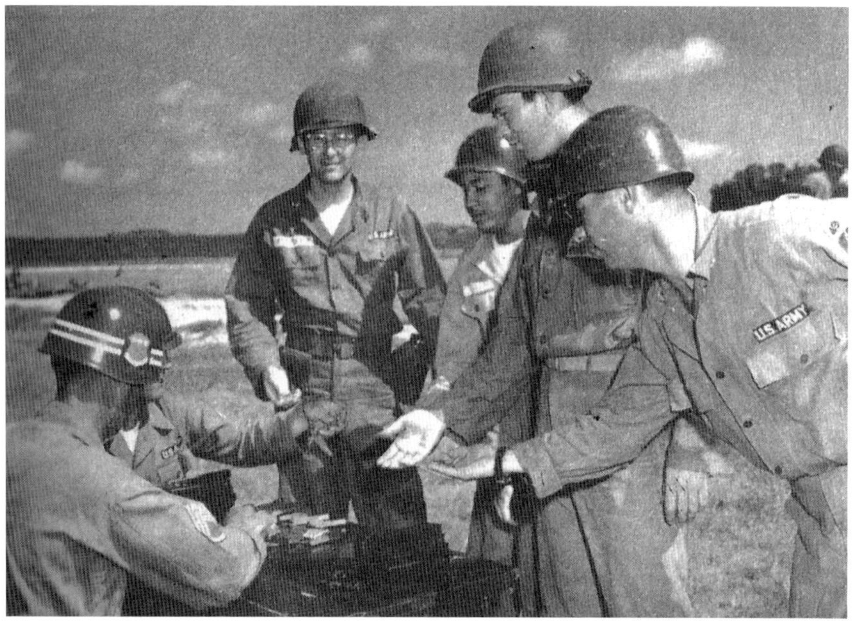

Drawing ammunition

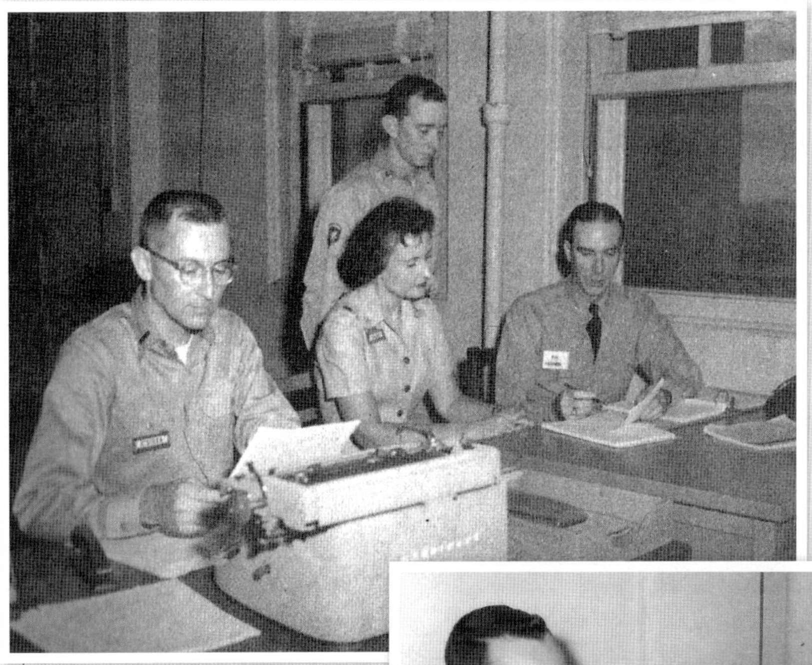

Administrative duties

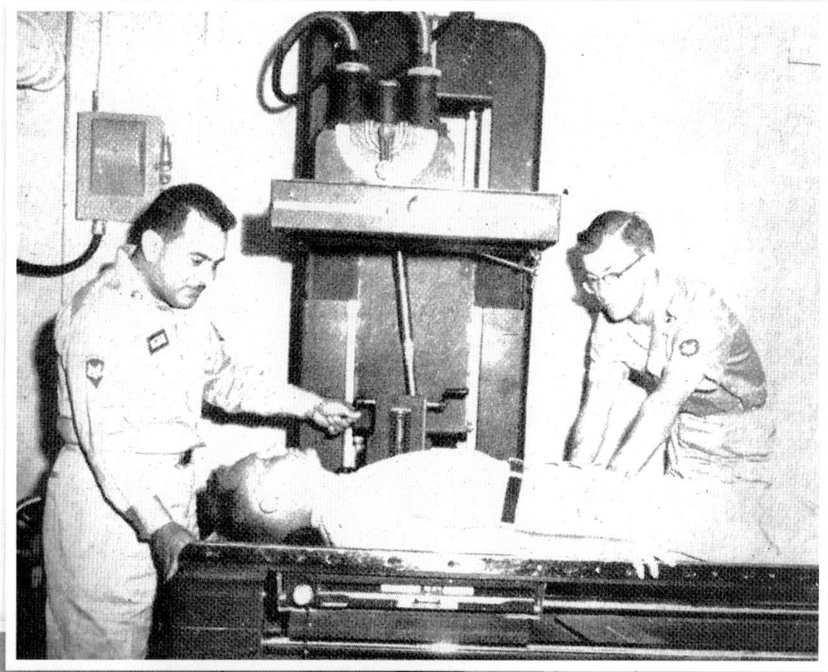

X-ray training

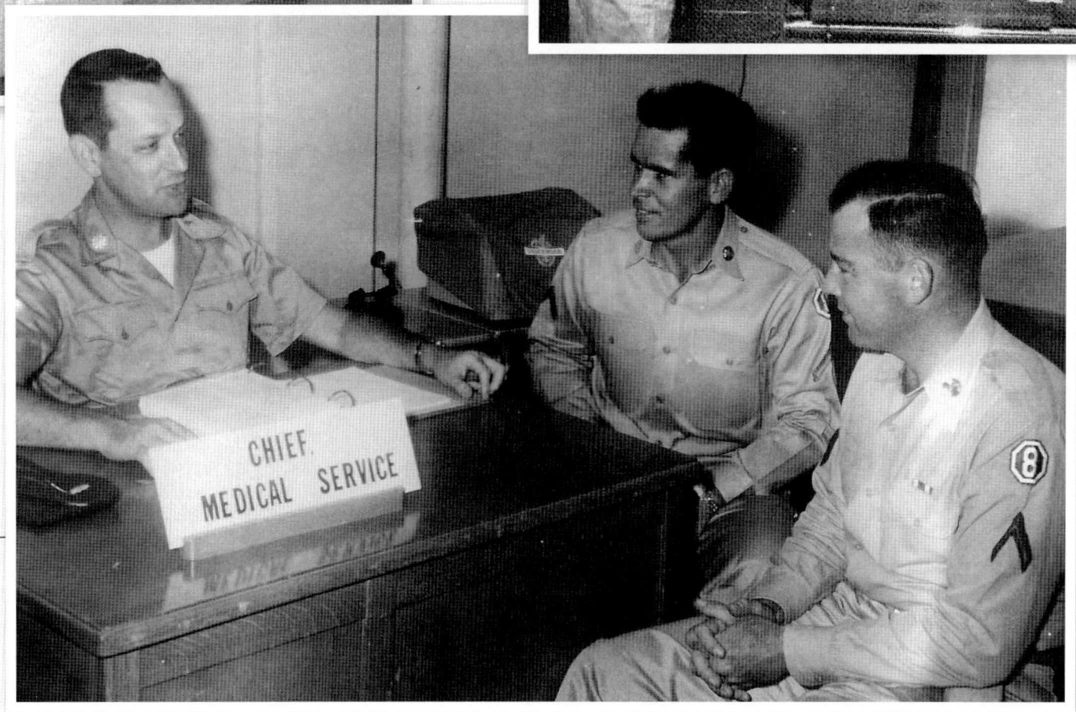

Briefing the chief

1959

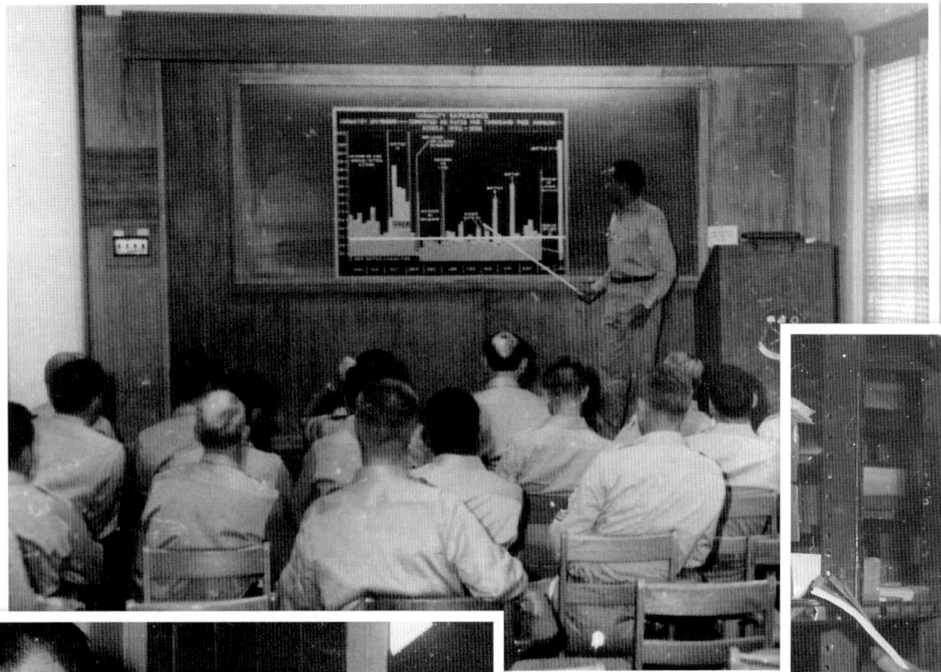

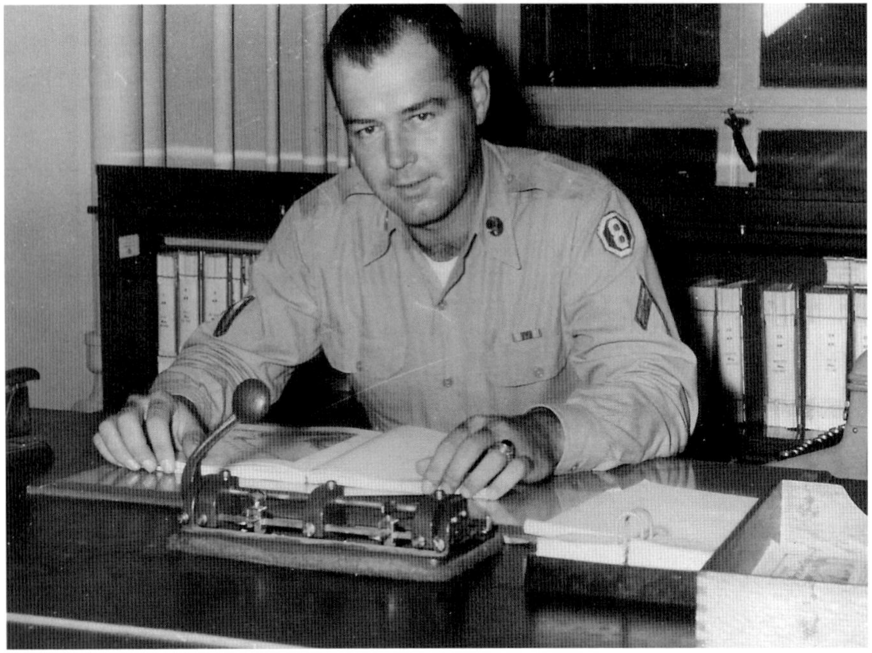

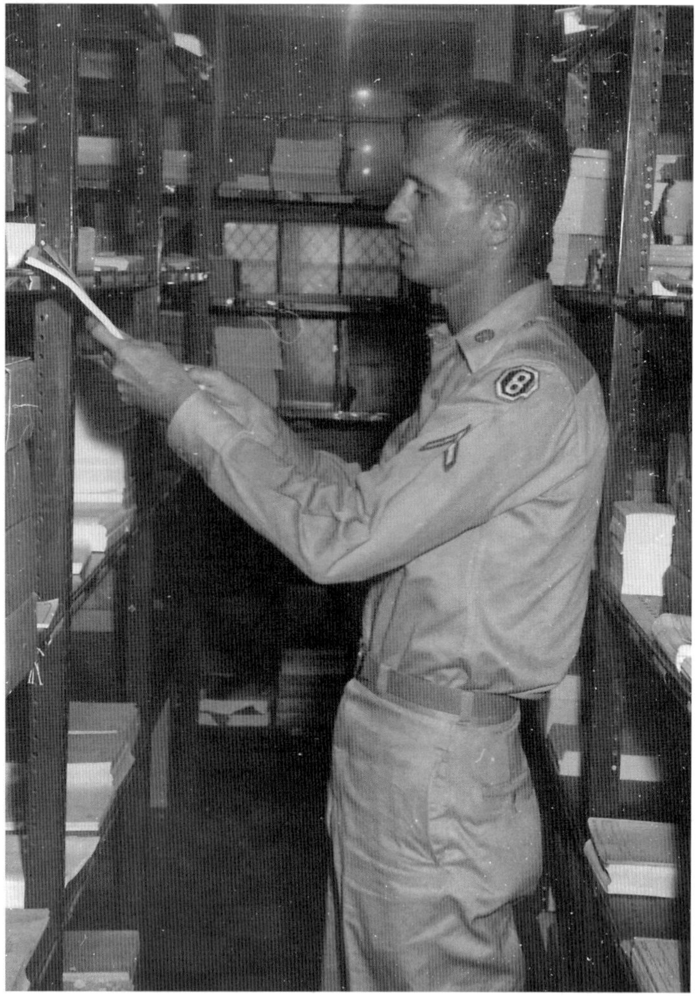

On-the-job training

(Photos from: 807th Hospital Center: Annual Active Duty for Training 1959, After Action Report, Stimson Library, Special Collections)

Saturday morning inspection

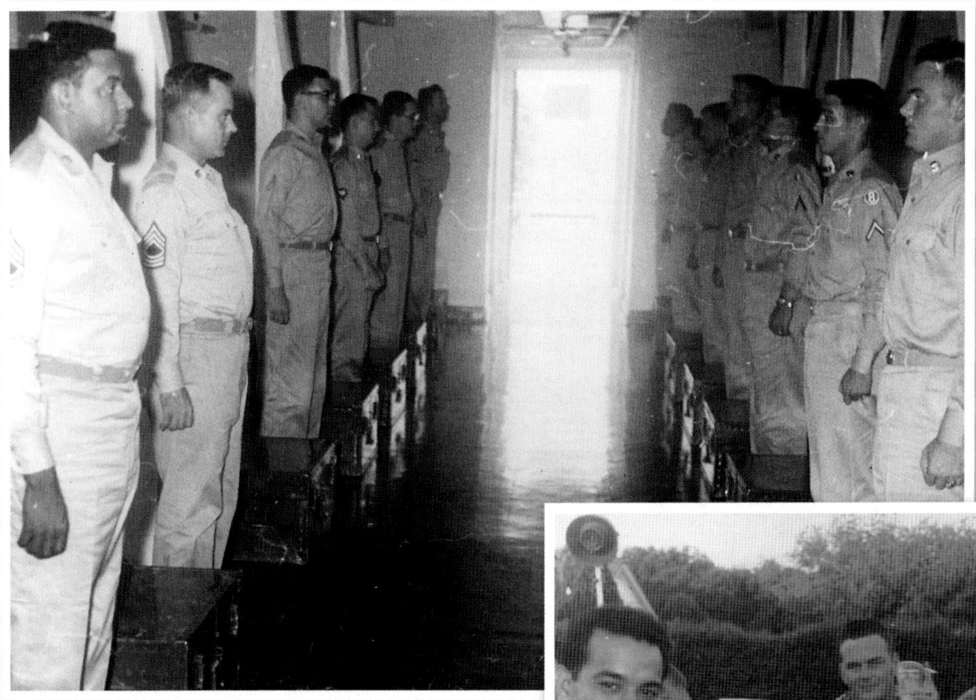

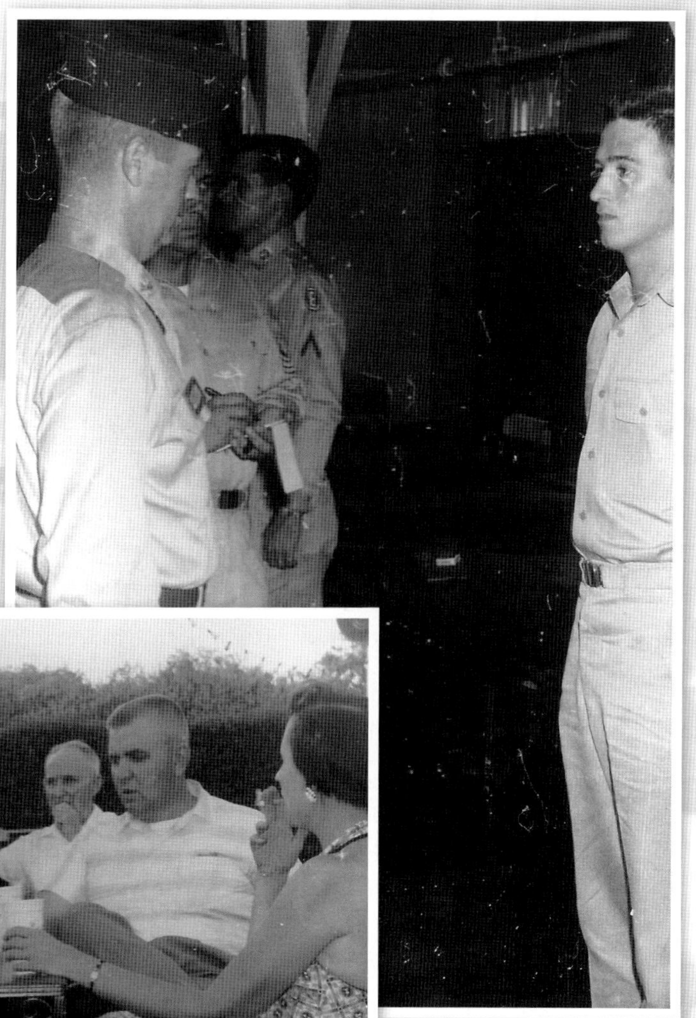

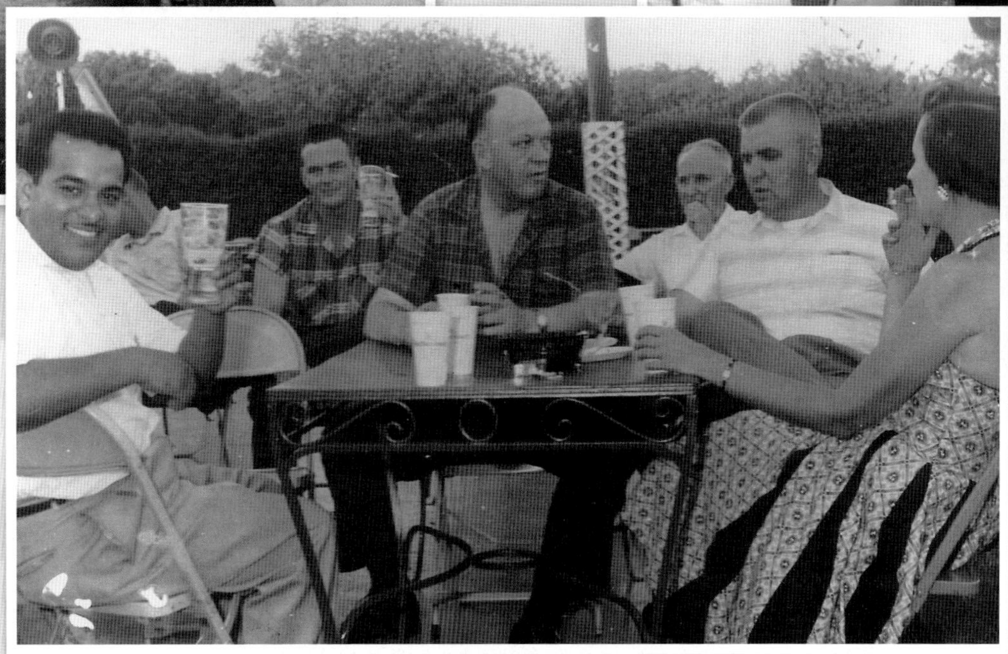

Recreation

1960 – 1969

Two Iranian officers become the first two allied officers to attend AMSS to study food inspection and food sanitation procedures.

("Iranians are First Allied Veterinary Officers to Train at BAMC," Talon, 21 Jan 1960)

The Brooke Army Hospital became Brooke Army University, a medical research and training center. The decision was made to permanently locate the Army's greatest facilities for medical treatment, education, training and research at Fort Sam Houston.

("Brook Army Hospital Becomes Brooke Army University," San Antonio Express, 9 Feb 1960)

"COL Pappas, Director of Supply at BAMC, predicts that the medic of 1974 may well be the glamour boy of the Armed Services. On the threshold of fantastic changes, he envisions medical teams using flying platforms or jeeps that will answer signals emitted from wounded soldiers. They will be in white uniforms capable of heat and carrying all supplies necessary. COL Pappas also stated that with hospitals being set up some 500 miles away, a guided missile cruising at a comfortable speed of 2000 MPH will transport patients to the hospital. An amazing number of hospital supply items will be disposable."

("Medic Envisioned as 1974 Glamour Boy," publication unknown, 17 March 1960)

The BAMC Float took Top Prize in the 1960 Battle of the Flowers Parade. Its theme was "Drama of Time."

("BAMC Float Takes Top Prize," Talon, 28 Apr 1960)

Birth of Prince

International relations at the AMSS in 1960 included celebrating the birth of the recently born Crowned Prince of Iran. Left to right are MG and Mrs. John F. Bojlender, Commander of BAMC; Mrs. Preston H. Dial, President of the San Antonio Council of International Relations; COL Chassem Nik-Nejjad, senior Iranian student at the AMSS; and BG and Mrs. James L. Synder, Commandant, AMSS.

("Friends, Classmates, and Instructors," Talon, 17 Nov 1960)

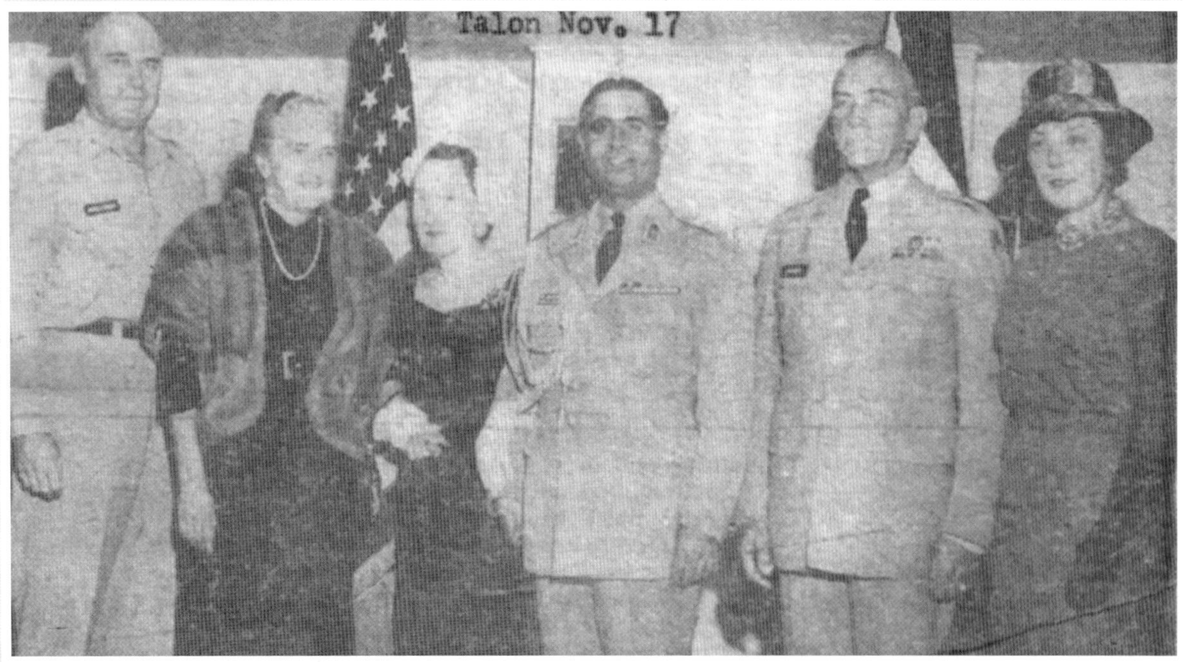

An Army Nurse Corps medal was authorized by the Office of the Surgeon General to be awarded to the most outstanding ANC student in each Advanced Military Nursing Class at the Medical Service School. The medal was a tribute from all members of the Corps interested in recognizing the professional standing of military nursing. The first recipient was CPT Angeline Hennick and was presented in June 1961.

("Outstanding Army Nurse Corps Student will Receive Newly Authorized Medal," Military Service News, 30 Sept 1960)

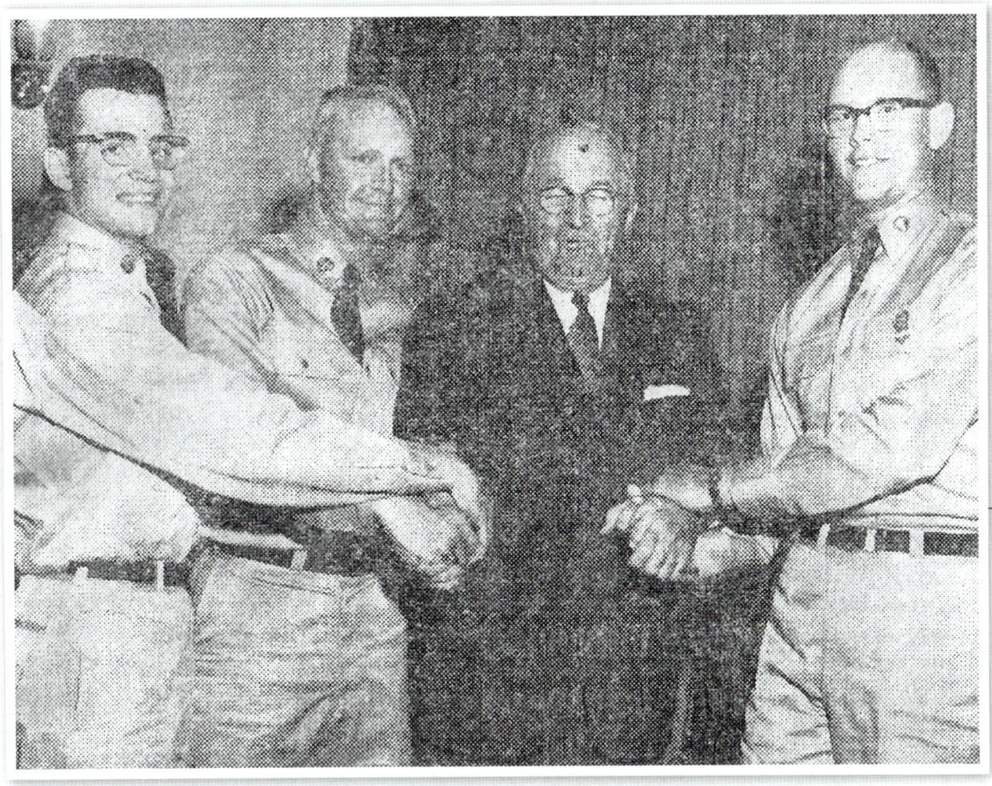

The AMSS Instructor's Training Unit trained students to become better instructors. By 1960 the Unit had trained 53% of all instructors assigned to the school. The Unit helped even seasoned instructors by conducting critiques of presentations as well as informing them of the availability of training aids, classroom equipment, or academic records.

("Students Become Teachers," Talon, 8 Sept 1960)

President Truman

Former President Harry S. Truman with three candidates of the AMSS "Citizen Soldier" Program. Left to right are PVT George Francis, PVT Ray Kaylor, and PVT Albert Woodward.

("Harry S. Truman Meets with MTC Citizen Soldier Nominees," Talon, 13 Oct 1960)

Fifty San Antonians presented a demonstration of emergency medical procedures in the Army Medical Service School Quadrangle. They cared for 150 simulated casualties to show how lives can be saved even though professional medical care personnel may not be available. These 50 people evacuated the pre-sorted casualties into 5 aid stations in the Quadrangle and demonstrated emergency life-saving procedures.

("Nonmedical Civilians To Test Emergency Medical Knowledge," Talon, 27 Oct 1960)

1961

On January 1961, the Army Medical Service School's name was officially changed back to the Medical Field Service School.

LTC George F. Rumer, Director of the Department of Medicine and Surgery at the MFSS, reported to a Congressional group in Washington, D.C., on the Army Medical Service Training in Care of Mass Casualities on 18 July 1961. The Congressional group, composed mainly of Congressmen holding commissions in the U.S. Army Reserves, heard Rumer discuss the "anticipated tremendous patient load" associated with nuclear warfare as well as the Army's emergency medical care program. He also presented a summary of the various levels of training received by all Army personnel.

("COL Rumer to D.C. Mass Casualties Report for Congressional Group," Talon, 13 July 1961)

The first enlisted pharmacy specialist course since 1953 was reinstituted.

("EM Pharmacy Courses Reinstituted at MFSS," Talon, 20 July 1961)

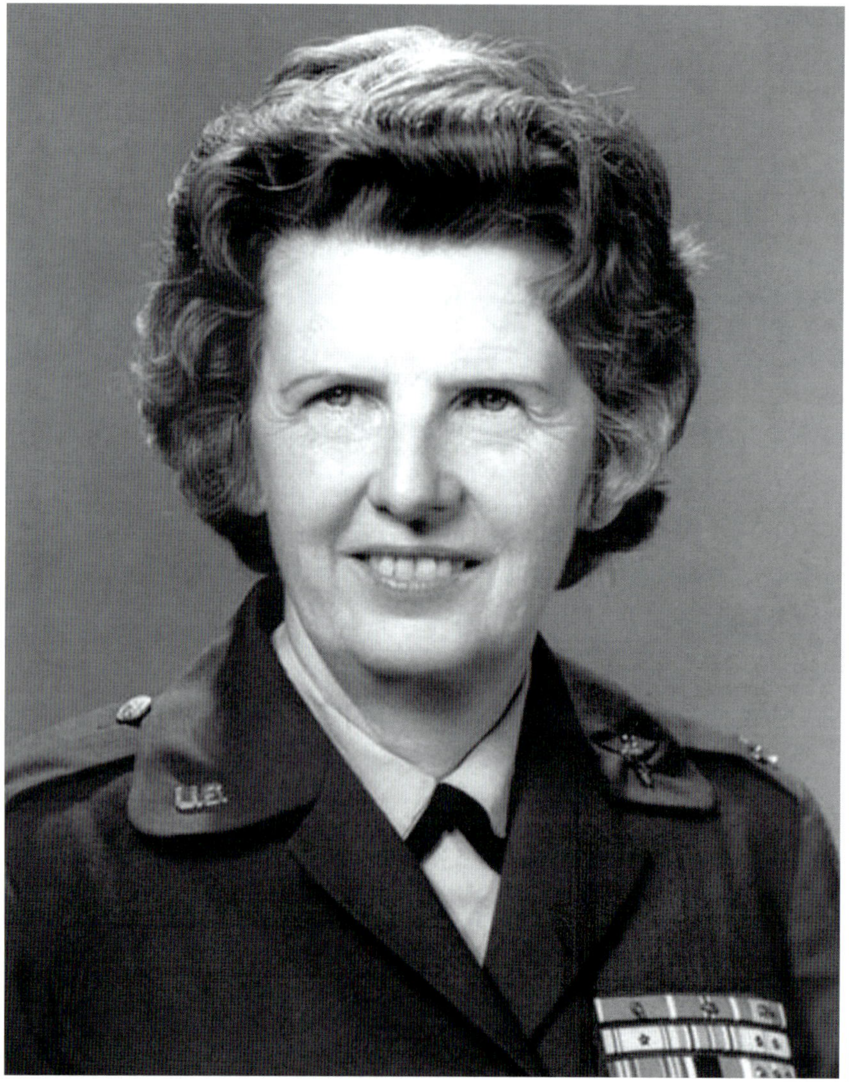

COL Ruby G. Bradley

COL Ruby G. Bradley, the Army's most decorated nurse, was assigned Director of Nursing Activities at Brooke Army Medical Center. Described in 1961 as "slight, graying, gentle-featured [and] soft-spoken," Bradley, an Army officer since 1934, was a nurse of steel and compassion, having accomplished her nursing mission as a Japanese prisoner of war in the Philippines during WWII and then in Korea, where she was one of the first combat nurses to arrive during the conflict. She was responsible for establishing nursing service for field and evacuation hospitals for the Army, and then, as Chief Nurse, Eighth Army, developing the Korean Nurses' Association to train Korean Nurses in American nursing methods.

("COL Bradley New BAMC Nursing Activities Director," Talon, 6 July 1961)

In anticipation of mobilization, the Medical Specialist Advanced Course was redesigned to open the course to more students, reduce training time, and raise standards by offering the course at other hospitals besides BAMC. By June 1961, Madigan and Womack Army Hospitals joined BAMC, Walter Reed, Fitzsimons, and Letterman General Hospital, where courses for advanced training had been taking place since 1955.

("Medical Advanced Course Now Open to Lower Grade," Talon, 29 June 1961)

Brooke General Hospital was named one of three new training sites for an advanced course for medical laboratory technicians by the Office of The Surgeon General.

("BGH Selected as Site for Advanced Med Lab Course," Talon, 27 July 1961)

The Entomology Branch of the Preventive Medicine Department of the MFSS made headline news multiple times in 1961 for publishing papers on antivenin, conducting a symposium at the 10th Pacific Science Congress in Hawaii, collecting mosquitoes and insects for study, and having been involved in toxicity studies of DEET (diethyl toluamide) from 1954-58.

("Antivenin Study in Health Periodical," Talon, 3 August 1961; "MFSS Entomology Instructor to Conduct Symposium at Science Congress in Hawaii," Military Science News, 11 August 1961; "New Insect Repellents Brings Fond Memories," Talon, 1 Aug 1961; "67th Med Group on Mosquito Hunt," Talon, 9 Nov 1961)

The largest single group of Army Veterinary Corps officers to train at the MFSS arrived in August 1961. Three BAMC field tents replicating a small animal ward were established at Camp Bullis. There, sentry dogs from Lackland Air Force Base played the role of simulated casualties for the veterinarians to work on.

("Three BAMC Field Tents Really Going to the Dogs," Talon, 10 Aug 1961)

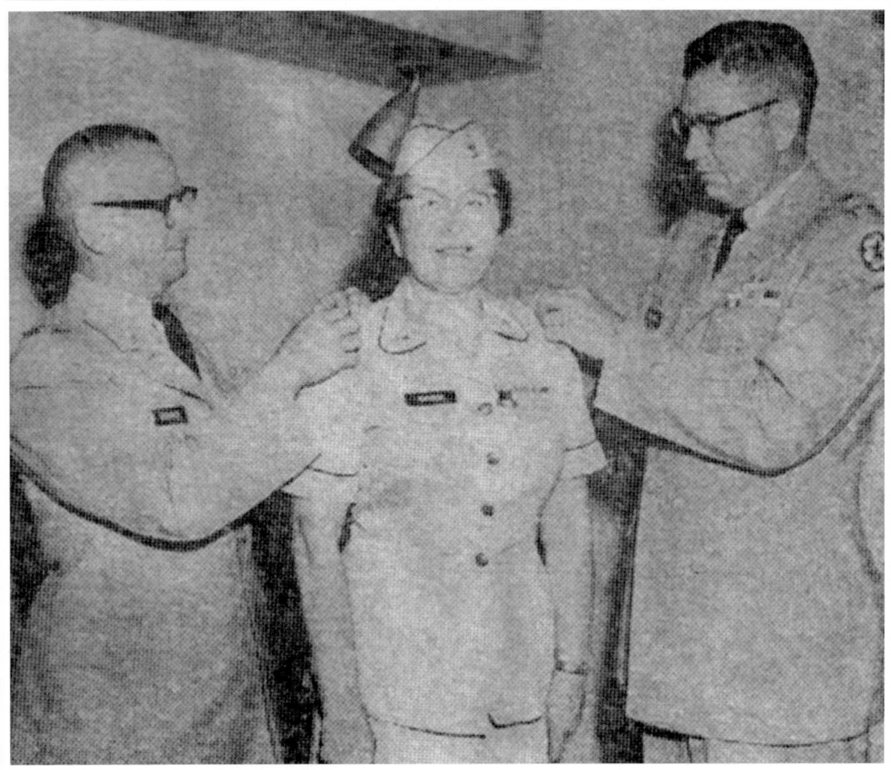

COL Clara Raven

COL Raven, "The first 'lady doctor' to wear the silver eagles of a full Colonel in the Army Medical Corps," was pinned at a ceremony at BAMC. COL Raven, pathologist, was the Chief of the Laboratory Service with the 323d General Hospital, a U.S. Army Reserve unit from Detroit, Michigan. The unit was at the MFSS for its annual two weeks training when her promotion was made during opening assembly. COL Raven was a woman of distinction. For six weeks, she was Post Surgeon at Camp Brackenridge, Kentucky, in 1959, making her possibly the first woman to command a medical unit. In her civilian life, she served in the capacity of the Deputy Medical Examiner for Los Angeles, California (1958), and then in the same position for Wayne County, Michigan (1959). At the time of her promotion, she knew of no other women conducting postmortem examinations and/or providing testimony and evidence in court from the results of their findings.

("Pathologist First Woman to Wear AMC 'Eagles,'" Talon, 24 Aug 1961)

1961

The 45th Surgical Hospital (Mobile Army), attached to the 67th Medical Group at BAMC, performed two missions: standing at ready to deploy on short notice and assisting in the training of students at the MFSS by demonstrating field medical procedures.

("45th Surgical Hospital's Reconstitution Underway," Talon, 2 Nov 1961)

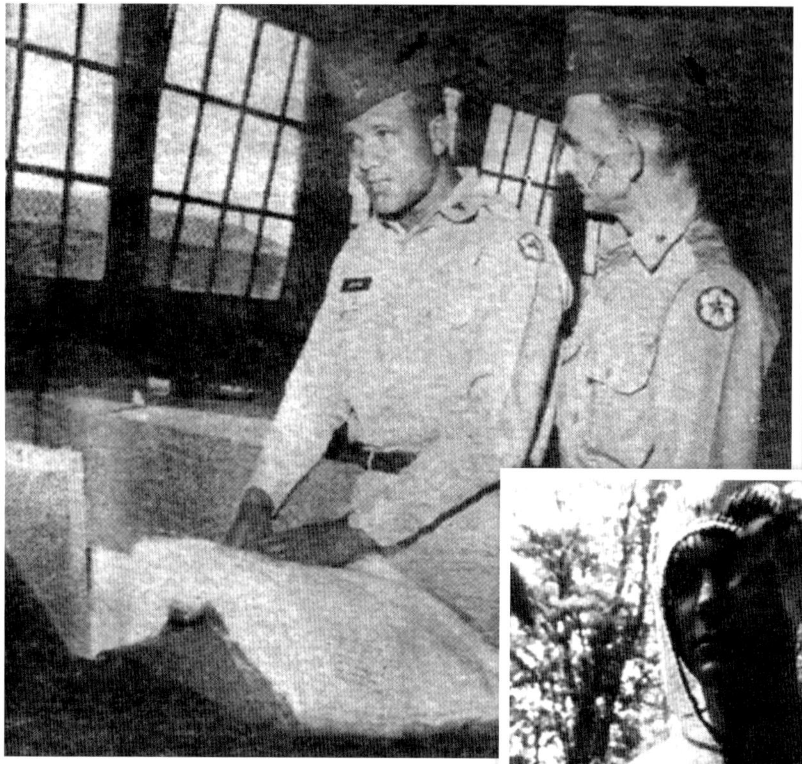

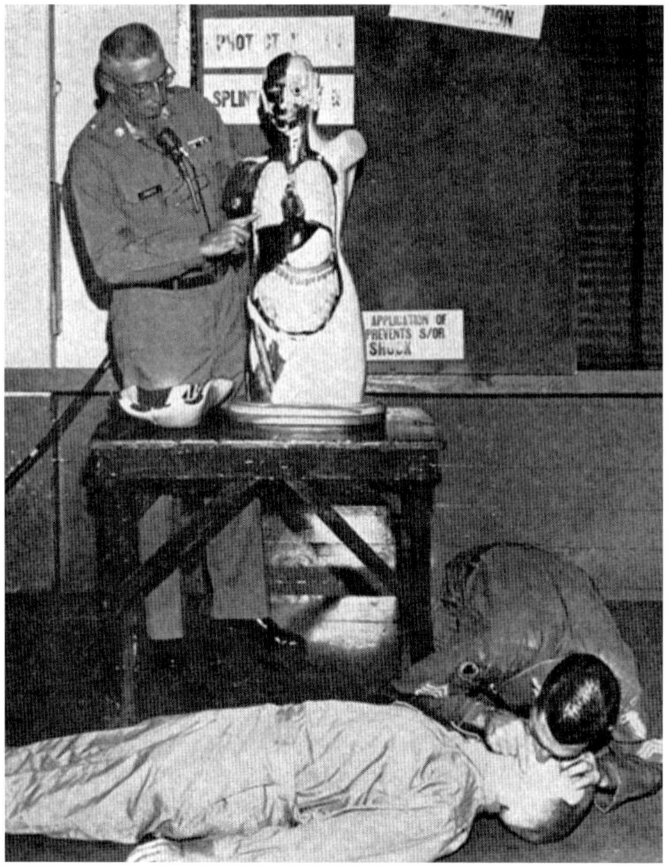

Practicing mouth-to-mouth resuscitation during classroom training for Army Medical Service enlisted men.

(U.S. Army Photo)

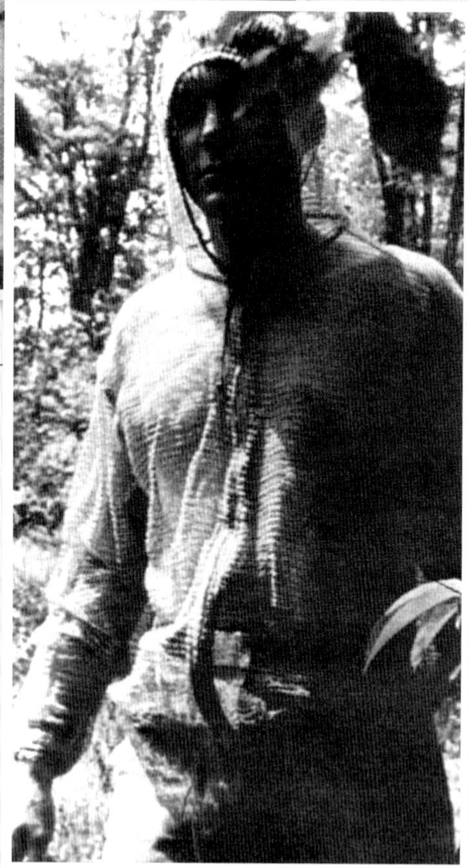

A DEET impregnated mesh protector suit worn by a volunteer.

(U.S. Army Photo, "AEHA Fights Pollution," Newsletter of the U.S. Army Medical Department, Vol I, Oct 1970, No. 3, p 82)

Dr. James W. Nixon, a San Antonio surgeon and Chief Surgical Consultant to the Office of The Surgeon General, discussed the quality of Russian physicians drawn from his own experiences performing surgery at Russian hospitals at an MFSS orientation course. The 350 students in attendance were probably most surprised to hear that 75% of the 18,000 Russian physicians trained per year were women, in comparison to the scant 7,000 women physicians graduated in the United States that year.

("Quality of Russian Doctors Discussed by San Antonio Surgeon," Talon, 31 Aug 1961)

For the first time, vehicles at BAMC and MFSS were equipped with seat belts.

("COL Pappas States: Sea Belts Promote Safety; Aid to Passenger Comfort," Talon, 5 Oct 1961)

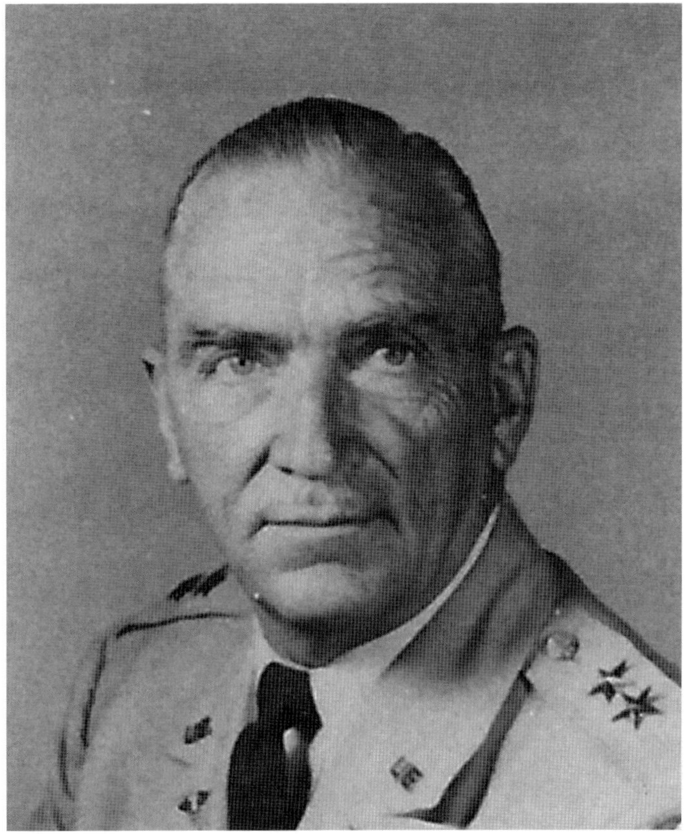

New commanding general of Brooke Army Medical Center
Major General James L. Snyder, Commandant of the Medical Field Service School, was promoted from the rank of Brigadier General in a ceremony at BAMC on 2 October 1961. Shortly thereafter, on 1 December, he succeeded MG John F. Bohlender, as commanding general of Brooke Army Medical Center.

("General James L. Snyder Receives Second Star," Talon, 5 Oct 1961; "Bohlender Will Retire," San Antonio Express, 1 Nov 1961)

1962

June 2, 1962: James T. McGibony, Commandant of the MFSS, was promoted to the rank of Brigadier General. BG McGibony assumed his position as Commandant of the MFSS on 1 March 1962.

("James T. McGibony Promoted to Brig Gen.," Talon, 5 July 1962)

CPT Alba F. Zanin, the first woman to complete the Army Dental Internship program, became the second woman dentist to enter the Army. In August of 1962, she was the only woman out of a class of 500 men to attend a basic military orientation course.

("Five Hundred Men - One Girl," Talon, 16 Aug 1962, p 3)

The "Documentaries Medical," a radio series of interviews with medical personnel, was broadcast every Sunday over the airwaves of Brooke General Hospital's radio station WOAI.

("Documentaries Medical," Talon, 5 July 1962, p 8)

The MFSS and all units with the Brooke Army Medical Center were assigned to the Fourth U.S. Army effective 1 July 1962.

("Fourth U.S. Army Gains 41 Activities, Unit," Talon, 5 July 1962)

The Medical Laboratory moved to Camp Bullis for five weeks of field testing. Conducted between 28 September and 3 November, the field test was a revision and shakedown inspection of inadequacies of organization and equipment, according to specifications drawn up in 1958.

("COL Lukeman, Commanding: Medical Lab Moves to Camp Bullis for Five Weeks Field Testing," Talon, 27 Sept 1962)

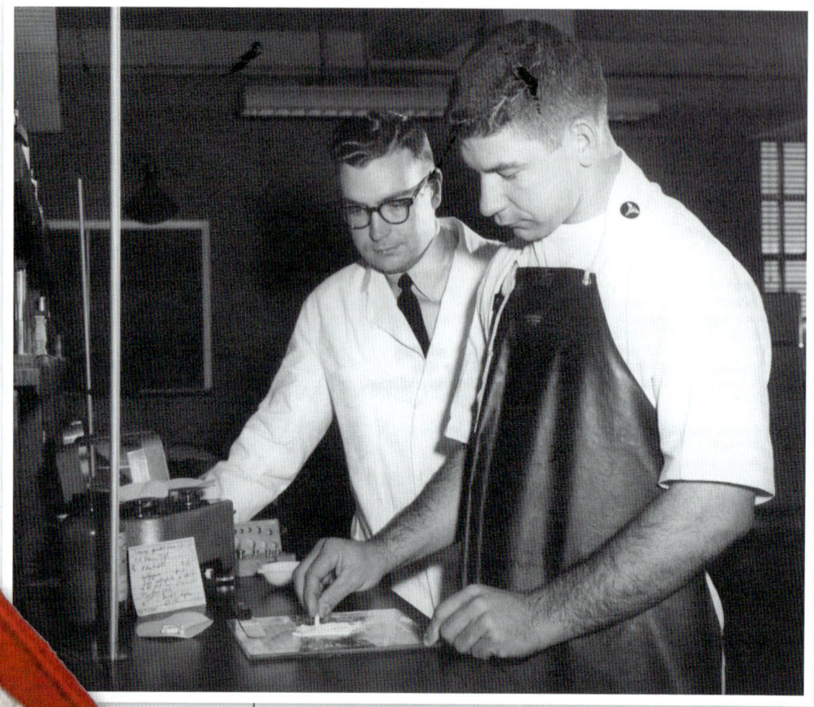

A student prepares a capsule as part of the Pharmacy Specialist Course. 5 Jan 1962.

(U.S. Army Photo, AMEDD Museum Photo Collection)

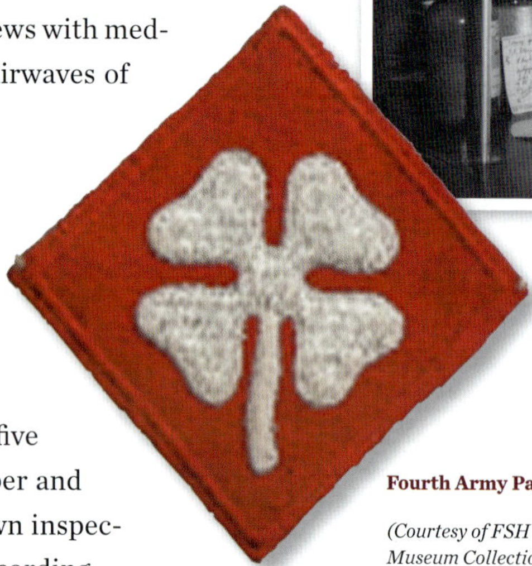

Fourth Army Patch

(Courtesy of FSH Museum Collection)

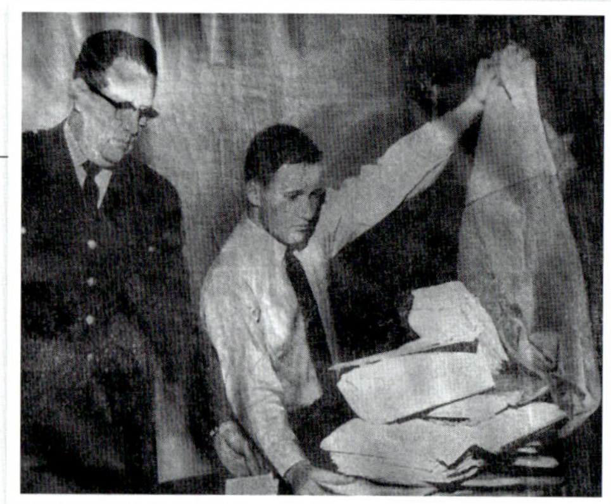

In 1962, the Non-Resident Instruction of the MFSS distributed educational material through correspondence courses and the U.S. Army Reserve School Program. COL Clayton views correspondence unsacked by SP4 Jack Skaggs. The department received an average of 3,000 pieces of correspondence a month.

("Education by Mail: Big Army Business," San Antonio Light, 6 Nov 1962)

The MFSS held its first course in Environmental Health Engineering.

("Medics Open New Environmental Study," Military Service News, 5 Oct 1962)

News articles throughout the year indicated how all elements of the MFSS were involved in planning and training for a potential nuclear blast. Researchers with the Department of Preventive Medicine prepared papers on "Providing Water Utility Operations After Nuclear Attack." Instructors and staff attended the Nuclear Weapons Medical Symposium to improve instruction for the Management of Mass Casualties Course. The Military Science Branch simulated nuclear weapons blasts for training exercises. The Training Aids Department focused its moulage techniques on specialized mock nuclear burns.

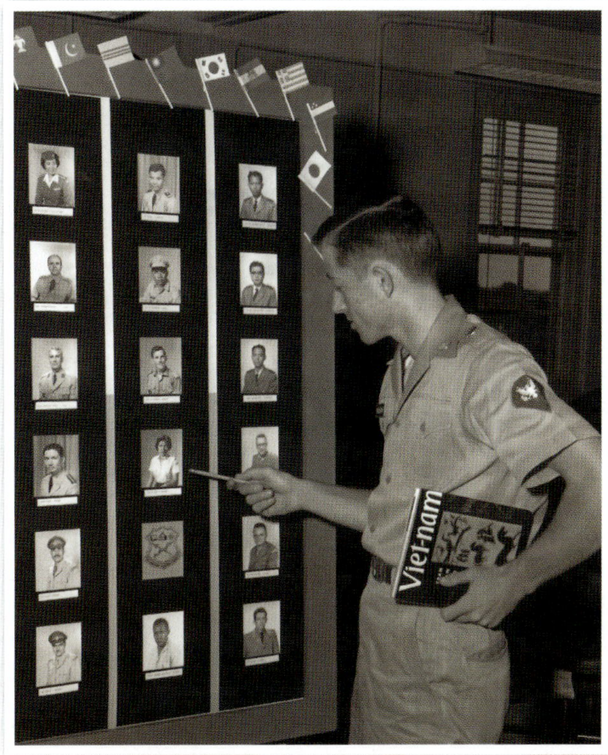

SP4 Dennis Przedzial locates an officer of Vietnam via a training aid called "One World-MFSS." The aid contained pictures of foreign officers attending courses at MFSS and was a precursor to the display located outside of the International Students Office at Aabel Hall.

(MFSS Scrapbook 1962, Stimson Library Special Collections)

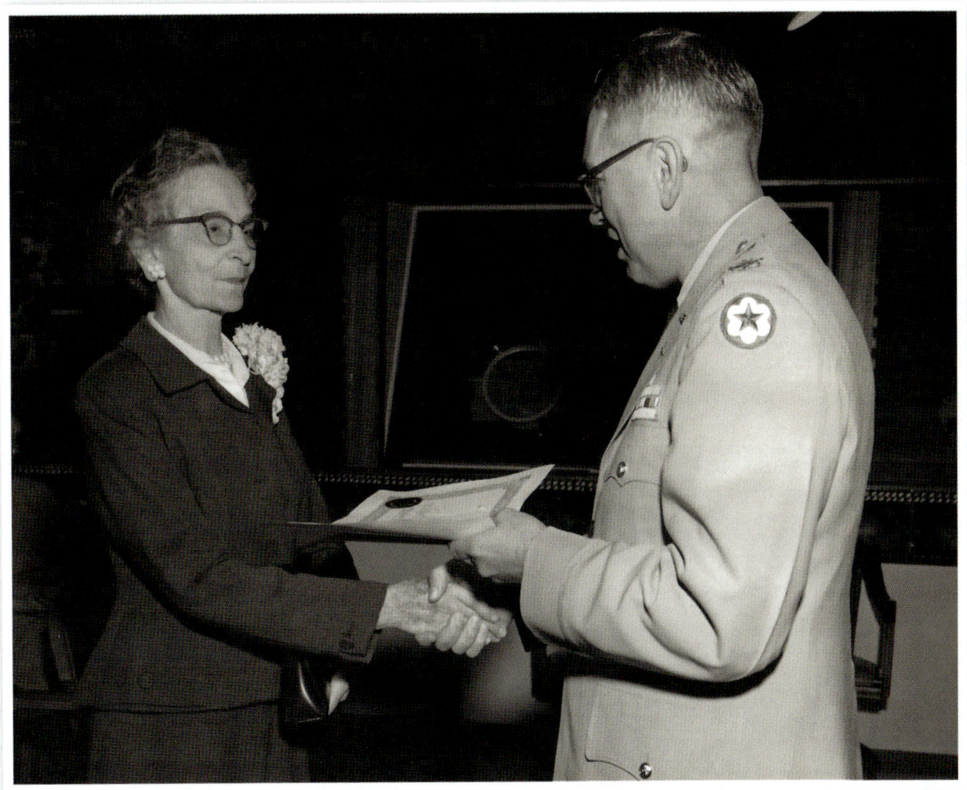

Mrs. A. L. Barlow, Stimson Librarian, is presented the Certificate of Achievement and Letter of Appreciation from BG James T. McGibony, Commandant, MFSS, upon her retirement. In 1962, the Stimson Library was considered one of the best medical libraries in the country, housing 30,000 volumes, including 10,000 medical works.

(U.S. Army Photo. "Stimson Medical Library One of the Best," San Antonio Light, 25 Oct 1962)

1963

In January of 1963, the MFSS started its second "Future War Medical Course" with approximately 25 senior Army Medical Service officers in attendance, including three Canadian, one Greek and two U.S. Air Force officers. The course was taught by LTC Jack C. Fitzpatrick, Director of the Department of Nuclear Science at the MFSS.

("Future War Medical Course Opens Here," San Antonio News, 16 Jan 1963)

COL Vincent I. Hack, Director of the Training Aids Department at FSH, delivered instruction to 200 Texas funeral directors at San Antonio College on their roles should San Antonio be struck by nuclear attack, 15 January 1963.

("Casualty Emphasize CD Points," San Antonio News, 15 Jan 1963)

The MFSS added a course for Medical, Dental, and Vet Corps Officers designed to acquaint newly commissioned officers with the problems of unit administration, personnel management, medical records and reports, and supply procedures. The course is given the tongue and cheek title of "In Basket Exercise (IBEX)."

("'Ibex' Aids MFSS Orientation Course," Talon, 7 Feb 1963)

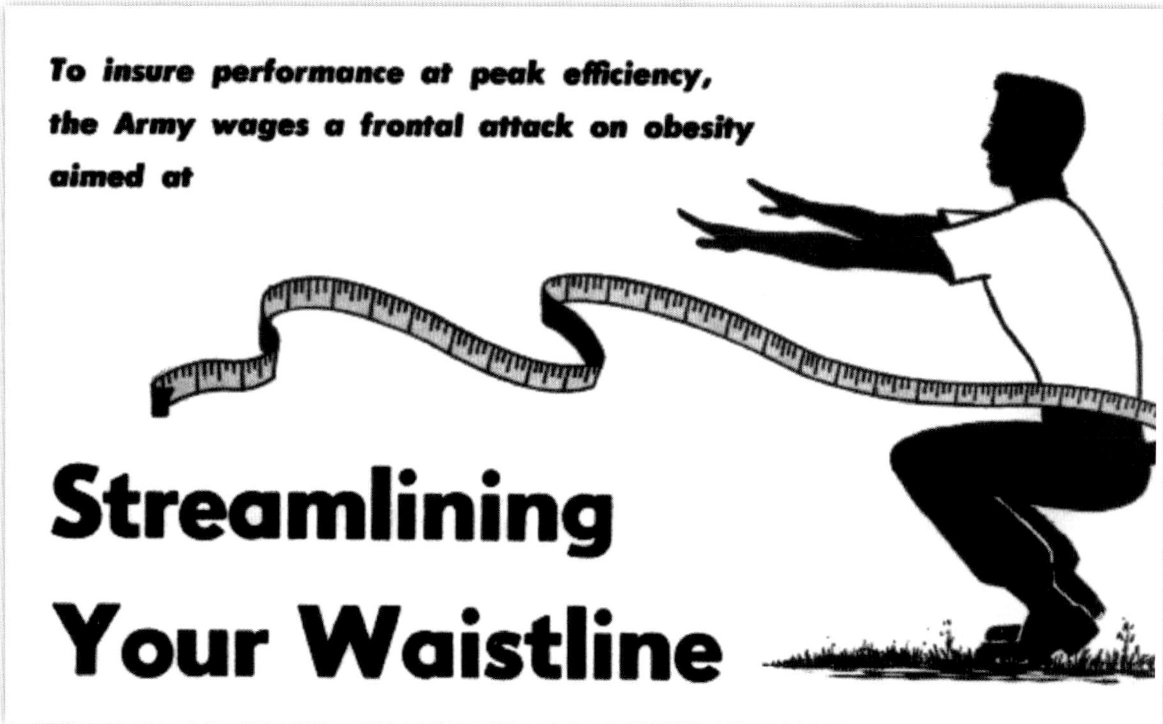

The Army's program against obesity was promoted at the MFSS. Images like the one at left were posted throughout the school.

("Streamlining Your Waist," by LTG Leonard D. Heaton, Army Information Digest, Jan 1963, p 31)

Five Marine Corps officers presented instruction to MFSS Service Career Course students on "Operation Sea Horse," an amphibious assault of the future, on 28 February 1963.

("Marines 'Land' As MFSS Instructors," Talon, 28 Feb 1963)

The Army's most decorated woman, COL Ruby G. Bradley, retired after 29 years in the Army Nurse Corps on 29 March 1963.

("Most Decorated Army Nurse Retiring," San Antonio Light, 28 March 1963)

From February to May 1963, televisions were placed in six classrooms as part of a feasibility study for the use of television as a training aid for instructional presentations.

(Annual Report of AMSS Activities, 1962, p 10)

The MFSS Wound Ballistic Laboratory was featured in the San Antonio Light. The lab was responsible for generating ballistic wounds studies, simulated wounds caused by various bullets.

("MFSS Course: Wounds Simulated," San Antonio Light, 3 May 1963)

Most Decorated Woman Retires

COL Ruby G. Bradley receives the Legion of Merit (Second Oak Leaf Cluster) from MG James Snyder, Commanding General, Brooke Army Medical Center. COL Bradley, the Army's most decorated woman, ended her Army career as Director of Nursing Activities at the center 29 March 1963.

(U.S. Army Photo, U.S. Lady, June 1963)

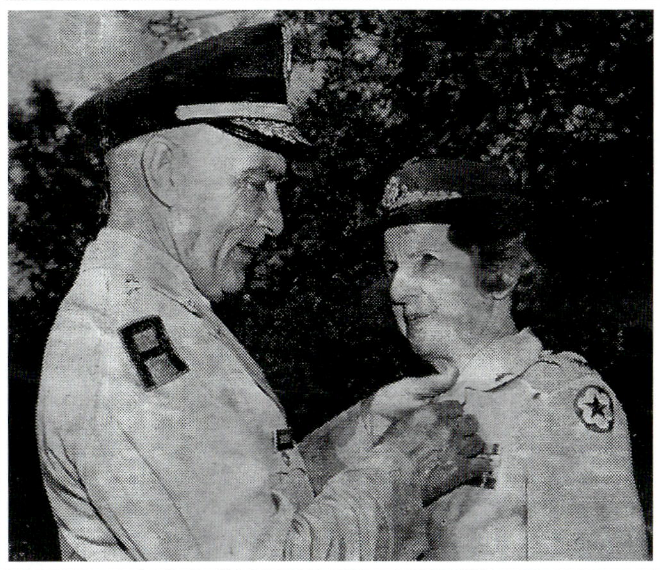

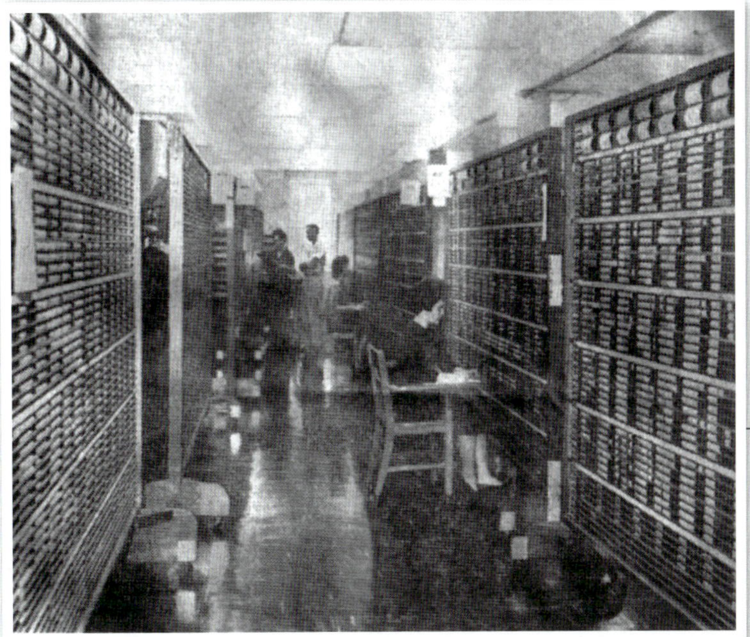

Giant floor-to-ceiling schedule boards are used for the tracking of all MFSS courses, instructors, and classrooms. (*"MFSS Has System: Planning Keeps Classes Efficient," San Antonio Light, 28 April 1963*)

1963

Representatives from the Armed Forces Radiobiology Research Institute briefed the staff of the Department of Nuclear Science on the Manually Operated Graphic Computer (GRACOMP) and presented the MFSS with a Radiac Fallout Simulator.

Two groups of civilian women were offered the opportunity to attend OPERATION BLOW UP at Camp Bullis, a dramatization of how an atomic attack would affect their community.

Fort Polk soldiers received moulage training from the MFSS. The Preventive Medicine Department published a study on the Common Cold.

(1963 MFSS Scrapbook, Stimson Library Special Collections)

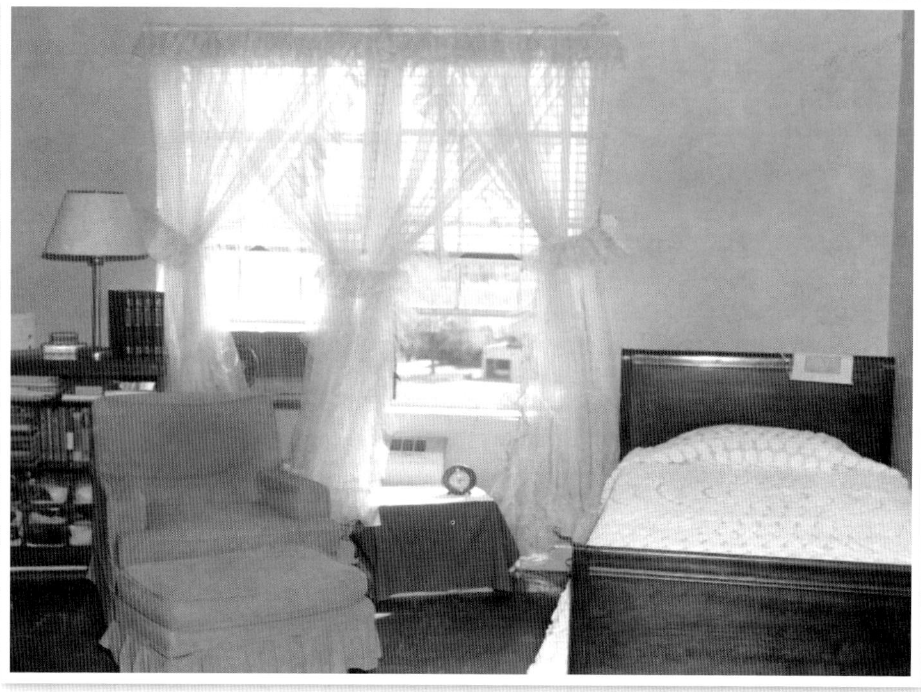

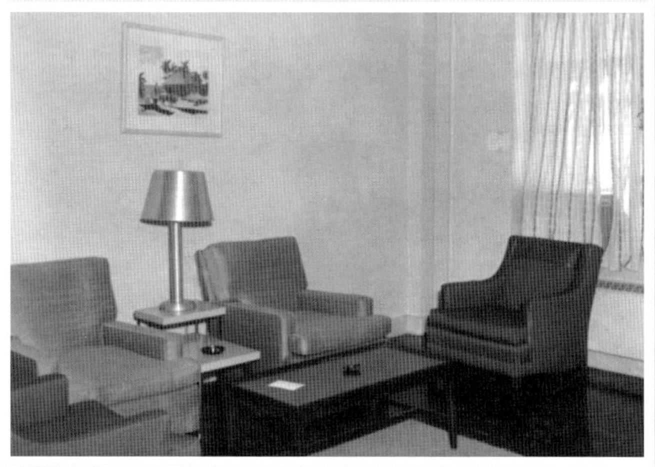

Home Sweet Home
Army Nurse Corps Quarters at Davidson Hall: homey touches, 12 March 1963.

(1963 MFSS Scrapbook, Stimson Library Special Collections)

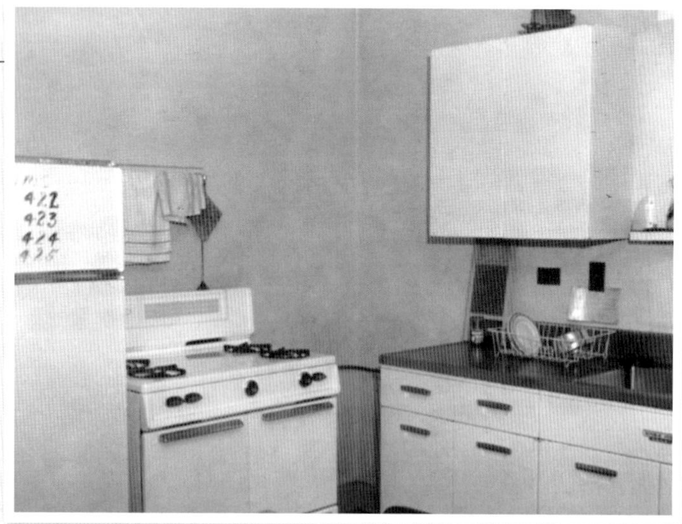

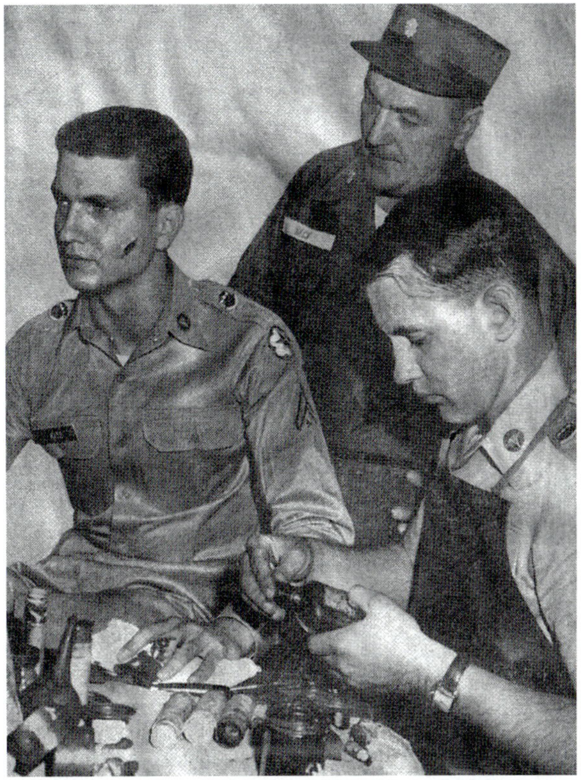

Moulages played an ever-increasing role as training aids in showing medical personnel what they would encounter in the field and hospital. LTC Vincent Hack (rear) adds realism to training. SP4 Robert C. Wells (right) applies moulage to PFC. Donald Kitz.

("Simulated Wounds: Moulages Horrify Observers," San Antonio Light, 28 March 1963)

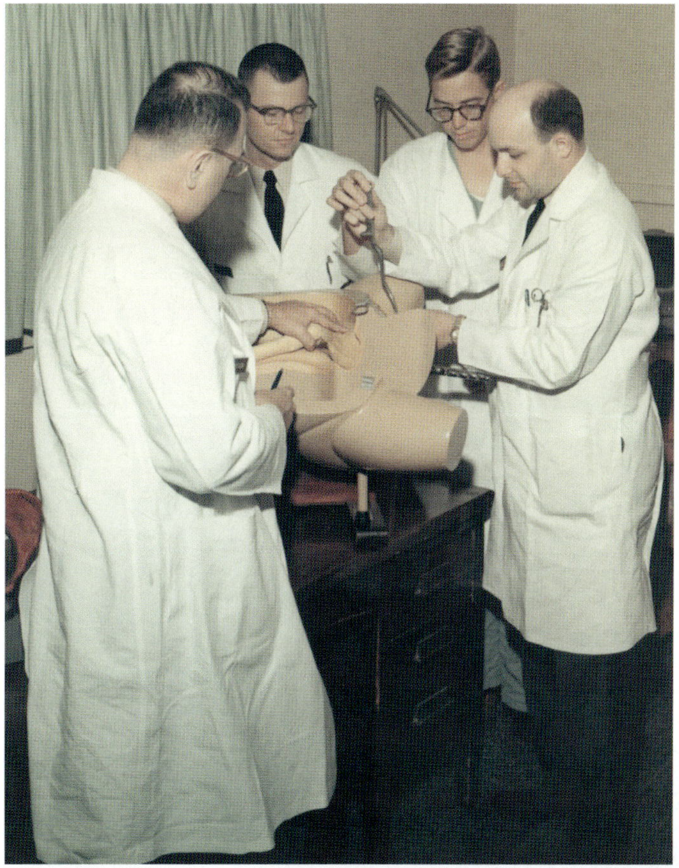

Students receive instruction in forceps delivery in May 1963

(U.S. Army Photo, AMEDD Museum Collection)

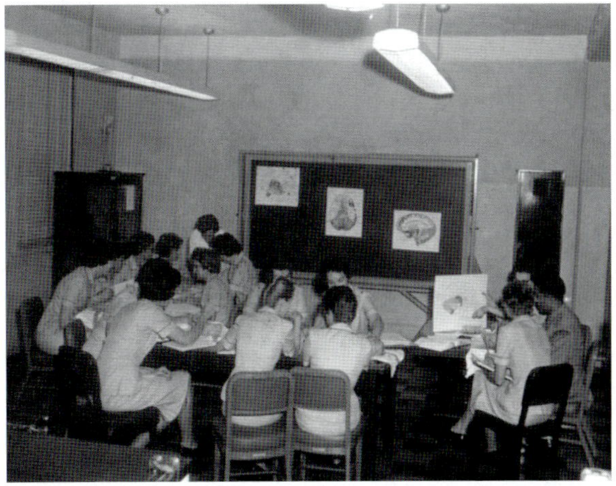

Dr. Virginia F. Harrison gives a class on gross anatomy to students in the Physical Therapy Course, 18 March 1963.

(U.S. Army Photo, AMEDD Museum Collection)

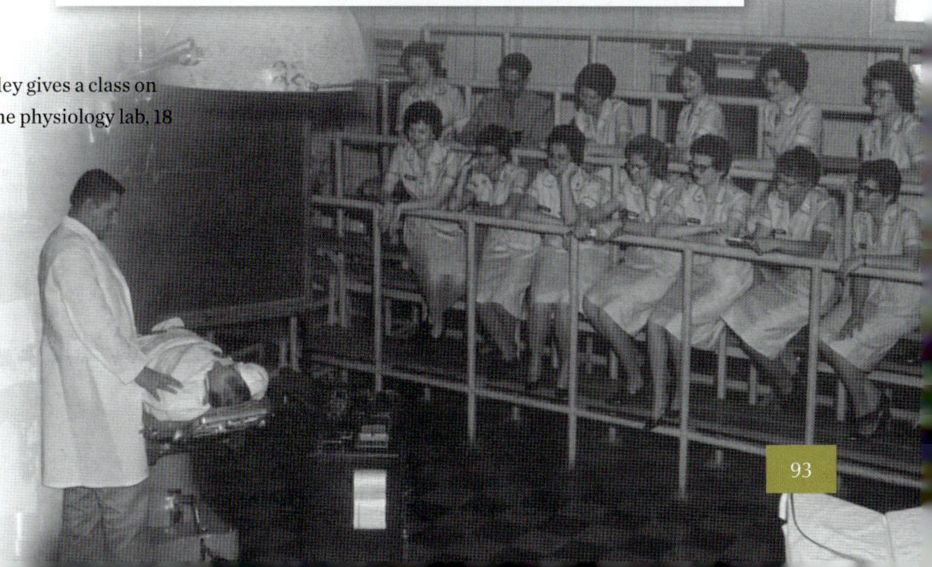

Physical Therapy

CPT John W. Lavalley gives a class on muscle science in the physiology lab, 18 March 1963.

(U.S. Army Photo, AMEDD Museum Collection)

1964

Designed to be as life-like as possible to evoke a shock reaction to medical responders in training, the first portable medical training dummy had a variety of simulated wounds, some of grievous character. The dummy could be operated independent of a base, allowing him to be placed in the field and in just about any position. It had a number of interchangeable moulages through which fake blood was pumped.

(United States Patent Office, Patent Number 3,027,655, patented April 3, 1962)

According to an MFSS inventory card, the dummy, donated to the AMEDD Museum in 1984, was in use at the school sometime between 1961 and 1963. It was invented by S.W. Alderson, inventor of the original aerospace crash-test dummies for NASA and the USAF in the 1950s. Alderson's work also included a CPR dummy nicknamed "Joe Blow," moulages worn by soldiers during medical training that oozed mock blood, and human-like figures called "medical phantoms" used to measure exposure to radiation.

("Obituary: Samuel Alderson, Crash-Test Dummy Inventor, Dies at 90," By Margalit Fox, The New York Times, 18 February 2005)

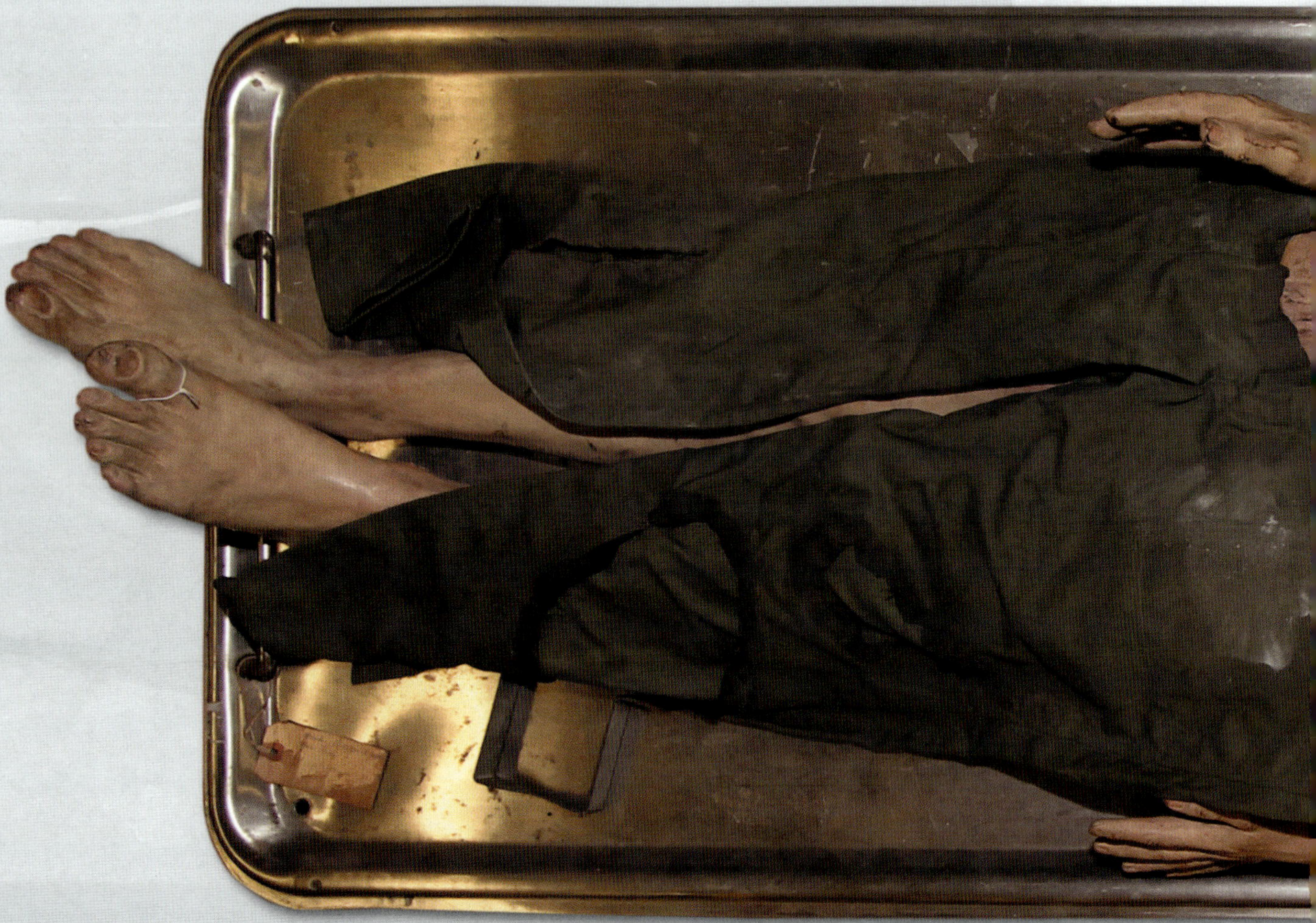

Twenty-seven nurses from the MFSS left BAMC early on a Sunday morning to participate in Operation Desert Strike, a massive U.S. Army maneuver being held in the deserts of California and Arizona. The three week exercise took place in lieu of their regular classroom training. They dealt with not only simulated casualties but also any real injuries that occurred during the extensive maneuver.

("MFSS Nurses to Join Desert Strike," Talon, 7 May 1964)

"Re-Teaching" sessions were adopted as a method of instruction at the MFSS, replacing the long used "critique" following examinations administered during a course. This type of session permitted the student to reinforce and clarify knowledge of principles when there was inadequate or incorrect understanding, and highlighted areas needing further study.

("MFSS Adopts New Teaching Method," Military Service News, 26 June 1964)

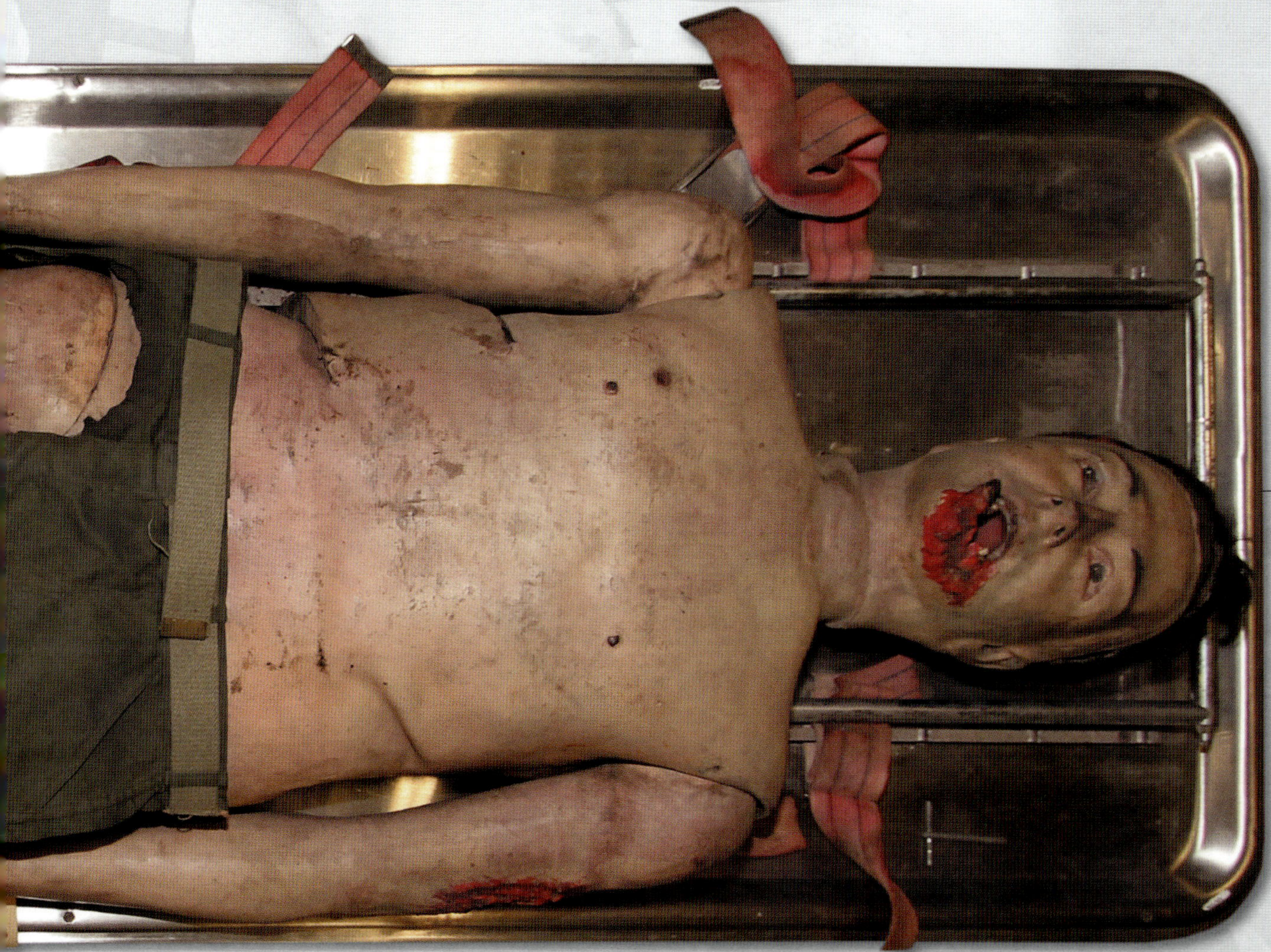

Synthetic Casualty
"PROTOTYPE MODEL 6910-M02-0001 (Male Body for First Aid Training). The original cost of the prototype was $18,300.

(U.S. Army photo, photo by Carlos Martinez; AMEDD Museum Collection)

1964

The 21st and 22nd Aeromedical Evacuation Squadrons of the 1st Aeromedical Group, Pope AFB, N.C., demonstrated the Tactical Aeromedical Evacuation System to students of the Army Medical Service Officer Career Course during a presentation given at Randolph AFB. The 1st Aeromedical Evacuation group was the only unit of its kind in the USA and supported both Army and AF exercises requiring the use of the "Casualty Staging Facility," which provided for the receipt, shelter, medical care, and processing of patients scheduled for movement by air.

("Angels of Mercy with Wings," Talon, 23 April 1964)

Seven special "study cubicles" to facilitate research and study were introduced to MFSS students and faculty members in August of 1964. Each cubicle, devoted to a specific disease entity and equipped with panels that detailed various aspects of each disease, was designed to decrease the time students would have to spend compiling data. They were installed in the library as a training aid for the Preventive Medicine Department.

("Cubicles Add Room for Study," San Antonio Light, 14 August 1964)

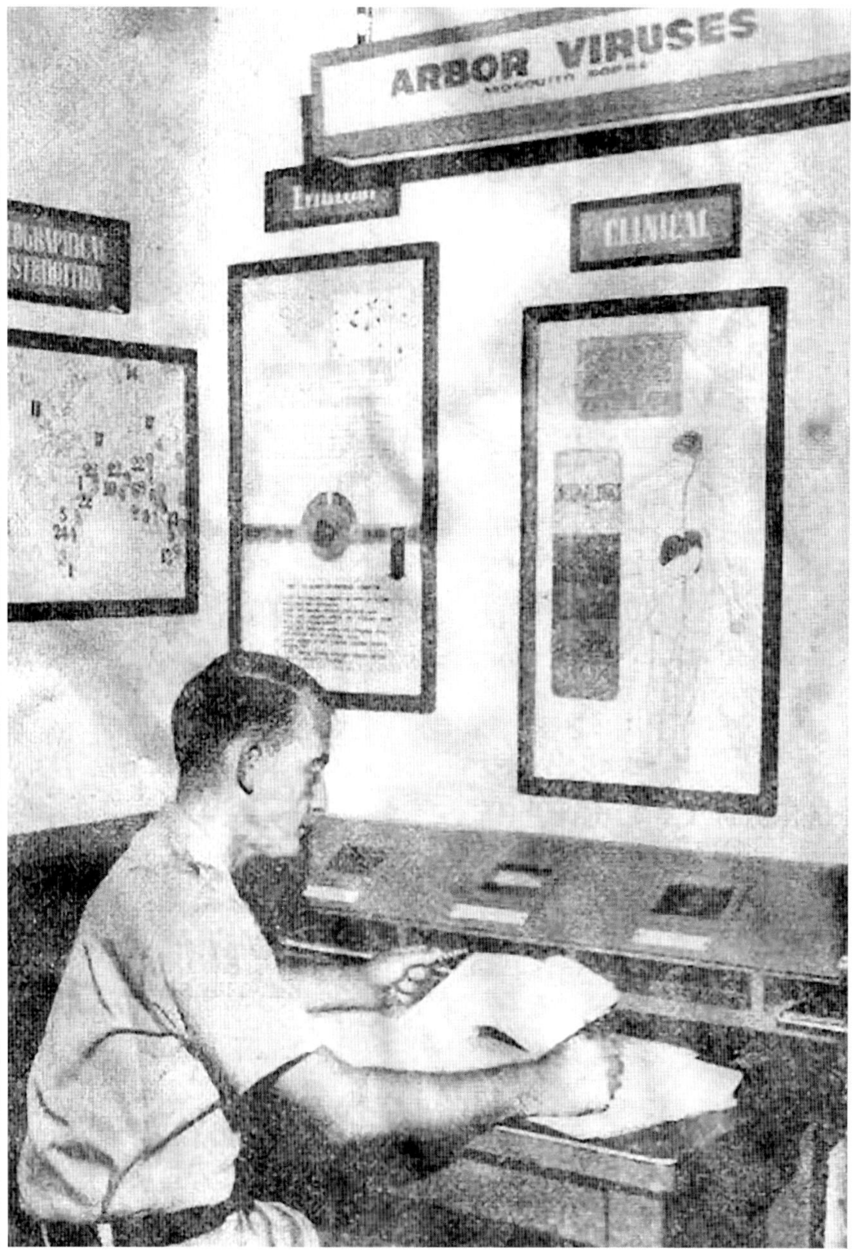

Arbor Virus Study Cubicle
One of the seven special study cubicles in Stimson Library.

(U.S. Army Photo)

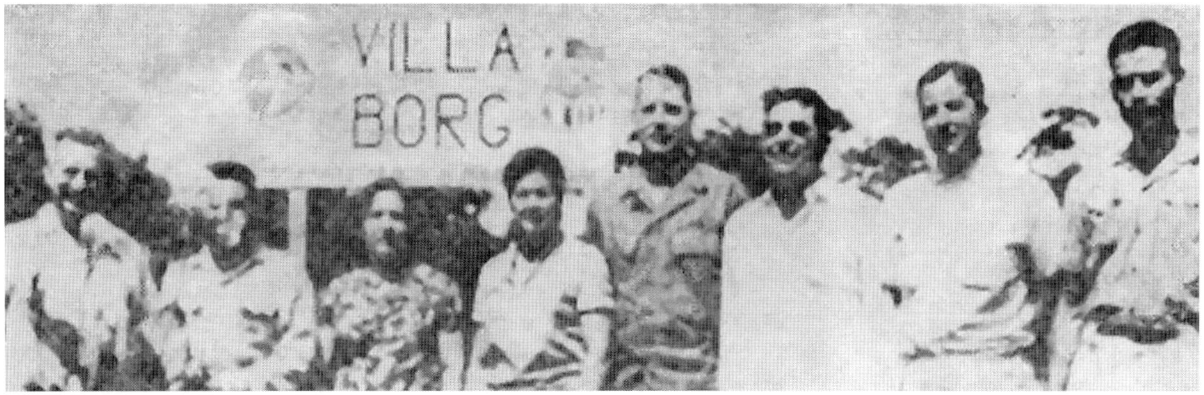

Villa Borg

Major Lavern P. Borg (fifth from the left) poses for a photo at the site of Villa Borg in Bolivia.

(U.S. Army Photo)

MFSS student Major Lavern Borg was the first Medical Service Advisor assigned to the Bolivian Armed Forces. Working through the Alliance for Progress Reform Program, the Bolivian Army requested U.S. help in setting up a medical service program. Major Borg was selected and he and his family moved to La Paz. There, he fulfilled his responsibility by coordinating, designing and implementating the Bolivian medical service program. At one point during his assignment, an outbreak of yellow fever occurred in the remote area of Alto Beni, resulting in 18 deaths. Through the combined efforts of Major Borg and other agencies, the outbreak was halted through immunizations and treatment. Grateful Bolivian settlers erected a sign for their town which read: "Another example of the Alliance for Progress" VILLA BORG.

("MFSS Student May Claim a First in Village Naming," Talon, 17 Sep 1964)

MFSS student, 2LT Stephen Richardson, was awarded the Soldier's Medal for Heroism by MFSS Commandant, BG James McGibony. 2LT Richardson was attending the U.S. Army Airborne School and was aboard an aircraft with other students to perform the first of five qualifying parachute jumps. Just prior to the approach to the jump zone, the aircraft developed engine trouble, crashed, and burned. 2LT Richardson escaped but re-entered the plane to rescue trapped students.

("Soldier's Medal Awarded Lieutenant," San Antonio News, 25 Nov 1964)

LTC Leo Osterhaus, a personnel management instructor in the Department of Administration, MFSS, explained the various techniques utilized at MFSS to "change dull subjects into pearls of knowledge," in the December issue of Adult Leadership Magazine, published monthly by the Adult Education Association.

("MFSS Officer Featured in Adult Leadership Magazine," Talon, 16 Jan 1964)

1965

In March 1965, the Army unveiled the first advance in field hospitals since the Civil War, the MUST (Medical Unit, Self-Contained, Transportable). Its basic features were mobility, short setup time, high reliability and efficiency, controlled environment, and the capability of maintaining all-weather operations.

(M.U.S.T. – Medical Unit Self-Contained, Transportable, developed for the U.S. Army Medical Service, A Garret-Airesearch Report, 1964)

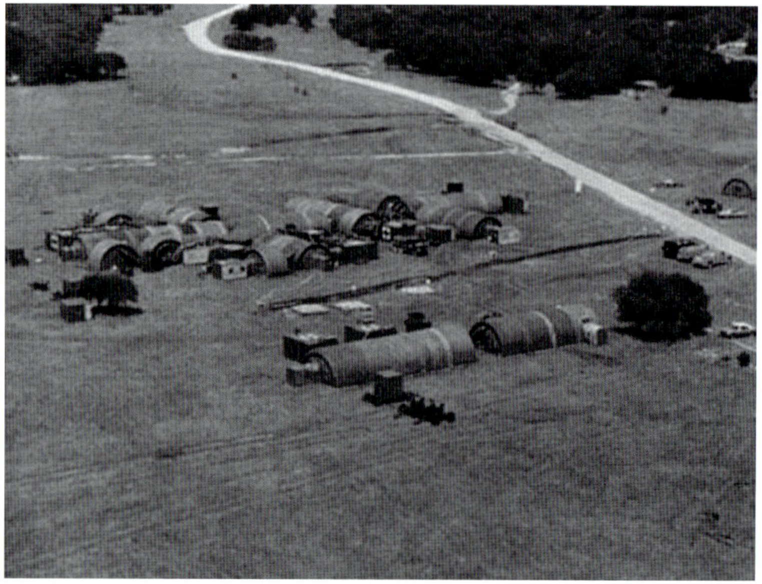

A 60-bed surgical hospital displayed the use of MUST (Medical Unit, Self-contained, Transportable) equipment in a demonstration at Camp Bullis in September 1968.

(U.S. Army Photo)

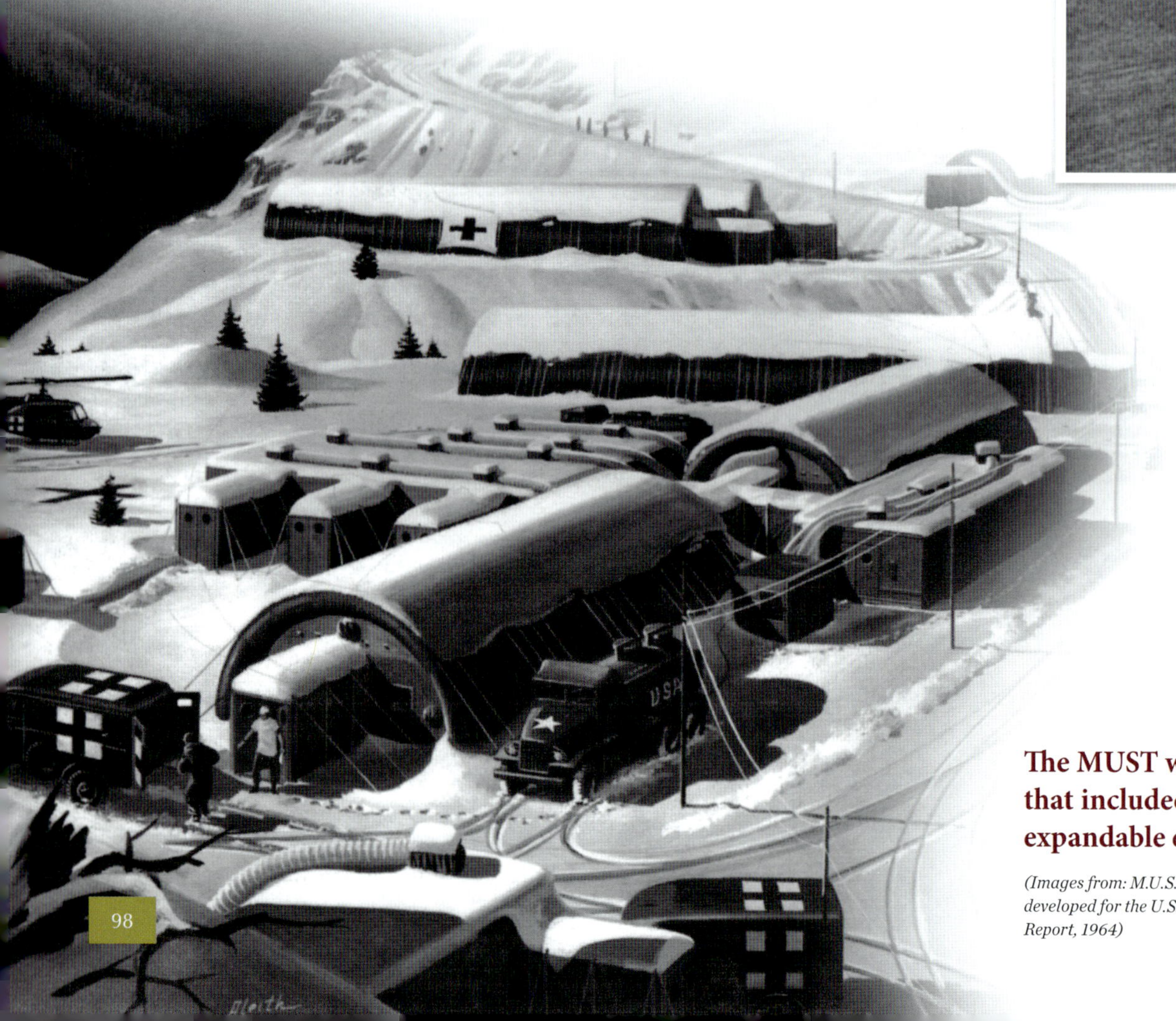

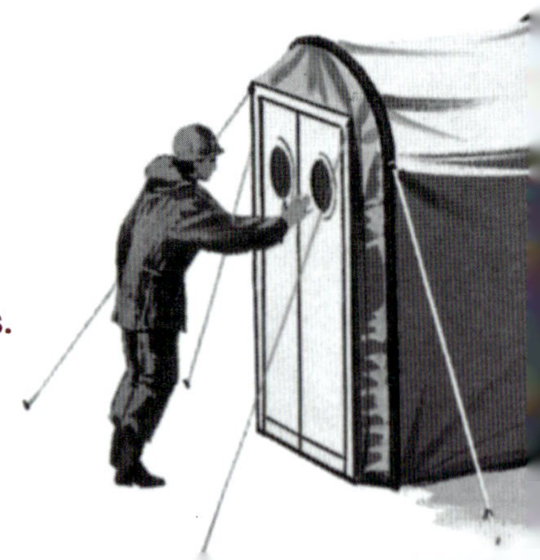

The MUST was a three-element system that included inflatable elements, expandable elements, and utility elements.

(Images from: M.U.S.T. – Medical Unit Self-Contained, Transportable, developed for the U.S. Army Medical Service, A Garret-Airesearch Report, 1964)

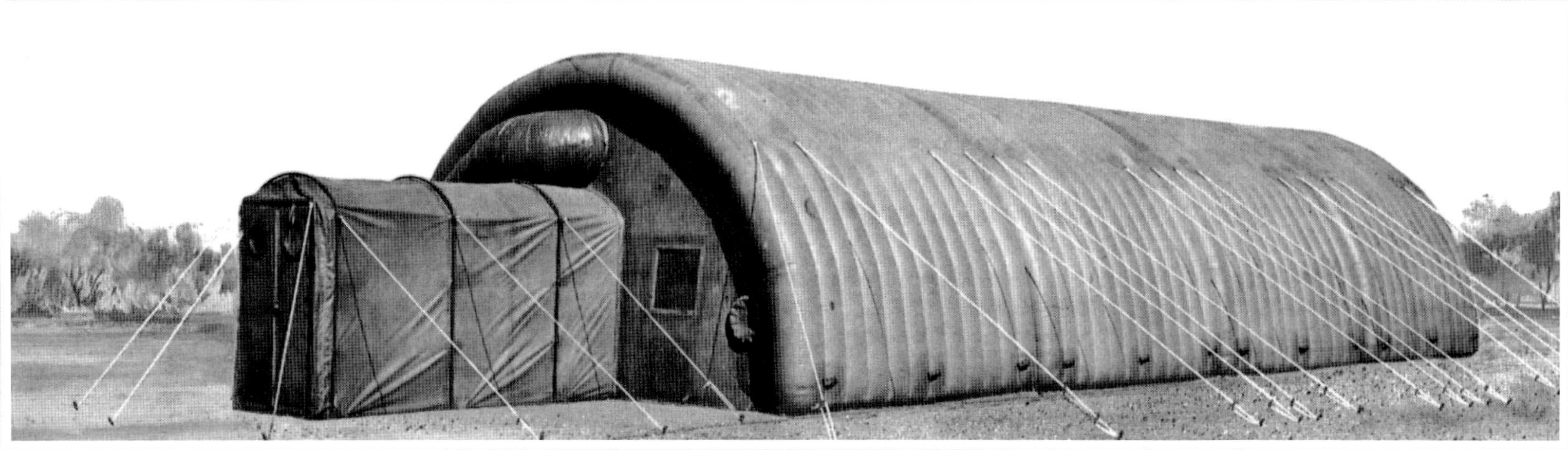

Inflatable elements

Double walled shelters that provided large free space areas used primarily as field hospital wards.

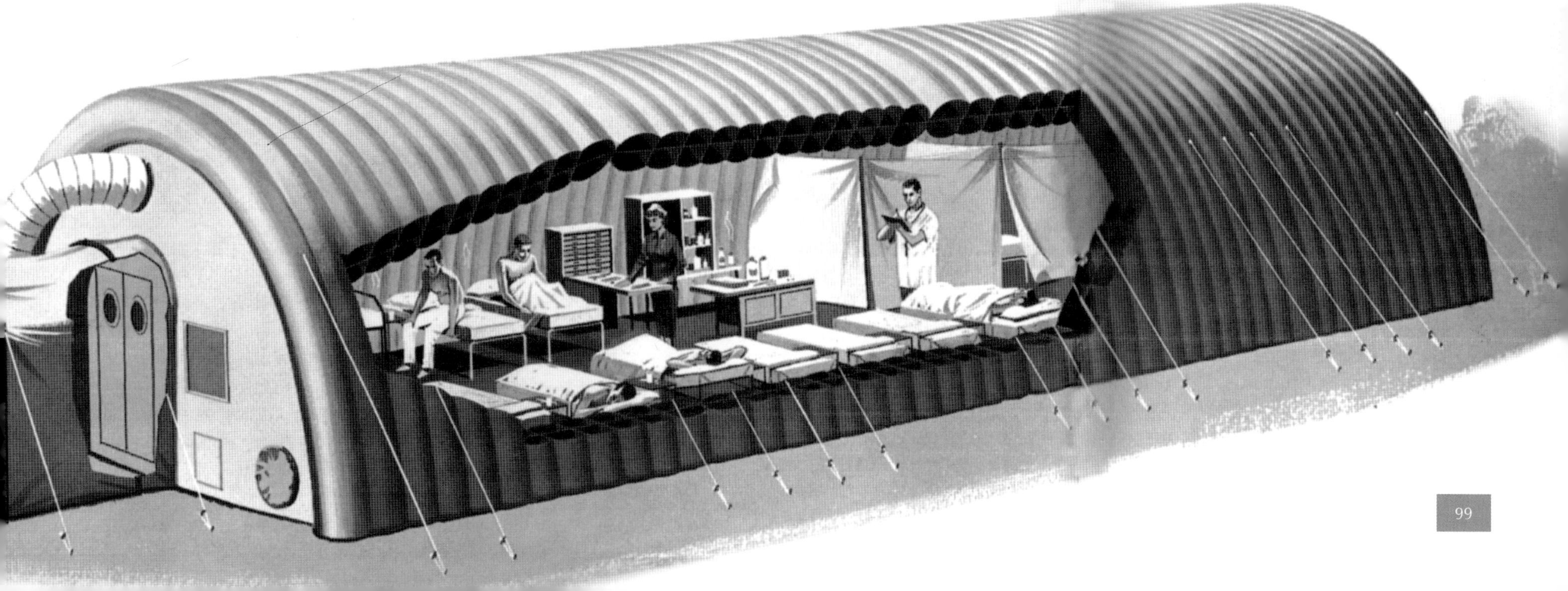

1965

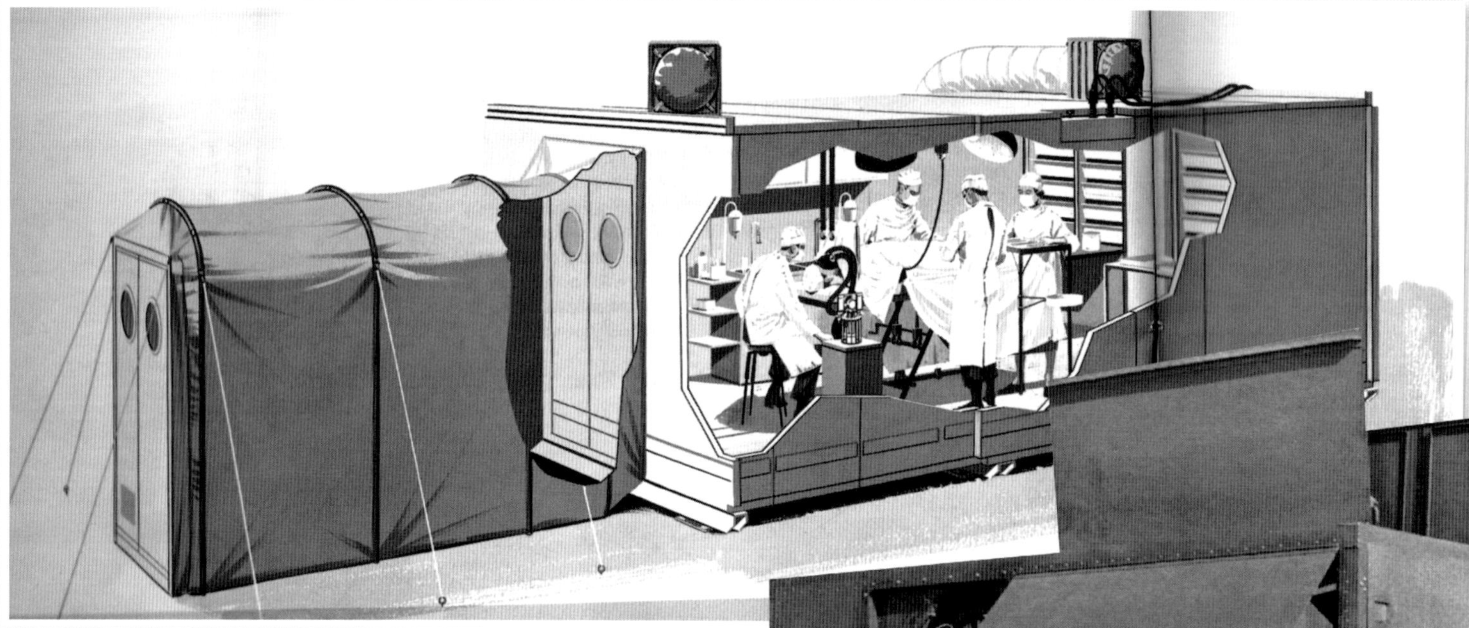

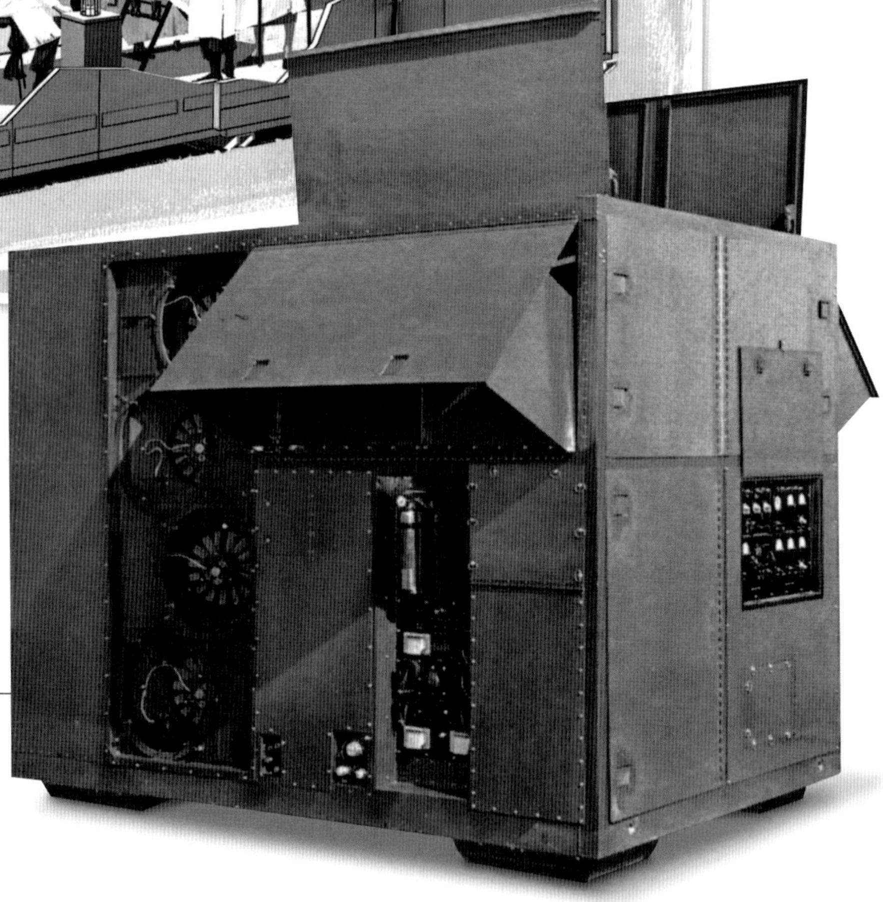

Expandable elements
Collapsible, rigid panel shelter that could be quickly opened and made ready within 30 minutes. Typical uses for these elements within a field hospital complex included surgery, sterile supply preparation, X-ray, pharmacy, clinical laboratory, central materiel supply, patient diet preparation, and dental facilities.

Utility elements
A power package that supplied refrigeration, air heating and circulation, water heating and pumping, air pressure, air pressure for the inflatable elements, and compressed air and suction.

Members of BAMC and MFSS assisted as part of the recovery team for the Gemini IV space flights in June 1965.

September 1965 marked the graduation of the 1,300th foreign student to have attended courses at the MFSS since 1946.

MFSS constructed and began utilization of special study booths that were considered miniature medical libraries, each devoted to a specific disease. The study booths were considered an outstanding teaching tool, enabling students to learn more quickly as their study materials were consolidated in one area.

A mock nuclear blast was conducted at Camp Bullis as part of the final stage of the Medical Management of Mass Casualties Course. Known as "OPERATION BLOW UP," it focused on casualty estimation, concepts of diagnosis, triage, prioritization and treatment.

MFSS celebrated its 45th anniversary in Salado Park with a BBQ picnic with service members and families.

(Annual Report of the MFSS, CY 1965)

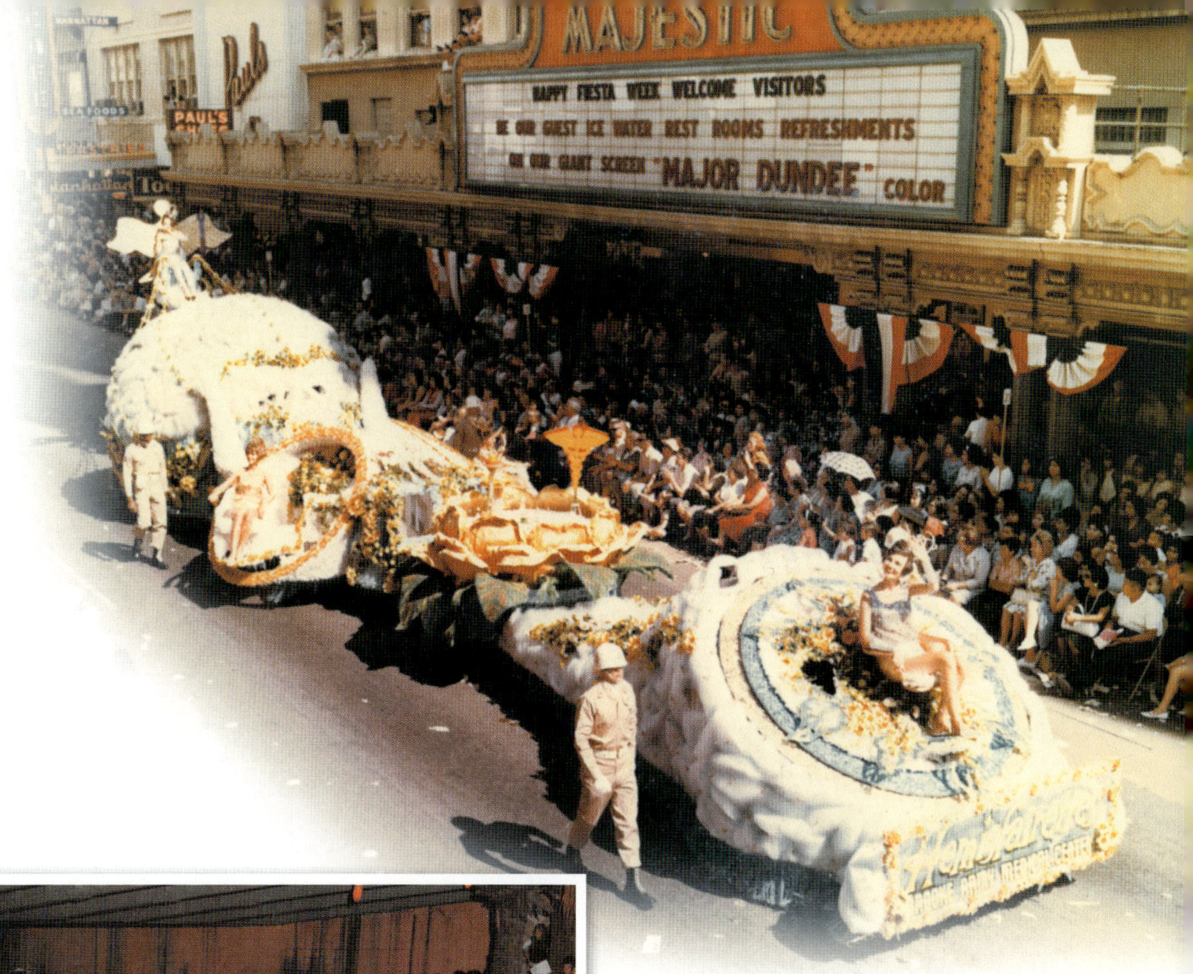
MAJESTIC
HAPPY FIESTA WEEK WELCOME VISITORS
BE OUR GUEST ICE WATER REST ROOMS REFRESHMENTS
ON OUR GIANT SCREEN "MAJOR DUNDEE" COLOR
PAUL'S

The 1965 BAMC Battle of the Flowers float.

(U.S. Army Photo, AMEDD Museum Photo Collection)

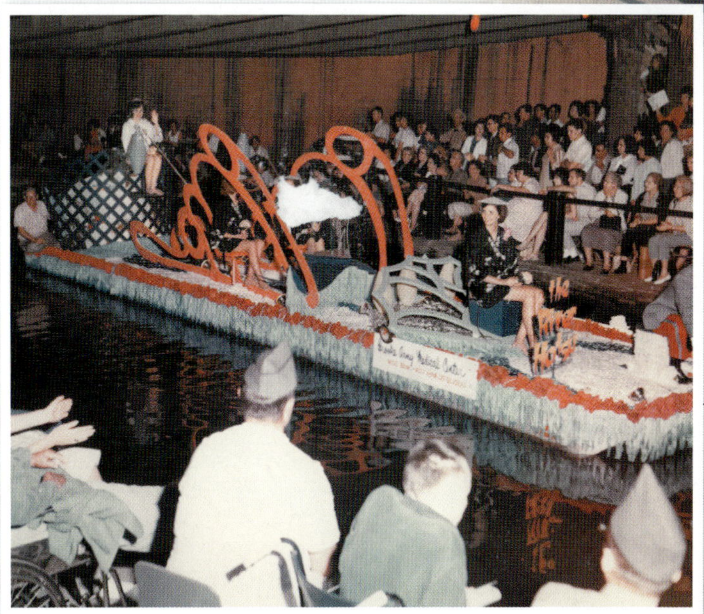

The 1965 BAMC float in the Texas Cavaliers River Parade.

(U.S. Army Photo, AMEDD Museum Photo Collection)

1966

The Department of Preventive Medicine investigated an epidemic of rubella that occurred at Fort Sam Houston the second week of February. The total number of cases within the MFSS was 87.

(Annual Report of the MFSS, CY 1966, p 24)

Camp Bullis hosted OPERATION BLOW UP, a demonstration of a mock nuclear blast for military and civilian personnel participating in the MFSS Management of Mass Casualties Course the second week of March.

("Camp Bullis Scene of Realistic Demonstration," Talon, 17 March 1966)

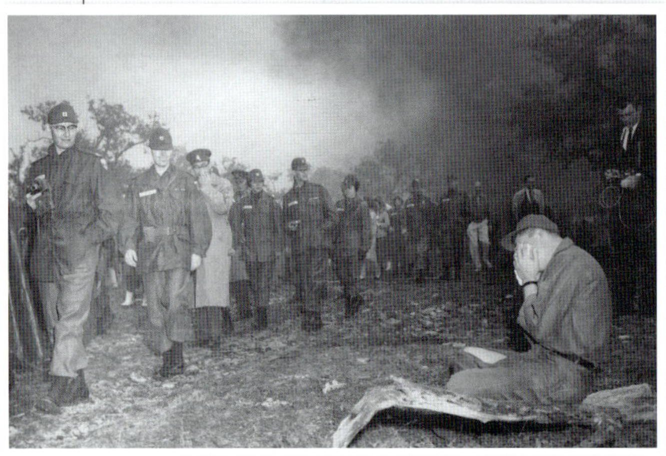

In a background of smoking debris, a simulated casualty sobs as he plays his role in OPERATION BLOW UP. 11 March 1966.

(U.S. Army Photo, AMEDD Museum Photo Collection)

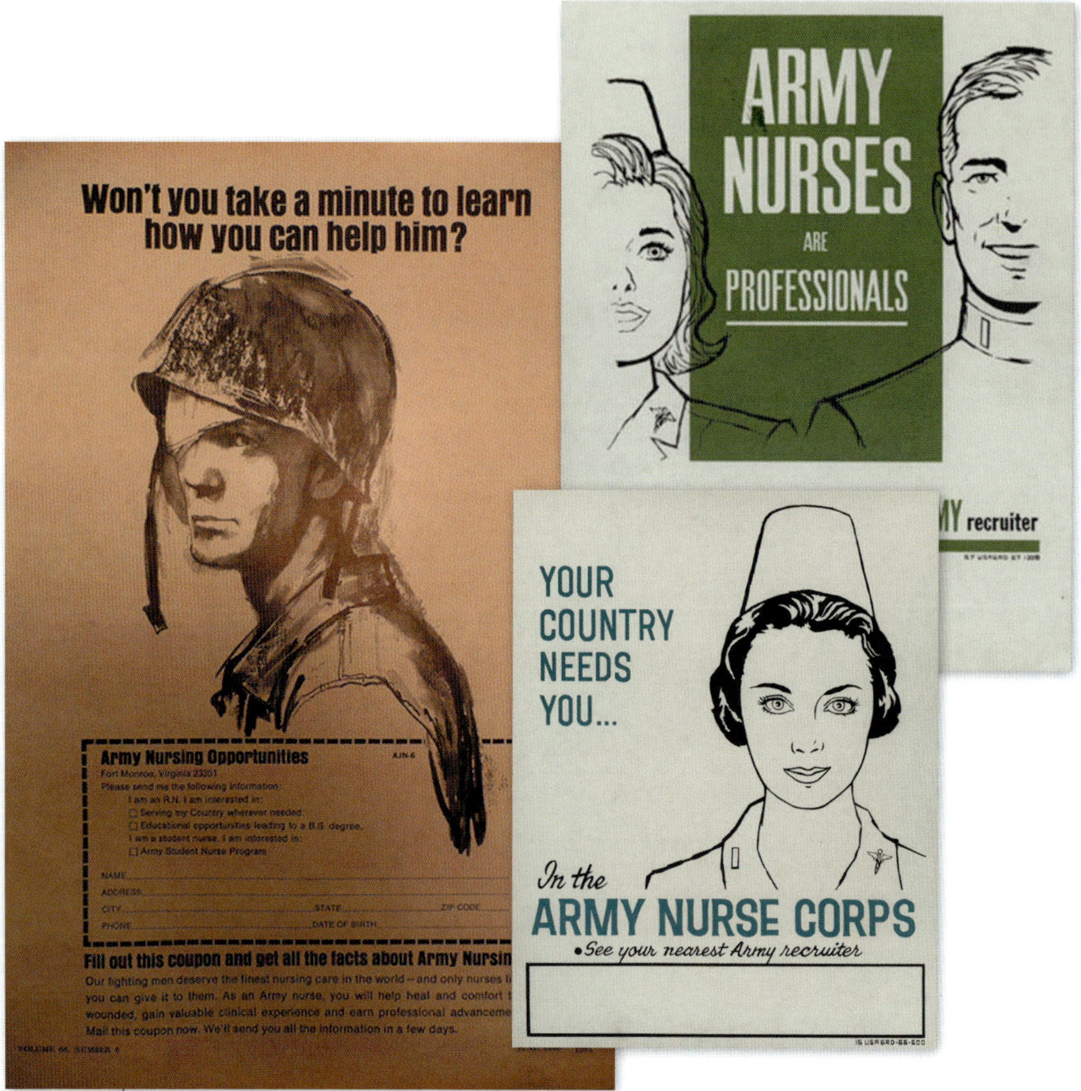

Forty-two nurses in the MFSS Army Nurse Corps Officer Basic Class volunteered for service in Vietnam following their 21 May graduation.

("42 Army Nurses at MFSS Volunteer for Vietnam Service," Talon, 12 May 1966)
(Army Nurse Corps Posters, AMEDD Museum)

Throughout the year, members of the Department of Veterinary Science, in cooperation with the Sentry Dog Training Center, Lackland Air Force Base, veterinary and trainer personnel, held sentry dog demonstrations at Camp Bullis for Veterinary Corps officer students in the Army Medical Service Officer Basic Course, 6-8-CZOA, and the Associate Army Medical Service Officer Career Course, 6-8-C23.

(Annual Report of the MFSS, CY 1966, p 19)

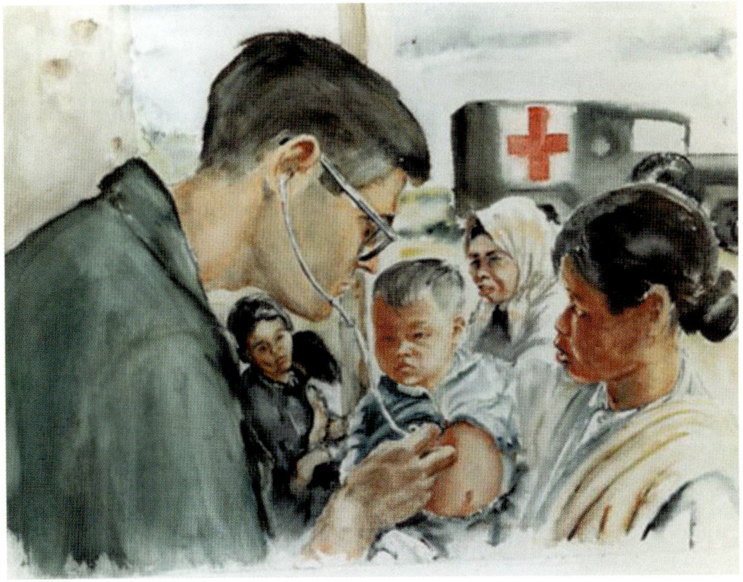

("American Doctor Examines Vietnamese Child," Samuel E. Alexander, CAT IV, 1967, Courtesy of the National Museum of the U.S. Army)

Six Army, Navy and Air Force mobile military medical teams, scheduled to serve in civilian provincial hospitals in Vietnam, were given two weeks training at the School in the Military Provincial Hospital Assistance Program (MILPHAP) at the MFSS. The teams were used to expand health and medical services for the Vietnamese civilian rural population.

(Annual Report of the MFSS, CY 1966, p 19)

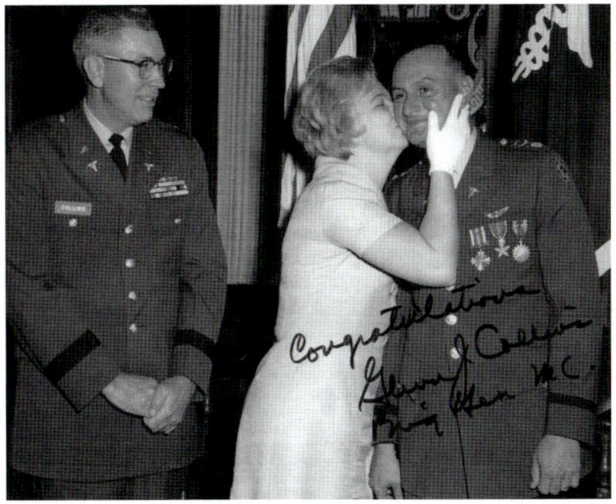

MAJ Francis A. Copeland, an instructor at the MFSS, former Commander of the 82nd Helicopter Detachment in Vietnam, received 23 decorations. BG Glenn J. Collins presented MAJ Copeland with two Distinguished Flying Crosses, the second through 19th Oak Leaf Clusters to the Air Medal and the Bronze Star Medal, on 24 June 1966. Nancy Copeland, his wife, is seen giving him a kiss.

(Photo courtesy of the Copeland family, "Fort Sam Officer Gets Decorations," San Antonio Express, 17 June 1966, p 2-F.)

The Television Division was established at the MFSS on 15 December 1966. Closed circuit television as an instructional medium had been evaluated at the School since 1953. After a study of closed circuit techniques from 23 February to 23 May 1963 by the U.S. Army Signal Corps Mobile Television Unit, the Office of the Surgeon General approved a permanent television system in 1966 and allocated $750,000 for the procurement and installation of a permanent closed circuit system for the School. A separate building was erected to accommodate the closed circuit instructional facility, along with four additional classroom buildings, along Patch Road.

(Annual Historical Report, MFSS, CY 1966, p ii)

Four video tape recorders were authorized for use by the Personnel Management Branch to improve oral communications for students in the Army Medical Service Officer Advanced Course and Hospital Administration Course. The recorders had instant playback capabilities to enable students to self-critique their performances.

(Annual Report of the MFSS, CY 1966, p 25)

1967

In July 1967, the Command Sergeants Major (CSM) Program was established by the Army Chief of Staff, General Harold K. Johnson. The program assigned a small group of selected sergeants major to all major commands of the Army. They were to serve as senior enlisted advisors and ombudsmen for all matters pertaining to enlisted members of their command.

1967 was a big year for BAMC and the MFSS with the dedication of the Charles L. Kelly Heliport, establishment of an efficient new blood donor center for the hospital, and installation of closed circuit television, which utilized the latest in color video equipment as a classroom teaching aid.

("BAMC Marks Anniversary," Military Service News, 28 Jan 1972)

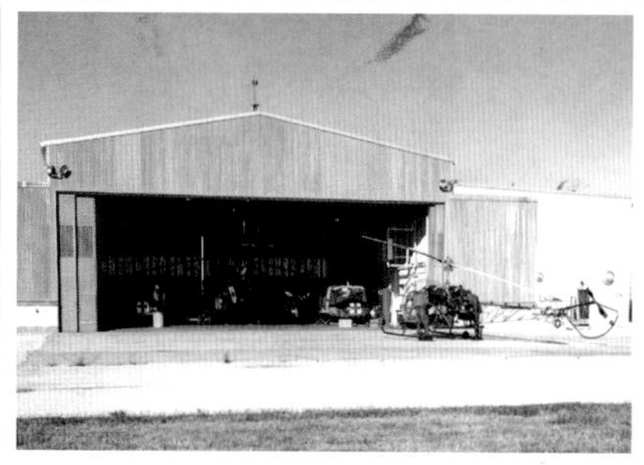

The Charles L. Kelly Heliport

(U.S. Army Photo, FSH Museum Collection)

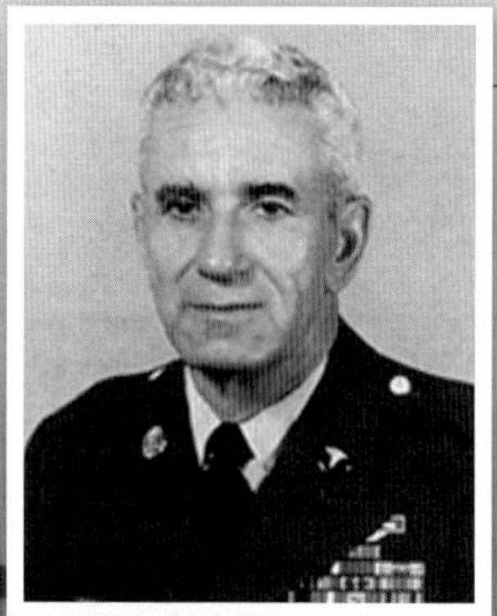

CSM Howard A. Tavernier, first CSM of the MFSS

(U.S. Army Photo, AMEDDC&S History Office files)

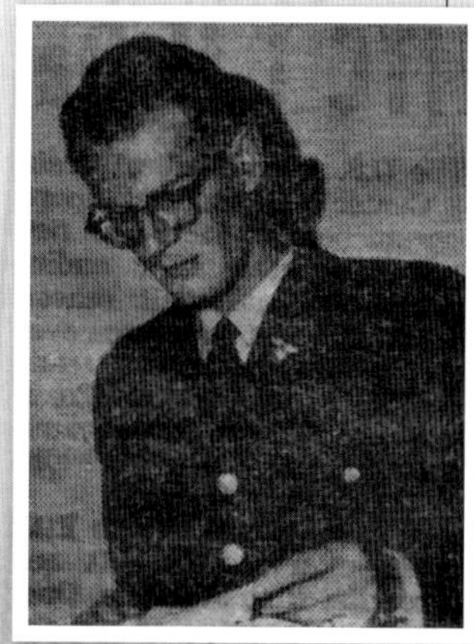

2LT Von Trapp studies during his MSC Officer Basic Course.

(U.S. Army Photo)

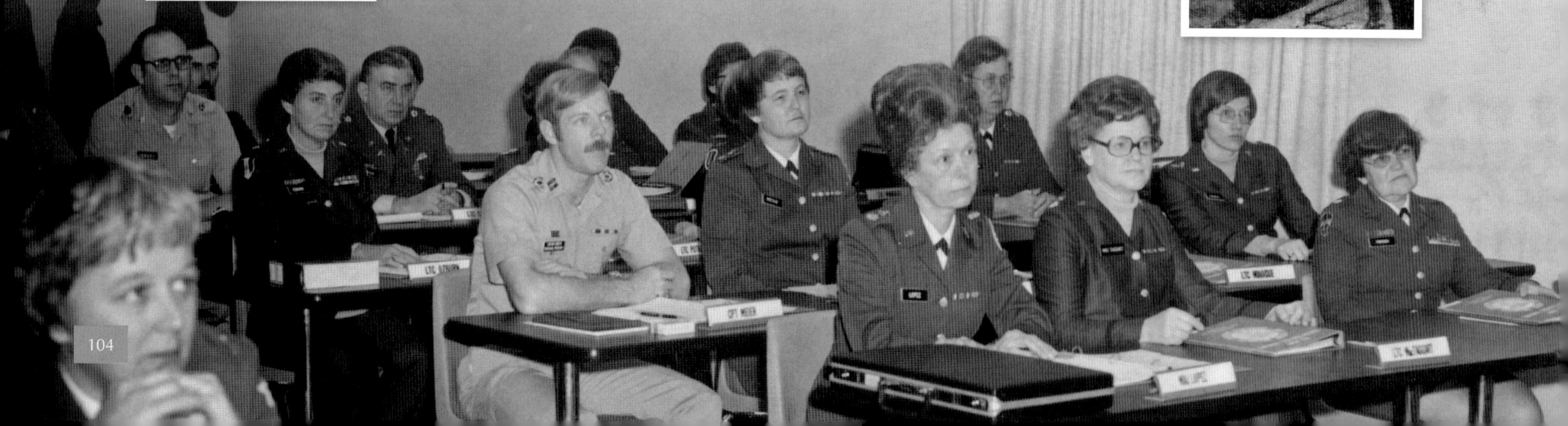

An unknown meeting in an MFSS classroom with newly installed closed circuit television monitor.

(U.S. Army Photo, AMEDD Museum Photo Collection)

2LT Johannes Von Trapp, the youngest member of the famed Baron Georg Johannes Von Trapp family (whose story was told in the motion picture musical, "Sound of Music") was interviewed while attending the MSC Officer Basic Course. 2LT Von Trapp was a member of the Vermont National Guard on active duty. After completing his military obligation, he hoped to return to college for his graduate degree.

("Von Trapp's Sound of Music Now Has A Military Rhythm," Talon, 9 Feb 1967)

By Fall 1967, the MFSS had the most modern and complete color closed circuit television system of any military establishment. The system was operated and maintained by a staff of 15, and nearly 300 receivers were installed in 100 classrooms as training aids for more than 15,000 military personnel annually.

("Medical TV Net Launched," San Antonio Express, 13 Aug 1967)

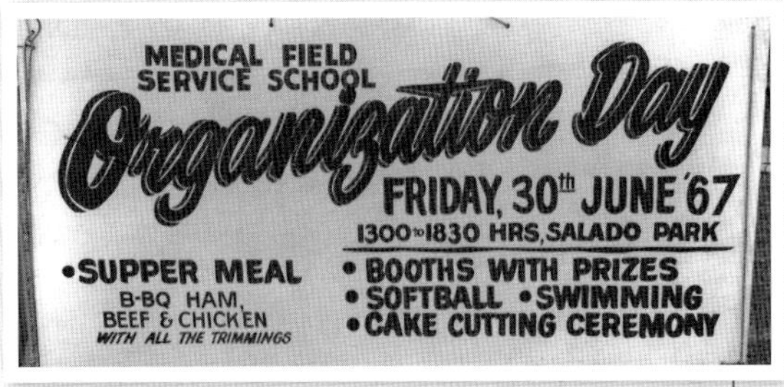

Organization Day 1967 included skydivers, a jump tower, balloon bust, and lots of good food.

(Organization Day 1967, AAR, Stimson Library Special Collections)

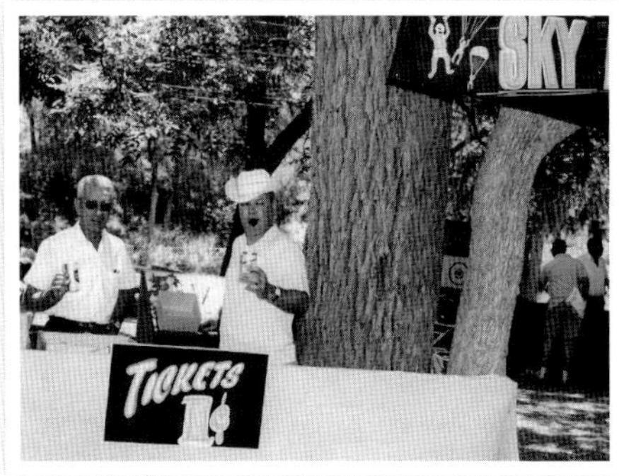

Ticket vendors toast the camera with Miller and Lone Star beer.

(Organization Day 1967, AAR, Stimson Library Special Collections)

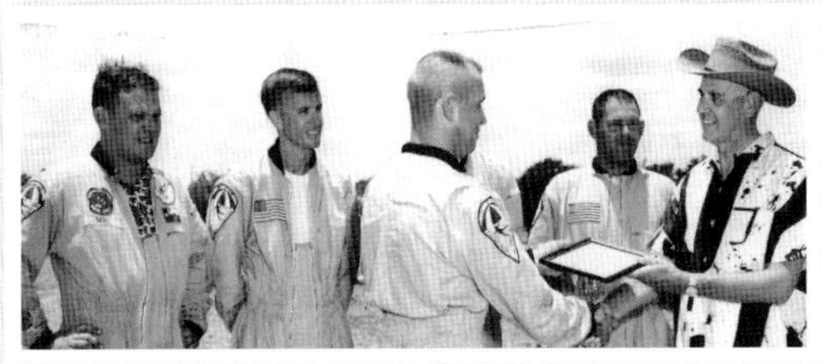

The skydivers gather after their jump. The one on the far left has a Hawaiian shirt beneath his jumpsuit. The skydivers appeared ready to stay and enjoy the celebration.

(Organization Day 1967, AAR, Stimson Library Special Collections)

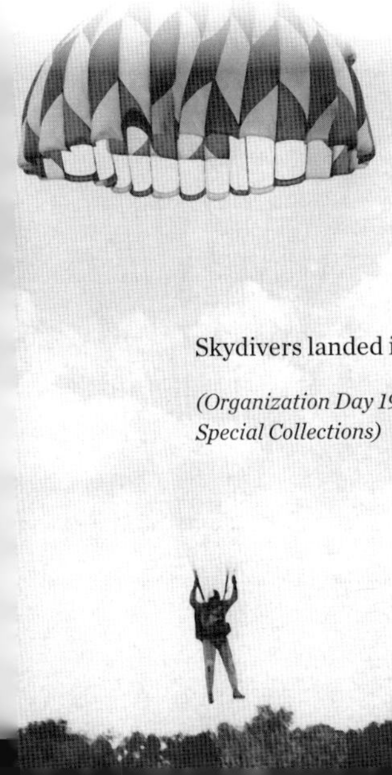

Skydivers landed in the midst of the celebration.

(Organization Day 1967, AAR, Stimson Library Special Collections)

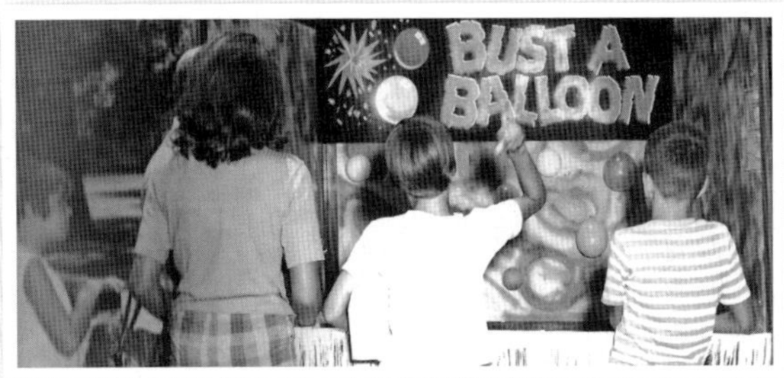

A "Bust a Balloon" booth for family entertainment.

(Organization Day 1967, AAR, Stimson Library Special Collections)

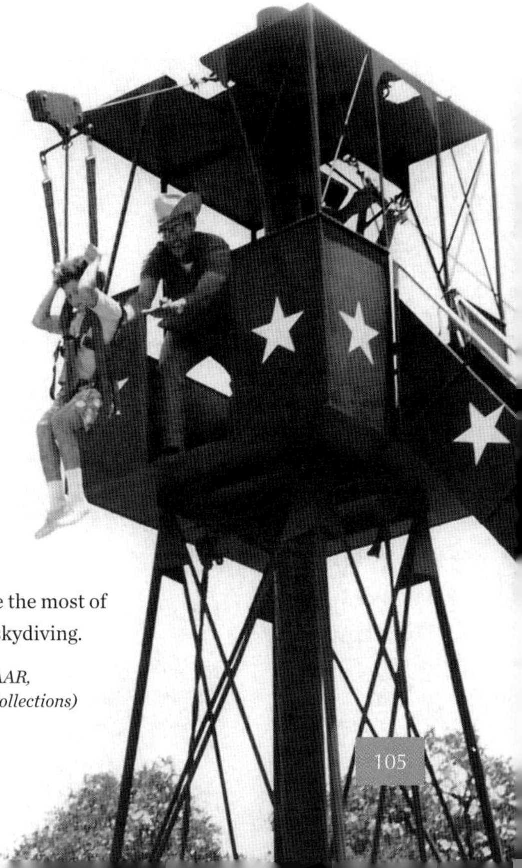

Family members make the most of an opportunity to try skydiving.

(Organization Day 1967, AAR, Stimson Library Special Collections)

1967

Not all California students were against the war in Vietnam. Four students at the MFSS joined the Army specifically to serve in Vietnam. All four were June graduates of the Los Angeles County General Hospital School of Nursing. They were a different breed from the students and non-students who made headlines with anti-war demonstrations at Berkeley.

("California WACs in S.A. Term Demonstrators 'For the Birds," San Antonio News, 20 Oct 1967)

2LT Thomas Bedick, an instructor at the MFSS, was one Army officer who got plenty of exercise moonlighting as a defensive back for the San Antonio Toros in the Texas Professional Football League. After most of personnel at the school went home for an evening of relaxation, 2LT Bedick headed for the practice field. A former player at Penn State, 2LT Bedick hoped for a major professional football tryout.

("MFSS Instructor Moonlights as Toro," San Antonio News, 19 Oct 1967)

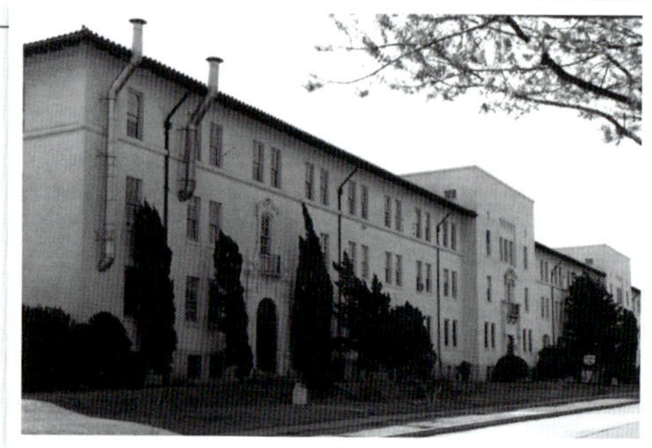

Building 2792 of the MFSS was well known to enlisted students as the location of many of their courses. Courses conducted in bldg. 2792 in 1967 included dental, operating room procedures, Special Forces Aidman, medical laboratory, pharmacy, and radiography.

(U.S. Army Photo, AMEDD Museum Photo Collection)

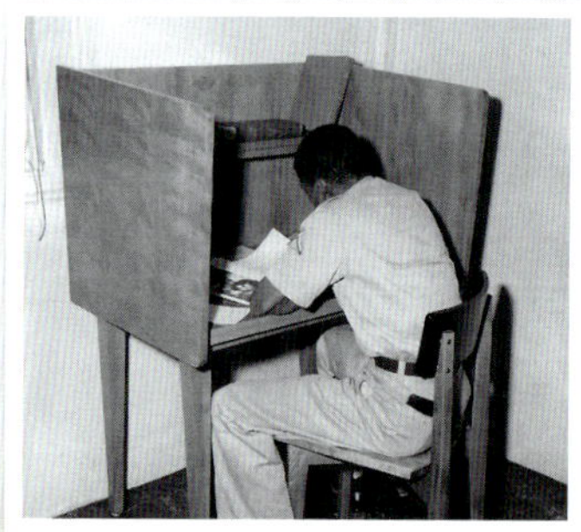

PFC Rochell Brown, MFSS student, uses one of four new carrels (study booths) given to Stimson Library by former students.

("New Carrels," Talon, 2 Nov 1967)

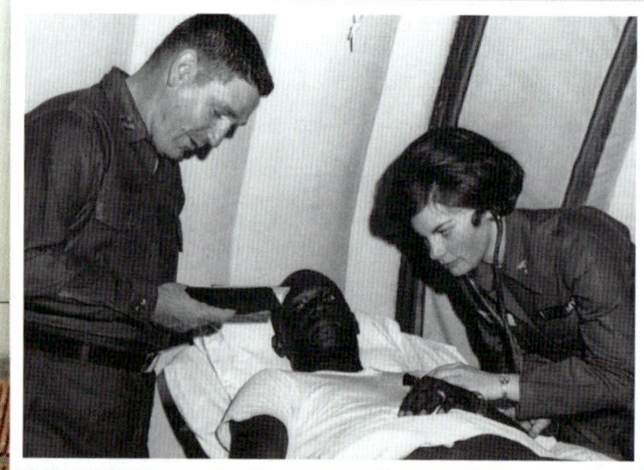

A Chaplain gives religious comfort to a patient while a student nurse works over her "patient" during field exercises in a MUST on 31 March 1967.

(U.S. Army Photo, AMEDD Museum Photo Collection)

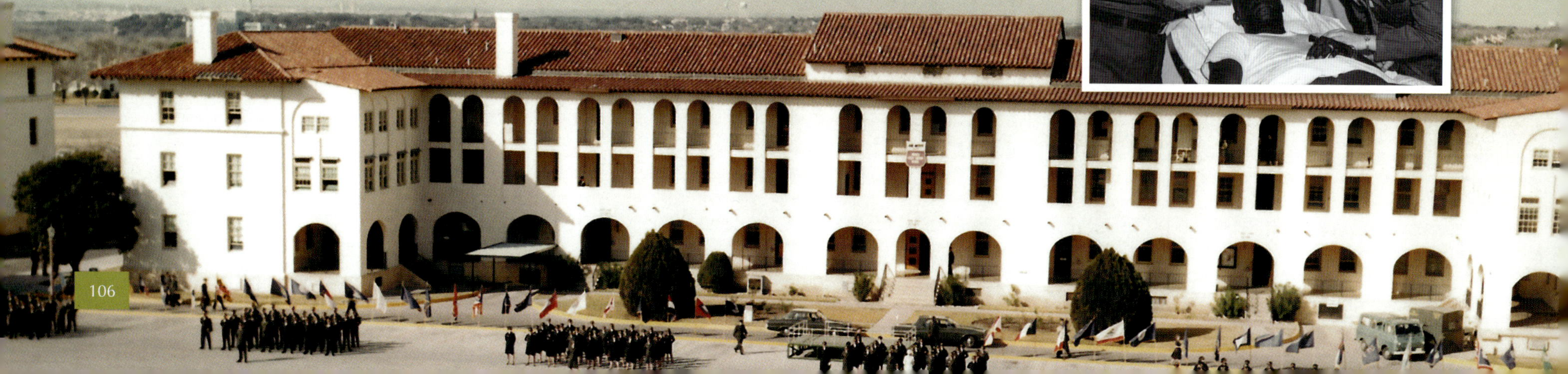

Students in the Army Nurse Corps Officer basic course at the MFSS prepare for dress blue inspection. Some of the nurses are in greens or whites because those going into Vietnam upon graduation were permitted to wait until return to the U.S. before buying dress blues.

(U.S. Army Photo, AMEDD Museum Photo Collection)

"Military nurses were more motivated and more likely to continue studying after they became nurses than their counterparts in civilian hospitals and institutions," according to the director of the division of nursing education at Teacher's College at Columbia University, Dr. Eleanor Lambertsen. Dr. Lambertsen also said that civilian hospitals and institutions would do well to adopt some of the military techniques – particularly in screening and selecting applicants for nurse training. "Military nurses are used to studying," she said. "In a civilian situation, there aren't compelling forces for nurses to keep studying."

("Nurse Program Praised by Columbia Professor," Talon, 7 Dec 1967)

A radiology resident demonstrates the injection of dye into the common carotid artery on 26 June 1967.

(U.S. Army Photo, AMEDD Museum Photo Collection)

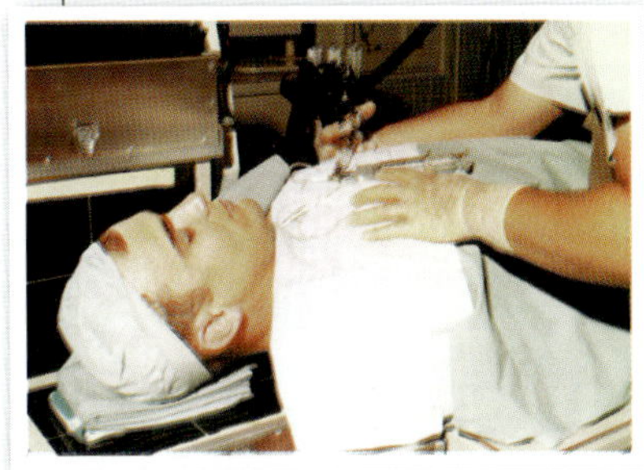

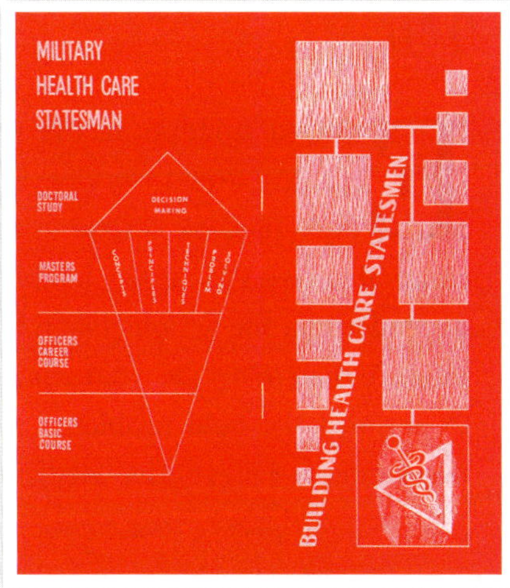

The Army-Baylor Program celebrated its 20th Anniversary of building "Military Health Care Statesmen."

("Building Health Care Statesmen," 1967, Stimson Library Special Collections)

A simulated Operating Room is set up at Camp Bullis during field exercises in October 1967.

(U.S. Army Photo, AMEDD Museum Photo Collection)

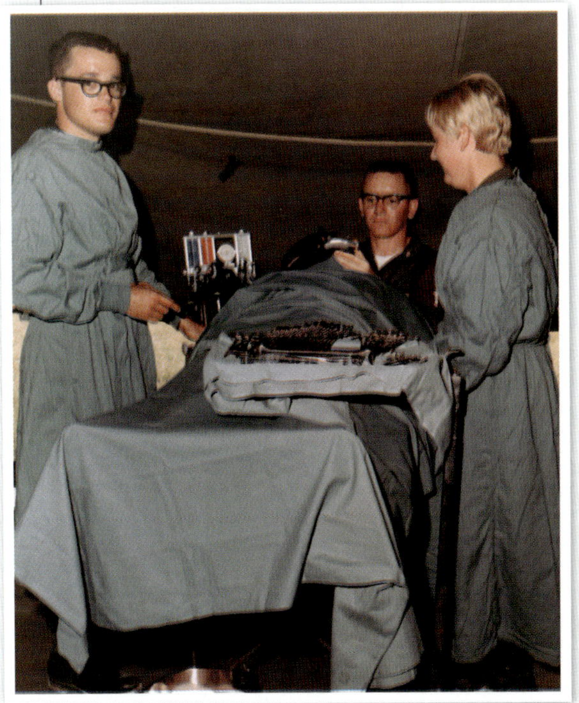

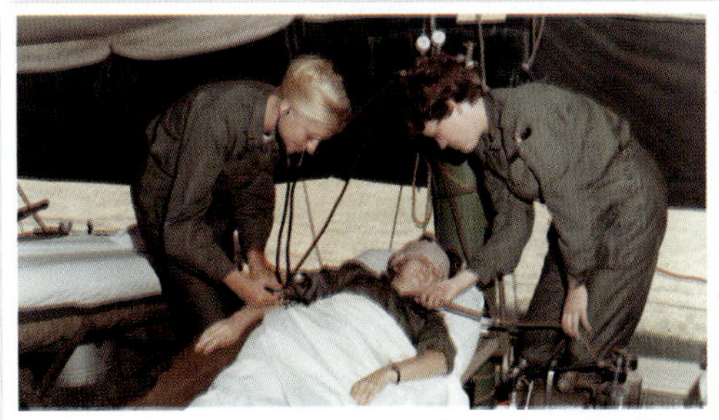

Officers Basic Course students treat a "patient" suffering from a skull fracture during field exercises at Camp Bullis.

(U.S. Army Photo, AMEDD Museum Photo Collection)

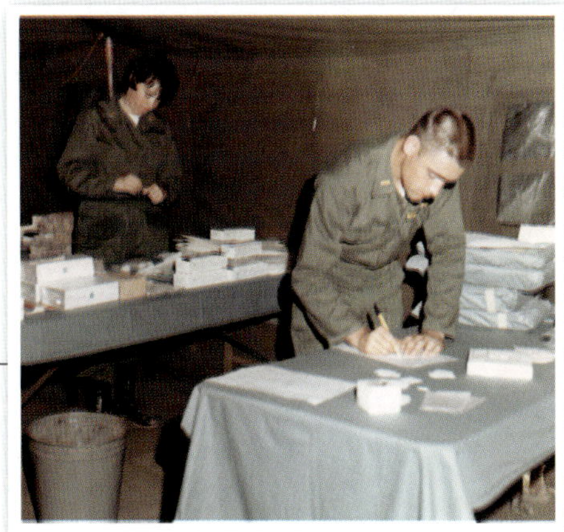

A simulated Operating Room is set up at Camp Bullis during field exercises in October 1967.

(U.S. Army Photo, AMEDD Museum Photo Collection)

1968

Enlisted students in the Preventive Medicine Course at the U.S. Army Medical Field Service School Advanced Course spent one week of their 16-week course in the field near Canyon Lake, Texas. "They do a comprehensive PM survey of the area to be occupied by troops. Everything is dependent on the actions taken by the students. They are given a situation and they are then to decide what equipment, vehicles, and supplies will be necessary to perform the field problem," said COL Jerome Greenburg, Director of the Department of Preventive Medicine.

("Week at Canyon Lake Part of MFSS Training," Talon, 3 July 1968)

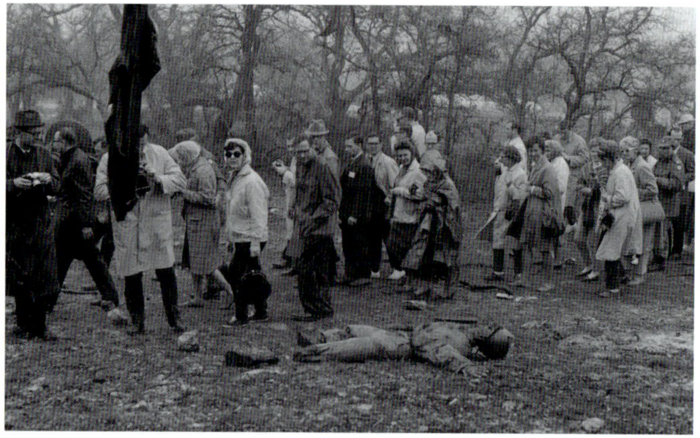

More than 600 persons witnessed OPERATION BLOWUP in March 1968. Photographers and spectators alike got a look at the "charred corpses" near the center of a simulated nuclear blast.

(U.S. Army Photo, AMEDD Museum Photo Collection)

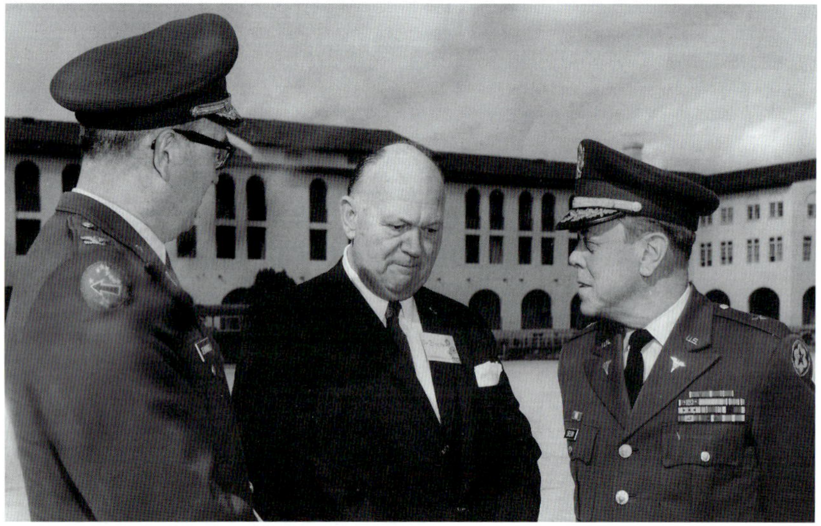

COL H. Jennings, Commander USAH, Fort Benning, Ga.; Dr. Truman G. Blocker Jr., President of the University of Texas Medical Branch (UTMB) at Galveston; and BG O. Elliot Ursin, Commandant of the MFSS, meet before their presentation to 135 UTMB students about to participate in OPERATION BLOW UP, a simulated nuclear blast designed as a training exercise in military and disaster medicine.

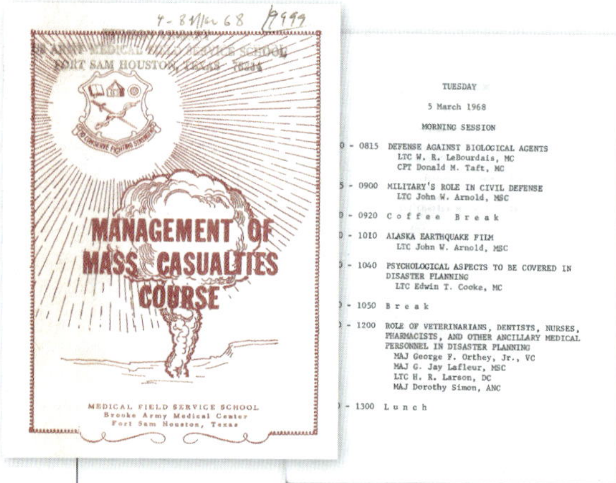

FORT SAM HOUSTON, TEXAS

MANAGEMENT OF MASS CASUALTIES COURSE

MEDICAL FIELD SERVICE SCHOOL
Brooke Army Medical Center
Fort Sam Houston, Texas

TUESDAY

5 March 1968

MORNING SESSION

- 0815 DEFENSE AGAINST BIOLOGICAL AGENTS
LTC W. R. LeBourdais, MC
CPT Donald M. Taft, MC

- 0900 MILITARY'S ROLE IN CIVIL DEFENSE
LTC John W. Arnold, MSC

- 0920 Coffee Break

- 1010 ALASKA EARTHQUAKE FILM
LTC John W. Arnold, MSC

- 1040 PSYCHOLOGICAL ASPECTS TO BE COVERED IN DISASTER PLANNING
LTC Edwin T. Cooke, MC

- 1050 Break

- 1200 ROLE OF VETERINARIANS, DENTISTS, NURSES, PHARMACISTS, AND OTHER ANCILLARY MEDICAL PERSONNEL IN DISASTER PLANNING
MAJ George F. Orthey, Jr., VC
MAJ G. Jay Lafleur, MSC
LTC H. R. Larson, DC
MAJ Dorothy Simon, ANC

- 1300 Lunch

Program from the 5 March 1968 Management of Mass Casualties Course.

(Stimson Library Special Collections)

A tour designed to emphasize career possibilities at Fort Sam Houston was conducted for 106 economically disadvantaged student aides hired at BAMC under the Youth Opportunity Program (YOP). Various stations located at BAMC, the MFSS, and other post departments offered a 30-minute orientation concerning their areas. The tour gave students the opportunity to look at various unfamiliar career possibilities.

("Career Possibilities Aim of BAMC YOP Tour," Talon, 29 August 1968)

A desire for diversification led a civilian medical social worker to become one of the few women among nearly 6,000 officers in the Army Medical Corps. CPT Myra Gulley, a student at the MFSS, was a medical social worker in Tulsa, Oklahoma, when she decided to make the change. She was seeking a place where work would be more diverse and she could do some supervisory work and have a chance to travel. She decided the Army Medical Service Corps offered the best possibility to achieve all of these.

("Desire for Diversification Leads Woman to MSC Commission," Talon, 7 November 1968)

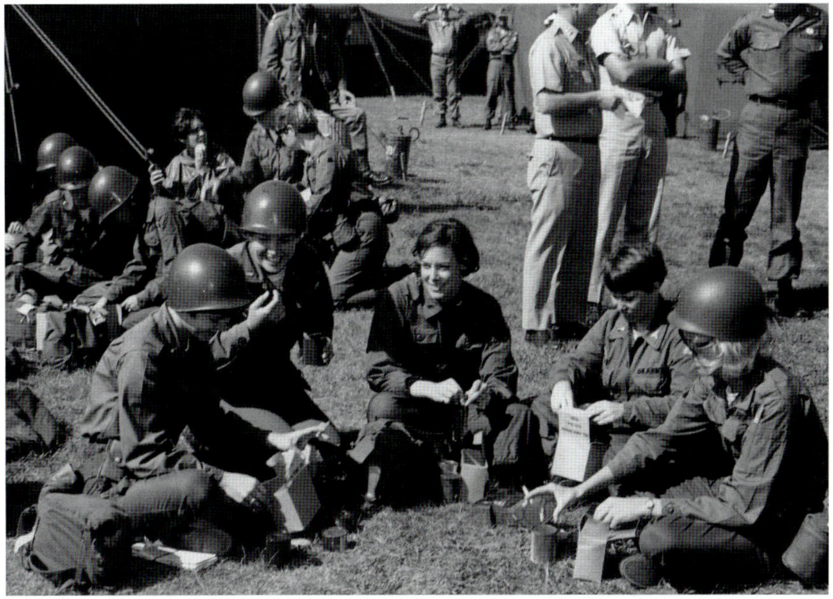

Army Nurse Corps students eat their C rations during field training at Camp Bullis, 18 Oct 1968.

(U.S. Army Photo, AMEDD Museum Photo Collection)

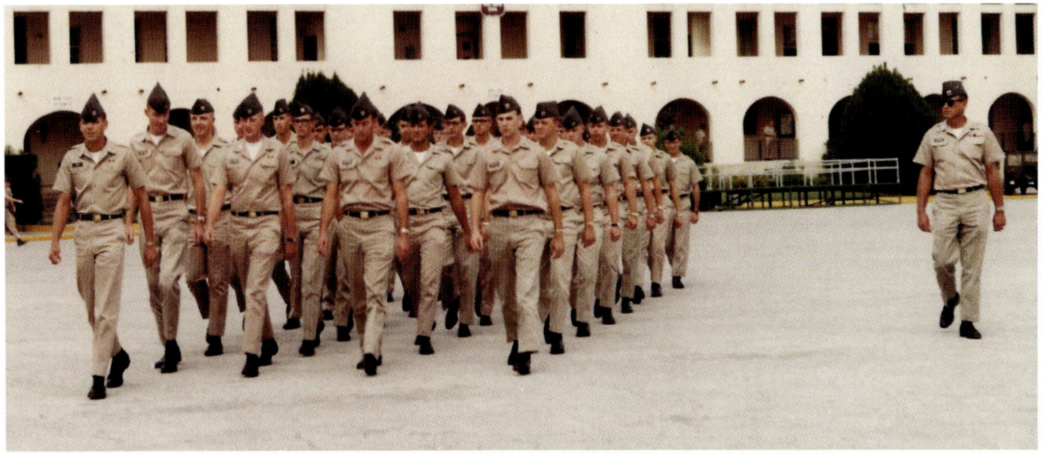

Veterinary Corps Officers attending basic course conduct drill and ceremony in the Quadrangle.

(U.S. Army Photo, AMEDD Museum Photo Collection)

1969

On 23 Jan 1969, the 323rd Army Band at the U.S. Army MFSS observed its 25th anniversary as the schoolhouse band. It was the only band assigned directly to an activity of the Surgeon General of the Army and had been proudly called "our band" by nearly every officer of the medical department for 25 years.

("Band Marks a Quarter-Century of Performance," Talon, 24 Jan 1969)

Graduation Exercises Program for the December 1969 MFSS Noncommissioned Officer Course.

(Stimson Library Special Collections)

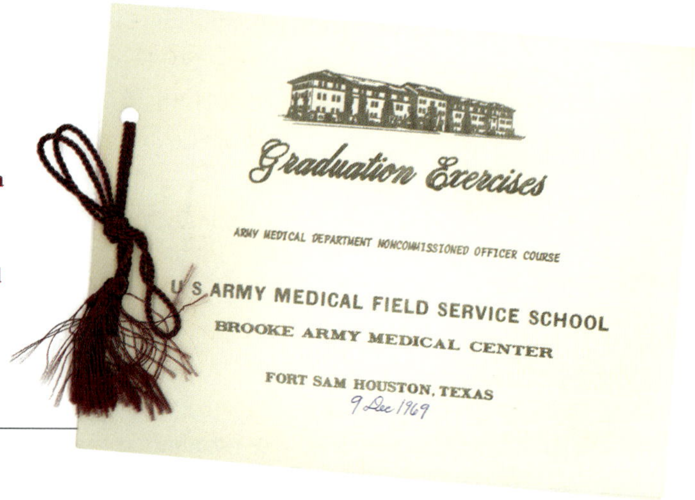

Designed to acquaint teachers with the equipment and explain the firsthand opportunities offered in the field of Army medical technology, the MFSS provided exhibits at Dunbar Junior High School in San Antonio in May 1969. It was the highlight of a gathering of the Science Teachers Association of Texas and lauded by those who attended.

("200 Texas Science Teachers See MFSS Exhibits; Get Picture of Medical Training Programs," Talon, 6 May 1969)

Less than 24 hours prior to their graduation from the Officer Basic Course, 64 Army Medical Officers, formerly citizens of 31 foreign nations, became U.S. citizens during a naturalization ceremony at the Federal Building in San Antonio on 5 May 1969. A total of 101 Medical Corps officers in the last two basic classes at the MFSS had been naturalized while attending school.

("MFSS Officers Become Citizens; 64 Naturalized in SA Ceremony," Talon, 8 May 1969)
("Band Marks a Quarter-Century of Performance," Talon, 24 Jan 1969)

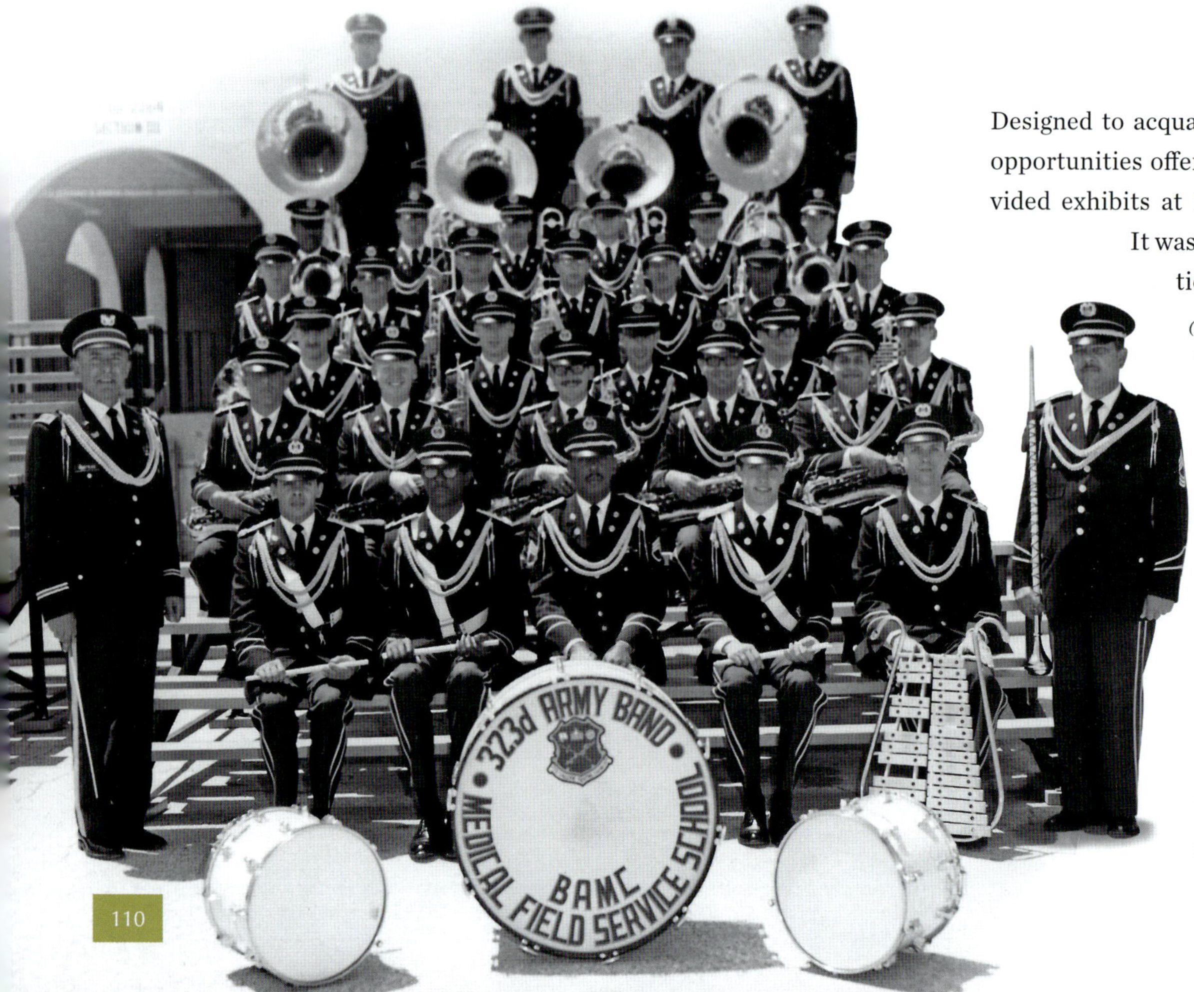

The 323d Army Band, 1969

(U.S. Army Photo, AMEDDC&S History Office files)

MSG Tanner, who served as a Special Forces instructor at the MFSS schoolhouse, was one of three military medical aidmen who served as an emergency response team during the launch at Cape Kennedy, Florida, in 1969. Stationed in three specially equipped armored personnel carriers, the members of the Pad Egress Team were there to respond to any fire or explosion that would have called for the rescue of the astronauts while on the launch pad.

("Ringside Seat for Apollo Launchings: MFSS Sergeant Serves Where the Action Is," Talon, 15 Aug 1969)

On 9 Oct 1969, MAJ Patrick H. Brady, Army Medical Department helicopter pilot and instructor at the MFSS, was awarded the Medal of Honor by President Nixon for his valorous action of January 1968. Already one of the Army's most decorated officers, he was the first officer in the MSC to be awarded the Medal of Honor.

("51 Lives Saved," Military Scene Magazine, December 1969)

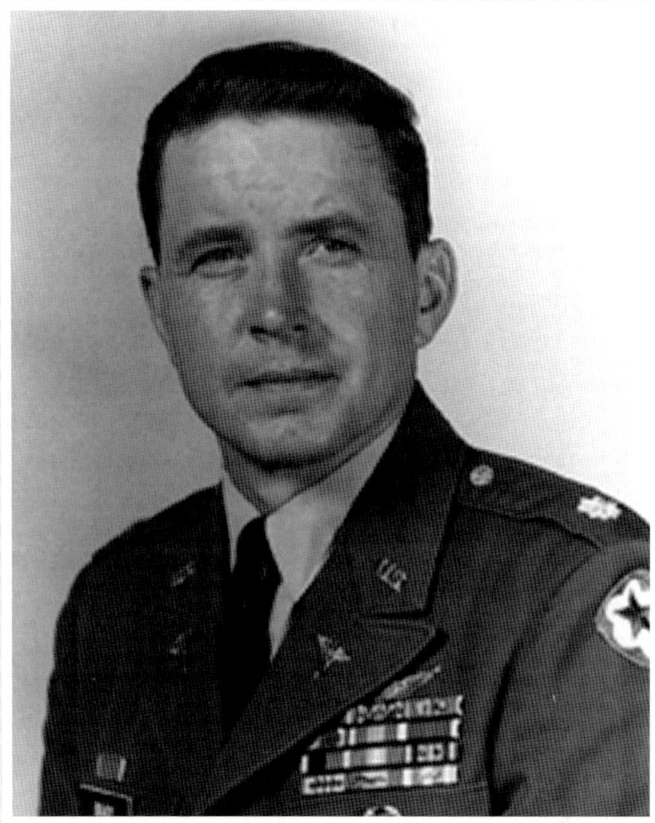

MAJ Patrick H. Brady

("51 Lives Saved," Military Scene Magazine, December 1969)

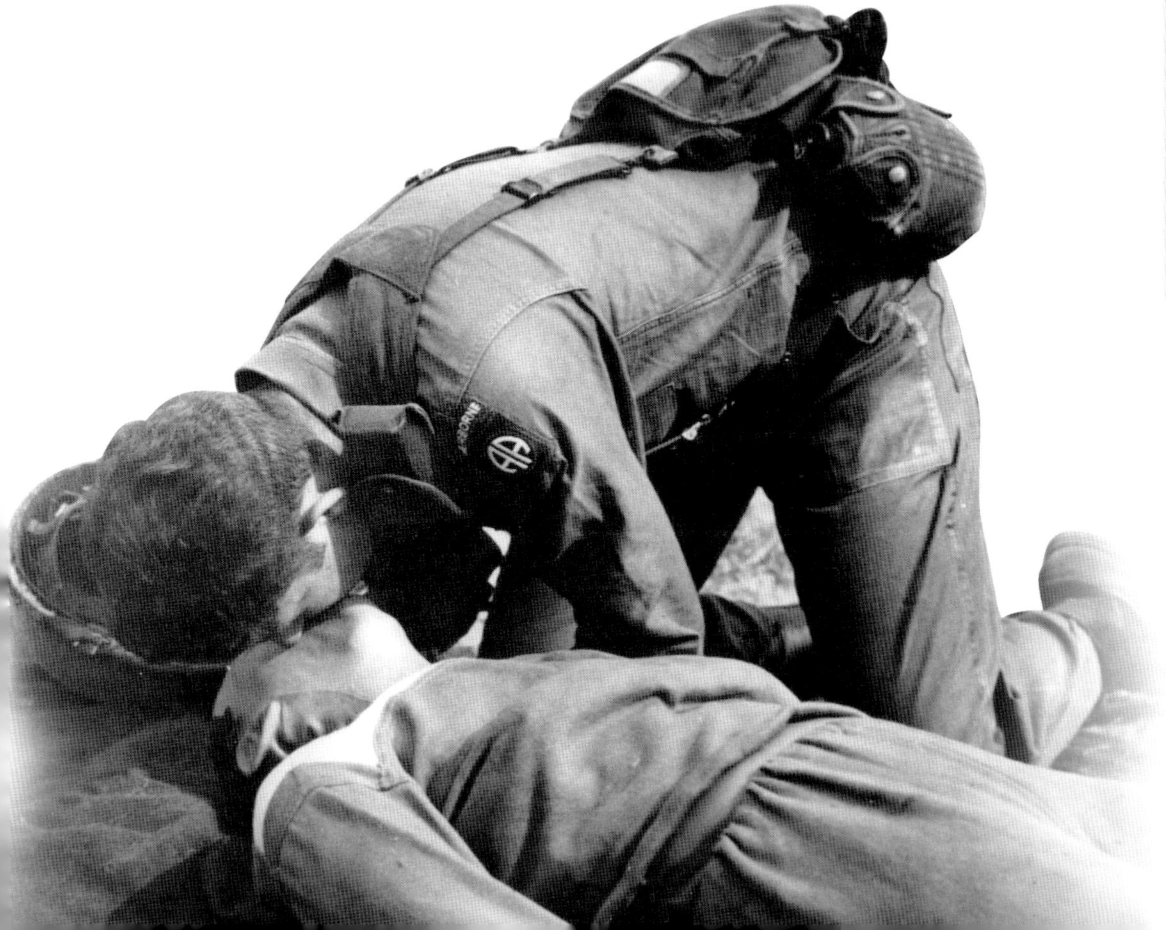

SP4 John W. Caddell demonstrates mouth-to-mouth on a mannequin during the Expert Field Medical Badge Test.

(U.S. Army Photo, AMEDD Museum Photo Collection)

1970 - 1979

Congress appropriated $9.8 million for the construction of the first building complex designed specifically for and to meet the needs of the MFSS.

The MFSS Social Work-Psychology Specialist Course was one of five selected from more than 600 mental heath programs nationwide to be showcased at the National Mental Health Association Convention in Washington, D.C., in February 1970. The course featured role-playing technique, closed-circuit television for immediate playback of observation and critique, peer teaching, group sensitivity training, case study methods, field studies, independent research, case conferences, and tutorial assistance.

("National Convention to Feature MFSS," Talon, 12 Feb 1970)

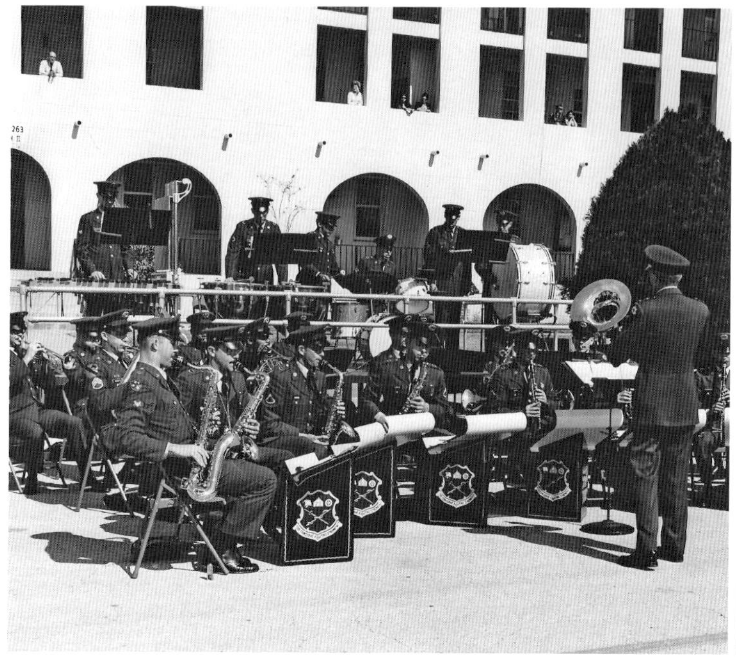

The 323rd Army Band played half-hour concerts in the Quadrangle of the School during the lunch hour
The band was under the direction of CWO Benjamin Cortese, Bandmaster.

(U.S. Army Photo, AMEDDC&S History Office Files)

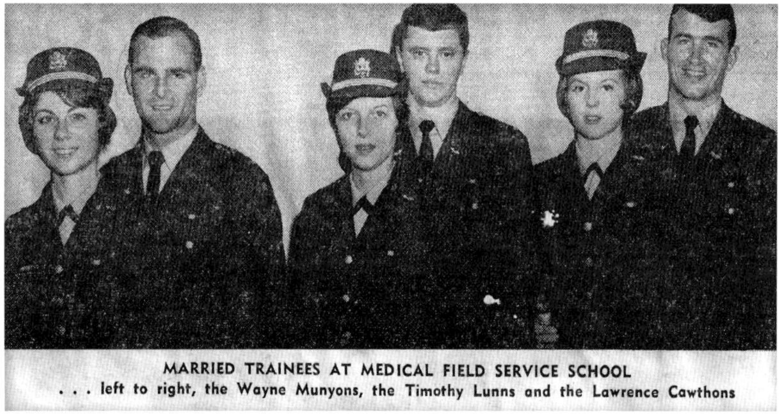
MARRIED TRAINEES AT MEDICAL FIELD SERVICE SCHOOL
. . . left to right, the Wayne Munyons, the Timothy Lunns and the Lawrence Cawthons

Six married MFSS couples attending the AMEDD Basic Course for Army Nurse Corps and Army Medical Specialist Corps Officers were featured in the Talon
The Army Medical Department was one of the only departments where dual careers were possible.

("MFSS Trains Couples: Med Officers Serve in Twos," Talon, 19 Feb 1970)

In 1970, many MFSS officers and soldiers returning from deployments in Vietnam were recognized in the local papers. An unusual one was Captain Gerald D. Poe. Poe, an MFSS Officer, served as a helicopter pilot in the Republic of Vietnam and was awarded the Navy Air Medal (Bronze Star in lieu of the First Award) for heroism on 15 February 1969, upon the recommendation of the Secretary of the Navy.

("MFSS Officer Gets Navy Air Decoration," Talon, 5 March 1970)

CPT Maria Dolores Martinez, a social worker originally from Puerto Rico, was the only woman in a class of 190 enrolled in the Officer Basic Course. She was also one of only three women social workers in the MSC at the time. Prior to joining the Army, she worked with prisoners in Puerto Rico, where she helped them establish a prison newspaper. Even after her departure to the U.S., her former patients continued to send her issues which she commented was "...satisfaction that you can't get with money!"

("Only Woman in Class of 190: Joined to Help People," Talon, 4 June 1970)

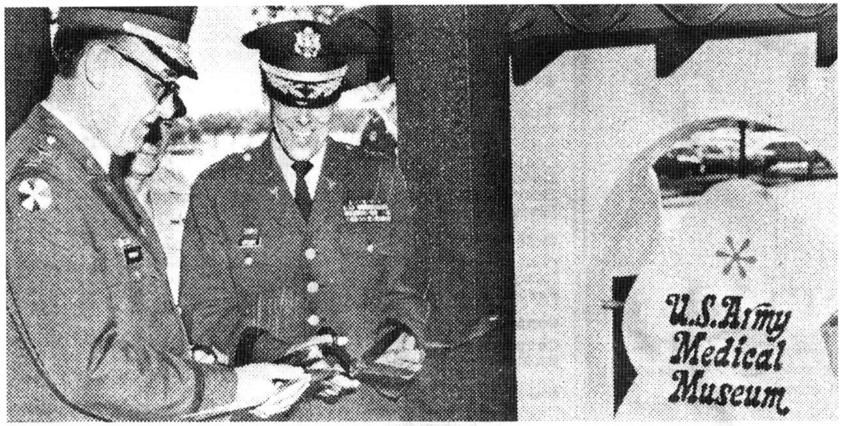

MEDICAL MUSEUM RENOVATION — COL Frank A. Neuman, left, commandant of the U.S. Army Medical Field Service School and MG O. Elliott Ursin, commanding general of Brooke Army Medical Center, cut the golden ribbon at the opening of the newly renovated Medical Museum at MFSS. The 50th anniversary of MFSS is next month and the museum opening is one of many events planned during the year.

In May 1970, the Army Medical Museum was re-opened with a ribbon-cutting ceremony. The museum, located in the basement of building 2264 (then called Blesse Hall), had occupied that location since moving to Fort Sam Houston with the MFSS from Carlisle Barracks in 1995. The renovated facility had 12,000 square feet of floor space plus an adjoining workshop.

("Army Medical Museum Re-opened with Ribbon-Cutting Ceremony," Military Service News, 22 May 1970)

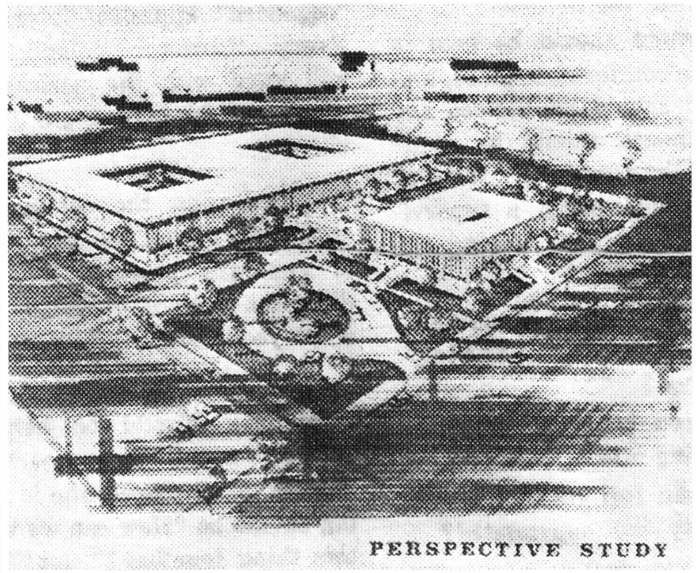

12 March 1970, the first architect's sketch of the new home of the MFSS appeared in the Talon

COL Anna Mae Hays, Army Nurse Corps, became the first woman promoted to the grade of brigadier general, making her the first woman general in the history of the Army Medical Department.

("Woman Nominated for BG," Patriot, 28 May 1970)

The MFSS observed its 50th anniversary with a huge open house celebration that included skydiving, a carnival, band concert, cake cutting, and history exhibit. Every department had an exhibit highlighting its recent achievements, which included a tour of a MUST hospital, Special Forces students treating patients in a field setting and mock field clinic, water purification equipment, and entomological control equipment demonstrations.

("MFSS Celebrates 50 Years," Patriot, 25 June 1970)

1970

In 1970, MG Kenneth D. Orr was dual-hatted, beginning in June as Commanding General of both BAMC and the MFSS.

("MFSS Welcomes New Commandant," Patriot, 25 June 1970)

At the end of the 1970 fiscal year (June 30), 1200 students completed training courses in Dental Specialist Basic, Dental Laboratory Procedures Basic, Dental Removable Prosthetics Specialist, Dental Fixed Prosthetic Specialist, and Dental Administrative Procedures.

("MFSS Trains Enlisted Dental Technicians: Program Prepares Students to Aid Dental Officers," Military Service News, 26 June 1970)

The Department of Nonresident Instruction was able to expand its extension services due to the introduction of a computer capable of grading exams and lessons, and record keeping. "Without the computer's assistance, we would soon be buried in piles of paper," said Colonel Larry W. Coker, the department director. The Department of Nonresident Instruction also relied heavily on instructional video tapes provided by the BAMC Television division (AMEDD TV).

("Extension Services to Expand," San Antonio Light, 28 June 1970)

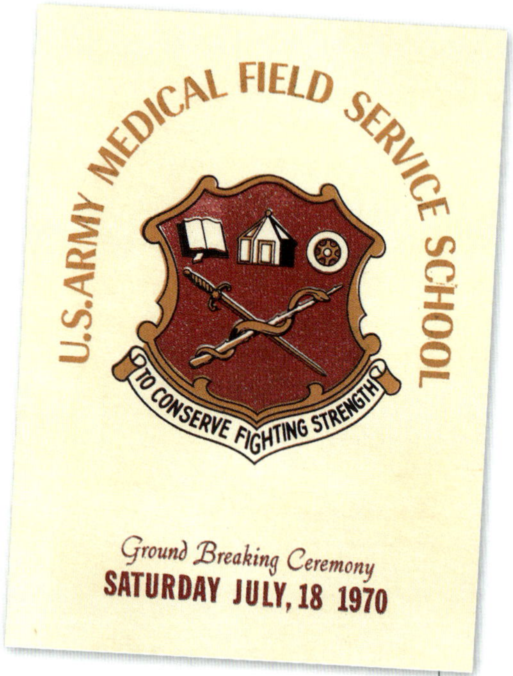

Program from the 18 July 1970 Ground Breaking Ceremony

(Stimson Library Special Collections)

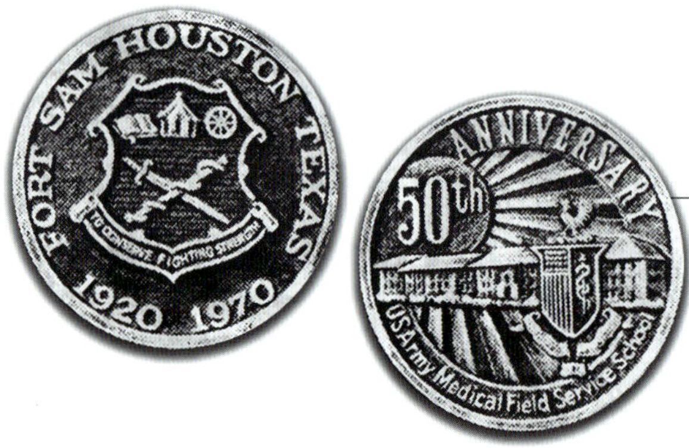

A special commemorative coin was minted for the 50th anniversary. One side bore the MFSS crest and the other contained the likeness of the old school building at Carlisle Barracks.

("Medal Minted," Patriot, 25 June 1970)

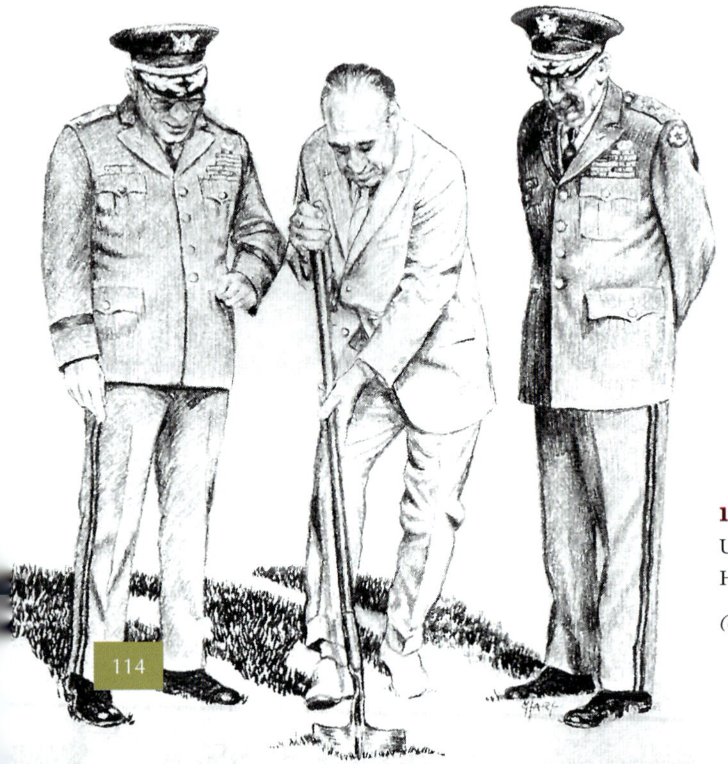

18 July 1970

U.S. Representative Henry B. Gonzales, left, breaks ground for the new MFSS to be built at Fort Sam Houston. MG Kenneth D. Orr, commanding general of BAMC and commandant of the new center, looks on.

(U.S. Army MFSS Dedication Ceremonies Program, 10 Dec 1972, Stimson Library Special Collections, p 4)

The MFSS sought to individualize instruction with television and computer-assisted instruction. The school began producing individual lesson plans that students could use at one of ten computer-assisted instruction stations. COL Frank Kellel Jr., Chief, Office of Educational Services, and his staff were involved in developing an exam that would test a student's knowledge upon arrival. This procedure allowed more advanced students to "test out" of a subject, saving both the school and student training time. A new learning center was in progress where students could work at their own speed using state-of-the-art learning tools, including audio tape machines, film strip projectors, and single-concept, sound-voice machines designed for individual use.

("Army School to Use Advanced Methods," San Antonio Light, 28 June 1970)

The first woman veterinarian in the Army since WWII, CPT Jean E. Hooks, attended OBC at the MFSS in October 1970.

("Lady Veterinarian Breaks into Male-Dominated Field," Patriot, 16 Oct 1970)

The MFSS embarked on the use of Computer Assisted Instruction (CAI). By November 1970, the MFSS had completed CAI courses in item analysis; systems engineering of training; selective grinding of dentures; anatomy and kinesiology of the knee; calculation of nuclear effects; arthropod identification; and medical patient management simulation. The school's CAI used an IBM 1440 system. Eleven IBM 1050 typewriters with audio-visual devices (the student terminals) were connected by cable to the IBM 1440 system located in the BAMC data processing complex. Eight of the terminals were in the main Quadrangle and three in the Schock Hall teaching annex.

("Computers Replace Instructors at MFSS," Patriot, 12 Nov 1970)

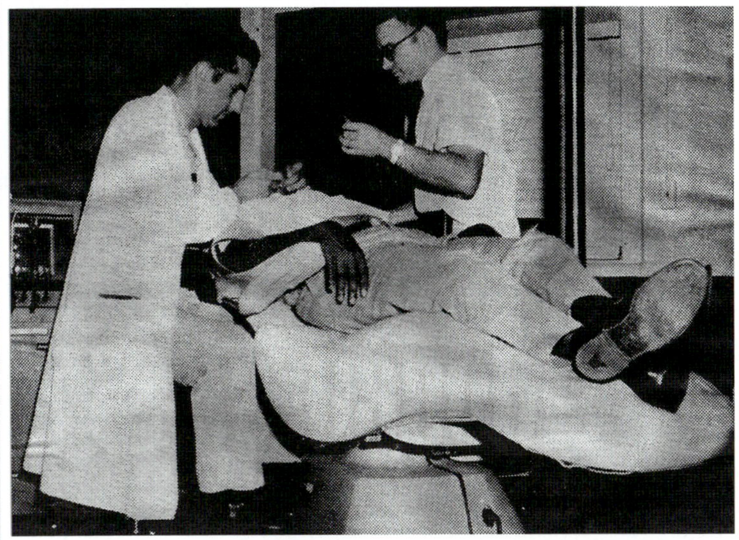

The Department of Dental Services of the MFSS debuted a new dental chair that gave patients the sensation of "floating on air." The chair, which could be moved easily, was supported on a column of air, greatly improving a dentist's efficiency. A hand-held, high-speed suction device that cleared oral cavities was introduced as a replacement for the old-fashioned cuspidor.

("Patients Float on Air in Dental Science Chair," Patriot, 1 Oct 1970)

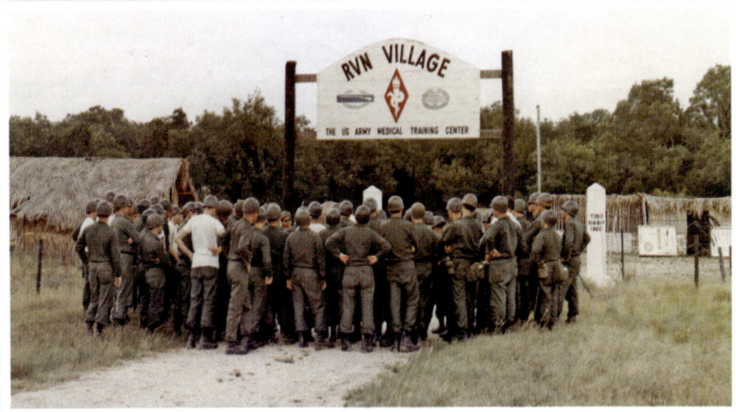

The mock Republic of Vietnam Village at Camp Bullis, originally built in 1965

(U.S. Army Photo, AMEDD Museum Collection)

1970

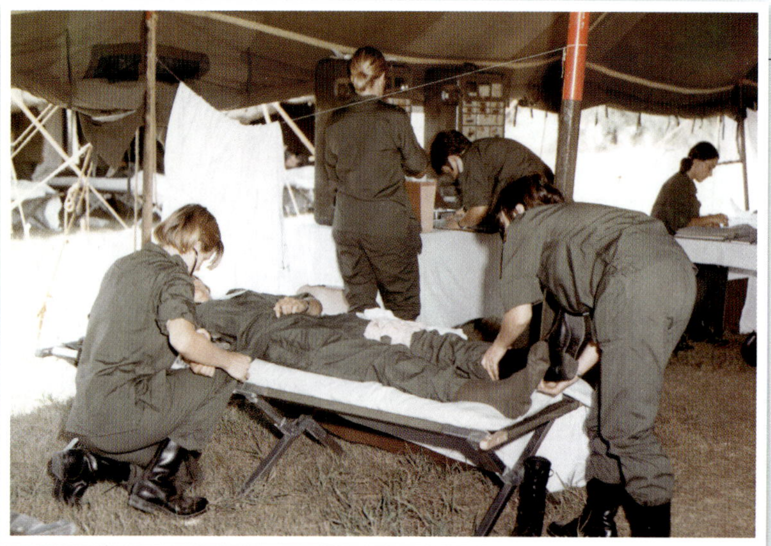

Field Exercises at Camp Bullis
ANC nurse takes a patient's pulse.

(U.S. Army Photo, AMEDD Museum Collection)

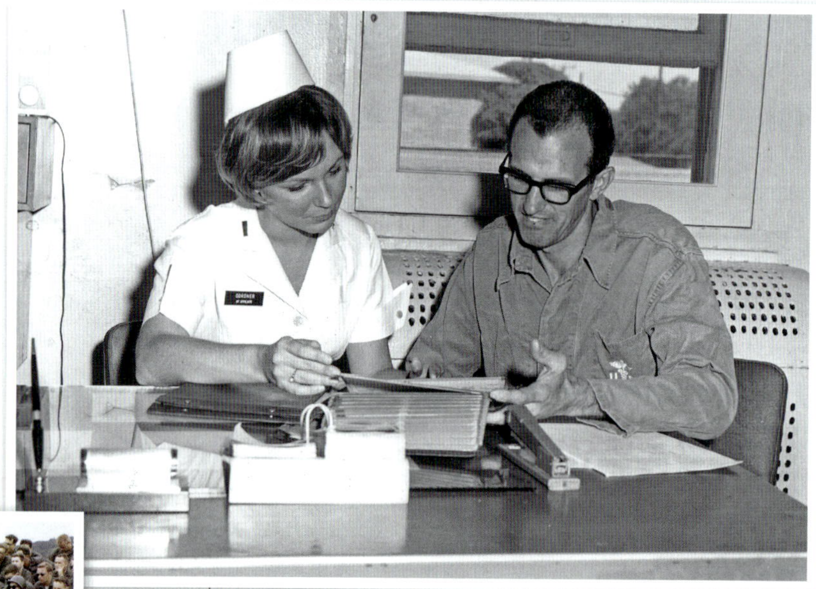

LT Gordner, OT Affiliate, and mock "psych" patient

(U.S. Army Photo, AMEDD Museum Collection)

Weapons familiarization

(U.S. Army Photo, AMEDD Museum Collection)

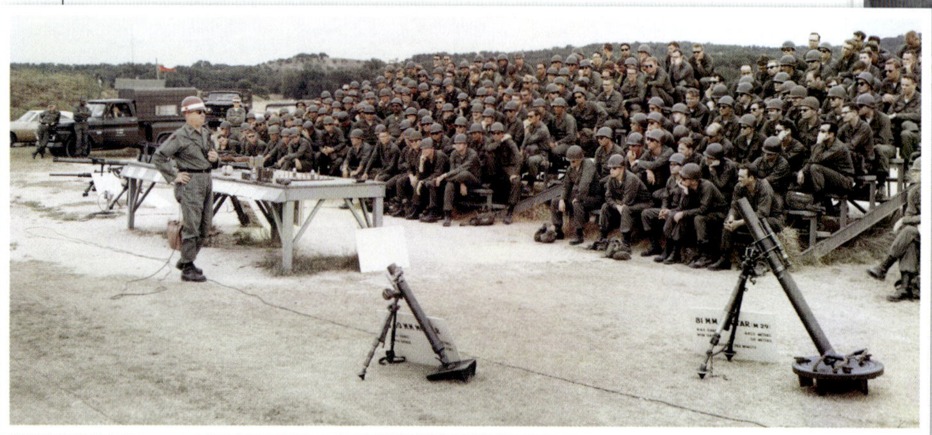

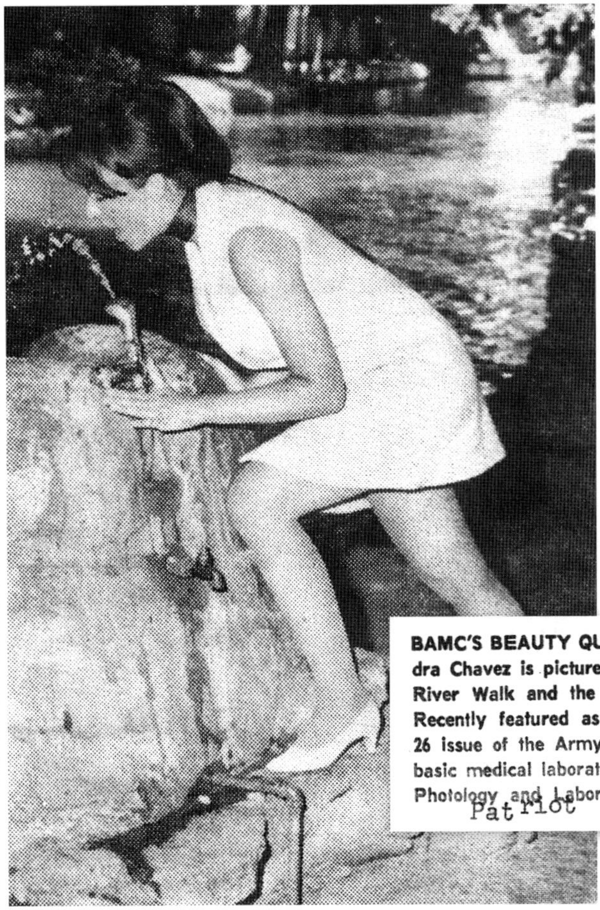

BAMC'S BEAUTY QUEEN — Miss BAMC 1970, SP5 Sandra Chavez is pictured above taking in the sights at the River Walk and the HemisFair Plaza in San Antonio. Recently featured as "Wac of the Week" in the Aug. 26 issue of the Army Times, Sandra is an instructor in basic medical laboratory chemistry in the Department of Photology and Laboratory Sciences at MFSS.

Patriot 17 Sept. 1970

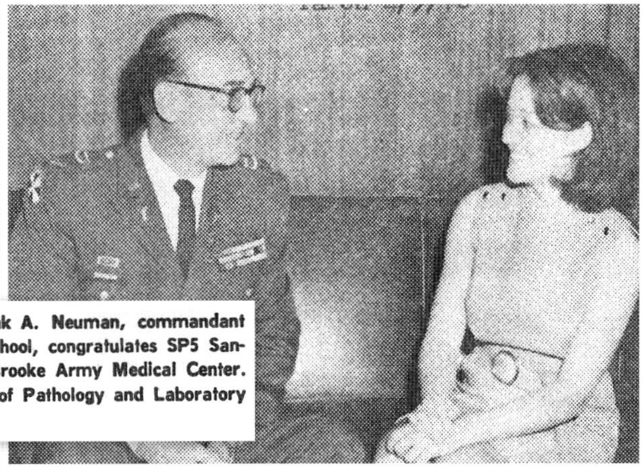

QUEEN CONGRATULATED — COL Frank A. Neuman, commandant of the U.S. Army Medical Field Service School, congratulates SP5 Sandra Chavez upon her being selected Miss Brooke Army Medical Center. SP5 Chavez is assigned to the Department of Pathology and Laboratory Sciences at the School.

Patriot April 30, 1970

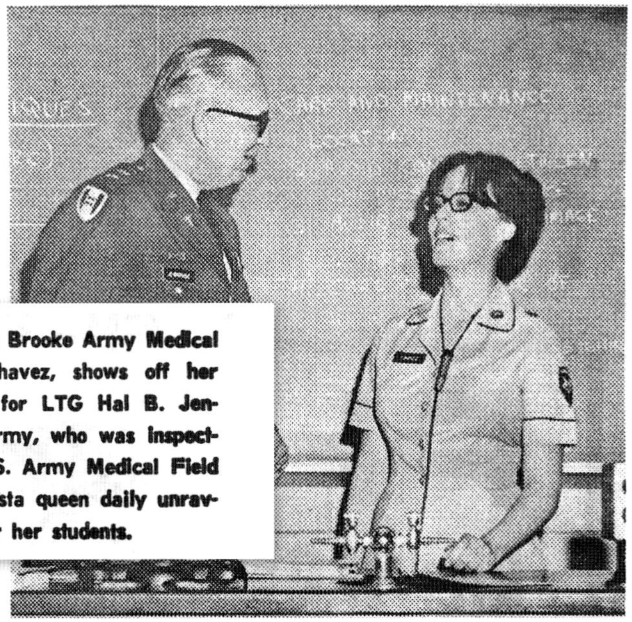

BEAUTY PLUS BRAINS — Miss Brooke Army Medical Center 1970, SP5 Sandra L. Chavez, shows off her knowledge of clinical chemistry for LTG Hal B. Jennings, Surgeon General of the Army, who was inspecting classroom facilities at the U.S. Army Medical Field Service School where BAMC's fiesta queen daily unravels the mysteries of chemistry for her students.

Miss BAMC 1970

While numerous MFSS women had won the title of Miss Brooke Army Medical Center over the years, Miss BAMC 1970, SP5 Sandra L. Chavez, an instructor of basic medical laboratory chemistry, was the first featured repeatedly in the Patriot as "Beauty Plus Brains."

("BAMC's Beauty Queen," Patriot, 17 Sept 1970; "Beauty Plus Brains," Patriot, 30 April 1970; "Queen Congratulated," Talon, 9 April 1970)

1971

In January 1971, the MFSS underwent a vast structural reorganization. Department, division, and battalion commanders, each responsible directly to the Commandant, Deputy Commandant, and Executive Officer, were organized into three major departments with specialized divisions. The reorganization streamlined the number of leaders reporting directly to the Commandant, provided them with better functional control, and eliminated overlapping responsibilities.

The first new department, the Department for Doctrine and Evaluation, incorporated newly-acquired Medical Department agencies, the Health Care Research Division, and the Medical Material Test and Evaluation Division, with the Training Literature Doctrinal Review Division (previously a part of the Department of Nonresident Instruction).

The second, the Directorate of Instruction, consisted of Medicine and Surgery, Pathology and Laboratory Sciences, Nonresident Instruction, Health Care Administration, Preventive Medicine, Educational Services, Mental Hygiene, Veterinary Sciences, Dental Science, Military Science, and Nursing Science.

These two departments were primarily responsible for the direct instruction of enlisted and officer students at the school.

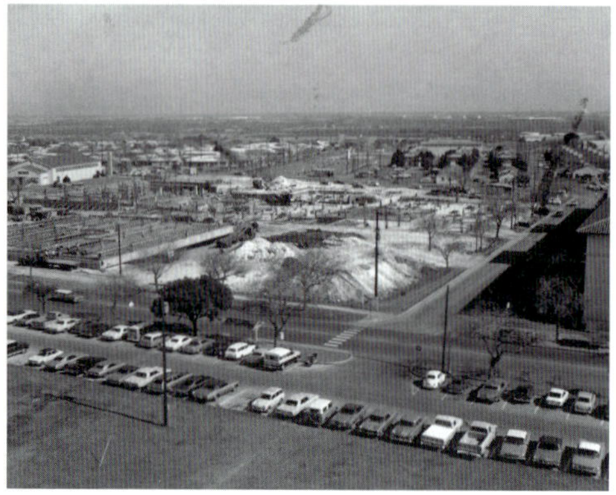

A view of the south side of the future Aabel Hall. The mound of dirt is the current location of Neel Plaza.

(U.S. Army Photo, AMEDD Museum Collection)

The east entrance of the future Willis Hall

(U.S. Army Photo, AMEDD Museum Collection)

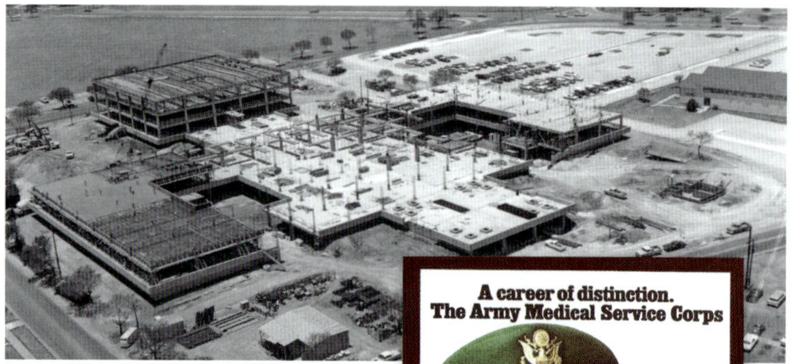

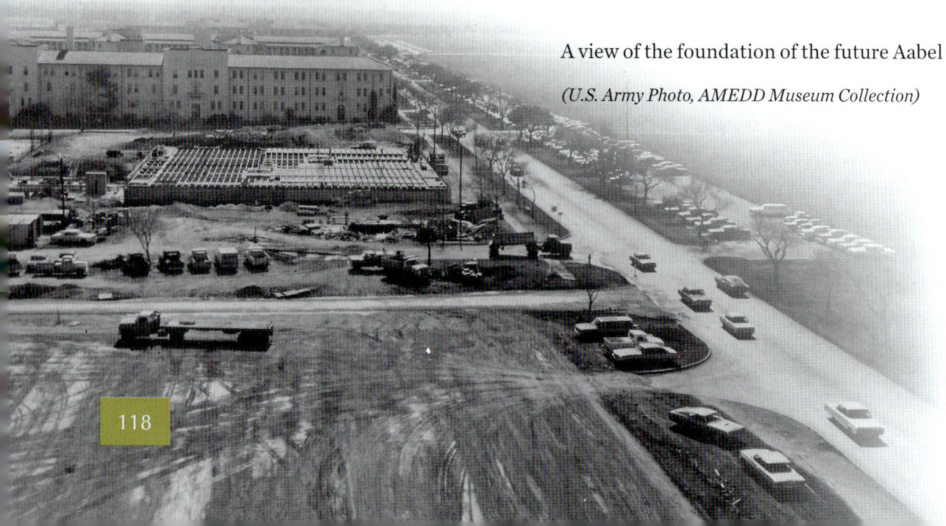

A view of the foundation of the future Aabel Hall.

(U.S. Army Photo, AMEDD Museum Collection)

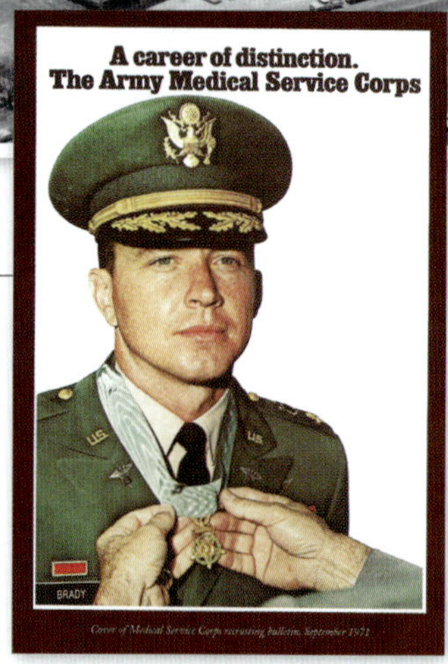

Medical Service Corps recruiting brochures featured a cover photo of Major Patrick H. Brady, MSC, receiving the Medal of Honor.

(AMEDD Museum, MSC Corps Collection)

The last department, the Support Services Department, included the Administration Division, Academic Operations Divisions, First Battalion (the cadre, 323d Army Band and enlisted), and the Second Battalion (officer students). Under the Administration Division were the Administrative and Classified Files Section, Mail and Distribution Section, Publications Section, Academic Records Section, Academic Records Branch, book store, library, museum, and Foreign Liaison and Protocol (formerly the Foreign Student Liaison Office). It also served as the liaison for the MFSS Officer's Open Mess and BAMC Headquarters elements such as the Management Division, Personnel Division, Public Affairs Office, and Legal Assistance.

(Patriot, 14 Jan 1971)

The Physician Assistant Branch was authorized and added to the Medicine and Surgery Division. The primary mission was to conduct the newly-designed Physician Assistant Course to provide warrant officers with a working knowledge of health care delivery techniques necessary to assist a medical officer. The initial screening for enlisted applicants for the new Physician Assistant Program began in October 1971.

("Physician Assistants Program: A new course at MFSS, A new job in the Army," Patriot, 21 Oct 1971)

The MFSS Physical Therapy Program was approved for a Master's Degree by Baylor University under the U.S. Army-Baylor University affiliation.

("Physical Therapy Course Gives Master's," Patriot, 26 Aug 1971)

In September 1971, all medical training of Special Forces Aidmen moved from Fort Bragg to the MFSS. The program, expanded from 10 to 13 weeks, consisted of six weeks of on-the-job training at various hospitals and seven weeks of advanced medical training at the MFSS. A number of changes were made to increase the clinical emphasis of the course.

("Green Berets Train at MFSS," Patriot, 9 Sept 1971)

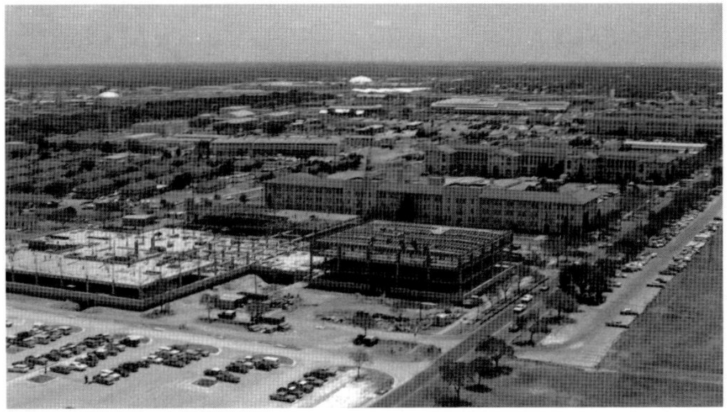

Construction at about 40% complete

(U.S. Army Photo, AMEDD Museum Collection)

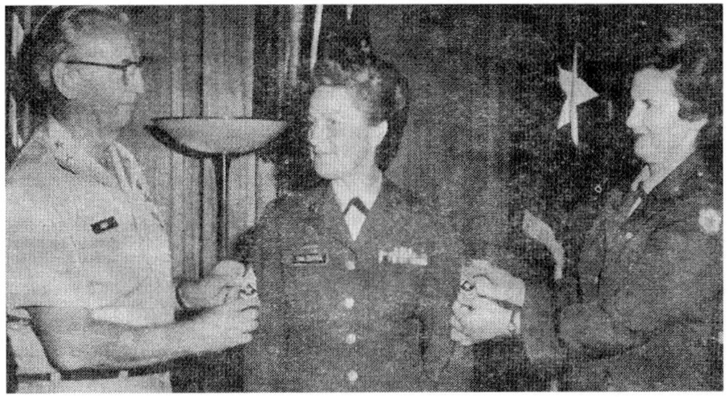

SGM Veva R. Halouska, assigned to the MFSS, became the first Women's Army Corps member in the San Antonio area to be promoted to the rank of SGM. SGM Halouska was the first woman test writer for the AMEDD, writing the annual test for all skill levels of dental assistants in the Army. Concurrent with her promotion, she was named Chief of the Military Occupational Specialty Test and Special Review Branch of the Department, becoming the first woman to hold this position.

("New Sergeant Major is a Lady," Patriot, 25 March 1971)

1972

In February 1972, the MFSS began its first Physician Assistant course.

The Army began giving maximum bonuses for re-enlisting in military occupational specialties (MOSs) with critical shortages. Military newspapers in 1972 featured images and amounts that service members received with the maximum re-enlistment bonus of $10,000 for re-enlisting for six years.

Coinciding with the Equal Employment Opportunity Act of 1972, MG Kenneth D. Orr appointed the first Equal Opportunity Officers (EOO) and Equal Employment Opportunity (EEO) Officers to BAMC. The two officers were assigned to ensure the fair and equal treatment and opportunity for all military and civilian personnel without regard to race, religion, sex or national origin.

("EEO, EOO Officers Named for BAMC," Patriot, 20 April 1972)

On 10 Dec 1972, administration building B-2840 and the primary academic building B-2241 of the MFSS were named in honor of COL Bernard Aabel, Medical Service Corps, and Major General John M. Willis, Medical Corps. During the building dedication, the Secretary of the Army, Robert F. Froehlke, announced that the MFSS name had been officially changed to the Academy of Health Sciences (AHS).

Constructed of reinforced concrete with precast native quartzite exterior panels, the 400,000 gross square foot complex cost some $11 million. Built by the Browning Construction Company, a locally based organization, the school was designed to house 48 classrooms with a seating capacity of 3,000.

("Modern New School Blends with Historical Buildings," Patriot, 10 Dec 1972)

MG Willis

A veteran of WWI, MG Willis commanded the MFSS from 1924-1934, developing the School into one of the most important agencies for the training of medical officers. He returned to the MFSS for two more years in 1938 and commanded the Camp Grant Medical Replacement Training Center during WWII. He was the first general officer to command BAMC in 1946. He retired from the Army in 1948.

("Surrounded by History," FSH Museum Publication, pp 41-42)

10 Dec 1972 Dedication Ceremonies Program cover

(Stimson Library Special Collections)

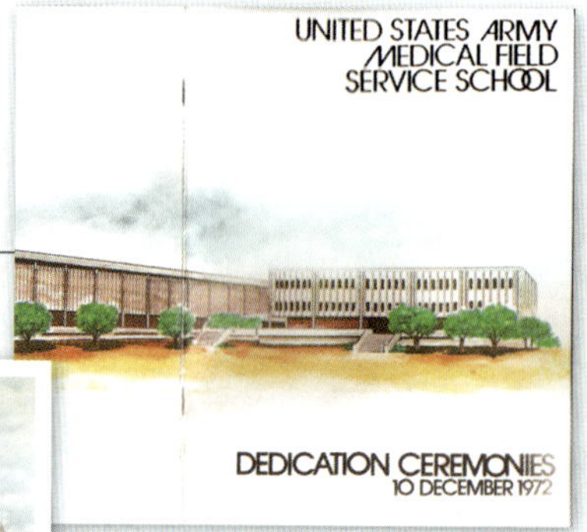

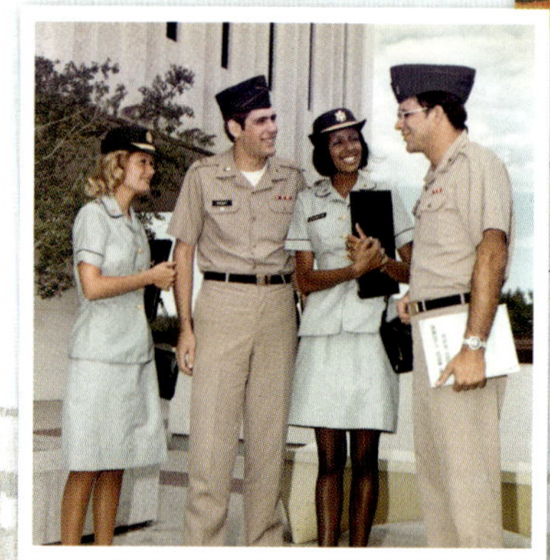

Photo taken for a Nurse Corps recruiting brochure in front of Aabel Hall, circa 1972.

(U.S. Army Photo, AMEDD Museum Photo Collection)

COL Aabel

Served through five campaigns in the European Theatre during WWII and was wounded in action. During the Korean War, he was Deputy Commanding Officer of the Medical Replacement Training Center, Camp Pickett. His service included duty with the Surgeon General's Office, as the Military Attaché to Finland and as Chief, MSC.

("Surrounded by History," FSH Museum Publication, pp 41-42)

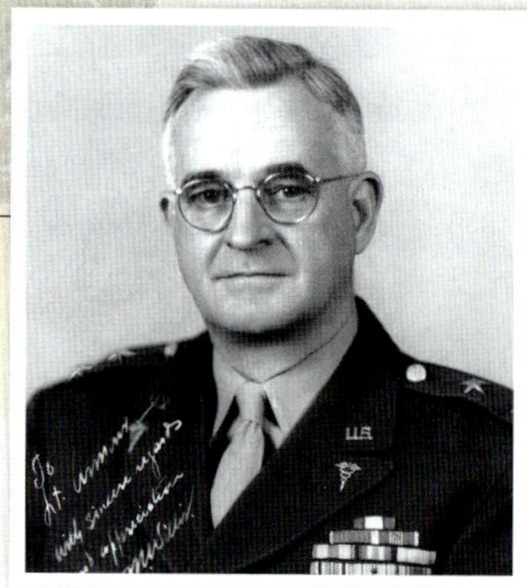

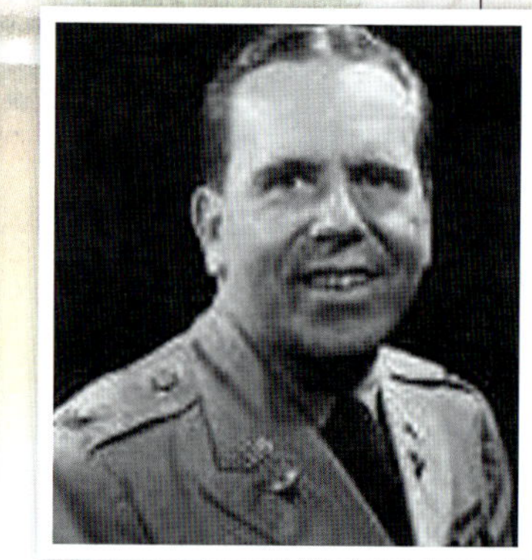

In October 1972, the MFSS conducted a two-week drug and alcohol education course, developed and funded by the DoD, for personnel involved in the Post alcohol and drug abuse program. The course was in response to the thousands of service members who returned from Vietnam with substance abuse problems.

("MFSS Fights Drug Abuse," Patriot, 5 Oct 1972)

The Army's first woman pharmacist, 2LT Verena A. M. Haynes, Army Medical Department, attended the Basic Course at the MFSS.

("First to Go," Patriot, 10 Aug 1972)

Everette R. Calloway, a Health Department sanitarian from Cabarrus County, N.C., became the first civilian to attend the Preventive Medicine Procedures Basic Course at the MFSS.

("Civilian Attends MFSS," Patriot, 7 Sept 1972)

Mrs. Alma Withrow, a civilian employee of the Andrew Rader Clinic at Fort Myer, VA, became the first woman and first civilian to attend the Patient Administration Course.

("Friends Meet Again in MFSS Classroom," Patriot, 5 Oct 1972)

More than 13,000 students were enrolled in correspondence courses through the Nonresident Instruction Division (NRI) of the MFSS. The correspondence courses were designed to make it possible for active duty personnel who were unable to attend resident courses at the MFSS to improve their military proficiency and potential by mail. Student enrollment had increased by 3,000 since 1969.

("Correspondence Courses Available at MFSS," Patriot, 10 Dec 1972)

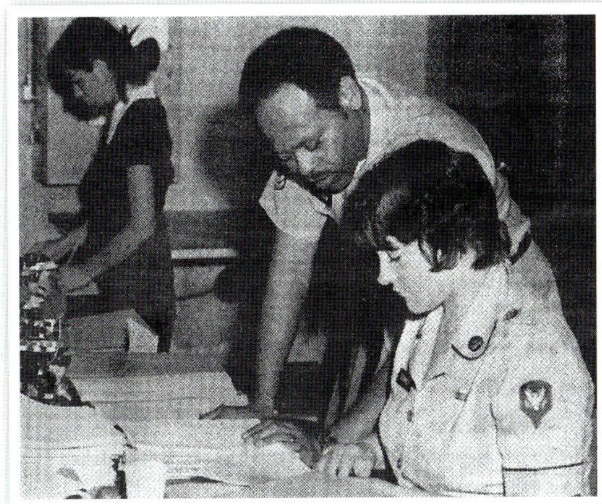

SFC John Clayton and SP4 Diane Schmidt work together to get instructional materials packed and sent at MFSS NRI. The mailroom handled some 200,000 separate pieces of material each month.

("Correspondence Courses Available at MFSS," Patriot, 10 Dec 1972)

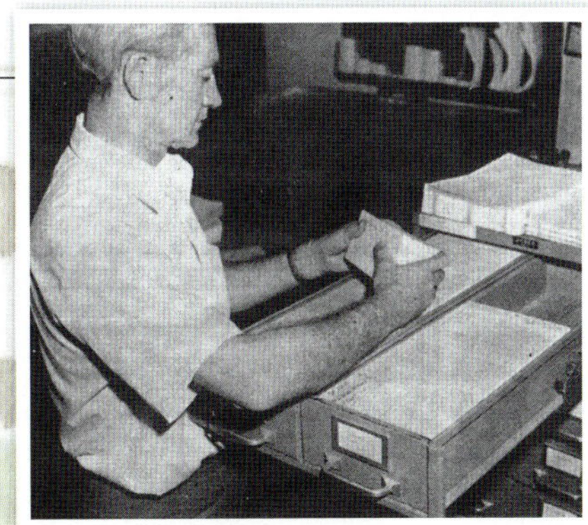

With MFSS NRI Division's enrollment hovering around 13,000 students, and with each student completing several lessons a week, NRI was faced with the mammoth task of correcting all the student's tests. An optical mark scoring reader does the job. Rudy Ochoa runs a handful of student answer sheets through the grader quickly and easily.

("Correspondence Courses Available at MFSS," Patriot, 10 Dec 1972)

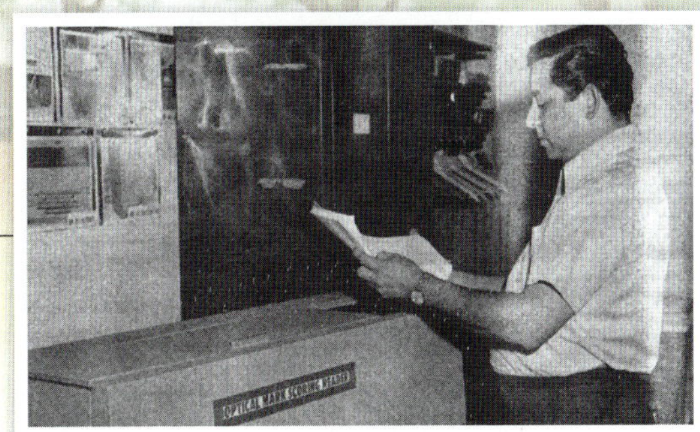

Every new student had a card and number, and someone at MSFF NRI Division kept track of the card. J.E. McElvy handled that work, filing the new enrollment cards as they were printed.

("Correspondence Courses Available at MFSS," Patriot, 10 Dec 1972)

1973

The reorganization of all Army medical activities was announced 11 Jan 1973, creating the U.S. Army Health Services Command (HSC). The Command was activated on 1 April 1973 and became fully operational on 1 July 1973. The Academy of Health Sciences (AHS) became a subordinate unit of the HSC.

The new Academy of Health Sciences incorporated all existing MFSS training and supervised all medical training previously conducted under the U.S. Army Medical Training Center (MTC) for enlisted medics, the Walter Reed Army Institute of Nursing, the U.S. Army Veterinarian School and the training mission of the Medical Optical and Maintenance Agency. The MTC formally deactivated and officially became part of the Academy of Health Sciences on 1 July 1973. The U.S. Army Medical Materiel Agency was also assigned to the AHS.

(General Orders Number 9, 8, 14 and 12, 1 Feb 1973.)

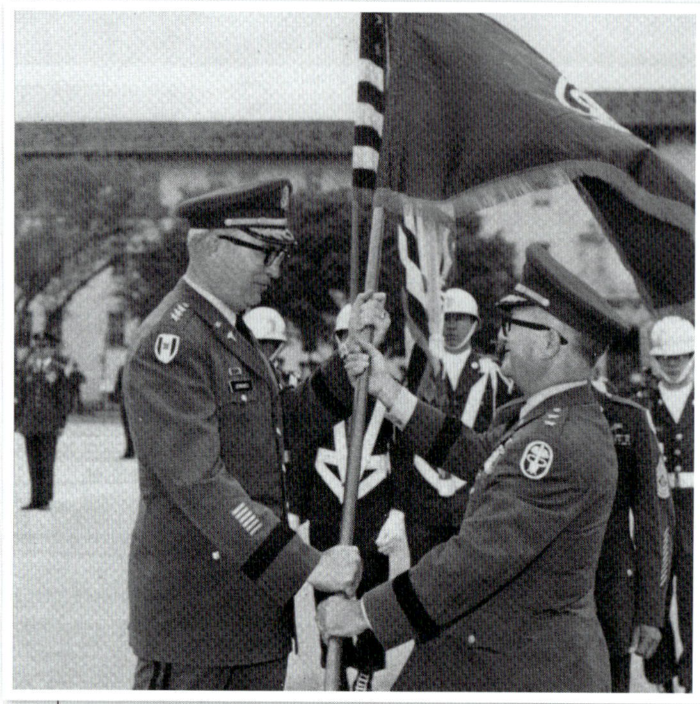

LTG Hal B. Jennings hands the command colors of the U.S. Army Health Services Command to MG Spurgeon Neel.

(U.S. Army Photo)

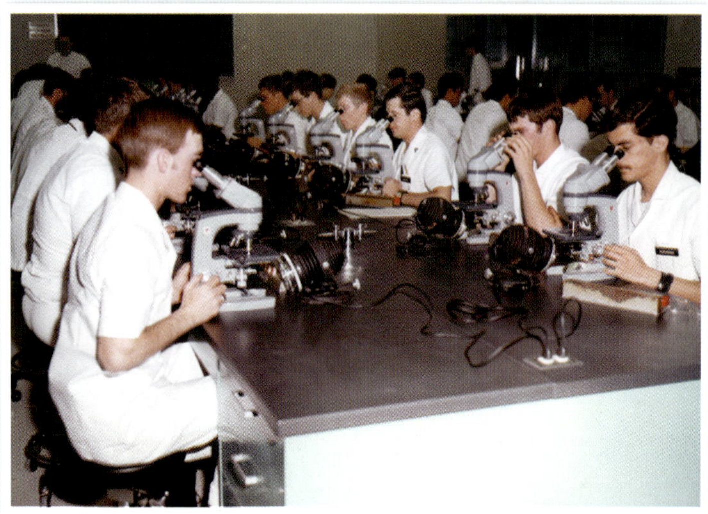

Students study parasitology in the Pathology and Laboratory Sciences Department.

(U.S. Army Photo, AMEDD Museum Photo Collection)

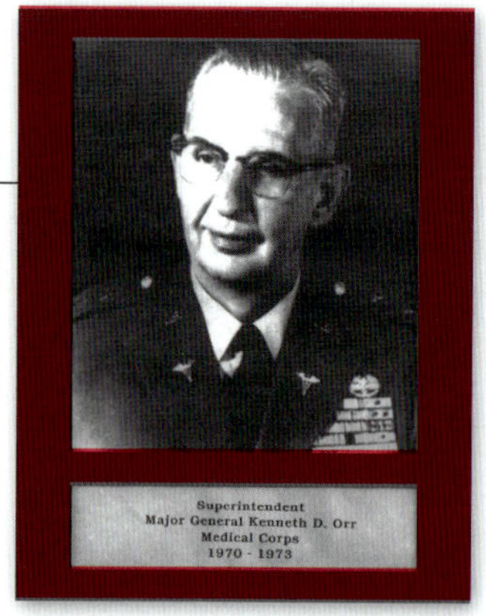

MG Kenneth Orr, former Commander of BAMC and first Superintendent of the AHS, retired on 30 June 1973.

(U.S. Army Photo, AMEDDC&S History Office files)

The Academy of Health Sciences completed the majority of moving operations into the new building complex of Willis and Aabel Halls in early January 1973. The first class to open in the new building was the Army Medical Department Noncommissioned Officer Course on 9 Jan 1973.

The first class of the Physician Assistant Course completed its didactic training at the Academy on 7 Feb 1973. After completion of Phase III clinical training at 14 outlying Army hospitals, the class returned to the school for graduation on 10 Aug 1973. The graduates were given Associates of Science degrees from Baylor University and appointed to the rank of warrant officer. The Physician Assistant Course was accredited by the American Medical Association (AMA) at its June 1973 meeting of the AMA Council on Medical Education.

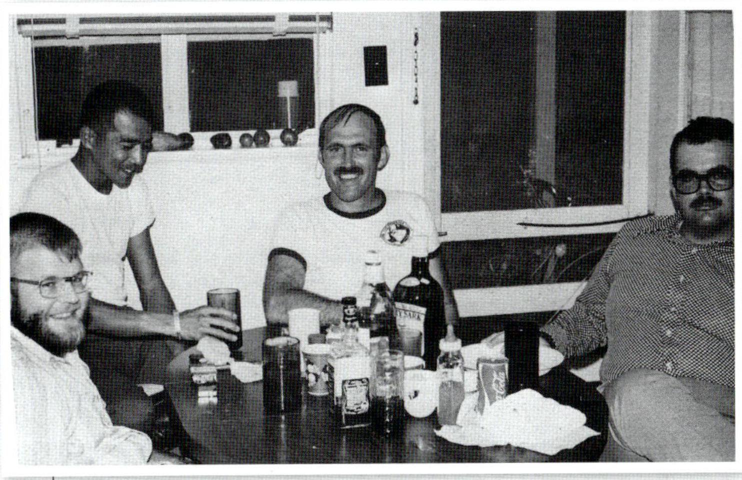

The first class of the Physician Assistant Course produced their own yearbook. The images suggest they earned bartending degrees along with Associates of Science.

(The First Physician Assistant Course Year, Stimson Library Special Collections)

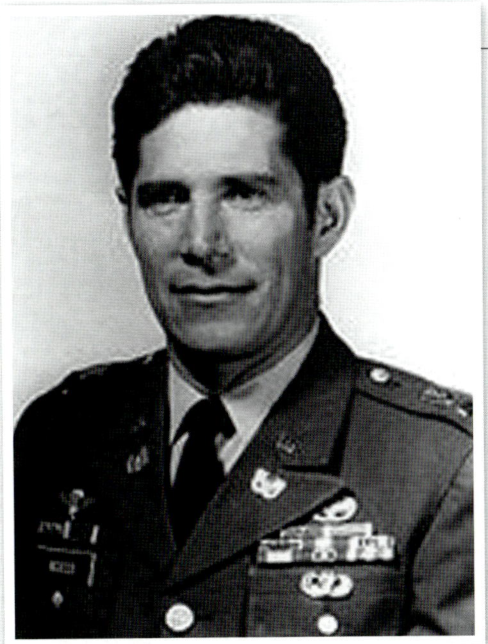

Louis R. Rocco, Medal of Honor recipient, was among the first class of Physician Assistants

(U.S. Army Photo)

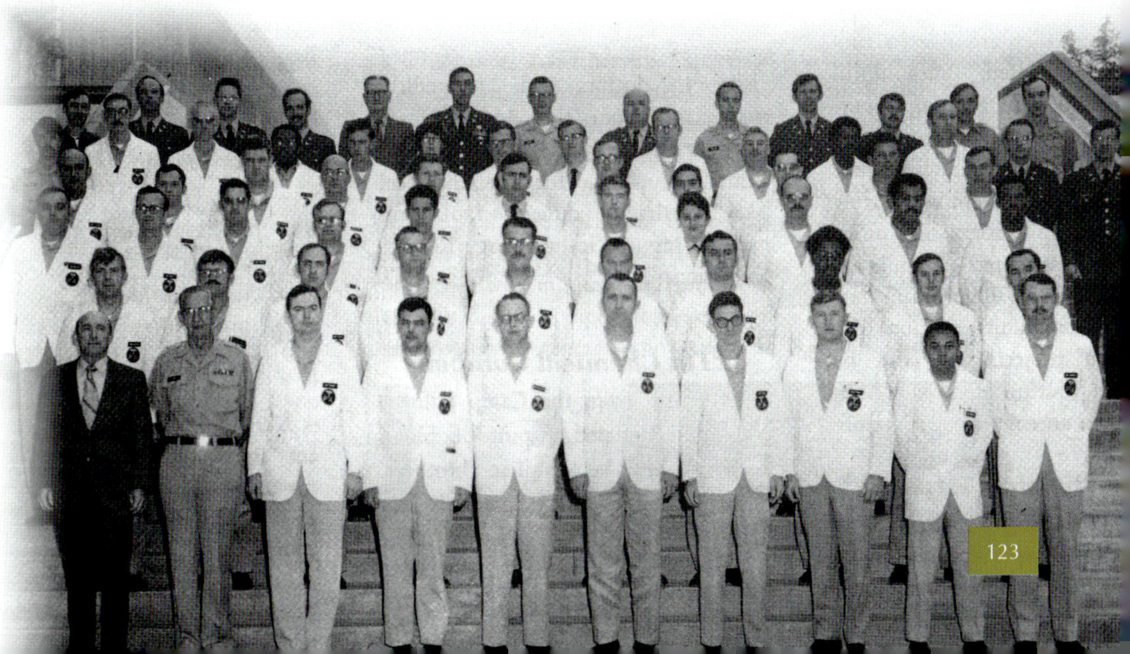

Warrant officer candidates attending the first class of the Physician Assistant Course pose along with staff and faculty members. The photo appears to have been taken on the northern steps of the causeway between Willis and Aabel Halls.

(U.S. Army Photo, AMEDDC&S History Office files)

1973

Enlisted students were first awarded an Associate of Science degree through the Academy of Health Sciences – Baylor University Enlisted Undergraduate Program in June 1973. Thirteen students were awarded the degree after completing a 50-week Advanced Medical Laboratory Procedures Course. This was the first occasion for civilian recognition of education received by enlisted service members at a military educational facility.

The Academy of Health Sciences Chapel was dedicated 26 Aug 1973. In attendance were the Superintendent, BG Edward Vogel Jr., and the Army Chief of Chaplains, MG Gerhardt Hyatt.

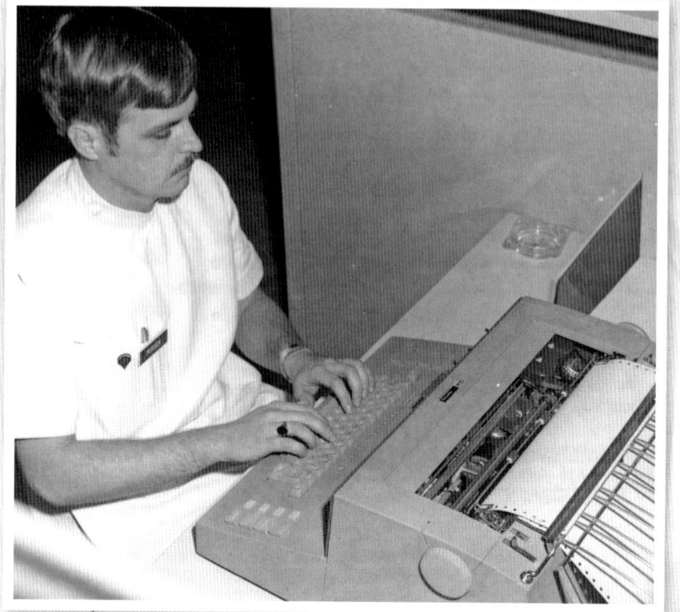

SP5 Persen navigates for information on a computer in the Learning Resources Library.

(U.S. Army Photo, AMEDD Museum Photo Collection)

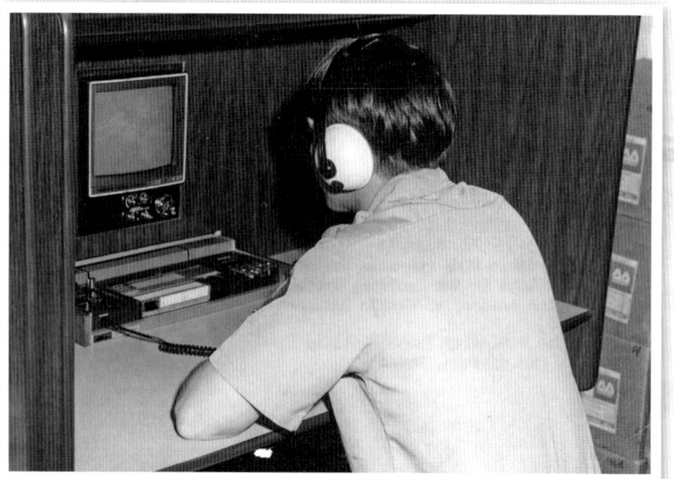

The Learning Resources Laboratory at AHS encouraged students to view instructional videos.

(U.S. Army Photo, AMEDD Museum Photo Collection)

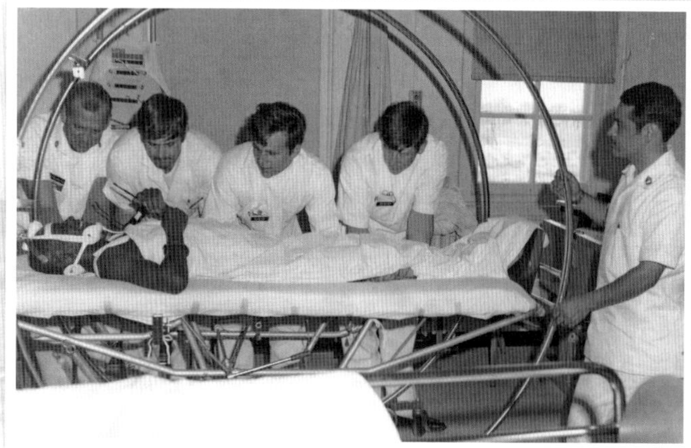

Instructors and students in the Clinical Specialist Course transfer a patient from a modified Stryker bed to a CircOlectric bed.

(U.S. Army Photo, AMEDD Museum Photo Collection)

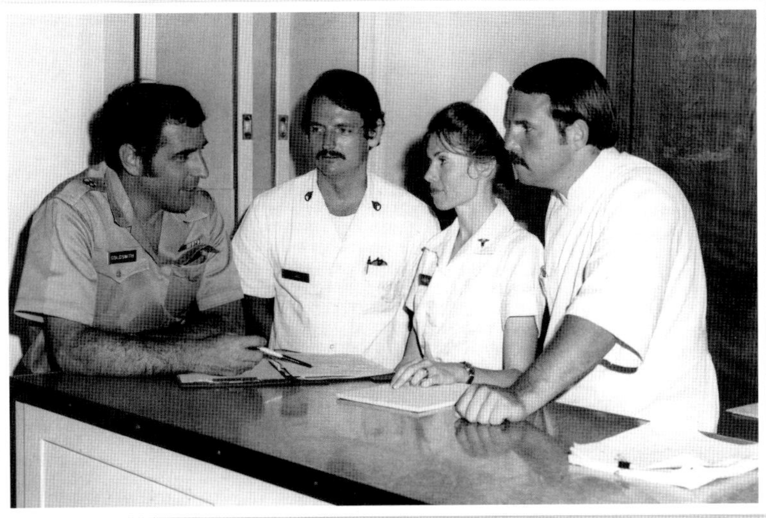

Members of the 143d Evacuation Hospital of Santa Monica, California. The National Guard unit was one of many to receive its annual summer training through the AHS and BAMC in 1973.

(U.S. Army Photo, AMEDD Museum Photo Collection)

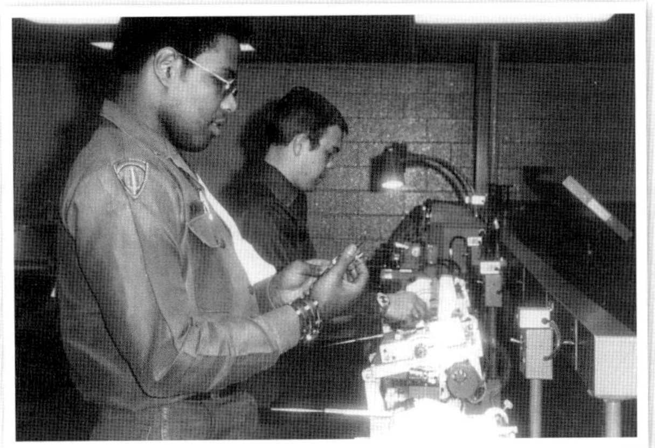

An Optical Fabrication Specialist (42E) hard at work.

(U.S. Army Photo, AMEDD Museum Photo Collection)

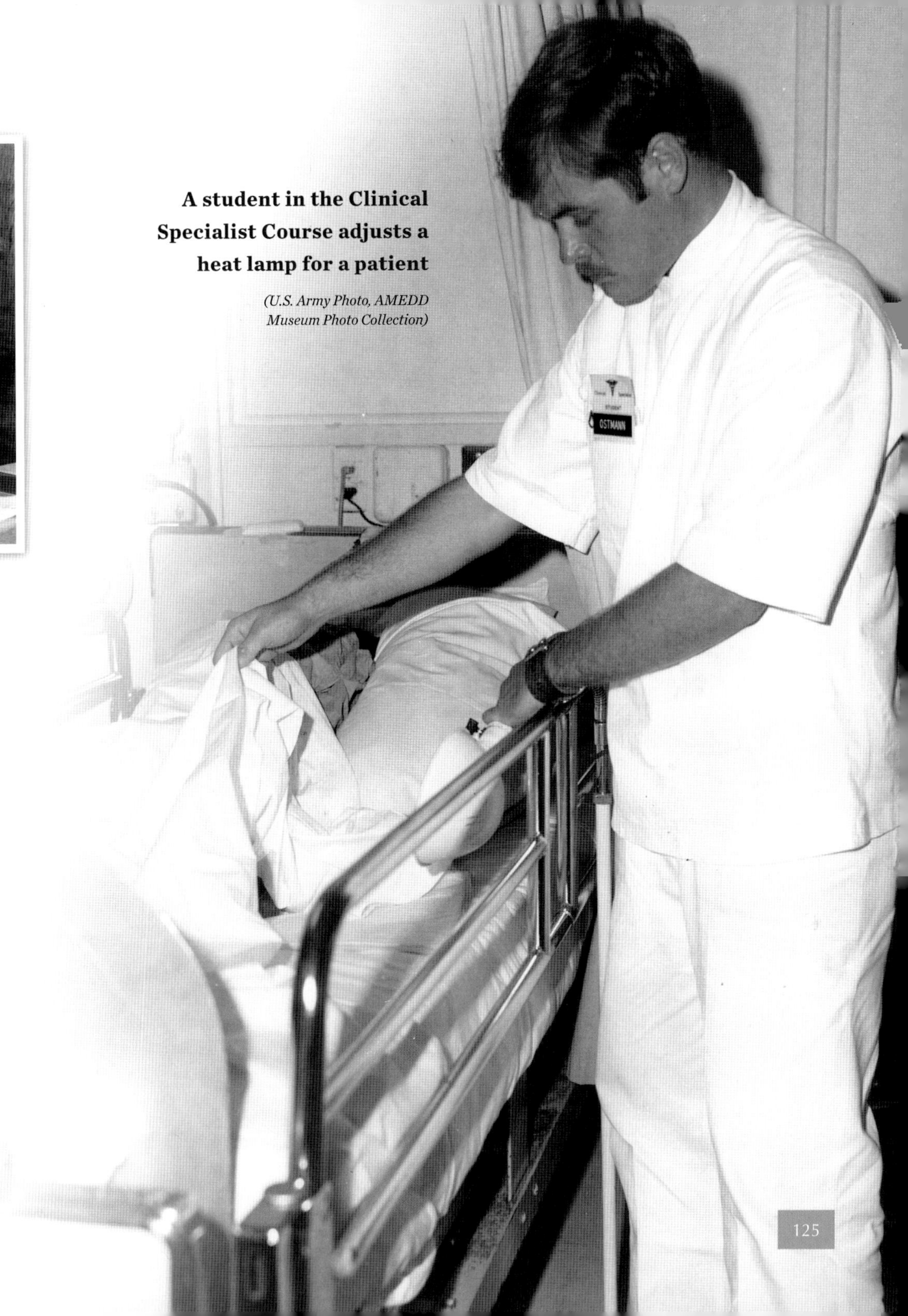

A student in the Clinical Specialist Course adjusts a heat lamp for a patient

(U.S. Army Photo, AMEDD Museum Photo Collection)

1974

The Occupational Therapy Specialist Program, in partnership with Baylor University, received approval for accreditation on 14 Jan 1974.

(AHS, CY 74, Annual Historical Review (AHR), p 13)

The AHS was accepted for membership into the Association of Schools of Allied Health Professionals, joining the ranks of higher education institutions such as Harvard, Yale, and Columbia University. The ASAHP is a not-for-profit association chartered in 1967 in response to an urgent need for an interdisciplinary and interagency association to improve the quality and quantity of the workforce in health occupations and professions.

("Academy Enters School Association," Patriot, 24 Jan 1974)

AHS observed Black History Week from 10 to 16 February. This appears to be the first AHS observance of Black History Week.

("BAMC and Academy Observe Black History Week," Patriot, 7 Feb 1974)

BAMC held a memorial service for the late Rev. Martin Luther King, Jr., at the AHS Chapel.

("BAMC Holds Memorial Services for Rev. King," Patriot, 24 Jan 1974)

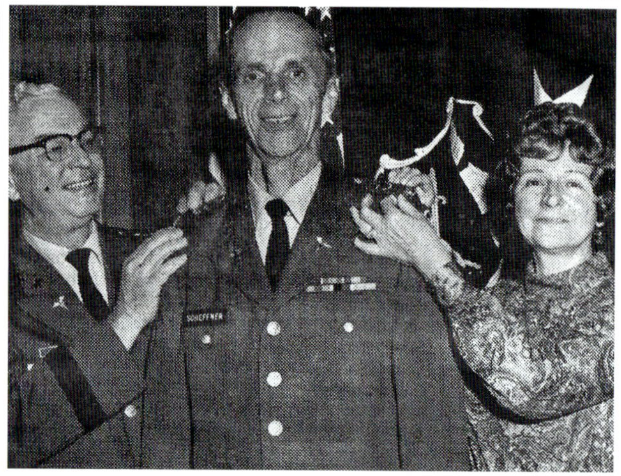

First Male Nurse Corps Colonel
COL Lawrence Sheffner, Organization Division at the AHS, becomes the Nurse Corps' first male colonel in April 1974.

("Nurse Corps Gets First Male Colonel," Patriot, 11 April 1974)

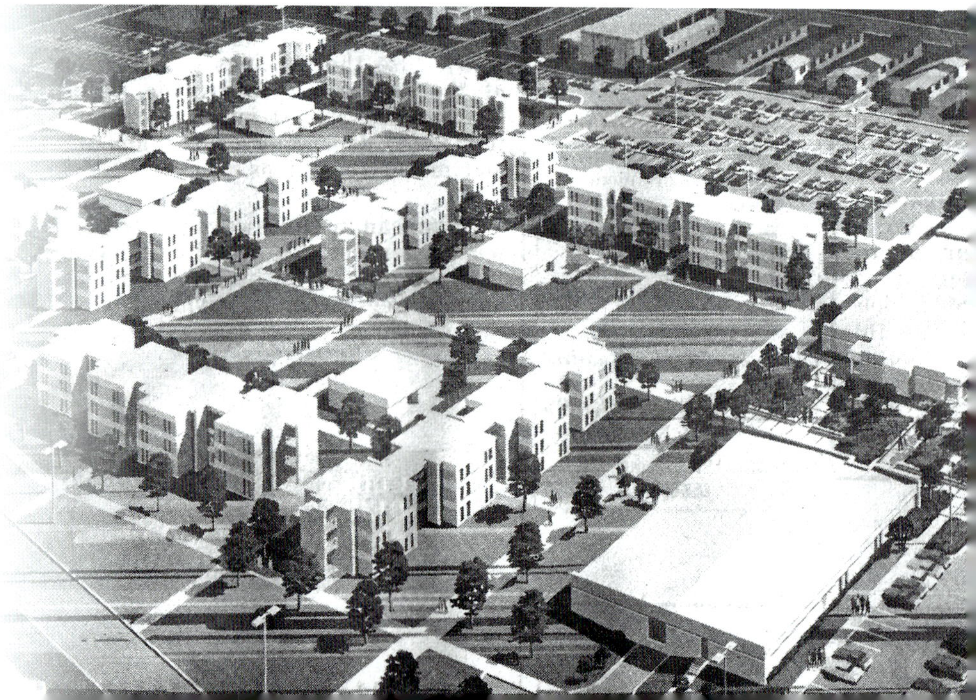

Construction on the $8.5 million enlisted barracks complex behind the AHS began in August 1974

("Barracks Complex Announced," News Leader, 25 July 1974)

The 323rd Army Band was officially assigned its first female band members. PVT Tanya Schroeder, clarinet; SP4 Sheryl A. Johnson, tuba; and PFC Frances San Soucie, flute, received their official orders within hours of one another. SP4 Johnson and PFC San Soucie had been playing with the band since the beginning of the year. The impact of the women's presence in the band was minimal — the only change behind the scenes, according to the Bandmaster, was that the men had to tone down their language somewhat.

("AHS Band Goes Coed," Military Science News, 31 May 1974)

In July of 1974, the Combat Development and Health Care Studies (CDHCS) activity was reorganized as a result of a direct manpower reduction. The resulting reorganization combined the Materials Division and Organization into the Organization & Material Division.

(Army Medical Activities Report for the AHS, CY 74, AHR, p 5)

Also on 1 July 1974, the Women's Army Corps (WAC) ceased to exist. All officers formerly assigned to the WAC were reassigned to a number of other branches on that date. The change of corps increased the number and type of assignment available to female officers.

("Women's Officer Corps Ceases to Exist," Patriot, 1 July 1974)

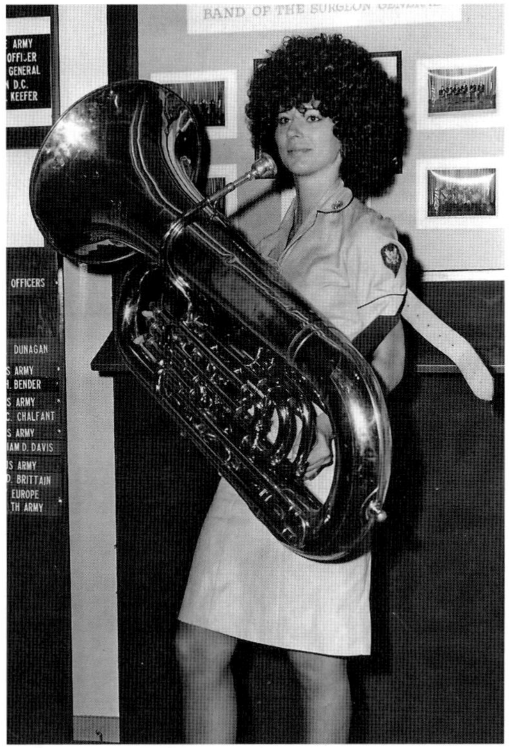

Tuba
SP4 Sheryl A. Johnson with her tuba. "Privates San Soucie and Schroeder do get suspicious of a man's real intentions when he asks to carry either the clarinet or flute for them, while Specialist Johnson says not too many offer to carry her tuba."

("Girls in the Band," typewritten article, 21 June 1974, Stimson Library Special Collections)

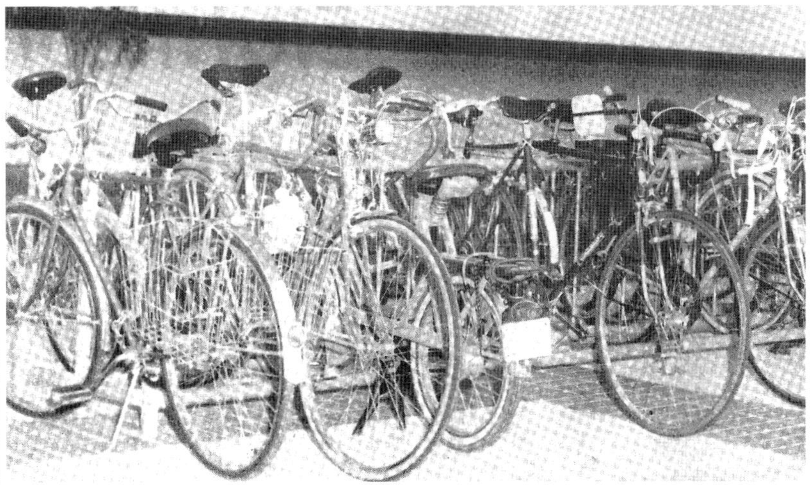

Rising price of gas prompts creative transportation
The price of gas drives AHS employees to develop a carpooling system. About 135 persons opted to participate in the program.

("AHS Personnel Participate in Fifty Carpools," Mil Service News, 3 March 1974)

1974

Effective 5 Sept 1974, the Basic Health Services branches were transferred from the Medicine and Surgery Division, Military Science Division, and the Nursing Science Division to the Basic Health Services Division.

(Army Medical Activities Report for the AHS, CY 74, AHR, p 5)

In November 1974, the functions of the AMEDD Veterinary School were transferred from Fort Sheridan, Illinois, to the Academy at Fort Sam Houston.

(Army Medical Activities Report for the AHS, CY 74, AHR, p 5)

The AHS Race Relations Council was formed to advise the Superintendent on matters of policy and procedure in the area of equal opportunity and race relations.

("BAMC and Academy Observe Black History Week," Patriot, 7 Feb 1974)

The Education Branch of the Equal Opportunity Office held its first Race Relations Seminar. By December 1974, 99% of all military and civilian personnel assigned to the AHS had attended 15 to 18 hours of mandatory Race Relations Education sponsored by the Equal Opportunity Office.

(Army Medical Activities Report for the AHS, CY 74, AHR, p 13)

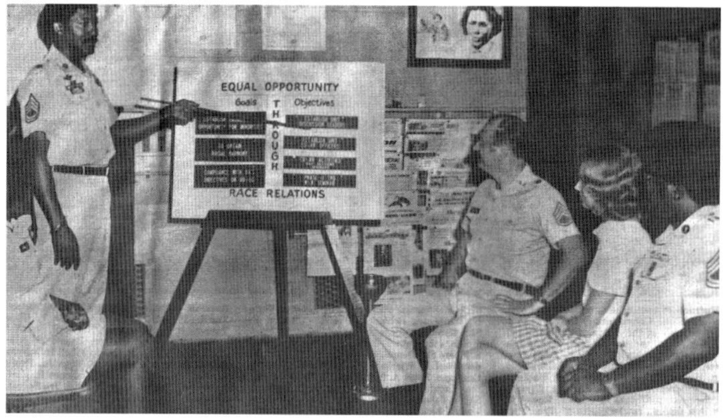

A Minority Information Culture Center was established in January 1974. The Center contained a collection of "race-related items: a Puerto Rican flag; African Liberation Movement flag; slave bracelets; a clenched fist; calendars featuring biographies of outstanding Blacks, Mexican-Americans, Puerto Ricans, and American Indians; a Quran; books on minorities; and literature on minority colleges."

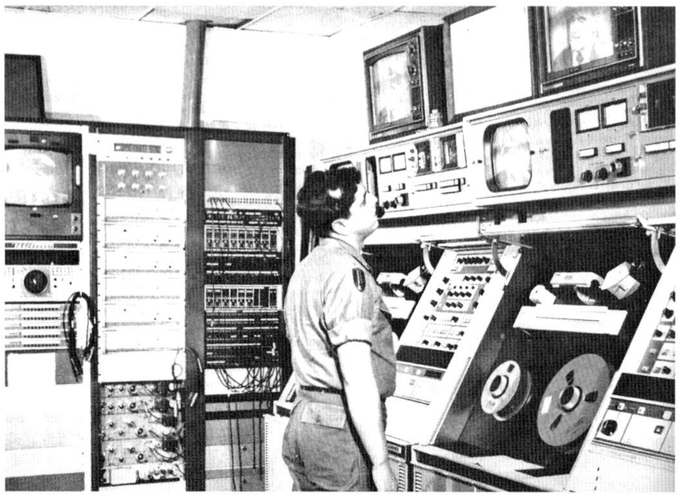

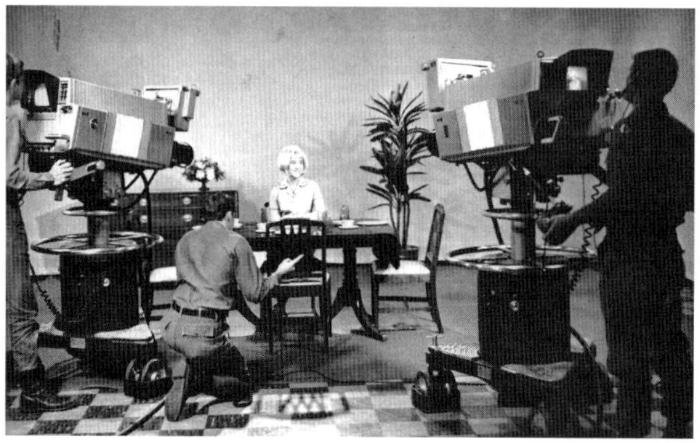

CPT Diana Barefoot, MSC dietician, discusses diet therapy for patients with renal disease for a "Continuing Medical Education" episode at the AHS Television studio.

("TV–Way to Go," Suzanne Ward, AMEDD Spectrum, Vol 1 No. 1, 1974, pp 48-53)

AVR-1 Ampex Quadraplex television recorders used by the AHS Television Studio in 1974

("TV–Way to Go," Suzanne Ward, AMEDD Spectrum, Vol 1 No. 1, 1974, pp 48-53)

The Academy of Health Sciences Television Division rivaled any major commercial TV station in equipment and expertise. It produced hundreds of instructional video TV programs each year. In 1974, it had a library with 900 master videotapes and loaned copies of its library contents world-wide. Its productions on the closed circuit system received an average of 290,000 views per year in the early 1970s. It had a complete production facility on wheels, a 30-foot van that toured the country wherever AMEDD news was being made.

("TV: Way To Go," Suzanne Ward, AMEDD Spectrum, Vol 1 No 1, 1974, pp 48-53)

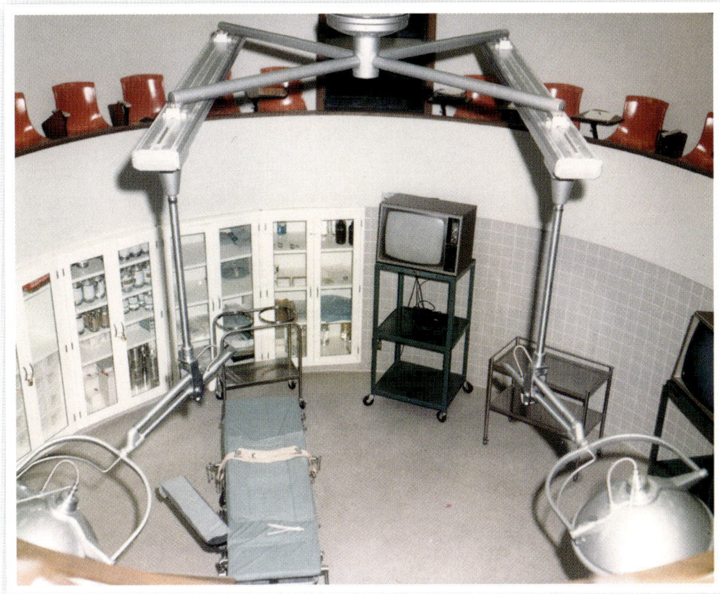

The Amphitheater, a mock operating room, at the AHS

(U.S. Army Photo, AMEDD Museum Photo Collection)

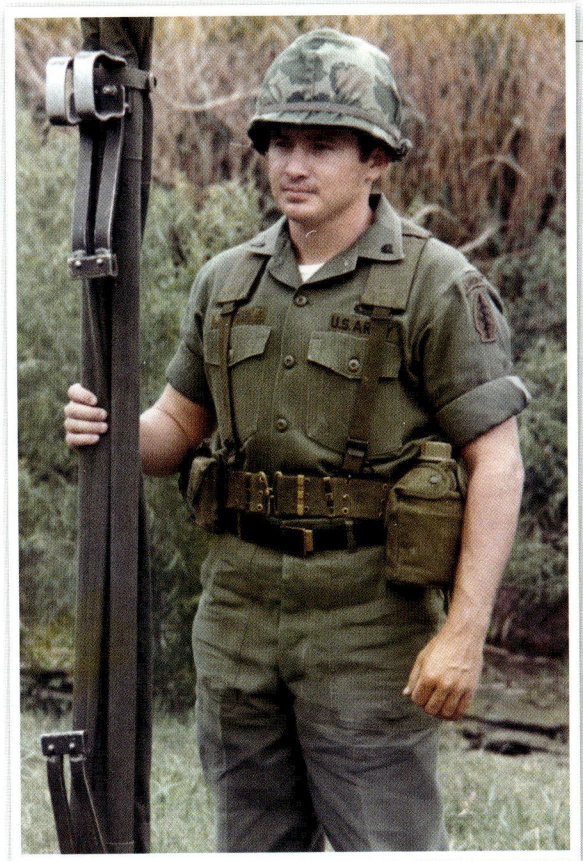

SP4 Sam Snyder
1st Battalion, Academy Brigade, demonstrates a litter carry.

(U.S. Army Photo, AMEDD Museum Photo Collection)

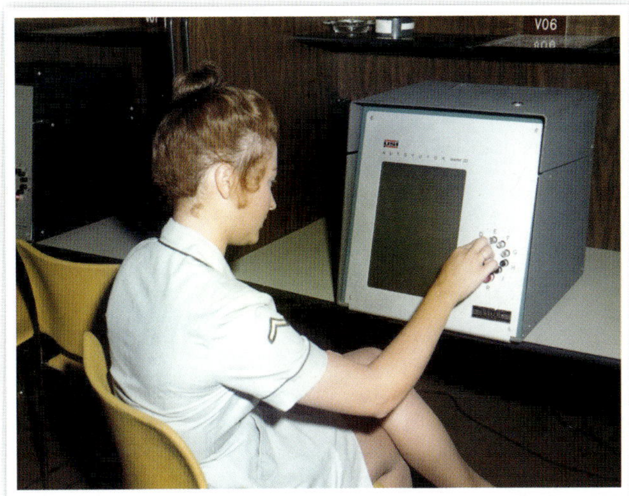

PVT Carol Strauss views a programmed instruction on a 35mm Autotutor at the Learning Resources Lab at the AHS.

(U.S. Army Photo, AMEDD Museum Photo Collection)

1974

Blesse Auditorium, 1974

(U.S. Army Photo, AMEDD Museum Photo Collection)

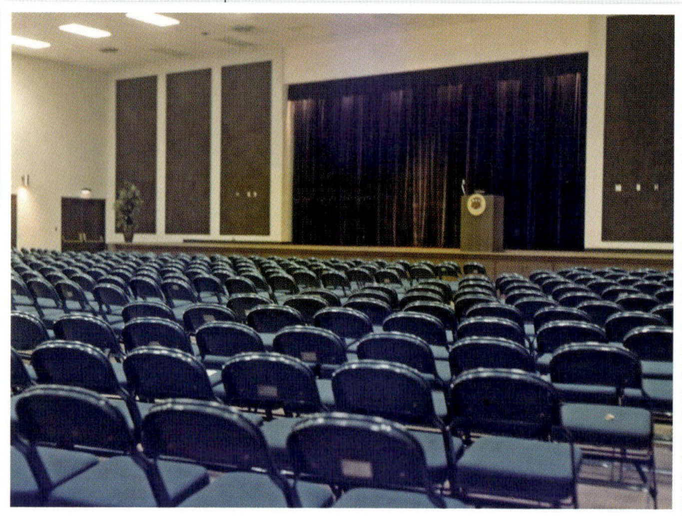

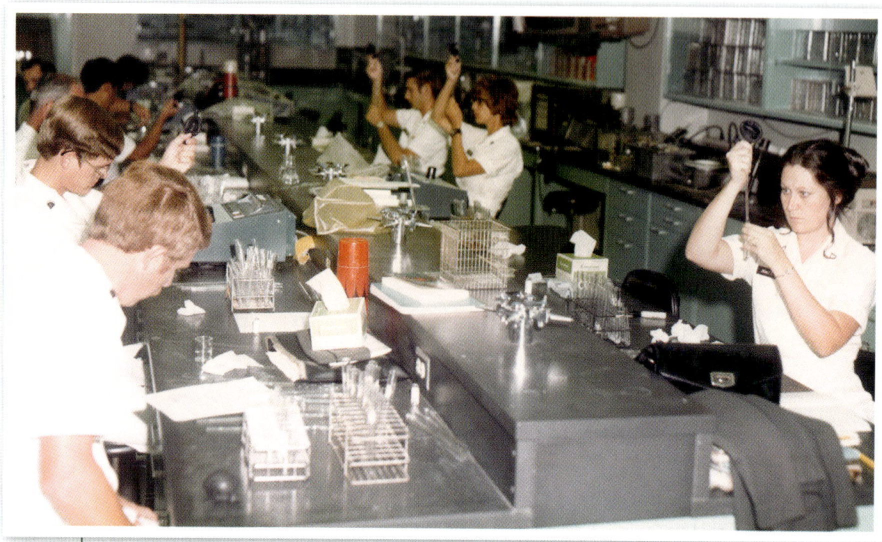

Advanced Medical Laboratory (92B30) students work in a chemistry lab in the AHS.

(U.S. Army Photo, AMEDD Museum Photo Collection)

Eye, Ear, Nose and Throat Specialist (91U20) students in the lab.

(U.S. Army Photo, AMEDD Museum Photo Collection)

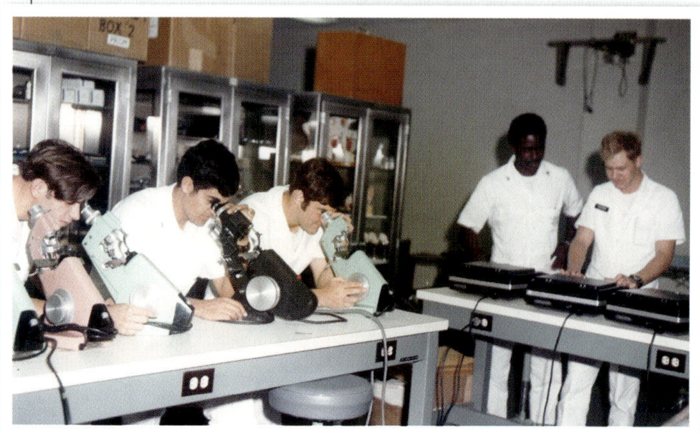

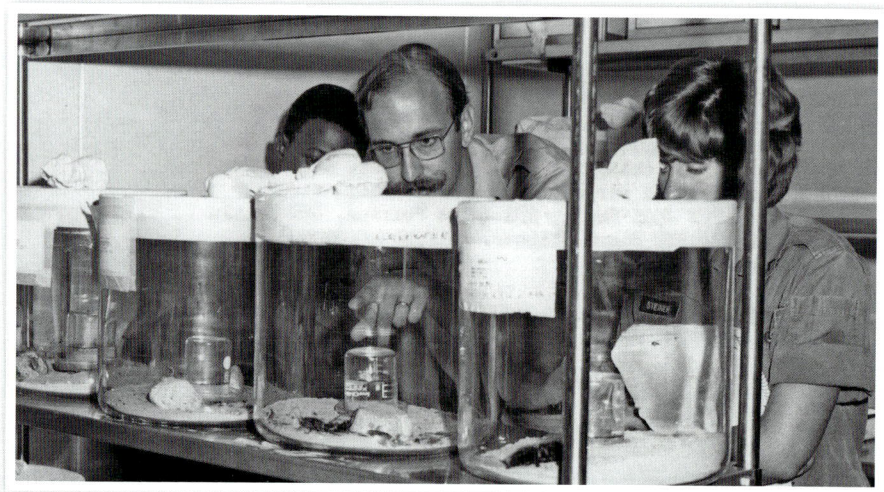

Students view spiders in the Entomology Department.

(U.S. Army Photo, AMEDD Museum Photo Collection)

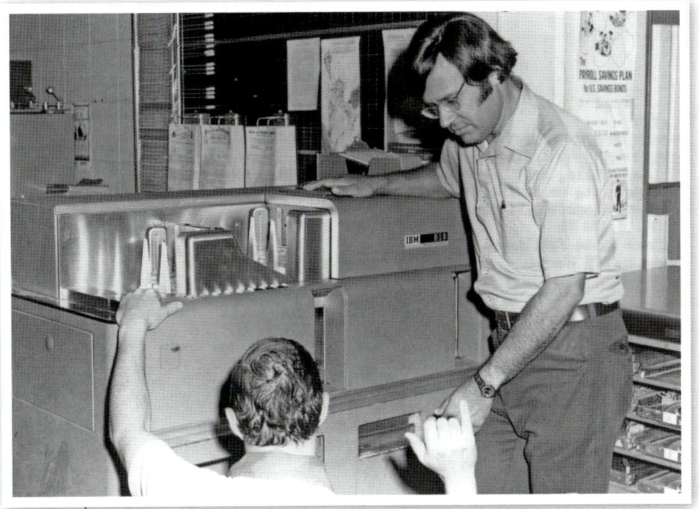

The IBM Reproducer allowed instructors to make instant copies of instructional materials.

(U.S. Army Photo, AMEDD Museum Photo Collection)

A spinal column in the Anatomy Lab is shown to attendees at the Army Midwest Regional Recruiting Nurse Team conference at the AHS.

(U.S. Army Photo, AMEDD Museum Photo Collection)

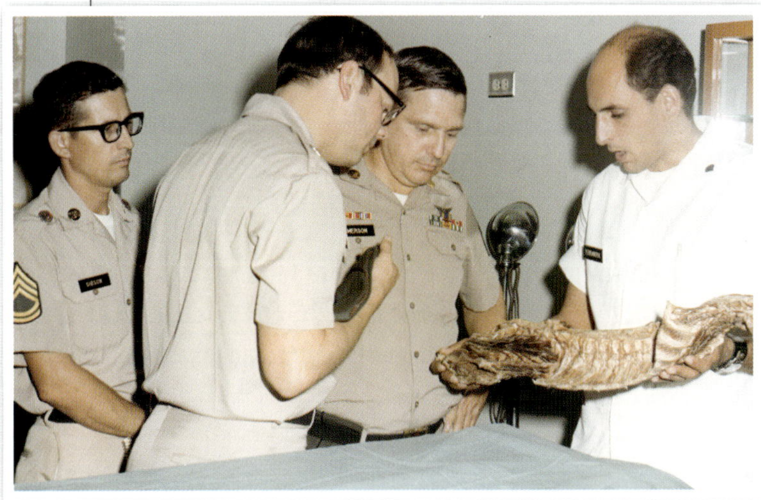

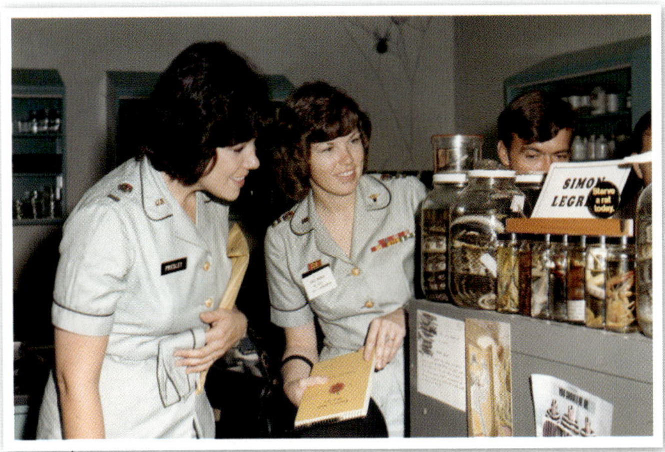

Nurses view the snake and insect specimens in the Entomology Lab during the Army Midwest Regional Recruiting Nurse Team conference at the AHS.

(U.S. Army Photo, AMEDD Museum Photo Collection)

A blood washing demonstration is checked

(U.S. Army Photo, AMEDD Museum Photo Collection)

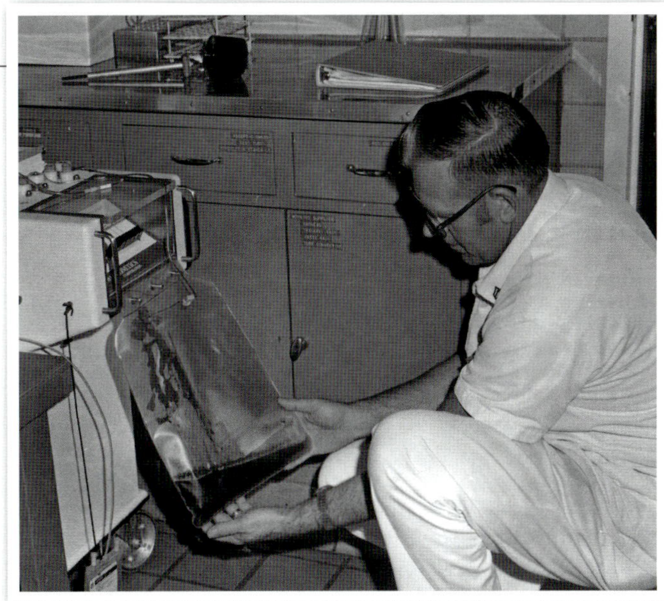

1975

In January 1975, SP4 Carolyn J. Walls graduated from the U.S. Army Medical Equipment and Optical School in Denver, Colorado, part of the AHS. SP4 Walls was the first female to graduate from the course in its 30 year history.

("First Woman Graduates as Army Biomed Tech," Patriot, 23 Jan 1975)

The Army Veterinary School physically moved to AHS in February after being located at Ft. Sheridan, Illinois, for 54 years.

("Army Veterinary School Comes to AHS," Patriot, 6 Feb 1975)

A WAC saved the life of a local woman. In her fourth week of the Basic Health Services Course, PVT Victoria Gwara saved the life of a woman at a local restaurant after the woman went into seizures. She attributes being able to perform these life saving techniques to her medical training.

("WAC Saves Life of Woman," News Leader, 20 Feb 1975)

The first grandmother to attend the Army Medical Basic Course. 1LT Lenoma Gray, 41, entered the Army as a nurse after being rejected twice before, first during the Korean War (for being married) and second during the Vietnam era (for having dependent children).

("First Grandmother to Attend Army Medical Basic Course," Patriot, 29 June 1975)

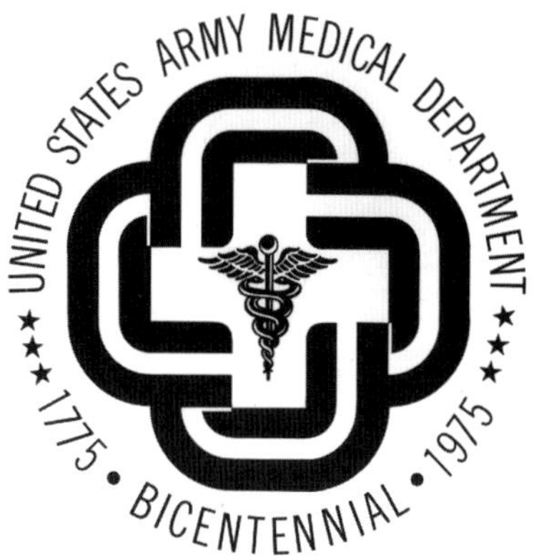

The AMEDD celebrated its 200th anniversary on 28 July 1975. The Color Guard of the Academy of Health Sciences displayed the U.S. Army Medical Department Bicentennial flag during the Bicentennial celebration.

(U.S. Army Photo, AMEDD Museum Collection)

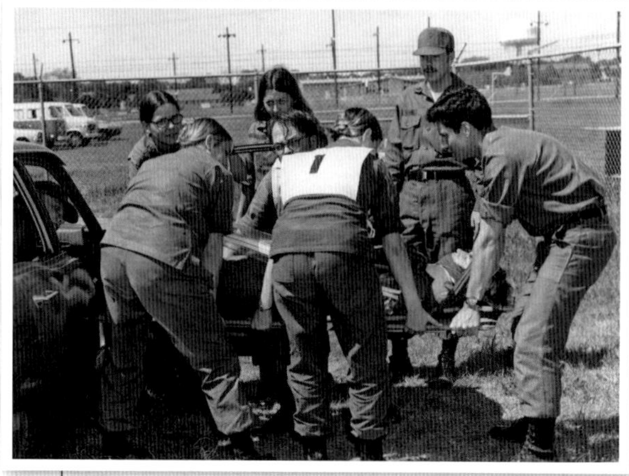

EMT students remove victim from a vehicle.

(U.S. Army Photo, AMEDD Museum Collection)

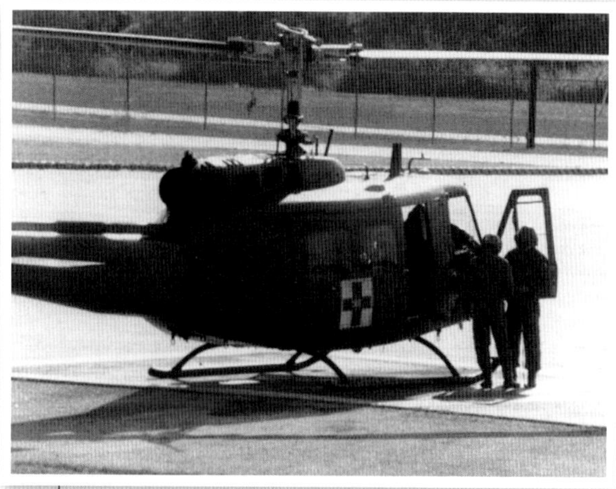

MAST crew boards the chopper to crank up for a rescue mission.

(U.S. Army Photo, AMEDD Museum Collection)

Jointly sponsored by AHS and the city of San Antonio, the Ethnic Expo took place in June at Fort Sam Houston with service members and local talent.

("Ethnic Expo '75," Patriot, 12 June 1975)

The AHS, in cooperation with the state of Texas, began its first course through which enlisted military personnel could eventually register as Emergency Medical Technicians (EMTs) with the state.

("Academy Program Leads to State Recognition as EMT Specialist," News-Leader, 9 Jan 1975)

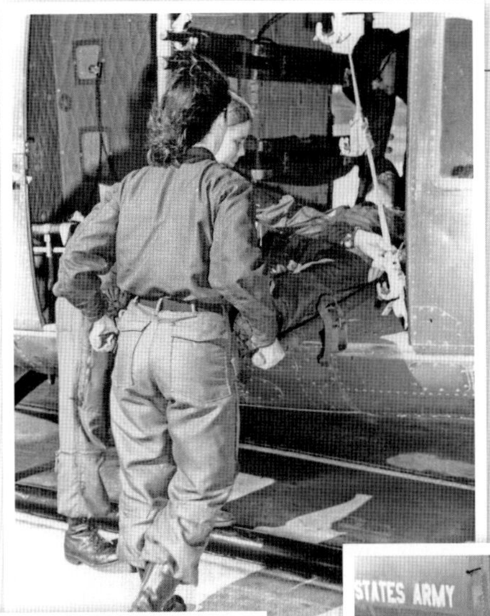

Female Medics with the 507th Medical Company assisted with MAST operations.

(U.S. Army Photo, AMEDD Museum Collection)

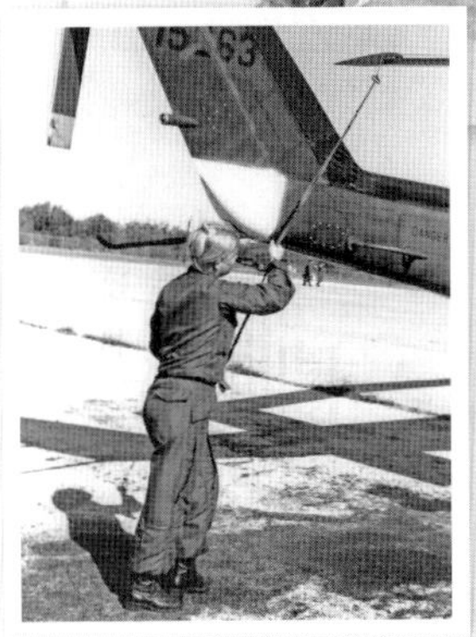

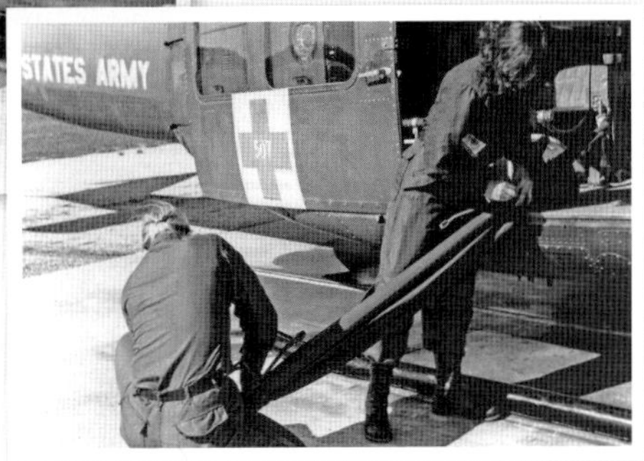

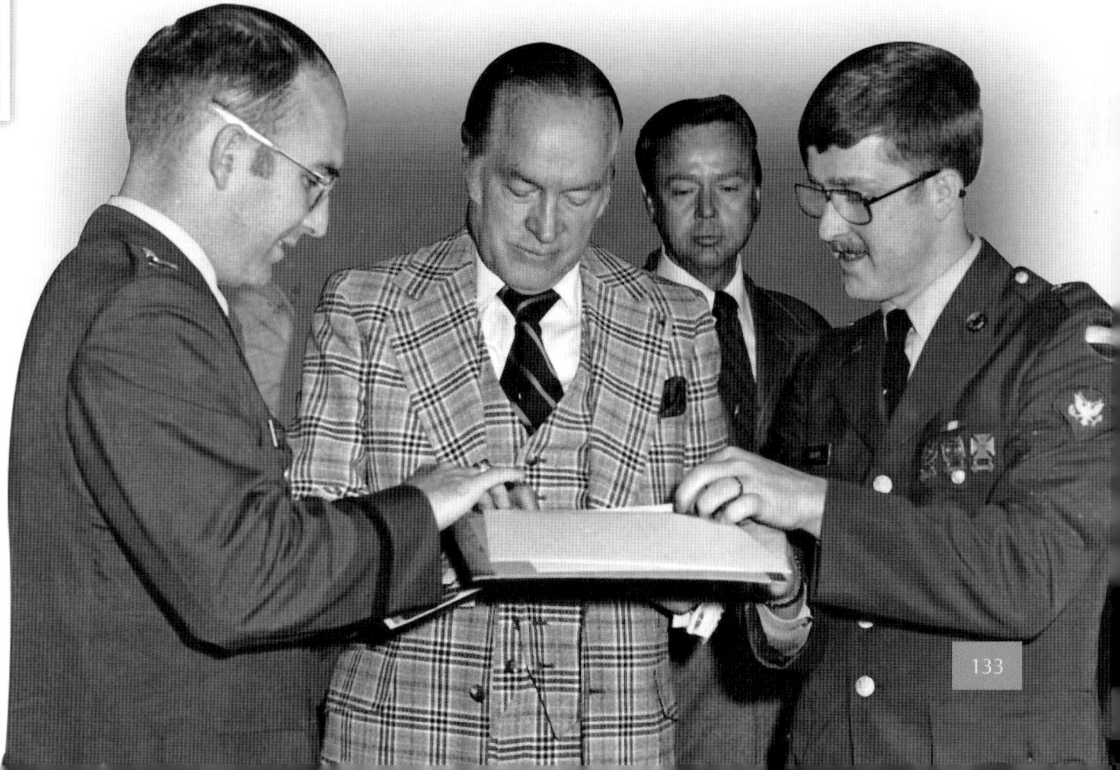

Bob Hope Visits
Medical Officers get autographs from world famous comedian and entertainer, Bob Hope, after his Christmas time performance at BAMC.

(U.S. Army Photo, AMEDD Museum Collection)

1976

The AHS won a silver medal from the International Film and Television Festival of New York for the production of "Centuries of Service: Army Medicine, An American Heritage." The production, narrated by actor Robert Young, was a 52-minute documentary that traced the history of the Army Medical Department from its establishment by the Continental Congress to 1976.

("TV Star Robert Young Receives HSMD Plaque," News-Leader, 13 May 1976)

Key personnel from the three newest and largest medical organizations of the Army National Guard (ARNG) arrived the week of 27 Feb 1976 to train at AHS. The ARNG requested the training in order to familiarize themselves with command and control procedures at the highest echelon of combat field medicine.

(Military Service News, 27 Feb 1976)

The AHS Color Guard carries the colors during the American Bicentennial celebrations at Fort Sam Houston on the 4th of July.

(U.S. Army Photo, AMEDD Museum Photo Collection)

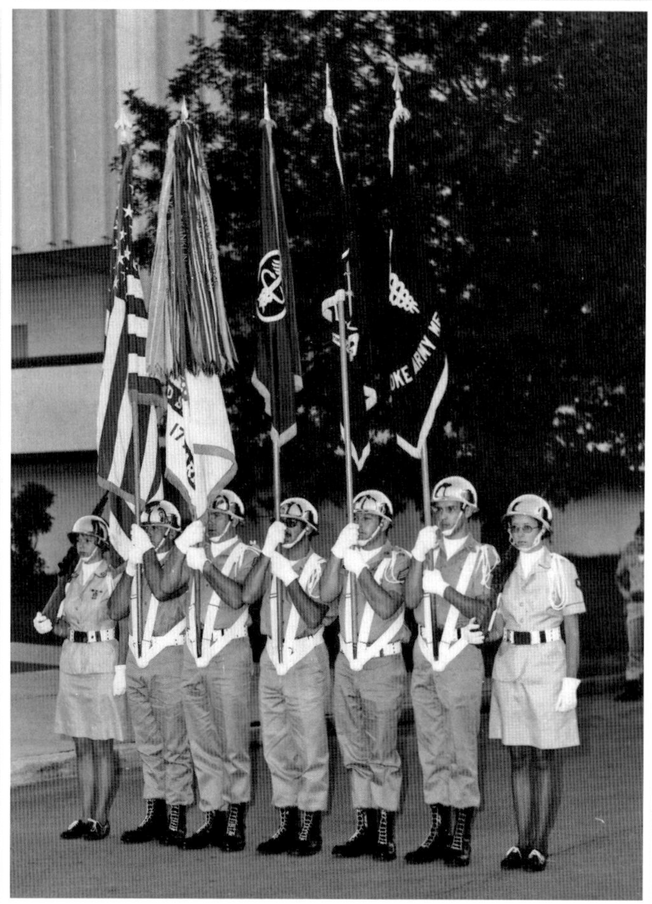

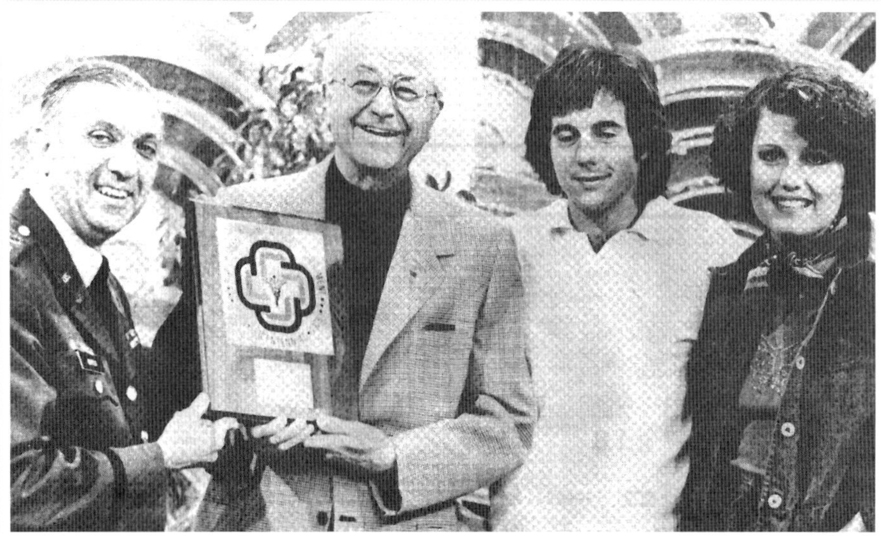

LTC Howard Gutin, Chief of Health Science Media Division at AHS, presents a plaque to actor Robert Young. Youthful stars Desi Arnaz, Jr., and Lucie Arnaz accompany Young as LTC Gutin presents the appreciation during the National Easter Seals Telethon in Los Angeles.

("TV Star Robert Young Receives HSMD Plaque," News Leader, 13 May 1976)

As part of a DoD initiative to save money, AHS began to offer additional interservice courses. Air Force, Navy, and Marine Corps personnel joined AMEDD soldiers for courses in Social Work and Psychology, Food Inspection Procedures, Physical Therapy Aids, and an Occupational Therapy Specialist course.

("To Save Dollars: AHS Consolidates Training Efforts," Patriot, 20 May 1976)

Basic general supply information training moved from Ft. Jackson, S.C., to AHS. The revised and expanded course tripled the normal class input.

("Course Expanded at FSH," Patriot, 3 June 1976)

The Army Reserve trained and qualified 200 Guard and Reserve medical specialists during two weeks of active duty, in a pioneering effort for the Army Reserve to conduct its own training. Led by MAJ Gloria Boudreaux, the training was taught by reservists for reservists to ensure that they receive more meaningful training and additional paraprofessional skills to perform as an emergency ambulance technician, dental hygienist, or x-ray technician.

("Army Reserves Pioneer in Conducting Their Own Training at AHS," Military Service News, 20 Aug 1976)

AHS partnered with the Fort Sam Houston Post Management Information Systems Office to develop a computer-assisted property management exercise reflecting increased automation in the medical logistics environment. The exercise involved students inputting and evaluating results for a simulated Hospital Property Management Account.

("Computer Assists," Patriot, 14 Oct 1976)

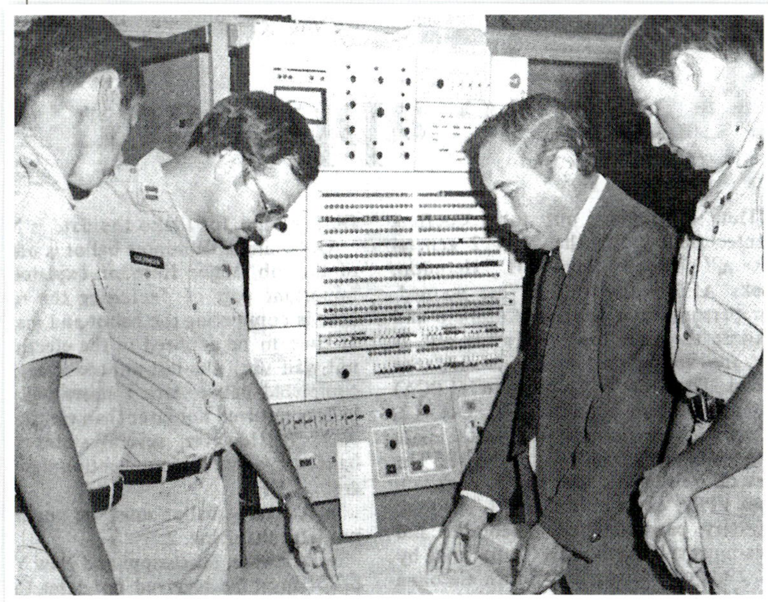

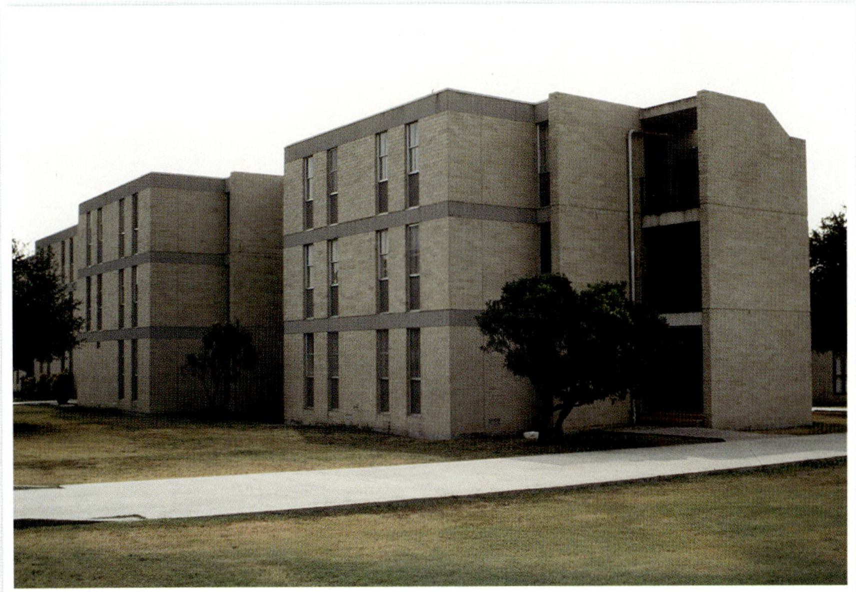

AHS students begin moving into the new $9 million complex of three-story barracks buildings next to Willis Hall in September 1976. The new barracks replaced the old "temporary" wooden barracks built during WWII. Constructed of masonry and air-conditioned, they were decorated with modernistic furniture and designed to give individuals as much privacy as possible.

("New Barracks Replace Old," Patriot, 2 Sept 1976)

1977

"Fetoscopy – A New World," a videotape produced by the AHS Media Division and BAMC Family Planning Department, wins national acclaim at the International Film and TV Festival of New York. The videotape showed imagery of a developing fetus through the combined use of a fetoscope and videography.

("HSC Film Wins National Acclaim," Patriot, 26 May 1977)

MG Pixley established the Directorate of Training Development and Evaluation, a centralized planning and instructional design activity. Its mission encompassed total analysis of AMEDD training needs to provide more comprehensive, life-cycle training support to Army Medical Department personnel worldwide. The Security Division, Management Information Systems Office, Logistics Division and the Army Medical Museum moved under the new Directorate of Support.

AHS and BAMC received four new commercial EMS ambulances to replace the Patient Transport Vehicles (PTV). Equipped with life support equipment that enabled patient treatment en route, the new ambulances were used solely for training.

("Ambulance Equipped with Life Support System," News Leader, 21 July 1977)

The first four civilians graduate from the AHS Medical Logistics Management Course on 28 July 1977.

("First Civilians Graduate," Patriot, 28 July 1977)

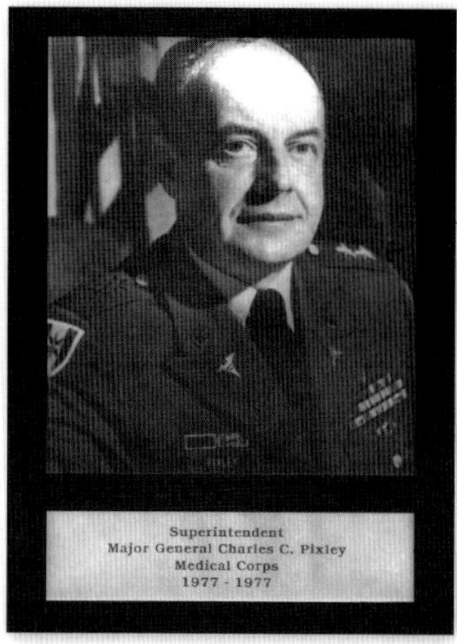

MG Charles C. Pixley
Superintendent of the Academy of Health Sciences on 6 Jan 1977.

(U.S. Army Photo, AMEDDC&S History Office files)

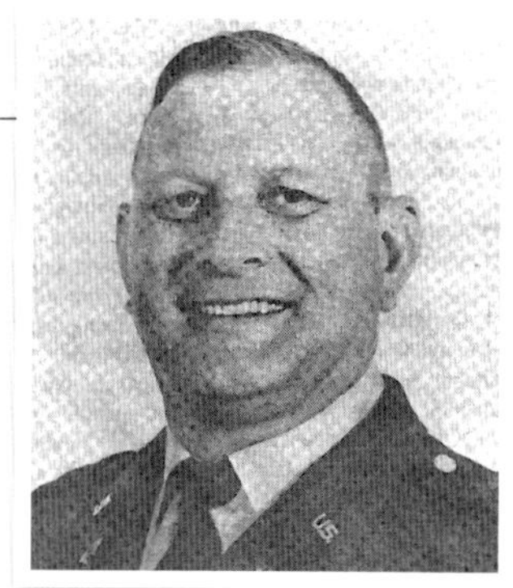

COL Robert E. Mathias
COL Mathias, Chief of the Concepts and Doctrine Division, Combat Development and Healthcare Studies, AHS, was inducted into the Infantry Officer Candidate Hall of Fame on 24 Feb 1977. COL Mathias, who entered the Army on 10 May 1948 and reached the grade of master sergeant, graduated from Officer Candidate School (OCS) in 1952. He also graduated from the Basic Course at the MFSS in 1952 and served a long and illustrious career with the AMEDD.

The AHS revised its Physical Fitness and Weight Control Program to comply with new Army regulations
The test for men included sit-ups; pushups; horizontal ladder; run, dodge and jump; and a mile run. For women, an 80-meter shuttle run and a stationary run replaced the mile run and horizontal ladder. Scoring was based on the participant's age.

("AHS Shapes Up for Army Regulations," Patriot, 24 Feb 1977)

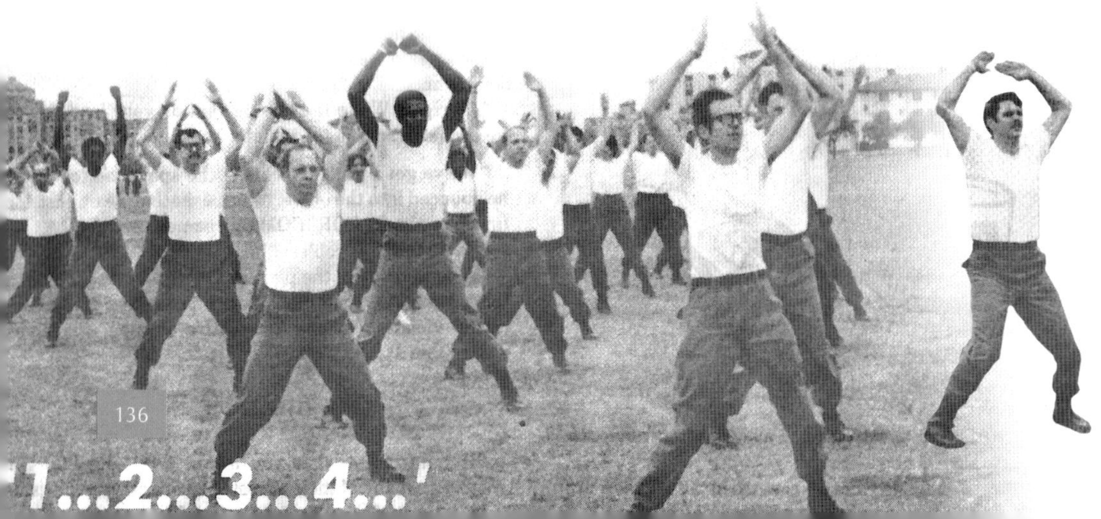

'1...2...3...4...'

For the first time, all faculty members and students at the AHS were required to receive training in cardiopulmonary resuscitation (CPR).

("At AHS: Training in CPR Begins," Patriot, 4 Aug 1977)

Dual careers are highlighted in news articles that mention simultaneous re-enlistments, receipt of ARCOM awards, and promotions.

("Husband, Wife Receive ARCOM," Patriot, 27 Oct 1977)

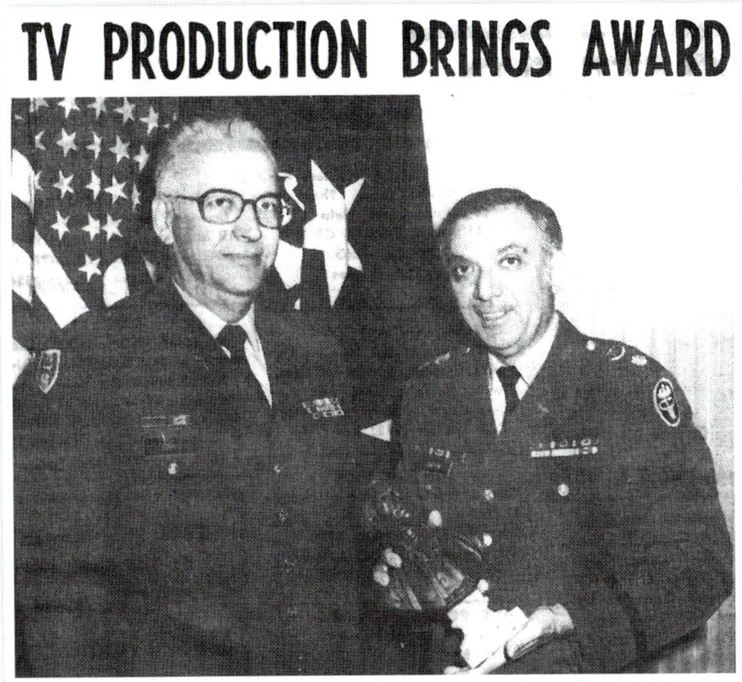

Television production of the video titled "Contraception" receives the Thomas Jefferson Award, the Department of Defense's highest award for military newspapers and electronic media.

("TV Production Brings Award," Military Service News, 10 March 1978)

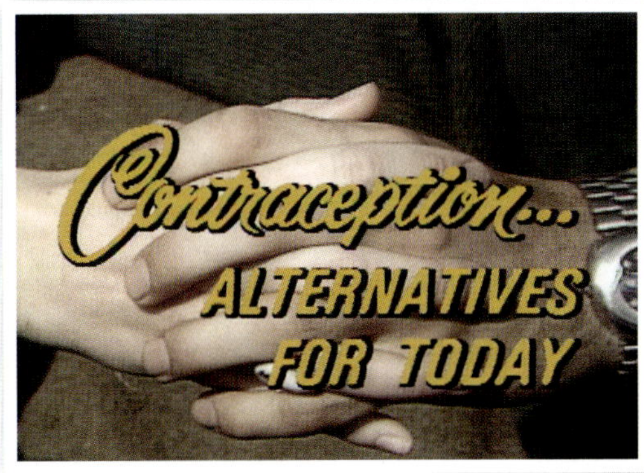

The AHS Media Division received the 1976 Keith L. Ware Award for the videotaped production "Contraception: Alternatives for Today."

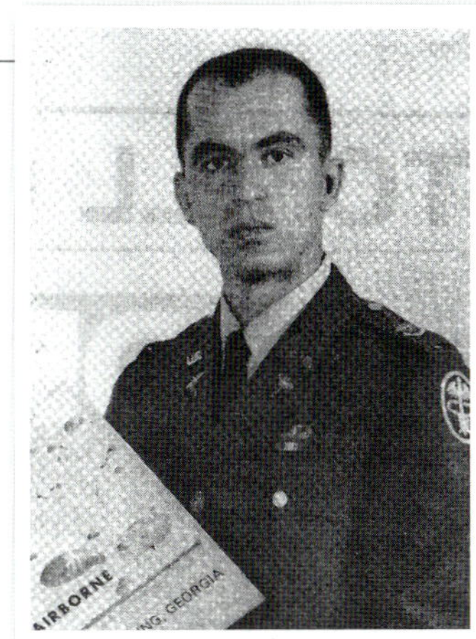

1LT Constantine G. Mourtous, Commander of Company C, 2d Battalion, AHS, received the "Iron Mike "award for being selected the Officer-NCO Honor Graduate of the Airborne School at Fort Benning, Georgia, in November 1977. 1LT Mourtous went on to become Executive Director of Memorial Hermann Healthcare System.

("Iron Mike," Patriot, 23 Nov 1977)

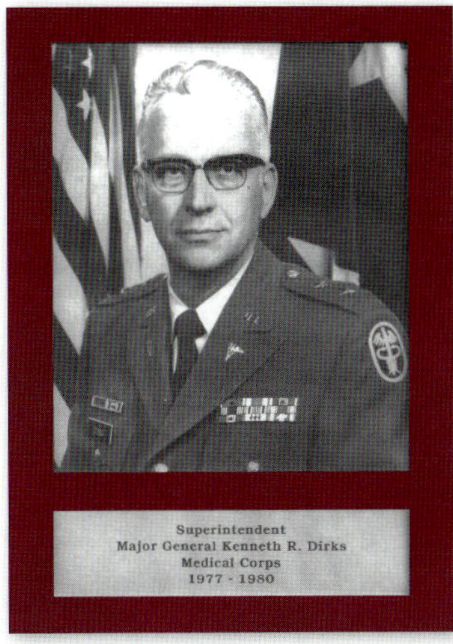

MG Kenneth R. Dirks became the Superintendent of the AHS on 17 Oct 1977, replacing MG Charles C. Pixley, who became the 34th Surgeon General of the United States Army.

(U.S. Army Photo, AMEDDC&S History Office files)

1978

Phase I of the two-year course Anesthesiology for Army Nurse Corps Officers was taught for the first time at AHS.

("Officers Begin Course," Patriot, 12 Jan 1978)

The Army Medical Department Museum Foundation was incorporated with the purpose of raising money to build a new Army Medical Department Museum at Fort Sam Houston. The Medical Museum, which traced its beginnings to the Medical Field Service School Museum at Carlisle Barracks, Pennsylvania, came to Fort Sam with the Medical Field Service School in 1946. It was renamed the U.S. Army Medical Museum in 1956 and was housed in the basement of building 2264, the old 9th Infantry Quadrangle.

Combat Medic Memorial

In 1977, under the leadership of LTC Richard J. Berchin, the Combat Medic Memorial Fund Committee was organized to construct a memorial to honor medics who went into combat to serve and save their fellow soldiers. The twice-life-sized figure of a combat medic giving aid to a wounded comrade was sculpted by Katherin Speed Ettl. The statue was placed in front of one of the last of two-story barracks on Fort Sam Houston, the location used by the Boy Scouts on Post until it was torn down for the new museum. The memorial was dedicated in 1979.

(News Leader, 14 July 1989, p 18)

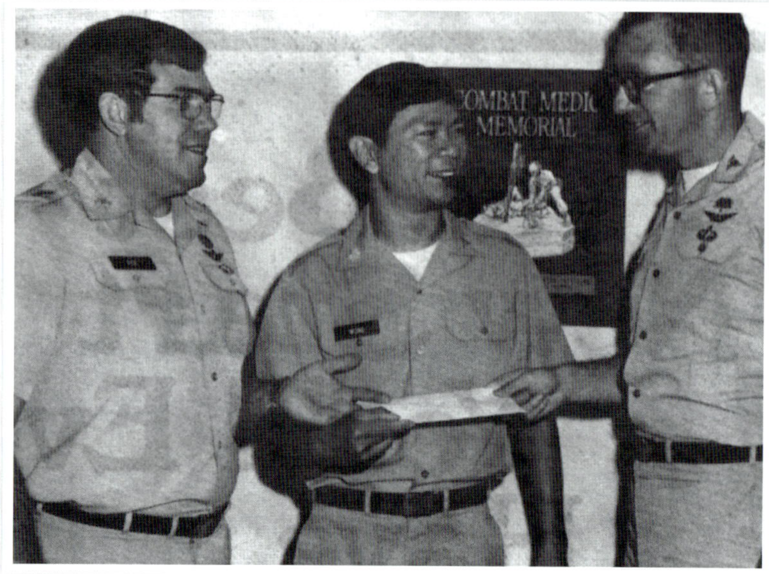

LTC Richard J. Berchin gathers donations for the erection of the Combat Medic Memorial Statue.

(U.S. Army Photo, AMEDD Museum Photo Collection)

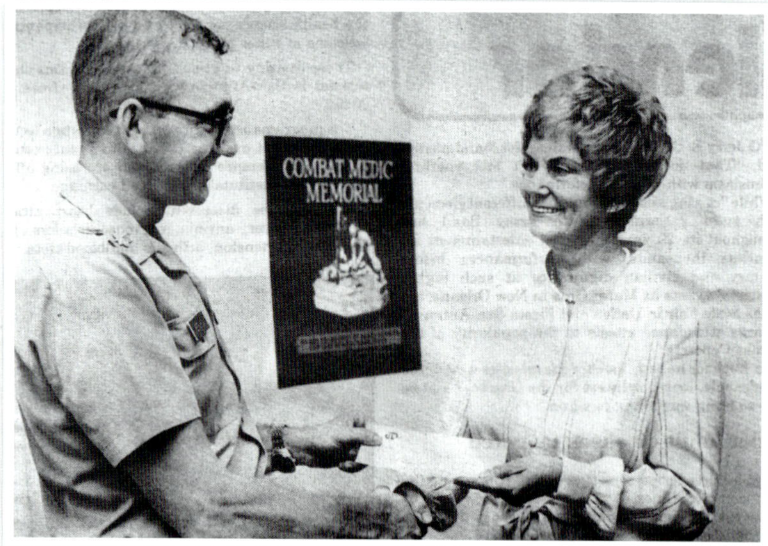

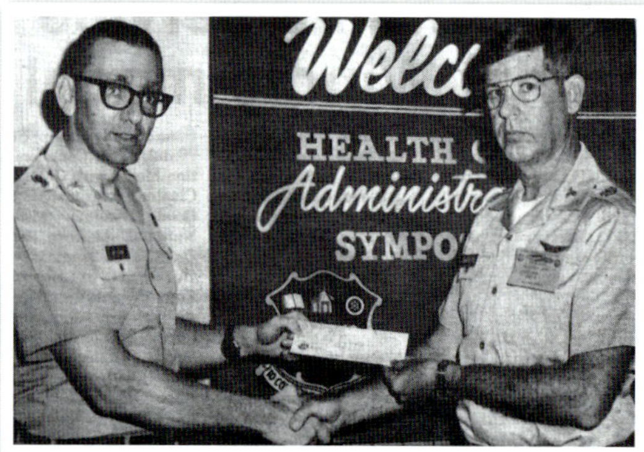

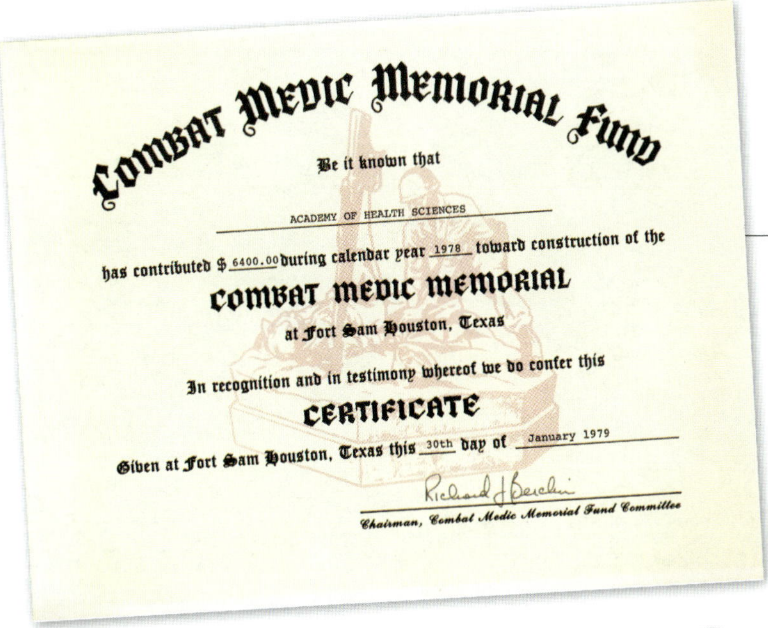

Combat Medic Memorial Fund

Be it known that

ACADEMY OF HEALTH SCIENCES

has contributed $ 6400.00 during calendar year 1978 toward construction of the

COMBAT MEDIC MEMORIAL

at Fort Sam Houston, Texas

In recognition and in testimony whereof we do confer this

CERTIFICATE

Given at Fort Sam Houston, Texas this 30th day of January 1979

Richard J Berchin

Chairman, Combat Medic Memorial Fund Committee

An acknowledgment certificate for monies donated by the AHS towards the Combat Medic Memorial Statue.

(U.S. Army Photo, AMEDD Museum Photo Collection)

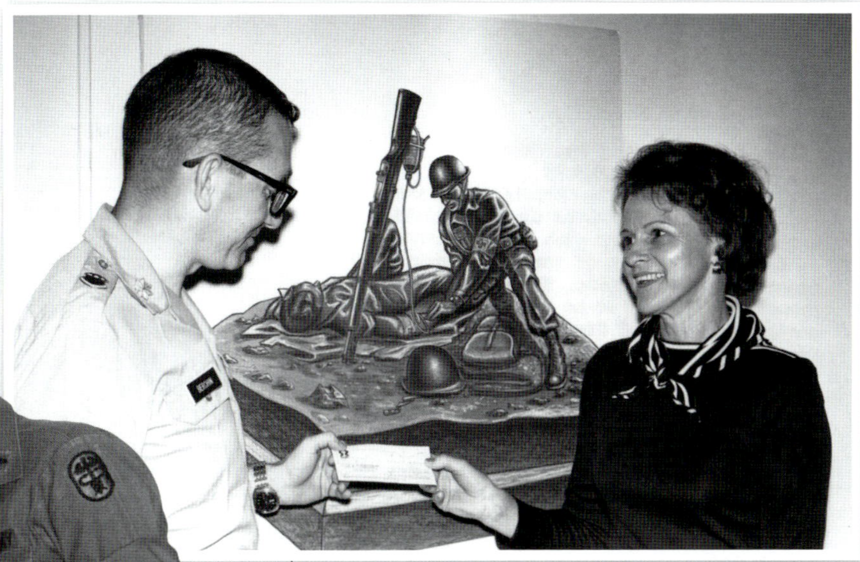

A Donation Check

In the background is one of the first artist concept sketches for the statue.

(U.S. Army Photo, AMEDD Museum Photo Collection)

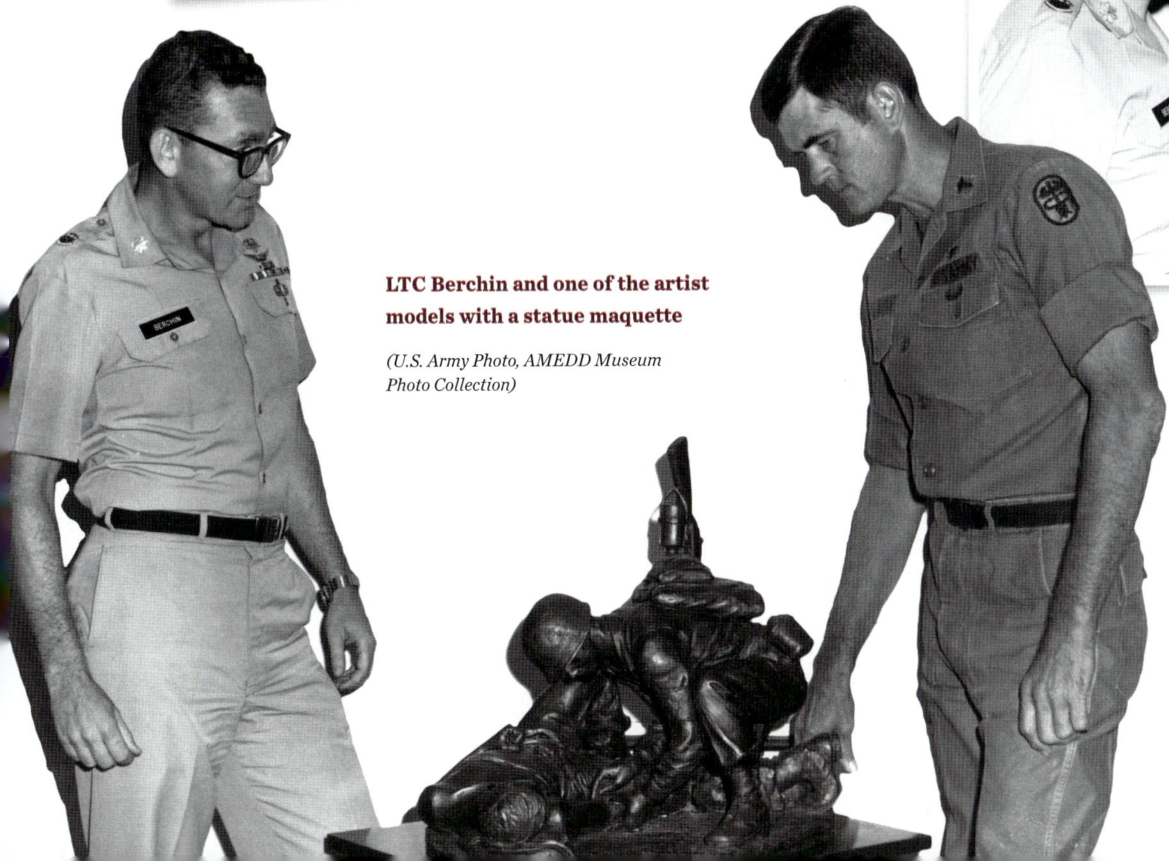

LTC Berchin and one of the artist models with a statue maquette

(U.S. Army Photo, AMEDD Museum Photo Collection)

1978

National Hispanic Heritage Week was featured in the pages of the *Medical Patriot* for the first time. Dr. Felix Almaras, Associate Professor of History at UTSA and Vice Chairman of the Bexar County Historical Commission, spoke on the "History of Hispanics," while mariachis serenaded AHS personnel throughout the third week of October.

("Hispanic Week Observers," Medical Patriot, 12 Oct 1978)

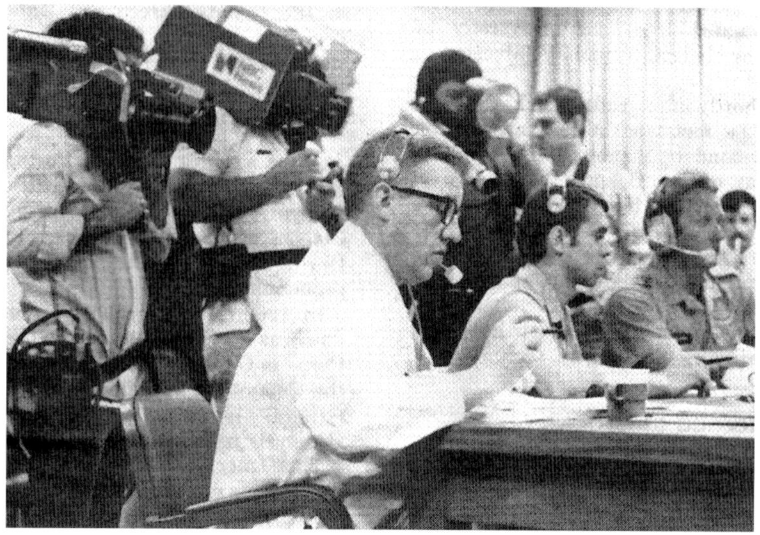

Television comes into its own during the 1970s as a teaching tool and for use in on-the-spot diagnosis. In May 1978, burn specialists from the Institute of Surgical Research (ISR) participated remotely in a simulated mass casualty exercise at the Baltimore-Washington International Airport by viewing and giving casualty care via live television coverage provided by national and local TV crews.

("Making History," Patriot, 25 May 1978)

Dynamic Duo

Husband and wife team, SSgt. Joseph A. Snyder and SP4 Beth A. Snyder, assigned to the AHS were awarded the Army Commendation medal for meritorious service at the same time.

("Husband, Wife Receive ARCOMs," Patriot, 2 Feb 1978)

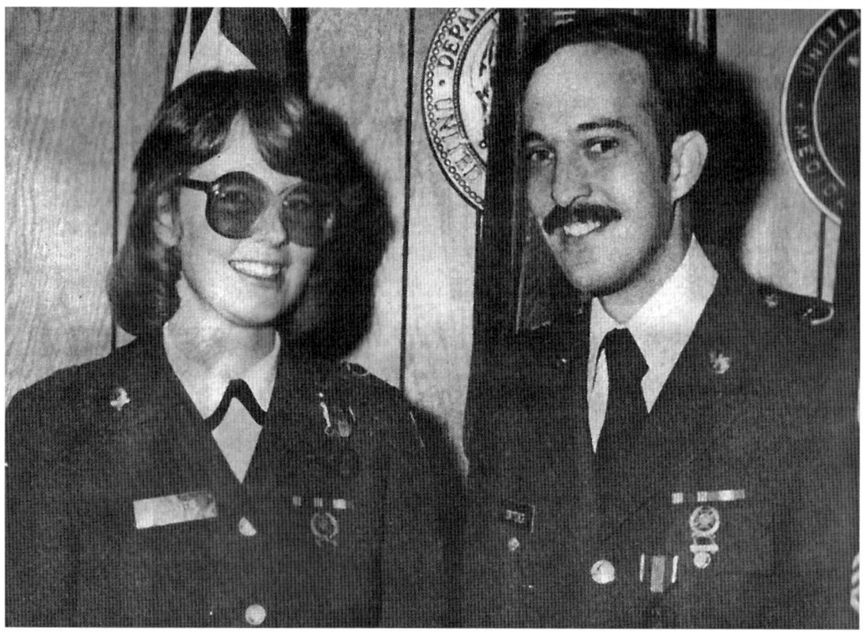

The U.S. Army Medical Equipment and Test Evaluation Division was redesignated as the Directorate of Medical Equipment Test and Evaluation and reassigned to the AHS.

(Permanent Orders 110-1, 1 Oct 1978)

The HSC medical education satellite program supported by AHS was launched 20 Nov 1979.

LTC Robert J. Jeffery of the Royal Australian Army Medical Corps became the first Australian Integrated Exchange Officer assigned to AHS in a staff capacity. LTC Jeffery served as the Executive Assistant to the Chief of the Concepts and Doctrine Division in the Directorate of Combat Development and Health Care Studies.

("Two-year Assignment: Australian Joins Academy Staff," Medical Patriot, 6 Dec 1979)

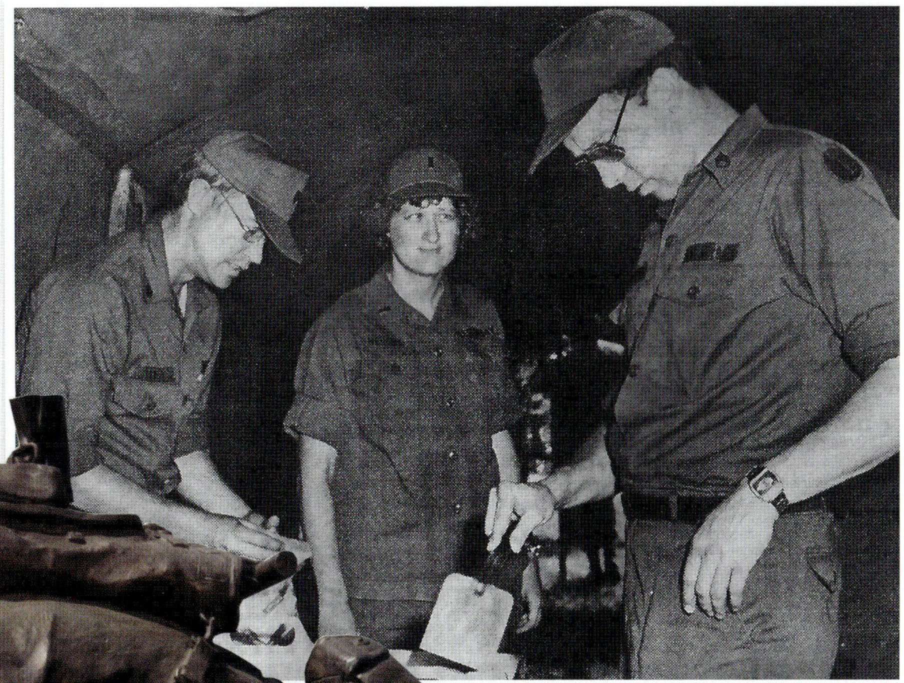

Reserve training activities at AHS increased and diversified in the post-Vietnam drawdown. Reserve training was divided into phases. Reservists with the 45th Station Hospital prepare garlic bread during field exercises for their Hospital Food Service Specialist Basic Course MOS.

("Garlic Bread," Patriot, 19 July 1979)

Dedication
The Combat Medic Memorial Statue, located on the corner of Stanley Road and Harry Wurzbach Road, was unveiled on 13 Dec 1979.

("Dedication," Medical Patriot, 13 Dec 1979)

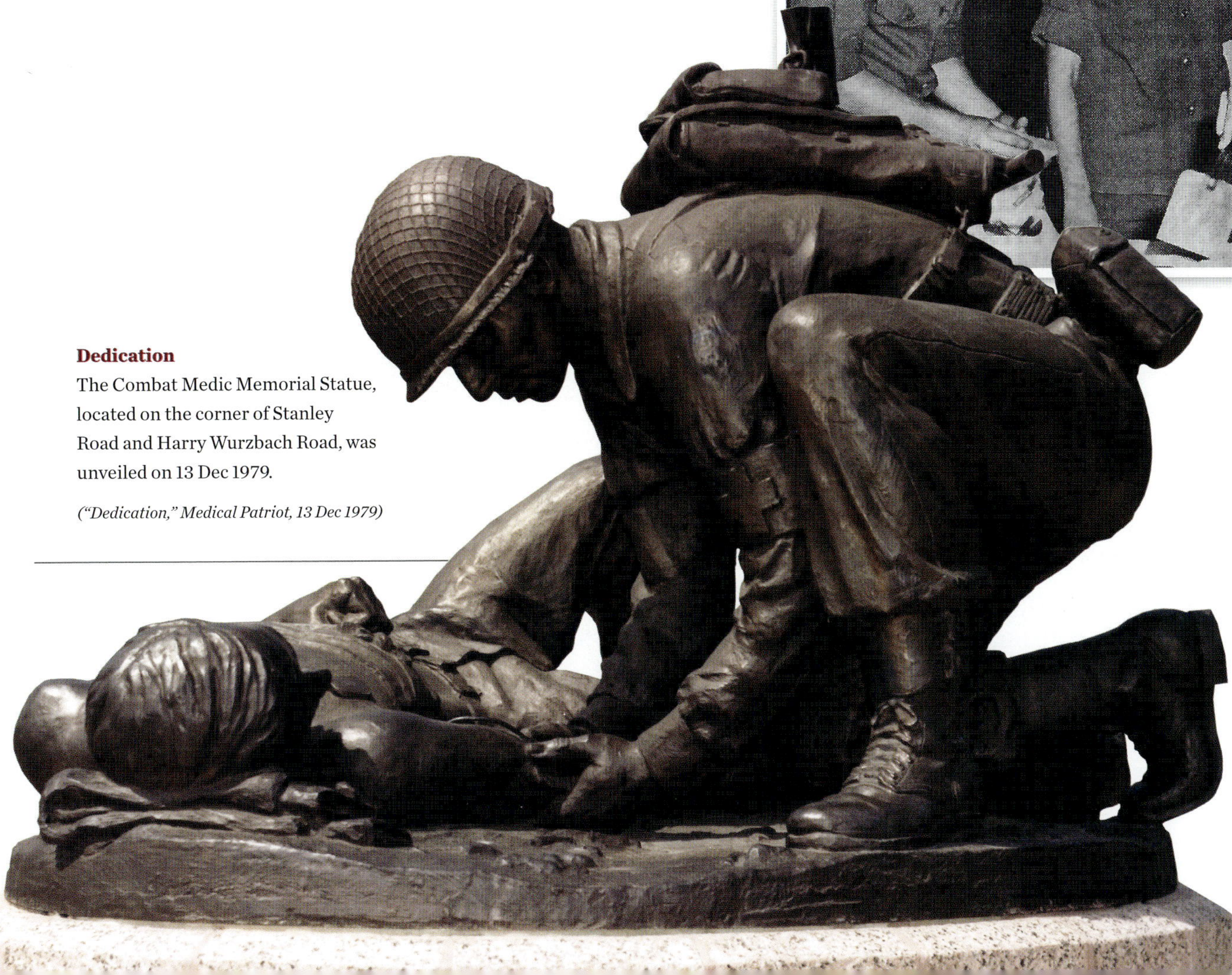

1980-1989

LTG Charles Pixley, the Surgeon General, announced planning for a tri-service combat training program for physicians throughout DoD. Developed under the academic auspices of the Uniformed Services University of Health Sciences, the Combat Casualty Care Course (C4), a graduate level course, would prepare health care professionals for direct support of combat operations. The first group began training 27 April 1980. AHS developed academic and logistics support for C4 at Camp Bullis.

("First C4 Class," AMEDD Mercury, 1 April 1980)

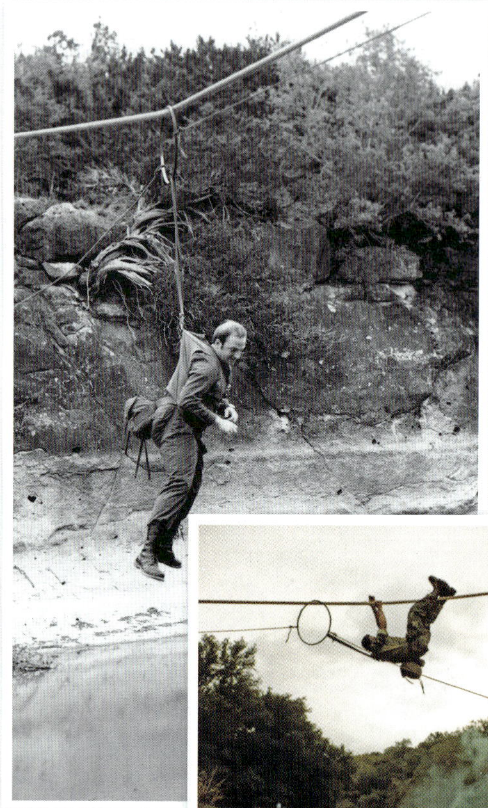

The "Slide for Life"
A trainee slides from one side of the creek to treat a patient on the opposite bank at Camp Bullis during the May 1980 C4. This soldier-physician appears to have gotten stuck mid-way.

(U.S. Army Photo, AMEDD Museum Photo Collection)

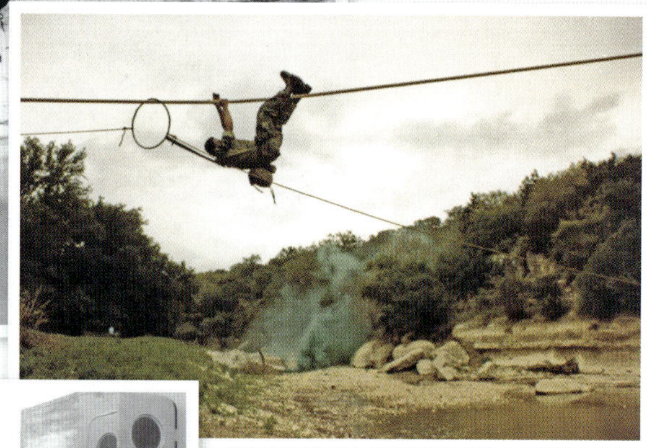

The proper technique to make the "Slide for Life"

(U.S. Army Photo, AMEDD Museum Photo Collection)

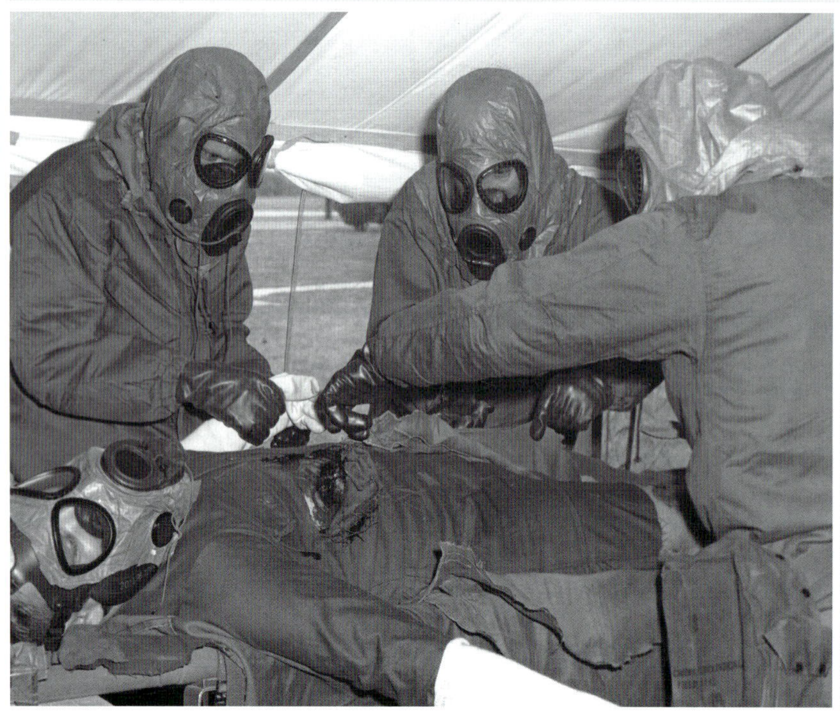

Medics treat a simulated casualty in a "dirty" decontamination tent before taking him into the clean surgery tent.

(U.S. Army Photo, AMEDD Museum Photo Collection)

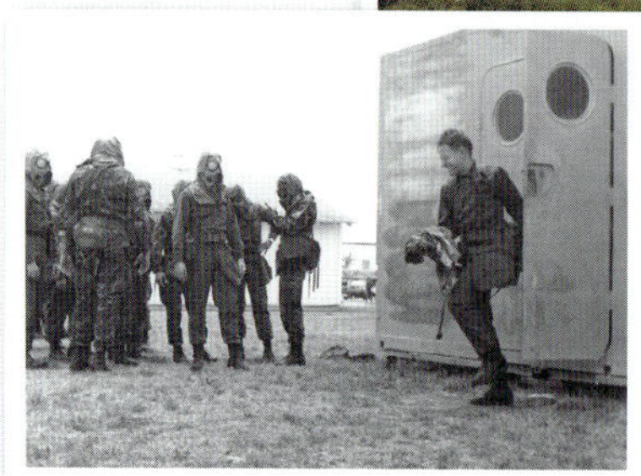

Trainees exit an improvised gas chamber at C4

(U.S. Army Photo, AMEDD Museum Photo Collection)

MEDEVAC landing amidst a smoke screen during C4 exercise.

(U.S. Army Photo, AMEDD Museum Photo Collection)

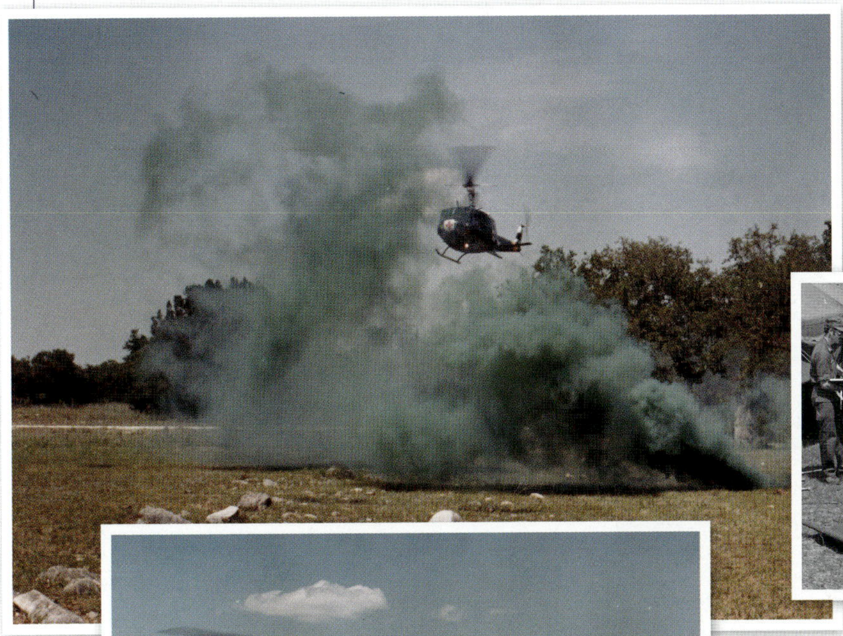

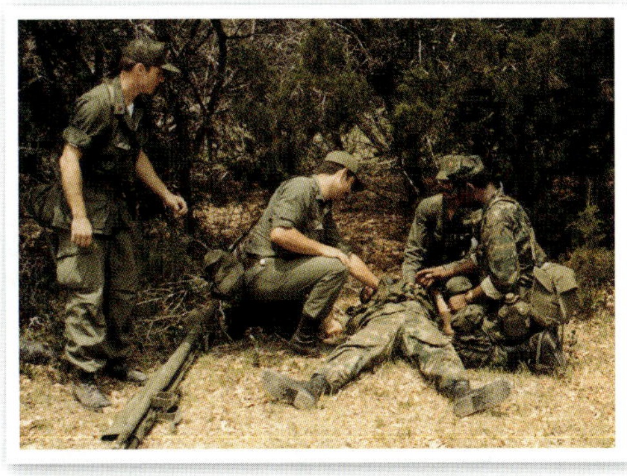

Military physicians assess a simulated casualty in the field during the C4.

(U.S. Army Photo, AMEDD Museum Photo Collection)

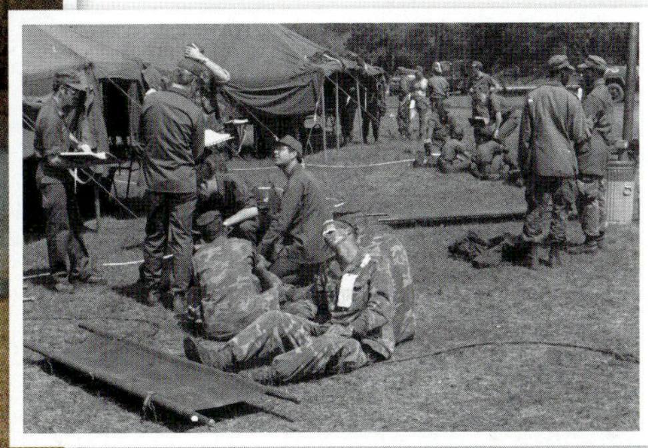

Initial triage lane at the Forward Operating Base (FOB)

(U.S. Army Photo, AMEDD Museum Photo Collection)

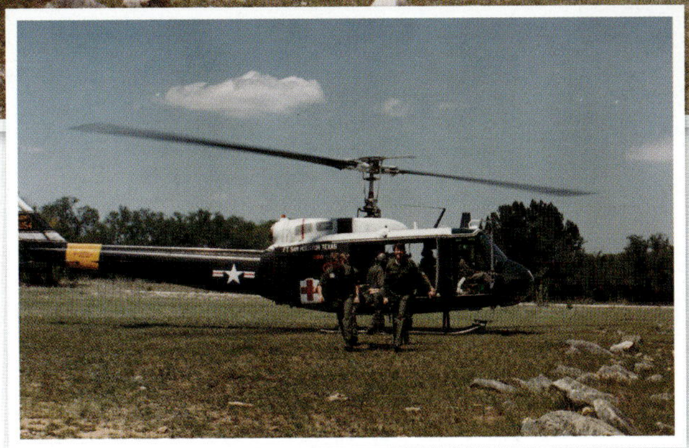

Medics practice loading and unloading patients from the MEDEVAC helicopter.

(U.S. Army Photo, AMEDD Museum Photo Collection)

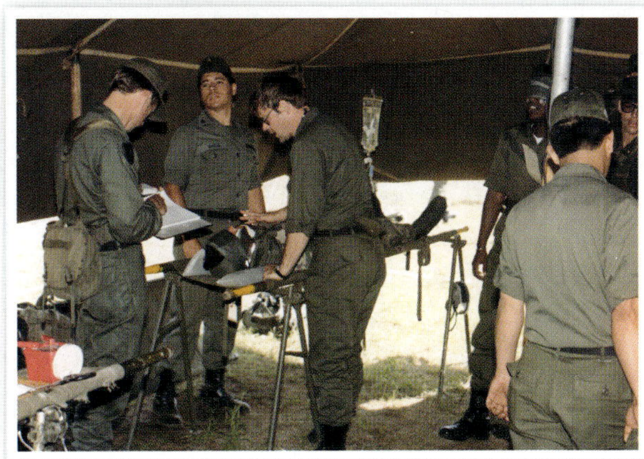

The field hospital during the C4 exercise.

(U.S. Army Photo, AMEDD Museum Photo Collection)

1980

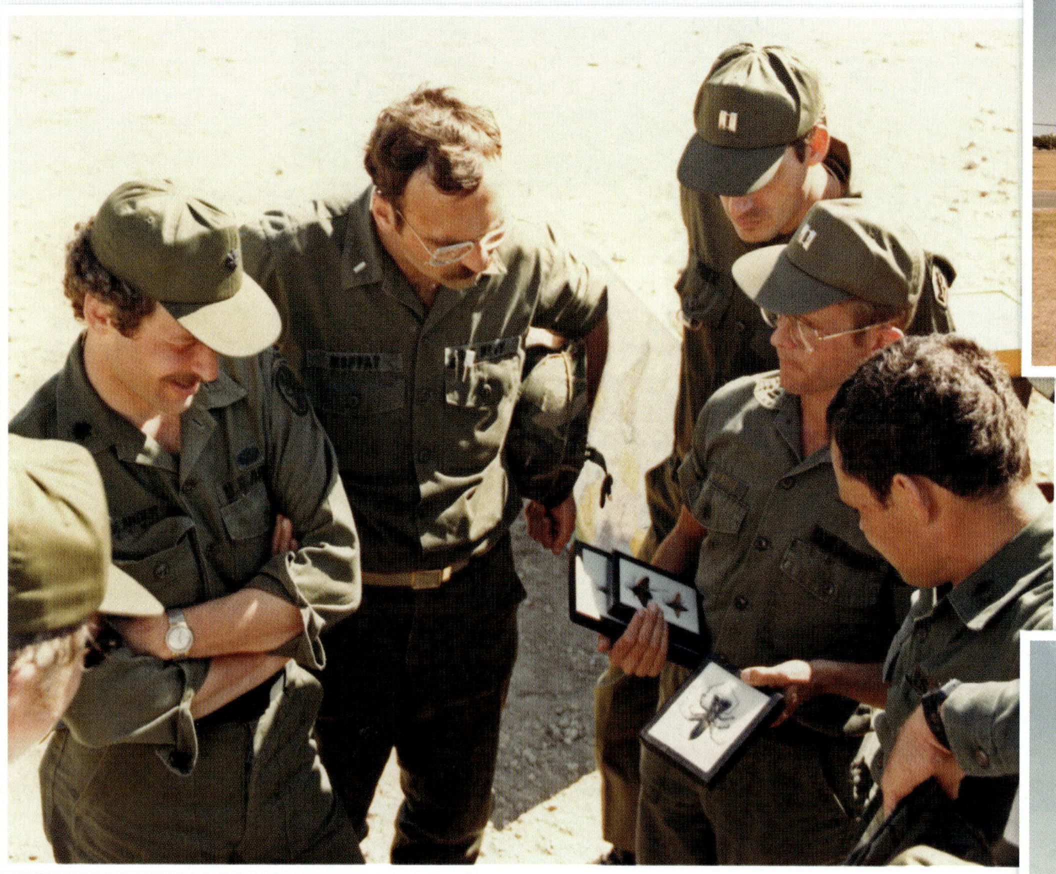

BUSHMASTER 1980

Uniformed Services University of Health Sciences students were exposed to entomological considerations they might find in a combat environment. The "bug" session is part of the preventive medicine training the soldiers received at Camp Bullis.

("BUSHMASTER Exercise with USUHS/AHS," Med Training 3-065-074, November 1980)
(U.S. Army Photo, AMEDD Museum Photo Collection)

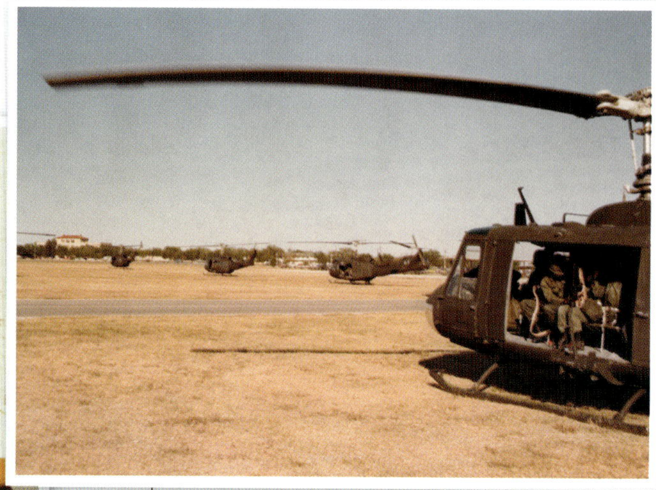

BUSHMASTER 1980

Participants are flown from the MacArthur Parade Ground to Camp Bullis by Ft. Hood's Aviation Battalion and 507th Med. Co. at Fort Sam Houston.

(U.S. Army Photo, AMEDD Museum Photo Collection)

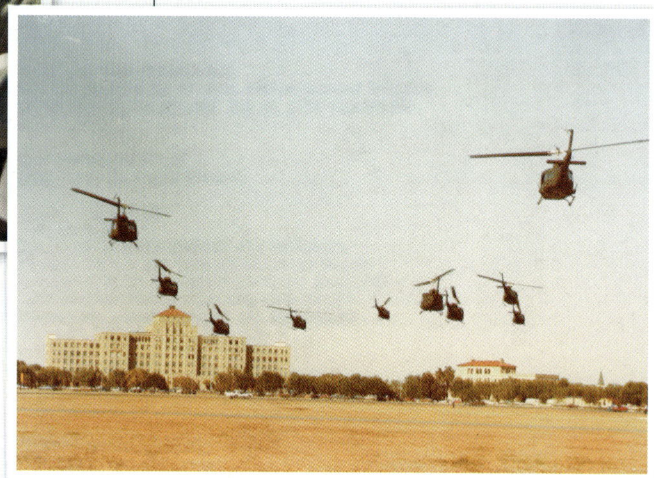

In 1980, the Air Force Veterinary Corps stood down and the Army became the executive agent for all DoD veterinary functions, resulting in the veterinary warrant officer program.

("Veterinarians Celebrate Their History," by MAJ Boris Brglez, The Mercury, Vol 37, No 7, June 2010: p 7) (USAF photo courtesy of the Lackland AFB History Office)

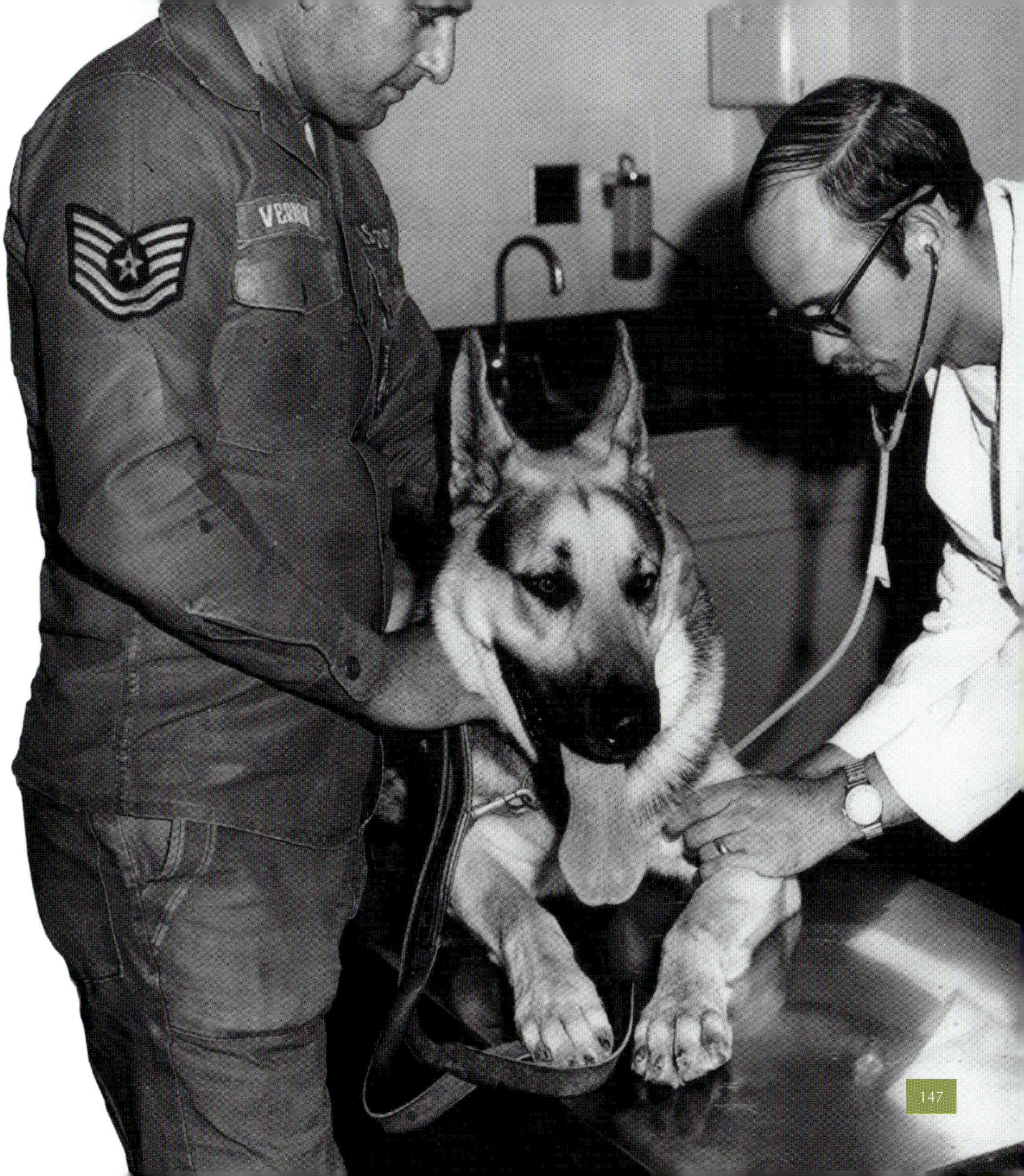

1981

A five-week Alternative ROTC Advanced Camp for nursing cadets was developed and designed to provide the nursing student with an experience that integrated clinical, interpersonal and leadership knowledge and skills. The concept was tested at four medical treatment facilities during the period 15 June to 17 July 1981 with 24 nursing cadets participating in the alternative advanced camp. Recommendations included the addition of field medical procedures, basic military skills training and more advanced clinical nursing skills. The program of instruction (POI) was implemented in the summer of 1982.

("5-week Alternative ROTC Advanced Camp for Nursing Cadets," AMEDD Activities Report, July 1981)

The first group of Army physician assistant students to become warrant officers during training graduated from AHS in 1981. The 55 students received the rank of Warrant Officer 1 (WO1) after completing their didactic training at the Academy. After another 12 months of on-the-job training (OJT), these graduates were given an option to select a four- or six-year obligation. Those who chose a six-year obligation were appointed to the Chief Warrant Officer.

("AHS Graduates 'Mister' Pass," AMEDD Mercury, August 1981)

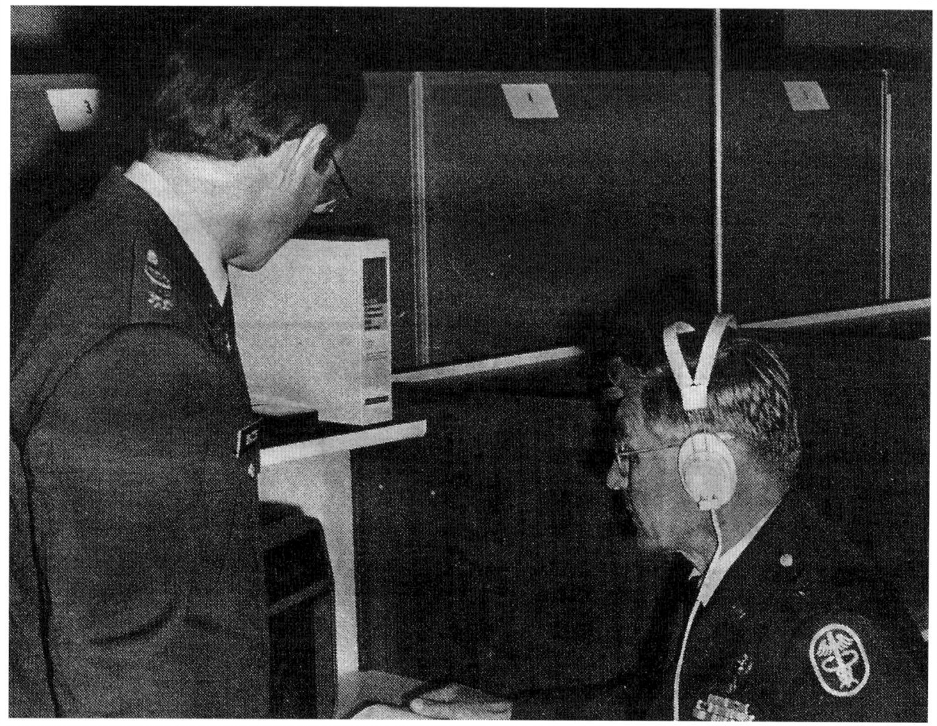

MG Quinn H. Becker, AHS commandant, uses a Kodak Ektagraphic 410 audio projector during the open house of the new revised Hospital Food Service Specialist Course at the AHS. Looking on is MAJ Roy S. Maize II, Chief of the Hospital Food Services Branch, Health Care Administration Division. The revised 10-week course is the first self-paced course instituted at AHS.

("Opening of Self-paced Course," Medical Patriot, 5 March 1981)

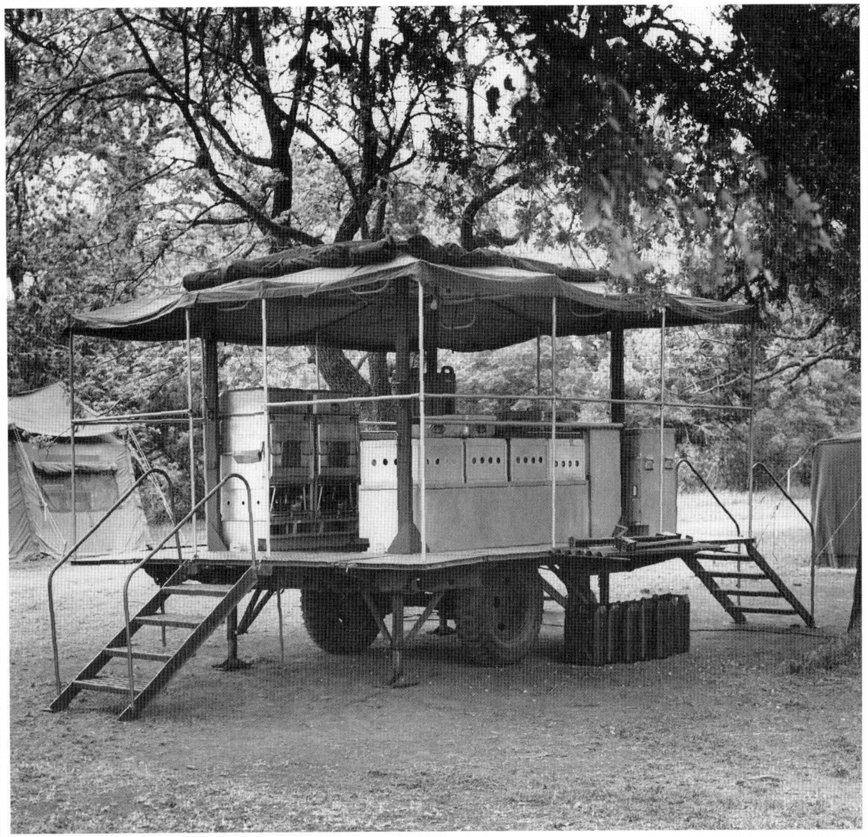

Mobile Kitchen
The complete Army kitchen of 1981 was an 8 ft. x 11 ft. trailer that included its own serving line, steam table and two field ranges. The kitchen could bake, roast, deep fry, boil, and griddle cook as well as serve as a portable ice chest. It was deployed by a four-person crew in about 30 minutes and fed a company-sized unit. AHS used its kitchen for training during the hospital food service course at AHS and field tested it at Camp Bullis.

("Release No 115, MOBILE KITCHEN," 24 April 1981, News Release: U.S. Army Health Services Command, Public Affairs Office)

The Military Science Division was among the AHS's major participants for a Department of Army (DA)-wide Logistics Exercise (LOGEX), conducted at Fort Pickett, VA, from 10 to 20 Aug 1981. The LOGEX was a Joint Command Services (JCS)-coordinated, DA-sponsored, Training and Doctrine Command (TRADOC)-directed, corps-level exercise (CPX), conducted primarily for Reserve Component units. Military Science (MilSci) developed the medical play, operational plans (OPLANS), and technical publications, and provided observer-controllers for the exercise.

("MilSci Participates in Army LOGEX," AMEDD Activities Report, August 1981)

The U.S. Army-Baylor University program in Physical Therapy (6H-65) class graduated on 21 November 1981. With this class, the U.S. Army-Baylor University program in Physical Therapy was terminated.

("Last Baylor PT Course," AMEDD Activities Report, November 1981)

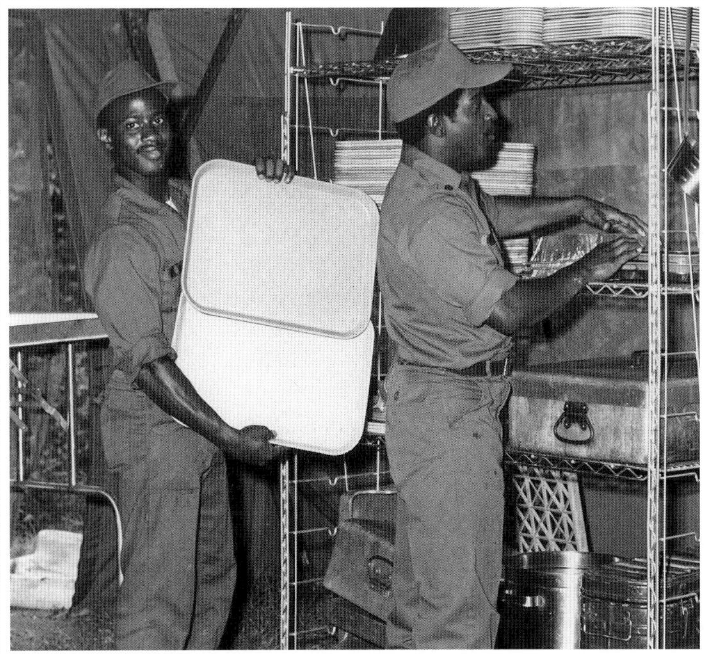

1982

The first iteration of the AMEDD Battalion/Brigade Pre-command, Phase II, Course was held 3 to 14 May. Phase II consisted of two weeks of an update on AMEDD doctrine, logistics, maintenance, and the Army Training Management System. A Medical Corps track was included for physicians. Several general officers were guest speakers, including LTC Bernard T. Mittemeyer, Army Surgeon General; BG France F. Jordan, Chief, Medical Service Corps; BG William E. Potts, Deputy CG, USA Missile Command; and BG Robert H. Buker, Commandant, AHS.

("AMEDD Bn/Bde Pre-Command Course 1," AMEDD Activities Report, May 1982)

The AMEDD Officer Advanced Course (OAC) underwent a major revision, developing a three-phased course consisting of 12 weeks of general professional military education and training required by all AMEDD officers, a seven-week period consisting of track instruction tailored to each individual officer's potential utilization, and a two-week phase consisting of sub-courses designed to train the officer for immediate signing following graduation from the advanced course. The first class under the new concept graduated on 15 Dec.

("OAC Revision," AMEDD Activities Report, May 1982)

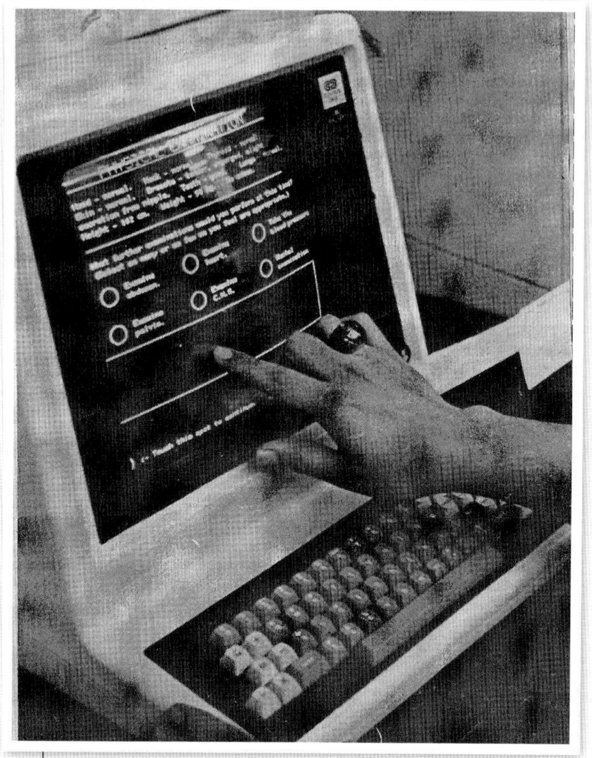

The Learning Resources Laboratory installed eight Programmed Logic for Automated Teaching Operations (PLATO) units. A computer-based education system, PLATO delivered as much as 6,000 hours of lessons. AHS PLATO programs were designed to prepare students for an Adult Basic Skills program that could prepare a student for the Graduate Equivalency Diploma (GED) exam.

("PLATO: Computer-Based Teaching Aid Makes Learning Enjoyable," News Leader, 26 March 1982)

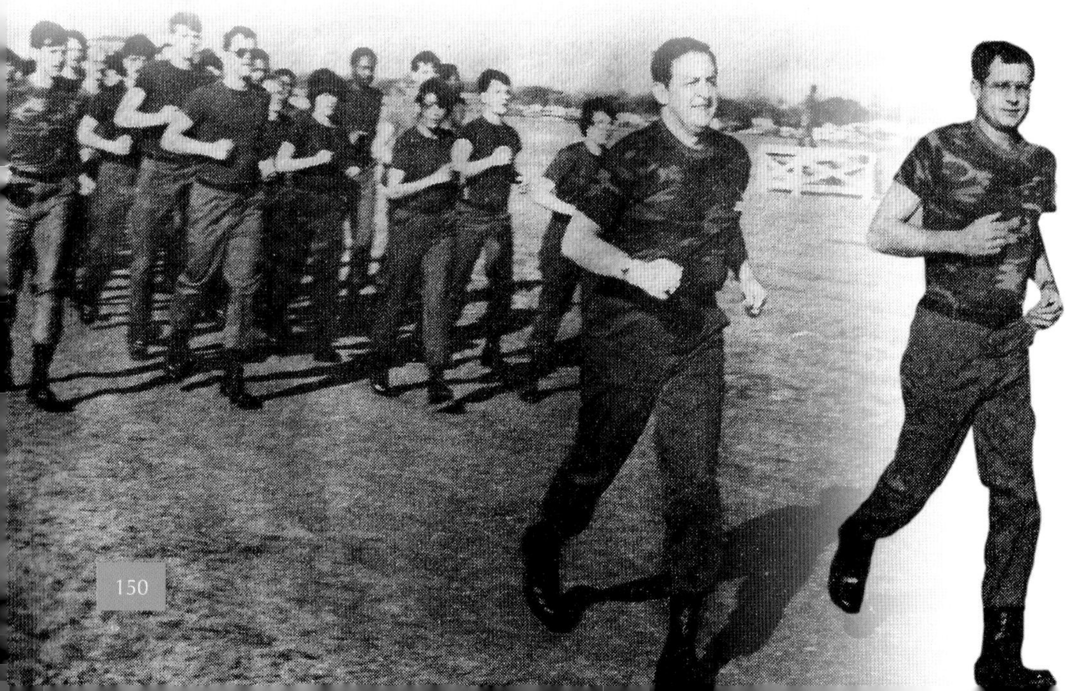

BG France F. Jordan, MSC Chief, runs with students in the AMEDD OBC at AHS

("BG Jordan Runs with OBC," AMEDD Mercury, May 1982)

Students attending the 48-week Dental Hygiene Course spent their final month at BAMC examining patients and offering preventive dentistry instruction. This new affiliation was structured to provide senior dental hygiene students with the opportunity to see patients by consult, one-half day per week, on selected wards at Brooke's main hospital and Beach Pavilion.

("BAMC, AHS Joining Forces for Dental Course," AMEDD Mercury, June 1982)

Graduate affiliation of the Anesthesiology for Army Nurse Corps (ANC) Officers Course with the State University of New York, Buffalo, was formalized in 1982.

("Graduate Affiliation with Nurse Anesthesia," AMEDD Activities Report, July 1982)

AHS began a revision of the 91B10 Basic Medical Specialist Course.

("91B, C Changes Start in October," AMEDD Mercury, August 1982)

The Health Research Activities Division completed its Long Range Planning System (LRPS). The intent of the OTSG-requested special unprogrammed study, "Long Range Planning System: The Medical Environment in the Year 2000," was to ascertain trends and describe the medical environment that could be reasonably expected to exist in the year 2000. The process forecast health status and expectations of the population at risk; anticipated presence/absence of disease by regions throughout the world; predicted clinical personnel requirements; and anticipated technologies affecting the practice of medicine, dentistry, vision, and clinical procedures.

("Long Range Planning System," AMEDD Activities Report, August 1982)

The first Urology Technician Course opens at the AHS in September 1982.

("First Urology Technician Course Opens at the Academy," Medical Patriot, 1982)

SSG Jasazai
NCO in charge of the AHS Urology Technician Course instructs new urology tech students.

(U.S. Army Photo)

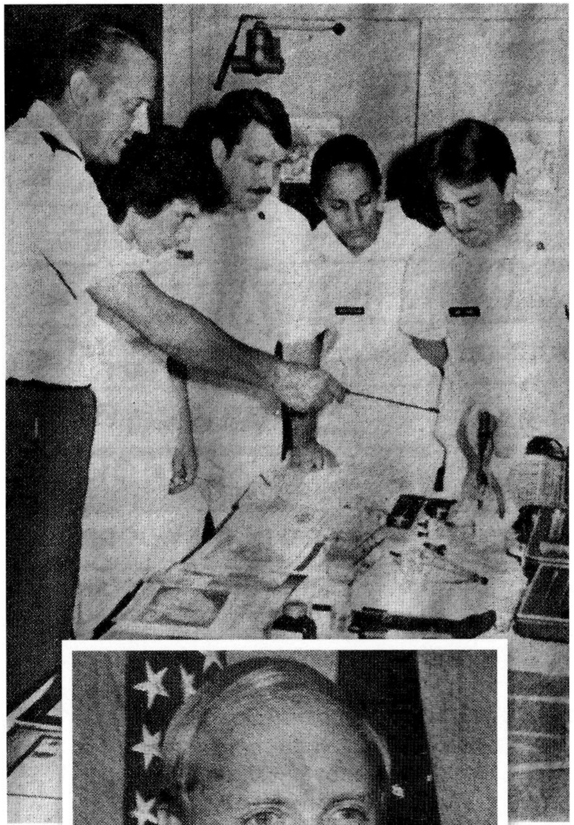

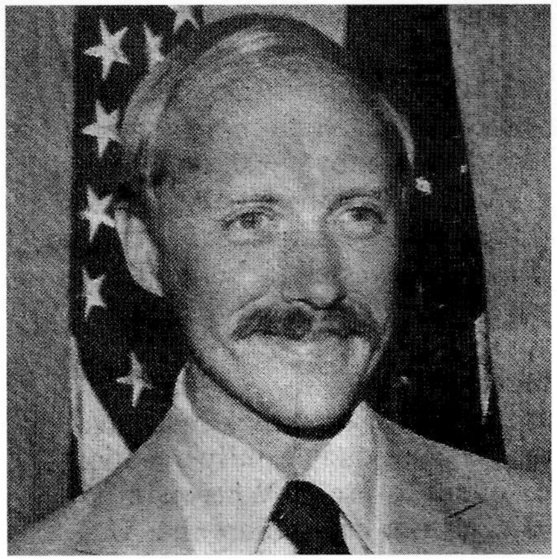

Dr. A. David Manglesdorff
Recipient of the American Psychological Association's 1982 Military Psychology Award for meritorious scientific and professional contributions to military psychology. At the time of the award, he served as a social science analyst with the Directorate of Combat Development and Health Care Studies.

("Psychologist Manglesdorff Receives Prestigious Award," Patriot, 14 October 1982)

1983

Combat Medic Specialist Division (CMSD) personnel participated in two iterations of paramedic training at the University of Texas Health Science Center San Antonio. This was in addition to the paramedic class that began in CY 82 and ended in January 1983. Approximately 40 members of CMSD were paramedic-certified.

("Paramedic Training," AMEDD Activities Report, January 1983)

The Behavioral Science Specialist Branch conducted the first "Annual Senior Behavioral Science Specialist Course" from 14 to 18 March 1983. The objectives were to provide an advanced management workshop, an advanced clinical skills workshop, and command consultation training. The course was also developed to identify and develop administrative and supervisory skills essential to the functioning of an NCOIC in a mental health, social work, or drug and alcohol setting. It provided an advanced combat psychiatry class to prepare the senior behavioral science specialist to perform his or her role in a combat environment.

("Behavioral Science Specialist Course," AMEDD Activities Report, March 1983)

The Military Subjects Branch developed a program for military history instruction in conjunction with the Uniformed Services University of Health Sciences, establishing a fellowship for one officer per year. Upon completion, the officer would return to the Military Science Division to teach military medical history to students of the AMEDD Officer Basic and AMEDD Officer Advanced courses.

("Military History Instruction," AMEDD Activities Report, June 1983)

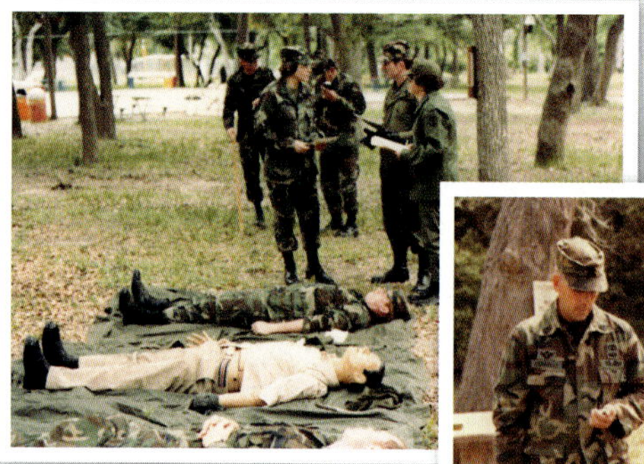

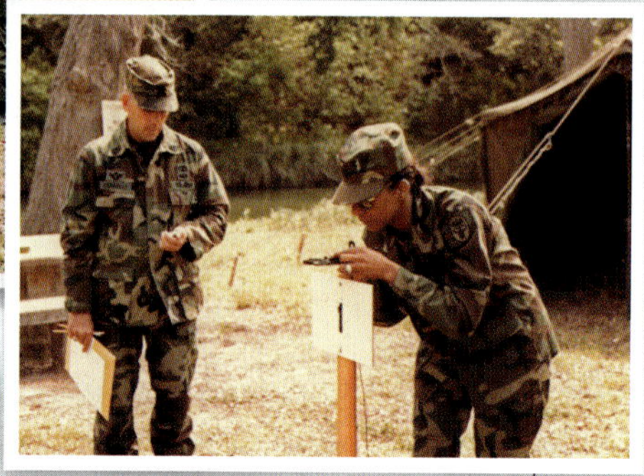

Competitors for the title of HSC's NCO and Soldier of the Year meet to compete in a command-wide competition on 5-6 April 1983. The competition included the APFT, completion of a map and compass exercise, break down and re-assembly of an M16 rifle, breaking down and familiarity with a protective mask, first aid demonstration, conducting drills, and personal interviews.

("NCO/Soldier of the Year Competition," Med Training 4-002, April 1983)

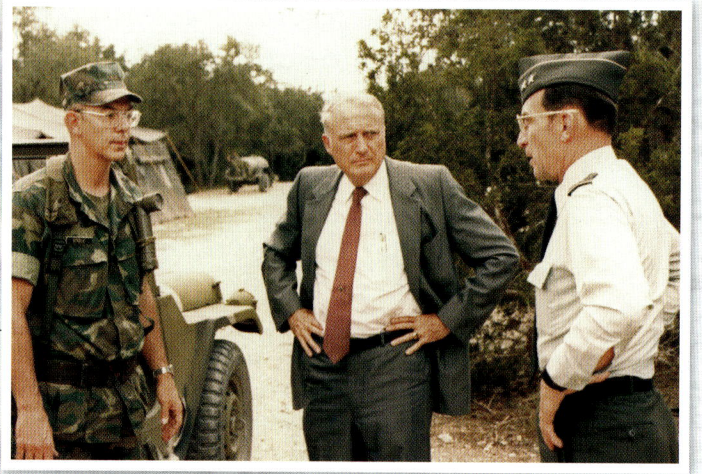

Secretary of the Army, John O. Marsh, Jr., discusses procedures of the C4 during a visit to Camp Bullis on 6 Oct 1983.

("Sec Army Visits Training," Med Training 4-027, October 1983)

The AHS re-implemented the U.S. Army-Baylor University Program in Physical Therapy after a one year hiatus. Three staff members received faculty appointments to assistant professor by the Baylor University Graduate School. All instructors in the U.S. Army-Baylor University Program in Physical Therapy received faculty appointments.

("PT Program Re-Implemented," AMEDD Activities Report, June 1983)

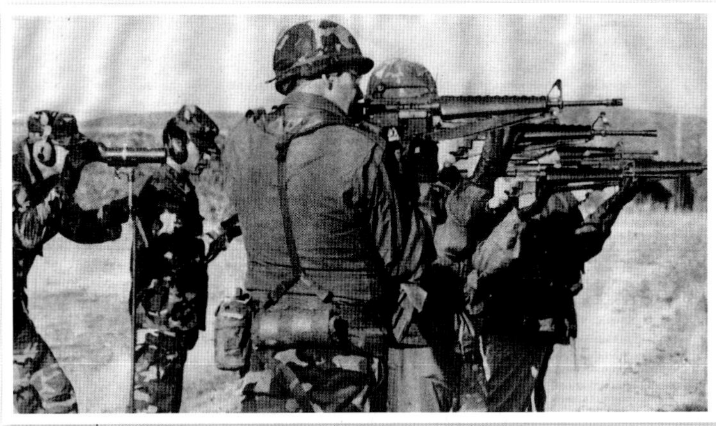

The AHS rifle team, the only team to enter the FSH Rifle Competition at Camp Bullis, won by default.

("Academy Rifle Team Takes Post Match," News Leader, 28 Jan 1983)

In October, the Army awarded the University of Oklahoma a contract of affiliation for the Army's Military Physician Assistant Course. This affiliation provided the PA students a bachelor's degree upon completion of two years of extensive training, which AHS expanded to include advanced cardiac life support, advanced trauma management review, and a CPR instructor's course.

("PA Affiliation with U of Oklahoma," AMEDD Activities Report, Oct 1983)

The new 16-week Advanced Medical Specialist Course started on 7 November. The student input was 100, with additional classes of 50 students scheduled to begin monthly.

("New 91B Course Trains NCO Medics," AMEDD Activities Report, Nov 1983)

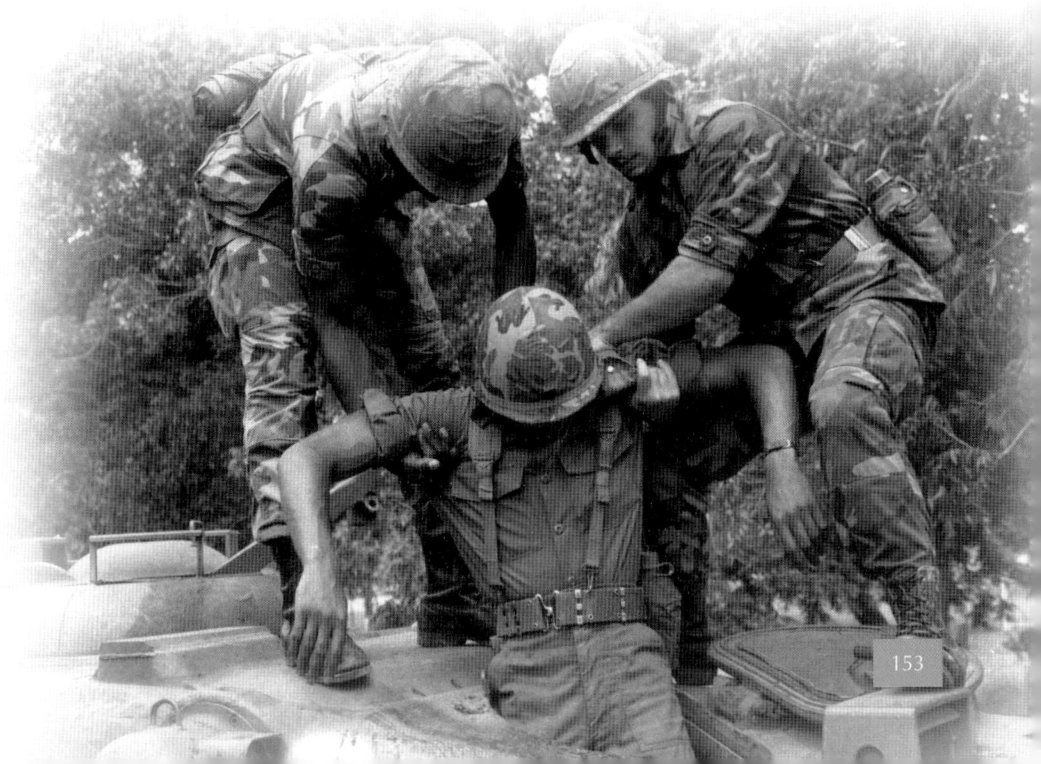

Students in the Combat Medic Specialist Course at AHS practice the extraction of a casualty from an M103A2 battle tank.

("Extraction From a Tank," Med Training 4-020, July 1983)

1984

An AMEDD professional post-graduate short course, Administration for Nutrition Care (Hospital Food Service) in Fixed and Field Hospitals, was conducted from 19 to 23 March 1984. The course was designed to provide practical information for nutrition care directors concerning the latest developments in the administration and management of Army nutrition care service systems and medical field feeding systems.

("Nutrition Care Short Course Begun," AMEDD Activities Report, March 1984)

Army, Navy, and Air Force healthcare professionals undergo the rigors of nuclear-biological-chemical training for the C4 at Camp Bullis on 18 May 1984.

("NBC Training at C4," Med Training 4-103, May 1984)

The U.S. Army Aeromedical Activity, U.S. Army Aeromedical Center, was redesignated as the U.S. Army School of Aviation Medicine (USASAM) and assigned to the AHS 1 Oct 1984.

(Permanent Orders 78-1, 1 Oct 1984)

The Directorate of Combat Development finalized the concept plan (Annex O) for Army 21 (Air Land Battle 2000).

("CONPLAN for ALB 2000 Finalized," AMEDD Activities Report, June 1984)

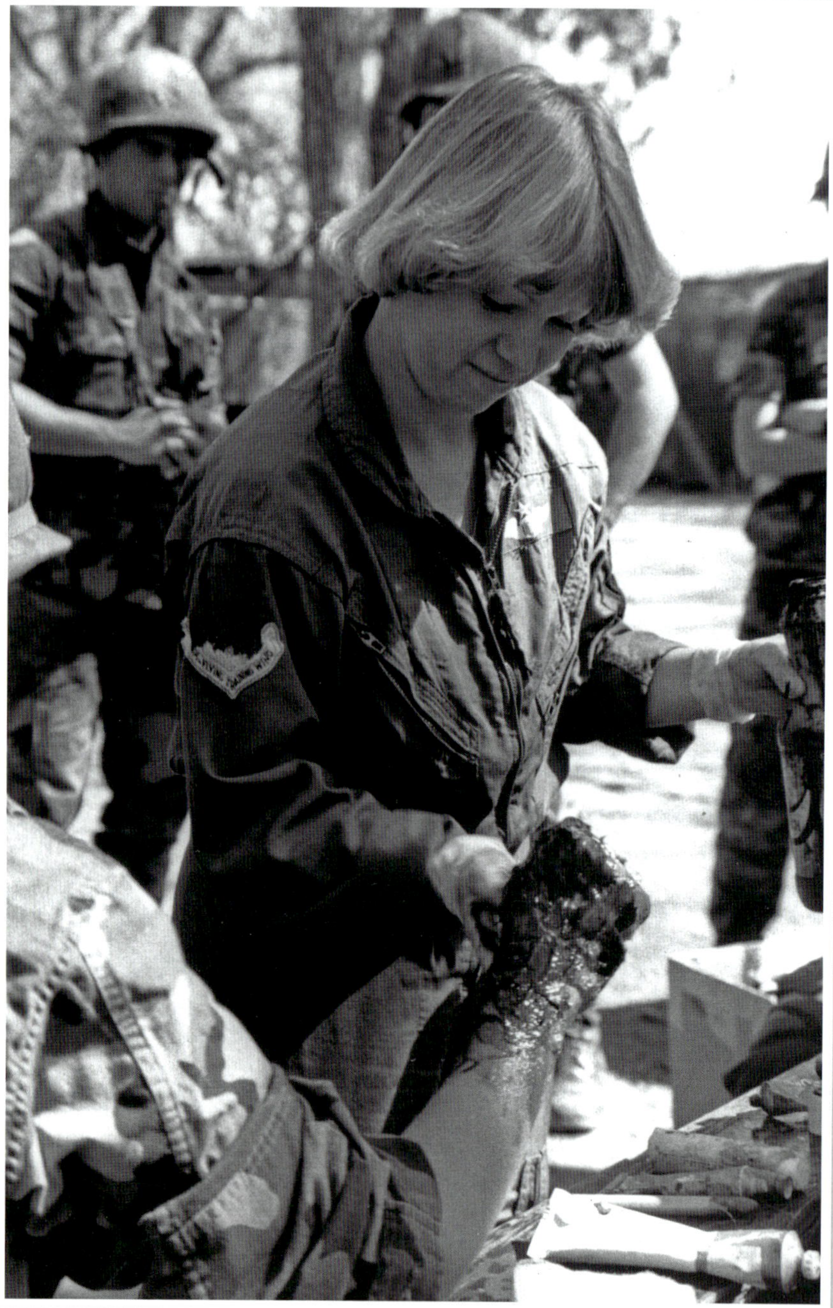

Instructors of the Combat Medical Specialist Course dress up students with fake wounds. This moulage makeup was applied to students acting as casualties during the course's FTX when they practiced what they have been taught about combat medicine. In this particular class, Army reservists from the 323d Medical Laboratory went through the FTX with the active duty trainees.

("Instructors Apply Moulage for FTX," Med Training 4-062, April 1984)

The Nursing Science Division developed an official Field Nursing Manual for Army Nurse Corps officers. The manual provided pertinent information regarding realistic field nursing expectations. A Field Nursing Survey was conducted to research the document. Combining the Field Nursing Survey results with the draft, a comprehensive Field Nursing Manual went to print in Jan 1985.

("Nursing Science to Develop Manual," AMEDD Activities Report, June 1984)

Stimson Library initiated an automated reference service with access to the databases of MEDLARS (National Library of Medicine), DIALOG (a global information database that includes federal research in progress), and DROLS (Defense Technical Information Center).

("Stimson Automated System," AMEDD Activities Report, July 1984)

The School of Aviation Medicine taught the first Aviation Branch Officer Basic Course to 70 students on 26 July 1984 and the first Aviation Branch Officer Advanced course to 80 students on 21 Aug 1984.

("School of Aviation Medicine OBC," AMEDD Activities Report, July 1984)

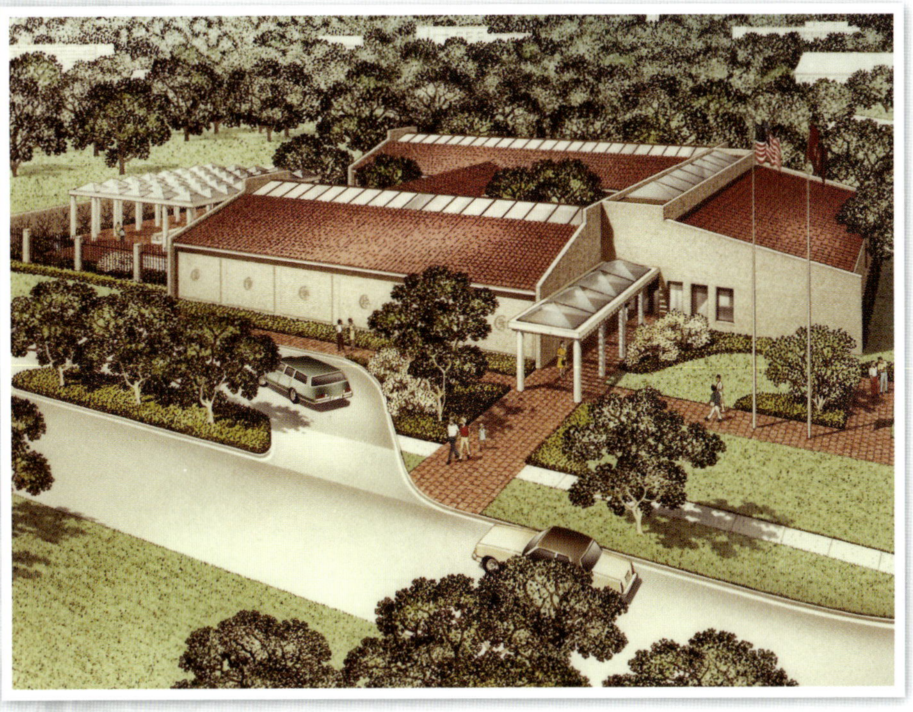

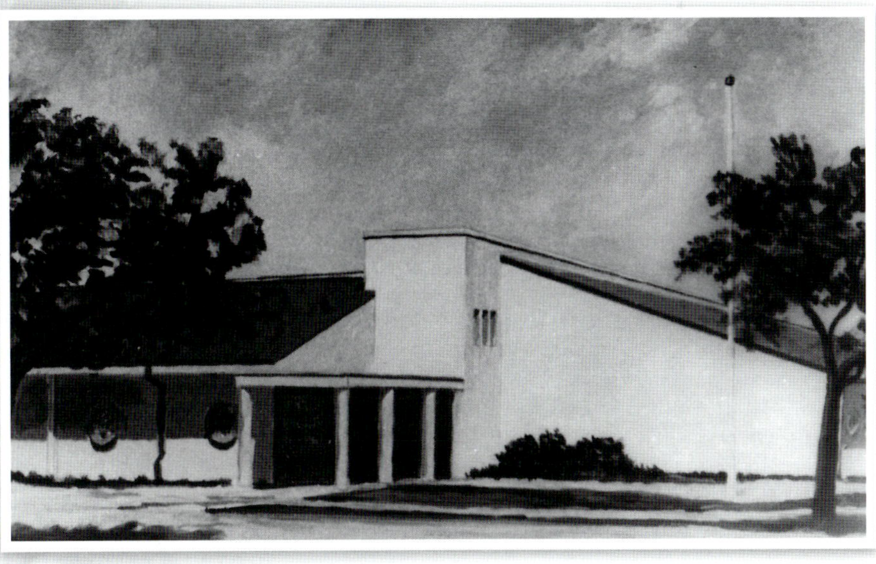

COL Archie D. Pollock, Jr., MSC, AHS, announced the groundbreaking of the AMEDD Museum in August 1984. Concept drawings of the building were released for viewing shortly thereafter.

(Letter to School Secretary (HSHA-SMM) from COL Archie D. Pollock, Jr., MSC, 13 August 1984; "Museum Donations," AHS, U.S. Army PAO Release, 4 May 1984)

1984

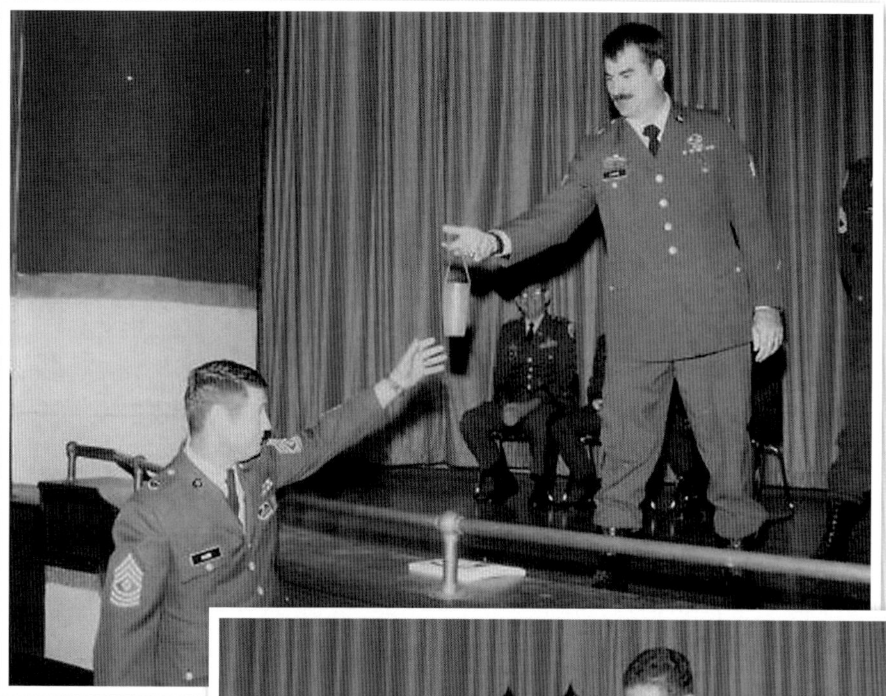

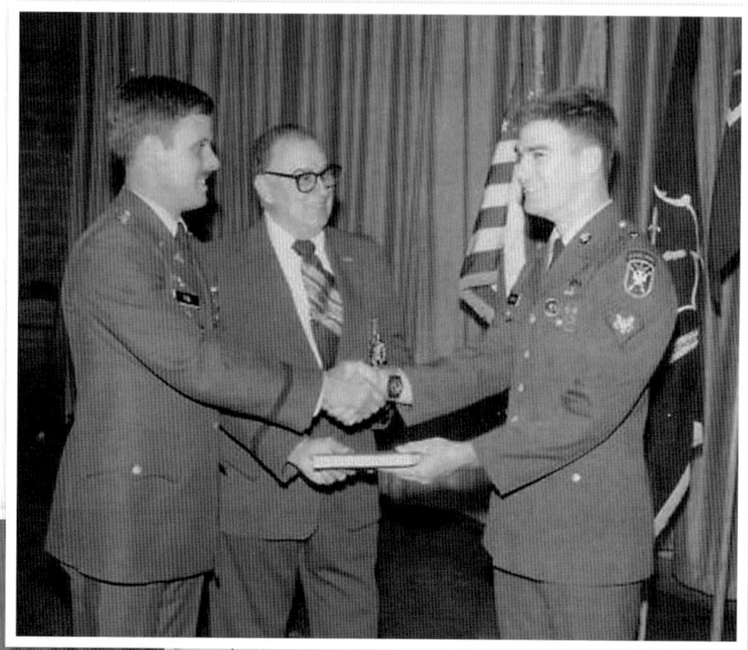

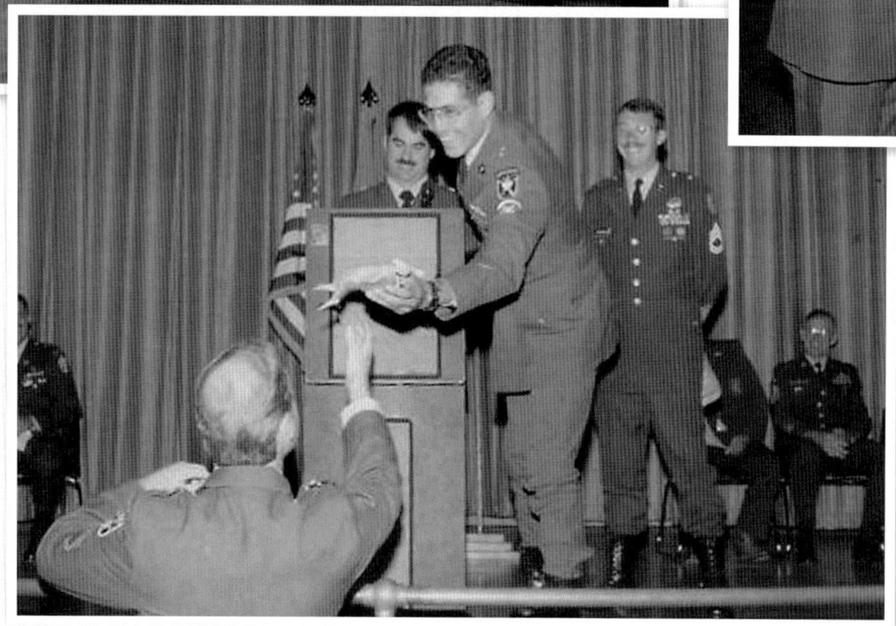

The first group of students to complete the new four-month Phase I of the Special Operations Medical Noncommissioned Officer Course at the AHS received "special" awards at their completion ceremony on 25 October.

(U.S. Army photo, TASC, FSH, TX)

The Low Intensity Conflict (LIC) Division was established on 14 June 1984 with the signing of a memorandum of agreement between AHS and the John F. Kennedy Special Warfare Center. The LIC Division was established to address Special Operations medical training and all other medical training needs for low intensity conflicts. As a result of intensified DoD concern over various aspects of LIC, such as terrorism and foreign internal defense operations, specific medical doctrine and training was anticipated.

("Low Intensity Combat Division Established," AMEDD Activities Report, June 1984)

AHS conducted a special FTX to study the effects of battle fatigue. Mental health officers who attended the AMEDD Officer Advanced course served in the capacity of medical personnel, while 91B10 students played the roles of emotionally overloaded soldiers, all in a combat-simulated environment. Behavioral science personnel conducted extensive studies of past wars to evaluate the extent of battle fatigue on the soldier. Studies included the experiences of the Israeli Defense Force in Lebanon and showed that the majority of battle fatigue casualties can be returned to their units and to their previous jobs within 72 hours, returning to be as effective as other soldiers.

("Special FTX Studies Battle Fatigue," AMEDD Mercury, August 1984)

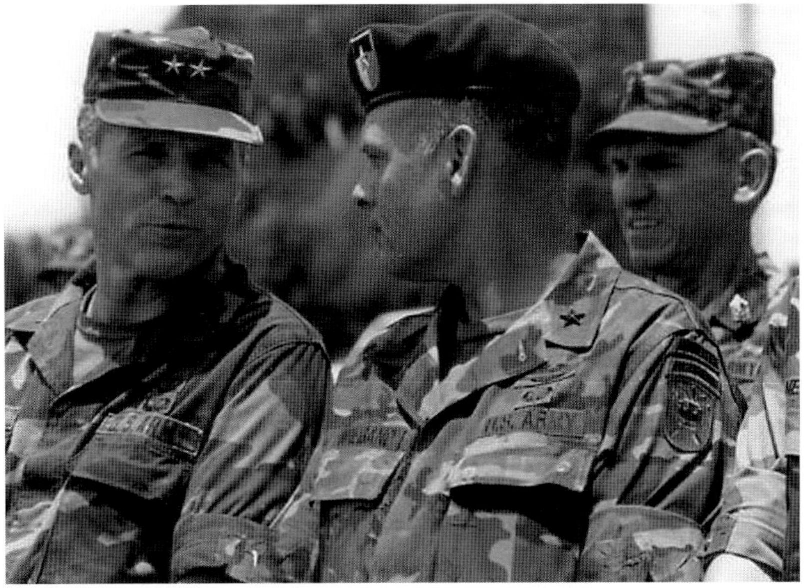

AHS Commander MG William P. Winkler, Jr., and BG Robert D. Wiegand, Commander of the U.S. Army John F. Kennedy Special Warfare Center at Ft Bragg, NC, confer at the activation of F Company (Airborne), 3rd BN, Academy BDE, Academy of Health Sciences, U.S. Army. As the leaders of the two institutions who cooperated in the formation of F Company, both generals spoke at the activation, which was held at the Academy in San Antonio, TX.

(U.S. Army photo, TASC, FSH, TX)

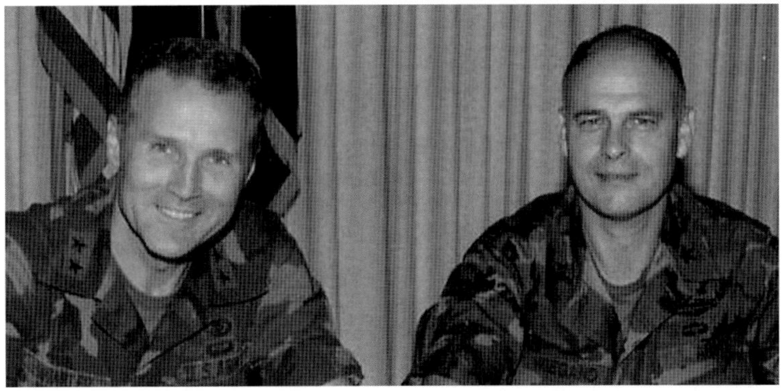

The commandant of the AHS, U.S. Army, MG William P. Winkler, Jr., and the commander of the U.S. Army John F. Kennedy Special Warfare Center at Ft Bragg, NC, BG Robert D. Wiegand, are all smiles after signing the document in which their organizations agree to a joint training program for the Army's special forces medics. The generals signed the memorandum of agreement 14 June at the AHS in San Antonio.

(U.S. Army Photo, TASC, FSH, TX)

1984

The Alcohol and Drug Abuse Prevention and Control (ADAPC) Program Course was established by the Behavioral Science Division, with the first iteration conducted on 14 Aug 1984. The two-week course was taught to active duty military members and civilians currently assigned as counselors in support of the Army's ADAPC Program.

("ADAPC Family Counseling Course," AMEDD Activities Report, August 1984)

AHS approved a proposal submitted by the Dental Science Division for a new 19-week Dental Laboratory Specialist Course, proposed to commence in July 1985. Course content encompassed the verbal and motor skills presently taught in the existing basic and intermediate Dental Lab courses.

("New Dental Lab Course Approved," AMEDD Activities Report, August 1984)

The AHS became accredited as an occupational education institution by the Southern Association of Colleges and Schools. The first class, consisting of 350 students, was registered to receive college credits in October.

("AHS Becomes Accredited," AMEDD Activities Report, September 1984)

Initial implementation of the Academy Locator and Academic Records System (ALARS) was accomplished in October 1984. This system was the first major in-house system installed on the AHS Burroughs computer. The initial capability provided for maintaining an AHS personnel master file, using Battalion PAC SIDPERS transactions routed through ALARS on their way to the SIDPERS Interface System.

("ALARS Implemented," AMEDD Activities Report, October 1984)

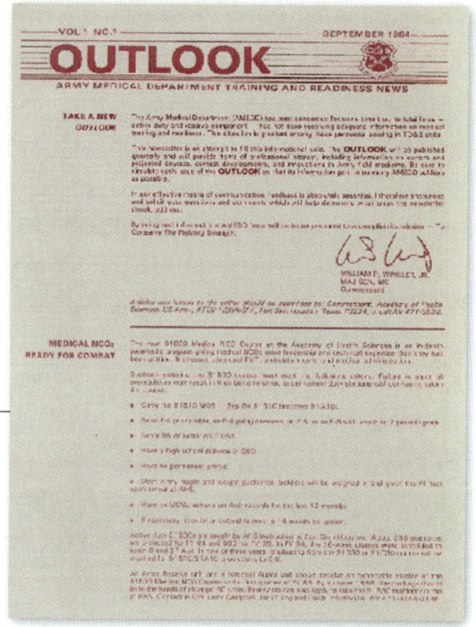
VOL 1 NO 1 SEPTEMBER 1984
OUTLOOK
ARMY MEDICAL DEPARTMENT TRAINING AND READINESS NEWS

The first issue of the Army Medical Department Training and Readiness monthly, The OUTLOOK, is published.

Following a tasking for the Army Vice Chief of Staff in December 1984, preparations were made for the development of DA-level documentation requirements for conduct of Force Development Test and Experimentation (FDTE) of Combat Support Hospitals (CSHs), Evacuation (EVAC) Hospitals, and a General Hospital configured with DEPMEDS equipment. These hospitals would be re-configured to replace the seven hospitals in the current force structure for combat zone and communication zone medical support. The CSH and EVAC hospitals were restructured to meet respective combat zone primary missions: 1) supporting return-to-duty patient populations in the CSH and 2) trauma stabilization in the EVAC for ultimate removal of such casualties from the theater of operations.

("AMEDD Activities Report," January 1985)

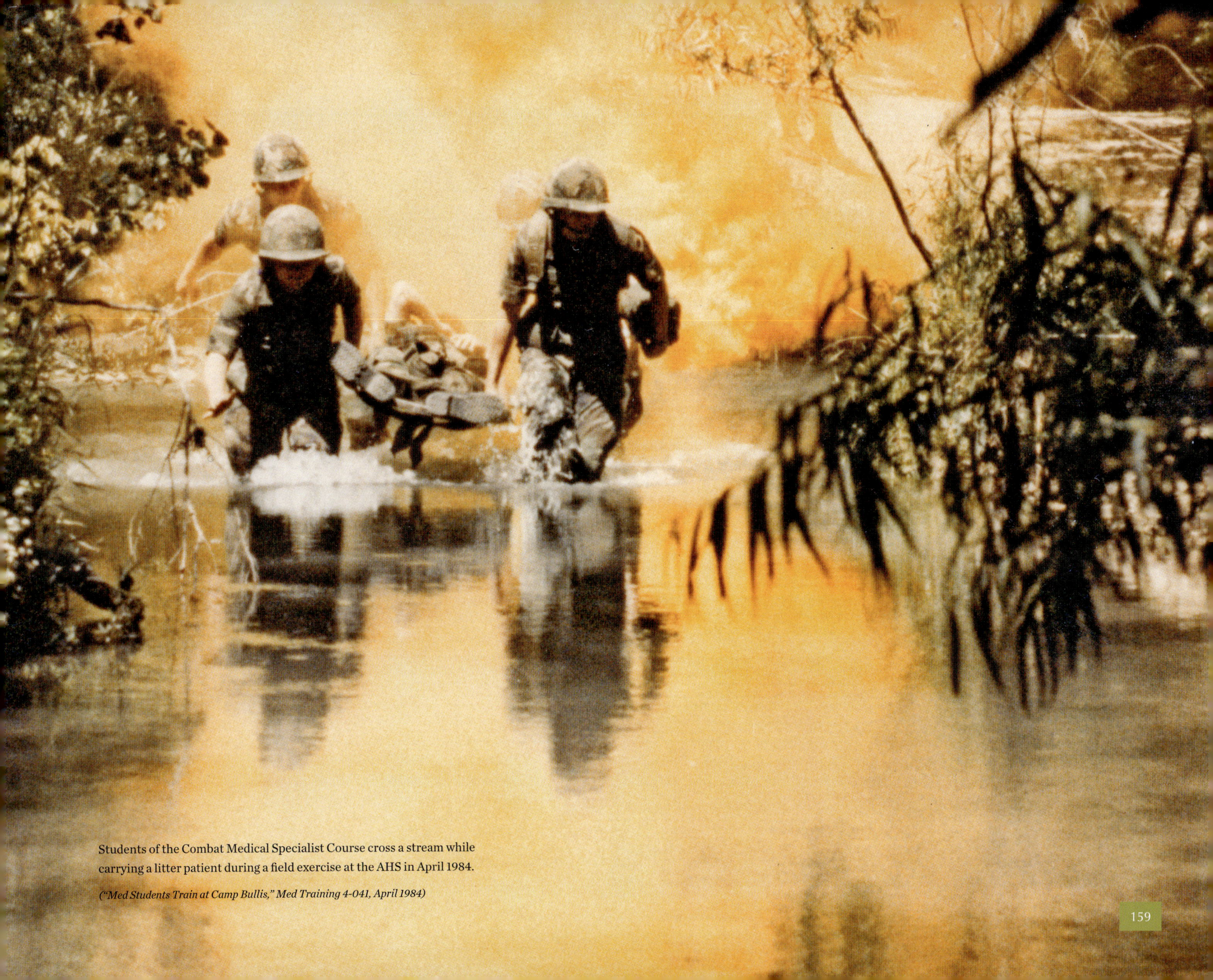

Students of the Combat Medical Specialist Course cross a stream while carrying a litter patient during a field exercise at the AHS in April 1984.

("Med Students Train at Camp Bullis," Med Training 4-041, April 1984)

1985

In the second quarter of FY 1985, MG Winkler decided to reduce the AMEDD worldwide Army Training Extension Course Program by four-fifths of its required staffing and workload. The remaining staff was tasked to review and revise field products.

(Command Performance Summary, AHS, U.S. Army, FSH, TX, 2Qtr FY 85 [Jan-Mar 85], pp 1.3-1.4)

The Health Care Administration (HCA) Division initiated a Pre-Command Course, as directed by OTSG, to help prepare senior Medical Corps (MC) and Dental Course (DC) officers for their duties as commanders of medical and dental treatment facilities.

("New Pre-Cmd Course from HCA," AMEDD Activities Report, January 1985)

NBC Sciences Branch established a laboratory for the Phase I training of health physics technicians. In addition, the U.S. Nuclear Regulatory Commission licensed AMEDD to use radioisotopes for health physics training.

("NBC Lab Training Established," AMEDD Activities Report, June 1985)

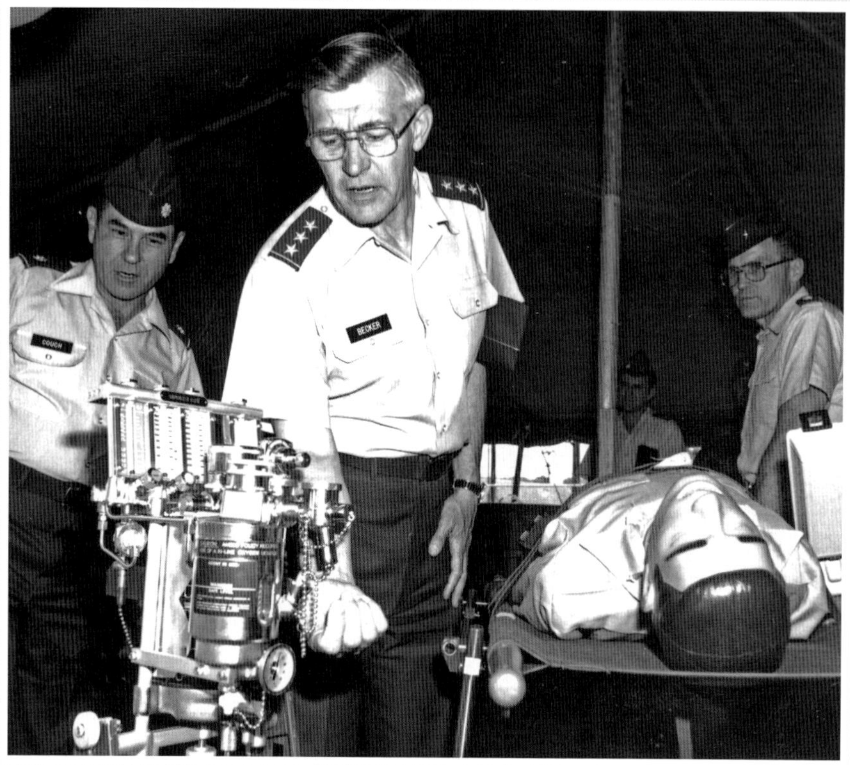

LTG Quinn Becker, Surgeon General of the Army, examines an anesthesia machine, a vital component in AMEDD's newly-developed surgical squad medical set. Becker reviewed several types of the new modular medical sets during his visit.

("TSG Visit to AHS," Med Training 4-128, May 1985)

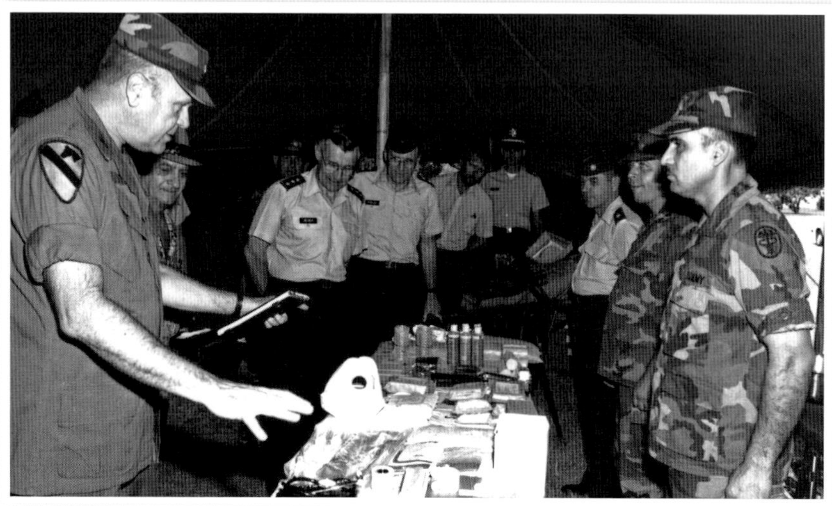

COL John D. Hayes, President of the AHS's Army Medical Board, explains the concept and details of the newly-developed modular medical sets to LTG Becker during his visit to AHS on 9 May 1985.

("TSG Visit to AHS," Med Training 4-132, May 1985)

The first Professional Postgraduate Short Course (PPSC) for field nutrition was held at AHS 16-20 Sep 1985. The Administration for Food Service in Field Hospitals Course provided current concepts and hands-on training for Army dieticians. It provided a forum for PROFIS designees in a field kitchen setting to have hands-on experience in revised medical field feeding concepts supporting the new Combat Field Feeding System.

("New Nutrition PPSC," AMEDD Activities Report, September 1985)

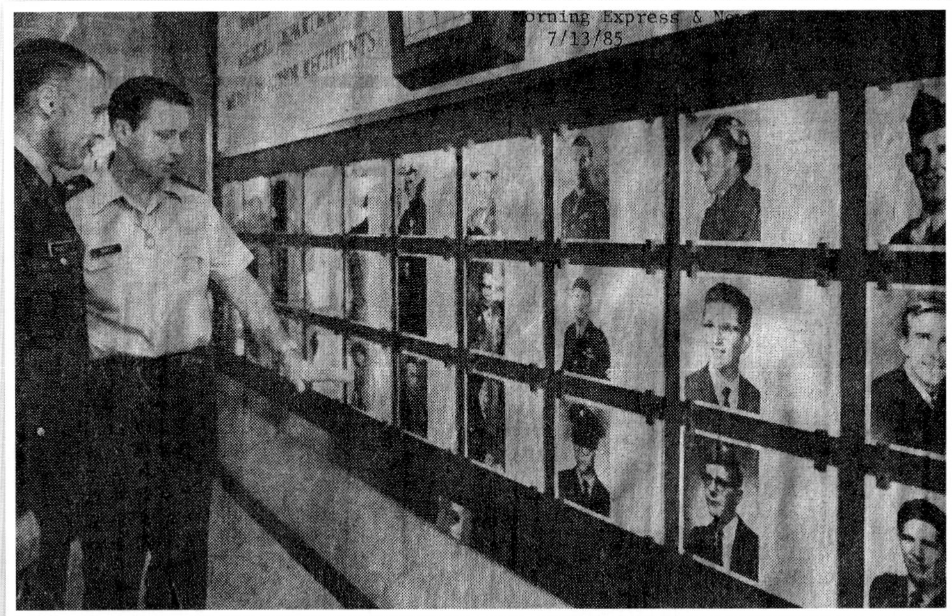

BG Patrick H. Brady unveils the Medal of Honor Wall in Aabel Hall in July 1985.

("Medical Medal of Honor Recipients Honored," Morning News Express, 13 July 1985, photo by Joe Barrera, Jr.)

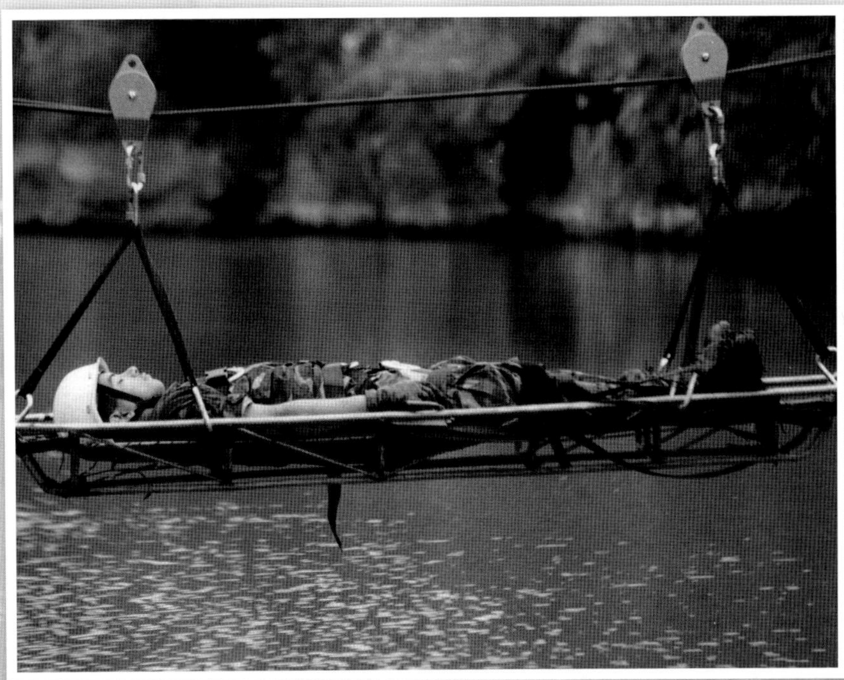

The U.S. Army Medical Board, AHS, tested vertical rescue techniques at Camp Bullis. A team of recent 91A10 (Combat Medical Specialist) graduates executed the test after one week of classroom study and one week of mountaineering training.

("Med Board Tests Vertical Rescue Techniques," Med Training 4-143, December 1985)

1985

The 16-week Medical Noncommissioned Officers (91B) Course at AHS formally began in 1983, but only in 1985 were its graduates circulating throughout the Army. This course was designed to prepare a soldier-medic to be well trained in first-line treatment of casualties and competent to function as a trainer and a leader. The main mission of these medics was to increase combat survivability by providing far forward care. Formerly, combat medics received no technical training after they completed AIT. Medical specialists (91A) provided first-line treatment on the battlefield as they literally worked beside combat soldiers. However, with the advent of the super 91B course, the basic medic received additional, advanced training to progress as a technician and a soldier.

("New 91B Course Trains NCO Medics," AMEDD Mercury, October 1985)

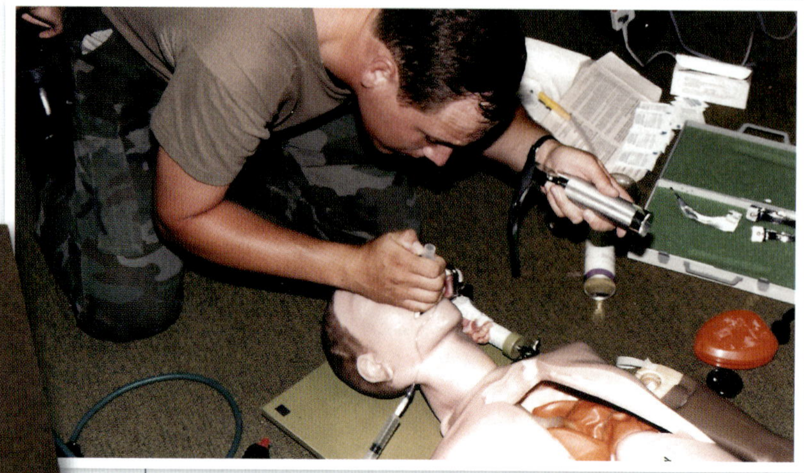

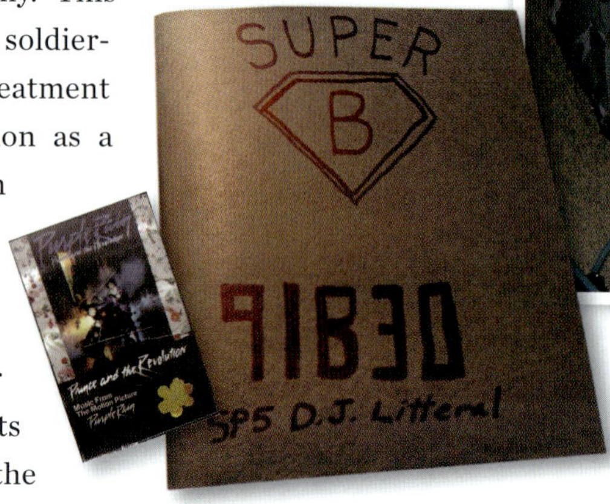

SP5 D.J. Litteral intubating a practice manikin known as "Fred the Head." At left, SP5 Litteral's study materials for the 91B course, which included Prince's *Purple Rain.*

(AMEDDC&S Photo)

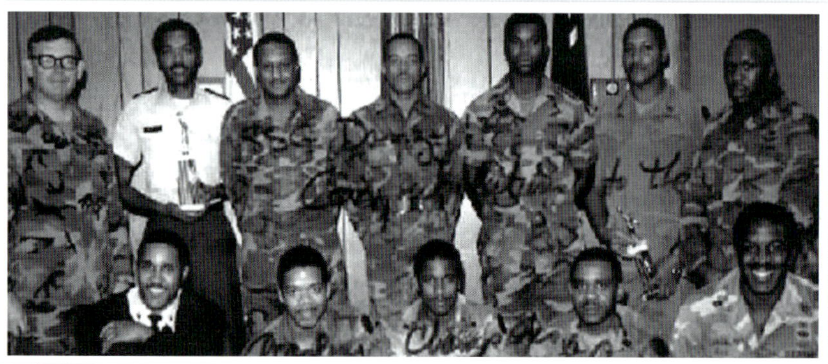

The 2D BN took the post-wide FSH Basketball Championship in 1985.

(AMEDDC&S Photo)

The Practical Nurse Course (91C20) achieved a significant reduction in attrition, advancing 176 of 187 students through the first of its two phases. They proceeded to three Phase II sites for further training.

("Practical Nurse Course," AMEDD Activities Report, October 1985)

Twenty-two Army Nurse Corps students began the Anesthesiology for Army Nurse Corps Officer's Course under its new affiliation with Texas Wesleyan College. As a pilot project, a fully-qualified certified Registered Nurse Anesthetist attended the course for degree completion. The student attended Phase I at AHS, and was awarded a Master of Health Science degree upon completion.

("New Nurse Anesthetist Course," AMEDD Activities Report, October 1985)

The U.S. Army School of Aviation Medicine installed the Army's first training hyperbaric chamber to provide training in hyperbaric medicine and clinical treatment of hyperbaric injuries.

("First Hyperbaric Chamber Installed," AMEDD Activities Report, November 1985)

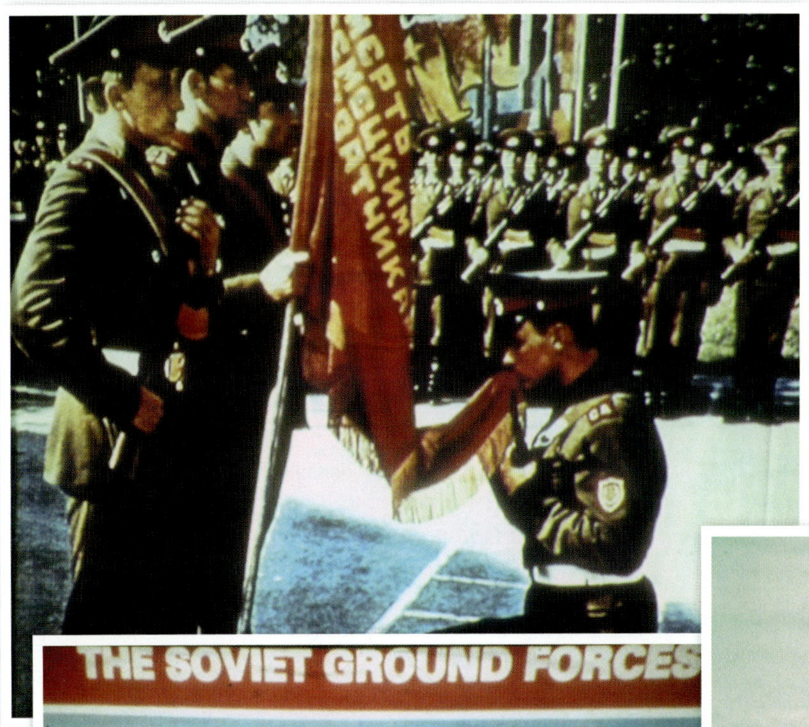

CPT Jeffrey L. McCollum taught a "Soviet Threat" course as part of OBC and CCC in the mid-80s. CPT McCollum on the right. Slides from his course to the left and below.

(Photographs courtesy of Jeffrey L. McCollum)

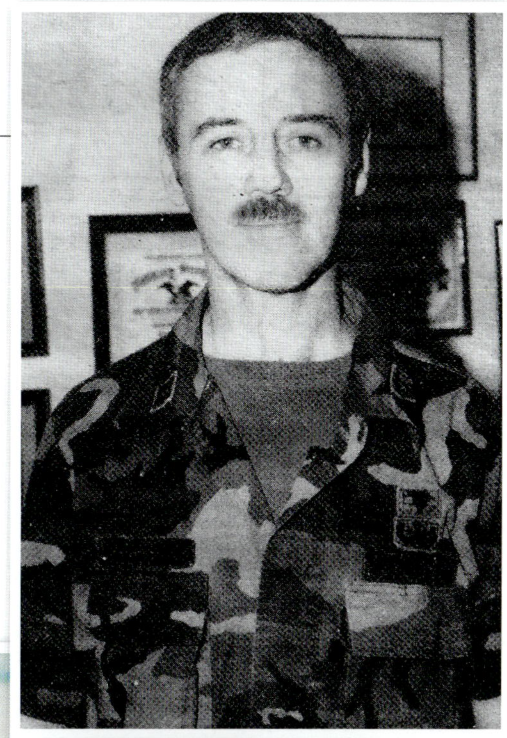

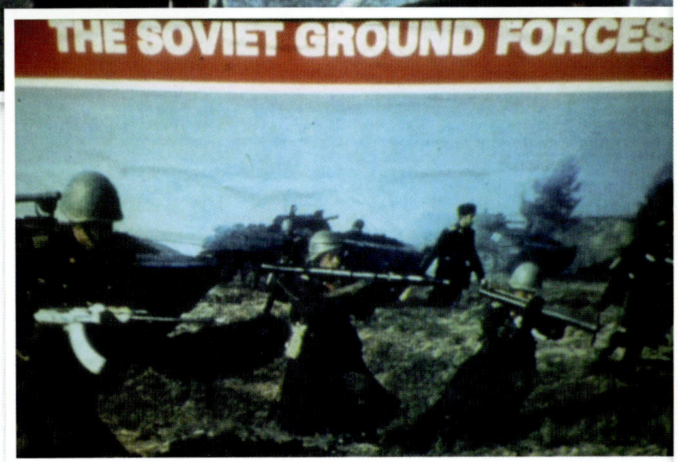

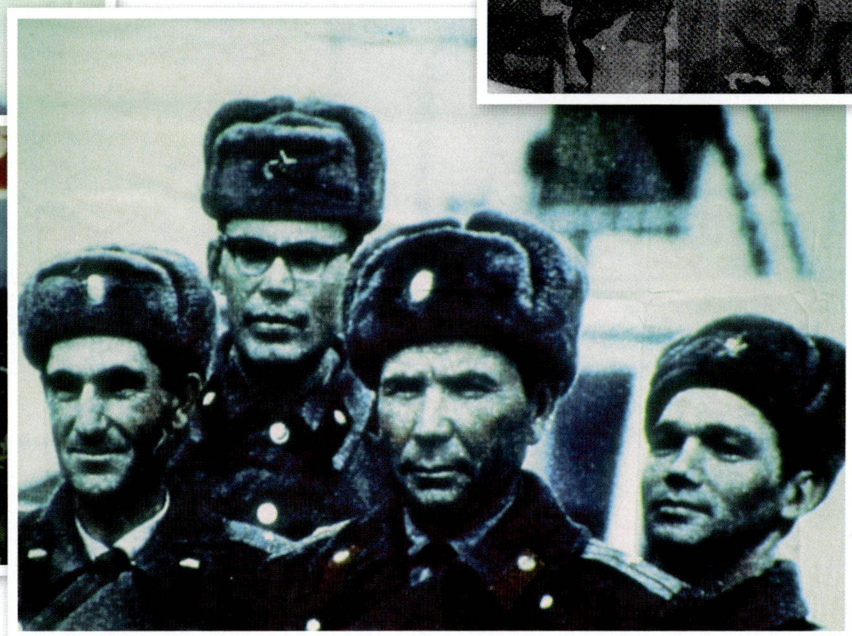

1986

Proclamation

San Antonio Mayor Henry Cisneros proclaimed July 27 to be U.S. Army Medical Department Regiment Day. COL Raymond Leahey, assistant commandant of the Academy of Health Sciences, and MAJ James Swain, regimental adjunct, receive the proclamation from City Councilwoman Helen Dutmer.

(Photo by Raymound Turner)

Proclamation

WHEREAS, THE UNITED STATES ARMY MEDICAL DEPARTMENT WILL BE ACTIVATED INTO THE ARMY REGIMENTAL SYSTEM, JULY 27, 1986, AND

WHEREAS, THE HOME STATION OF THE ARMY MEDICAL DEPARTMENT REGIMENT, WHICH HOUSES THE COLORS AND CREST, IS THE ACADEMY OF HEALTH SCIENCES, U.S. ARMY, FORT SAM HOUSTON, TEXAS, AND

WHEREAS, THE REGIMENT WILL BE THE SOURCE OF THE HISTORY, TRADITION AND LINEAGE OF THE ARMY MEDICAL DEPARTMENT, AND

WHEREAS, THE ARMY MEDICAL DEPARTMENT REGIMENT'S MISSION IS TO PROVIDE THE HIGHEST QUALITY OF HEALTH CARE SUPPORT TO THE FIGHTING FORCES, AND

WHEREAS, ITS PERSONNEL STAND READY TO DEPLOY AND SUPPORT THE ARMY IF CALLED TO COMBAT, WHILE PROVIDING DAY TO DAY HEALTH CARE TO ALL BENEFICIARIES, AND

WHEREAS, JULY 27TH MARKS THE 221TH ANNIVERSARY OF MEDICAL SERVICES TO THE U.S. ARMY, AND

WHEREAS, THE ARMY MEDICAL DEPARTMENT REGIMENT HOME STATION IN SAN ANTONIO FORMALIZES SAN ANTONIO AS HOME STATION OF ALL MEDICAL SOLDIERS.

NOW, THEREFORE, I, HENRY CISNEROS, MAYOR OF THE CITY OF SAN ANTONIO, IN RECOGNITION THEREOF, DO HEREBY PROCLAIM SUNDAY, JULY 27, 1986, AS

"ARMY MEDICAL DEPARTMENT REGIMENT DAY"

IN SAN ANTONIO, TEXAS, AND I URGE ALL CITIZENS TO RECOGNIZE THEIR NEIGHBORS AND FRIENDS WHO ARE MEMBERS OF THE UNITED STATES ARMY MEDICAL DEPARTMENT REGIMENT.

IN WITNESS WHEREOF, I HAVE HEREUNTO SET MY HAND AND CAUSED THE SEAL OF THE CITY OF SAN ANTONIO TO BE AFFIXED THIS 17TH DAY OF JULY, 1986.

Henry Cisneros

HENRY CISNEROS

MAYOR

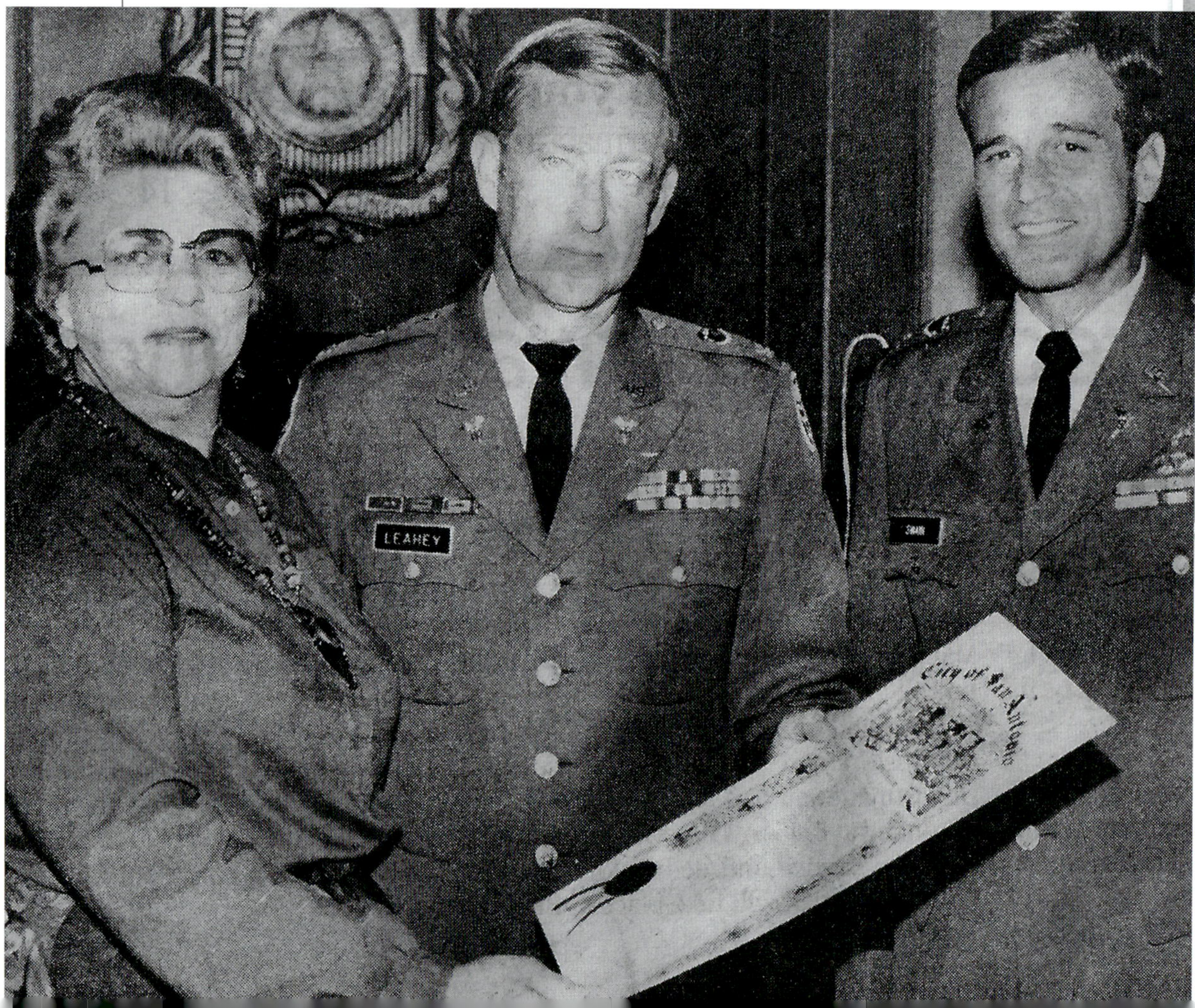

Father of the Army's Combat Lifesaver Program

Dr. Robert Howard Mosebar (COL, Ret) served the Army for 60 years as an active and reserve duty officer and then as a civilian. After seeing a soldier bleed to death early in his career, it became his passion to equip combat soldiers with advanced medical skills. In 1986, he took the lead in launching the Army's Combat Lifesaver Program, designed to train non-medic soldiers with moderate emergency medical training to provide care at the point of wounding.

("Mosebar developed lifesaver training for GIs," San Antonio News Express, 28 August 2011; Photo courtesy of Dr. Larry Johnson, AMEDDC&S, FSH, TX)

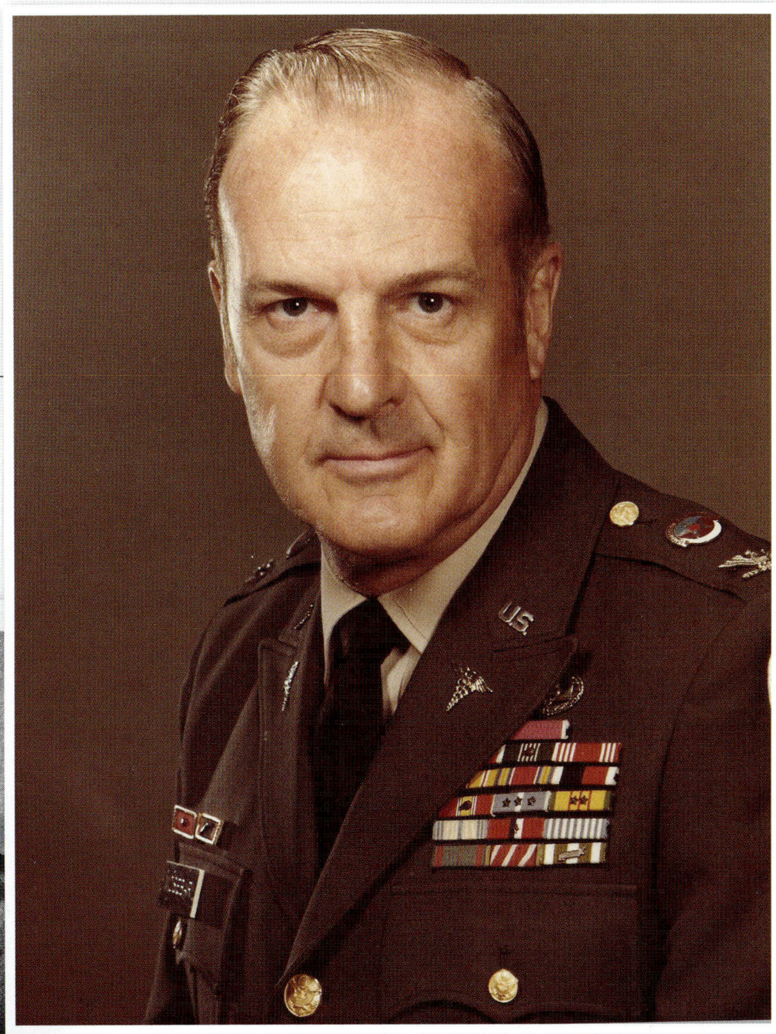

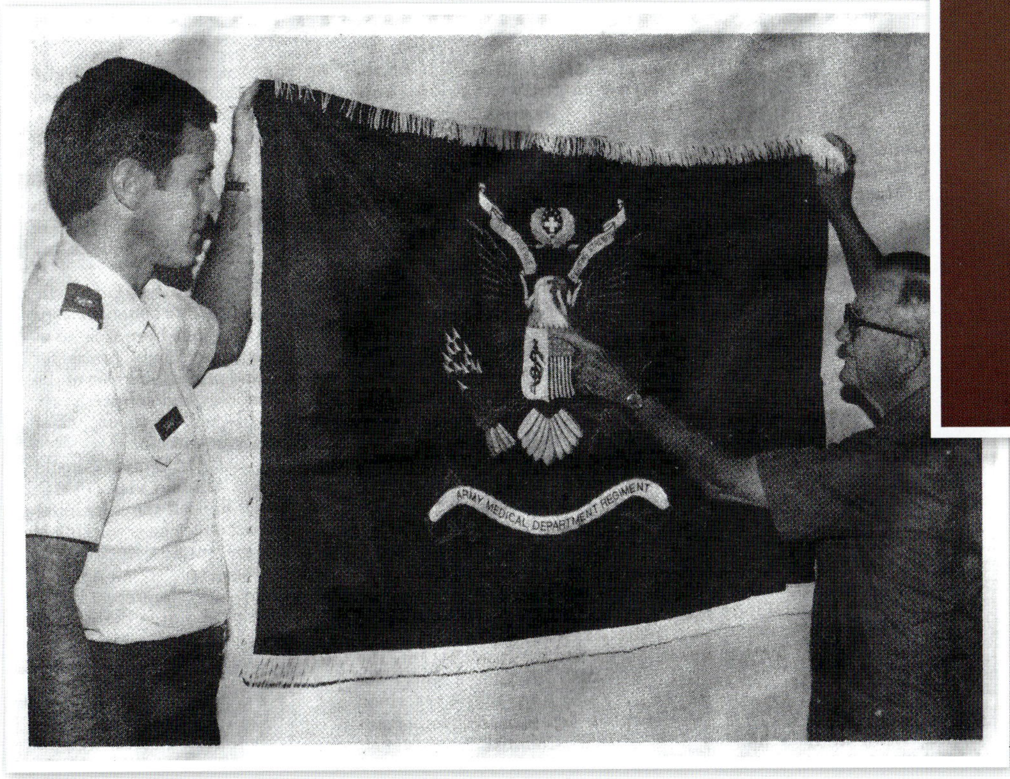

The AMEDD was activated into the Army Regimental System on 27 July, the anniversary of the Medical Department. The activation parade and unveiling occured on 28 July. AHS was selected as the home station for the AMEDD Regiment and MAJ James H. Swain became its first adjutant. Honorary officers selected were MG Spurgeon Neel, Jr. (Ret) and CSM George J. Pierce (Ret).

("Medical Department Joins Regimental System," AMEDD News Leader, July 1986)

1987

The first group of NCOs at the AMEDD's new NCO Academy began training. The school for Army medical enlisted leadership training finally became a reality, after nearly six years of planning.

("New NCO Academy Begins Training," AMEDD Recorder, April 1987)

AHS set up a field feeding facility for the Combat Field Feeding System Test. More than 500 students, faculty and staff members, and visiting dignitaries viewed the activity. Conducted by the AMEDD's Medical Board, the exercise tested the concept of providing hot, nutritious meals to patients and medical staff in a combat situation with new technological developments in food service equipment and techniques.

("Academy Simulation Tests Feeding System," AMEDD News Leader, June 1987)

The Academy Brigade's 1st Battalion and 2nd Brigade were redesignated as the 187th Medical Battalion and 232nd Medical Battalion effective 27 July 1987.

The original 187th was formed in New York during the late summer of 1943, and took part in the Rhineland campaigns. Following the war, the unit was inactivated at Camp Swift, Texas, on 17 Oct 1945.

The 232nd Medical Battalion was originally activated in Italy the summer of 1944 as the 232nd Medical Composite Battalion, and it was later redesignated as the 232nd Medical Service Battalion. It took part in the Rome-Arno campaign, serving in Italy until it was inactivated on 1 May 1946. Five and a half years later, the 232nd was reactivated in Korea. It participated in the UN Summer-Fall Offensive, Second Korean Winter, Korean Summer-Fall 1952, and Third Korean Winter campaigns.

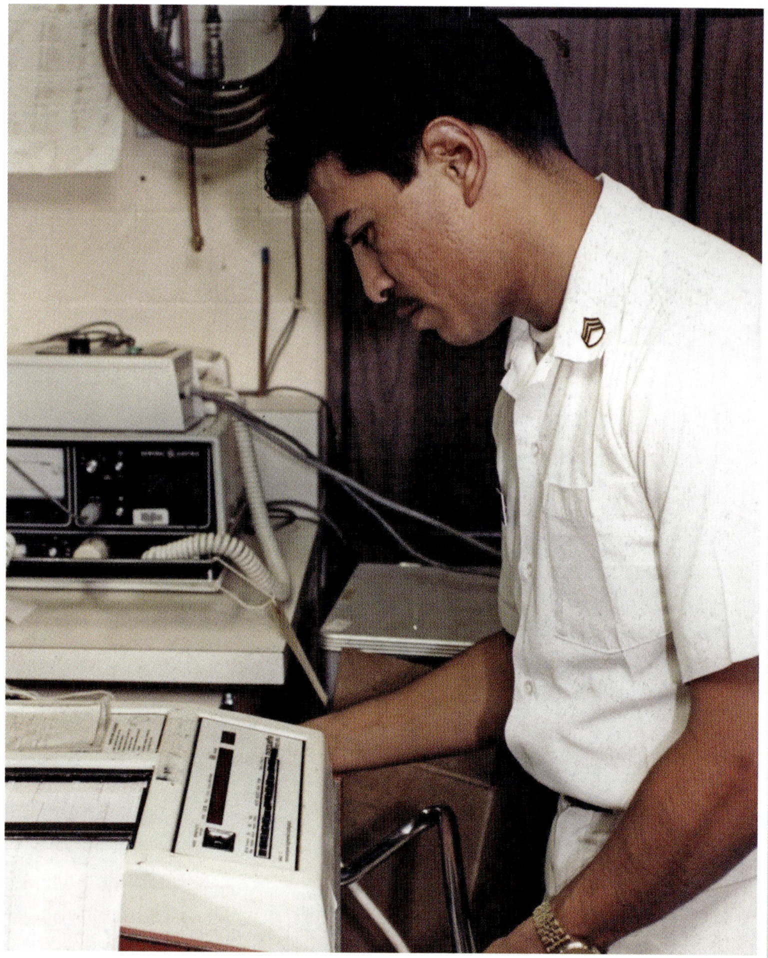

A student at the respiratory therapist course at BAMC, 25 Aug 1987

(U.S. Army Photo, AMEDD Museum Photo Collection)

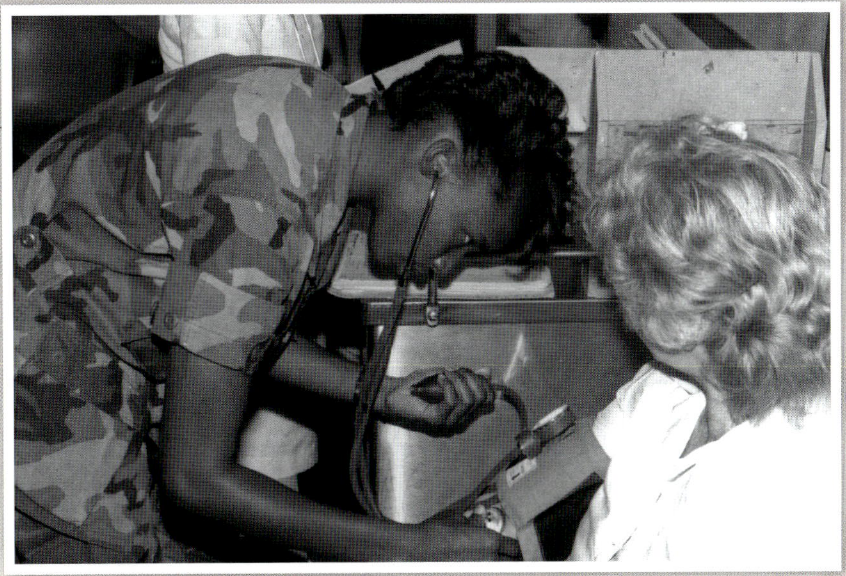

A student at the respiratory therapist course at BAMC, 25 Aug 1987.

(U.S. Army Photo, AMEDD Museum Photo Collection)

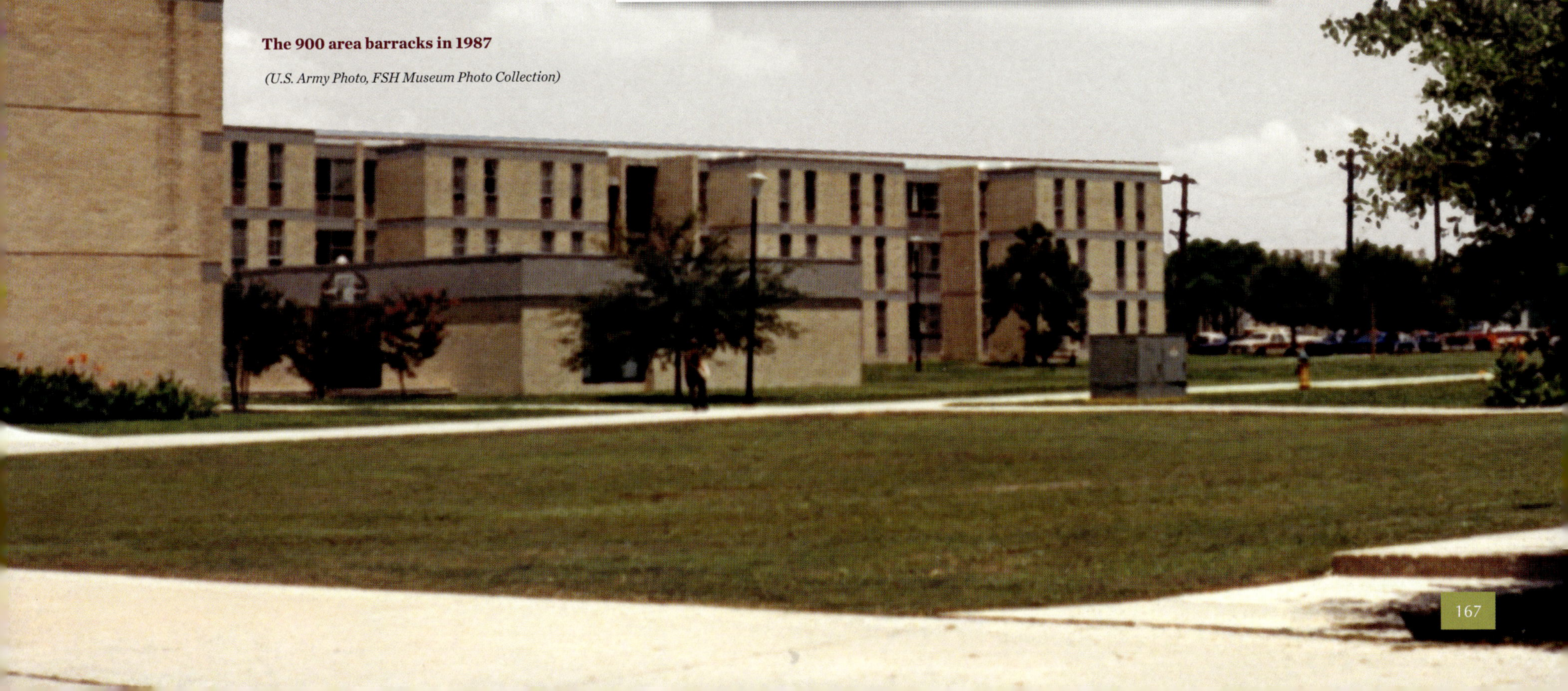

The 900 area barracks in 1987

(U.S. Army Photo, FSH Museum Photo Collection)

1988

The AHS formed a proponency analysis cell in January of 1988 that assumed the role of analyzing AMEDD officer personnel needs and policies. A cell for enlisted personnel already existed.

("Academy of Health Sciences Commandant discusses analysis of AMEDD officer needs," by Jerry Harben, HSC Mercury, January 1988)

Cpl. Larry O. Frances, an AHS student studying vocational nursing at St. Philip's College in San Antonio, through an Educational Services Agreement Program between the college and the AHS, was included in the 1988 edition of *Who's Who Among Students in American Junior Colleges*.

("Academic Who's Who inducts Academy soldier," by Ron Fellows, News Leader, 16 January 1988, p 6)

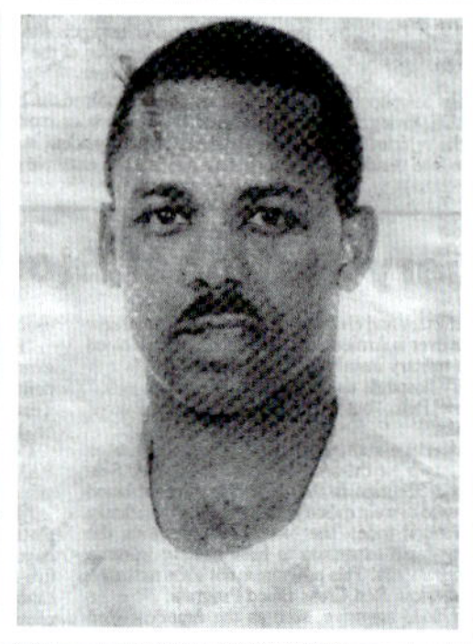

Who's Who

Cpl. Larry O. France, 1988 *Who's Who Among Students in American Junior Colleges* inductee.

(U.S. Army Photo)

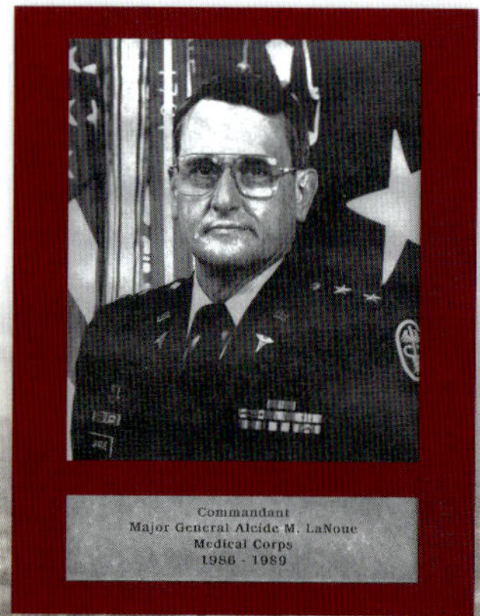

BG Alcide M. LaNoue, orthopedic surgeon and commandant of the AHS, was nominated for promotion to major general by President Ronald Reagan in June of 1988.

("AHS Commandant picked for second star," News Leader, 10 June 1988)

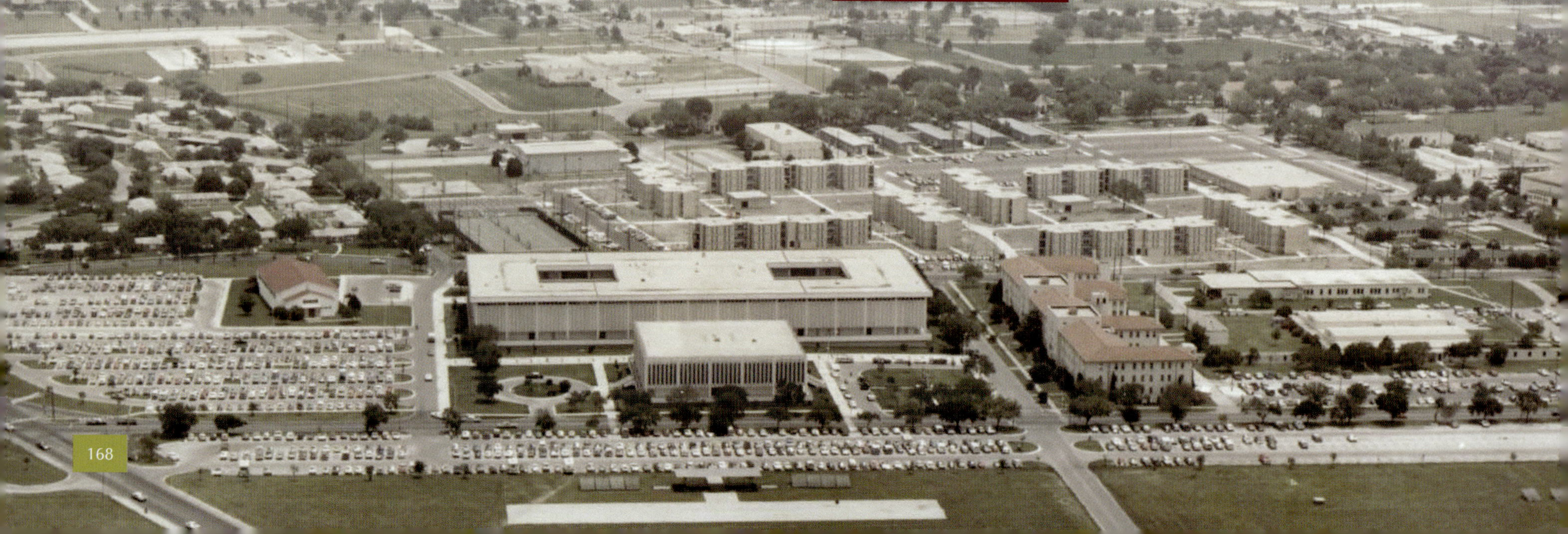

AHS campus, circa 1988

(U.S. Army Photo)

SFC Rafael Ruiz, combat medic instructor assigned to B-3, AHS, made the All-Army Track Team in January of 1988. At 30 years old, Ruiz was the second oldest runner on the Army team and was working to qualify for the Central American Games as a representative of the Puerto Rican National Team.

("Academy runner makes All-Army Team," by Fred Laureles, News Leader, 22 January 1988)

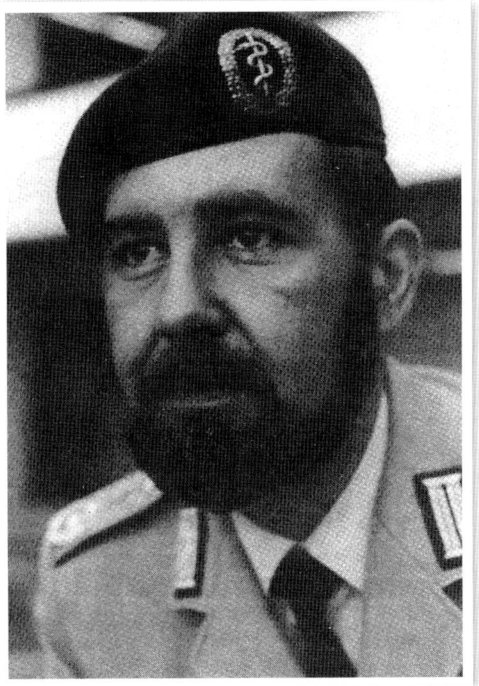

Permanent Exchange Program

Oberfeldarzi Wolfgang U. Weinert, the first German officer in the Permanent Exchange Program, joined an AHS team to review the medical field systems and the identification of medical and surgical treatment of casualty procedures for the Assistant Commandant's office in 1988.

("A Touch of Gemuetlichkeit...German Doctor Joins Academy of Health Sciences at Ft Sam," by Pat Davis, Flying Times/Military Service News, 5 February 1988)

The X-ray Branch of the AHS hosted its annual continuing education seminar in April. Subjects covered included: Infection Control Practices in Departments of Radiology; Pediatric Radiography; and Overviews of Angiography.

("AHS to host radiologic seminar," Patriot, 30 March 1988)

LTC Diane K. Corcon, deputy chief of the nursing science division of the AHS, was presented the prestigious Dr. Anita Newcomb McGee Award for outstanding service at the annual Daughters of the American Revolution Meeting. The award is presented each year to an Army nurse who has demonstrated outstanding service and performance over an extended period of time.

("Lt. Col. Corcoran presented most prestigious award in Washington," Flying Times, 6 May 1988)

Golden Knights

The Army's Golden Knights performed during the "Medics on Parade," event during the 1988 Fiesta celebration.

(U.S. Army Photo)

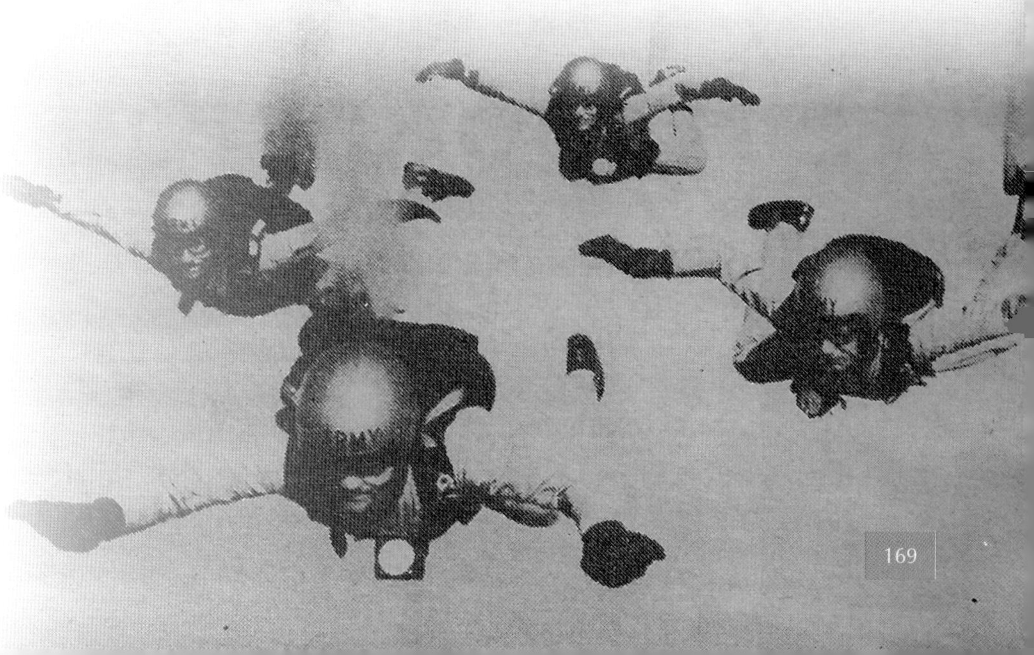

1989

The newly-completed AMEDD Museum had its opening ceremony on 26 July 1989. Media coverage included seven TV stations, nine radio stations, and three newspapers. San Antonio Mayor Lila Cockrell read the proclamation and Dr. Michael DeBakey of Baylor University School of Medicine was the guest speaker for the well-publicized event.

("Opening of New AMEDD Museum," AMEDD Activities Report, July 1989)

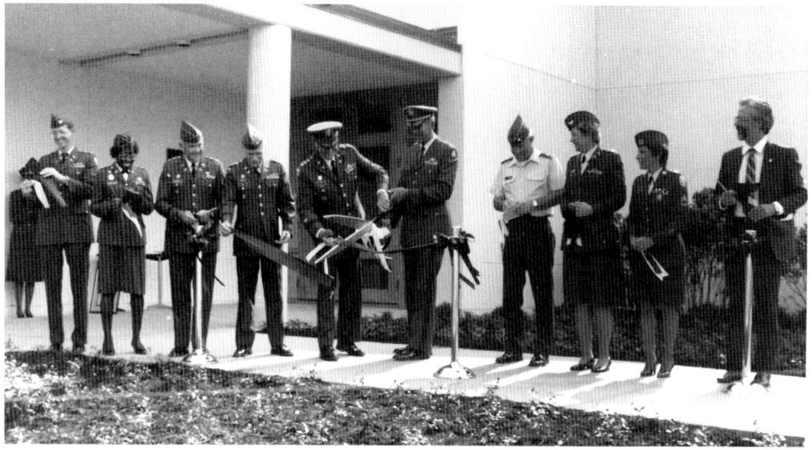

After the ribbon cutting ceremony, the AMEDD Museum is officially opened on 24 July 1989.

(U.S. Army Photo, AMEDD Museum Photo Collection)

A revised 91A10 Medical Specialist Course was developed and approved to incorporate EMT training that was recognized by the National Registry of Emergency Medical Technicians (NREMT). Upon completion of the 91A10 course, soldiers faced the challenging NREMT written exam.

("91A10 Medical Specialist Course Developed," AMEDD Activities Report, November 1989)

During 1989, the Directorate of Combat Developments completed the design for the four Theater Defense Brigades: Caribbean, Iceland, Panama, and the Aleutians. The redesign of the MASH was also completed.

("Design of Theater Defense Brigades," AMEDD Activities Report, December 1989)

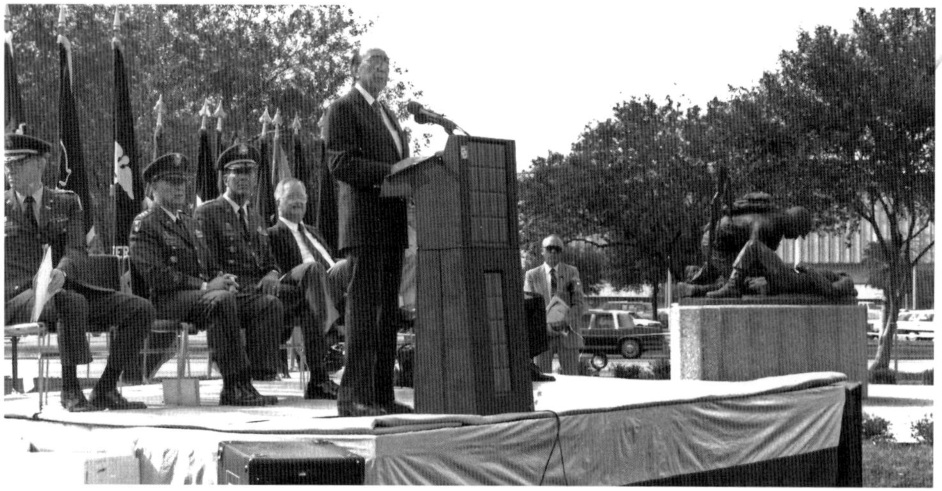

Famous cardiologist Dr. Michael DeBakey of Baylor University School of Medicine, guest speaker, during the museum opening.

(U.S. Army Photo, AMEDD Museum Photo Collection)

AHS created the office of the Deputy Commandant for Training and Clinical Affairs under the provisions of a working Table of Distribution and Allowances (TDA), and included the placement of the AHS/HSC Command Historian.

("Establishment of Department Commandant for Training and Clinical Affairs," AMEDD Activities Report, December 1989)

With approximately 37,000 resident students hosted in courses from one week to two years, and another 28,000 students enrolled in correspondence courses, the Academy of Health Sciences was declared the world's largest health care training center.

("World's Largest," San Antonio Express-News, 25 June 1989)

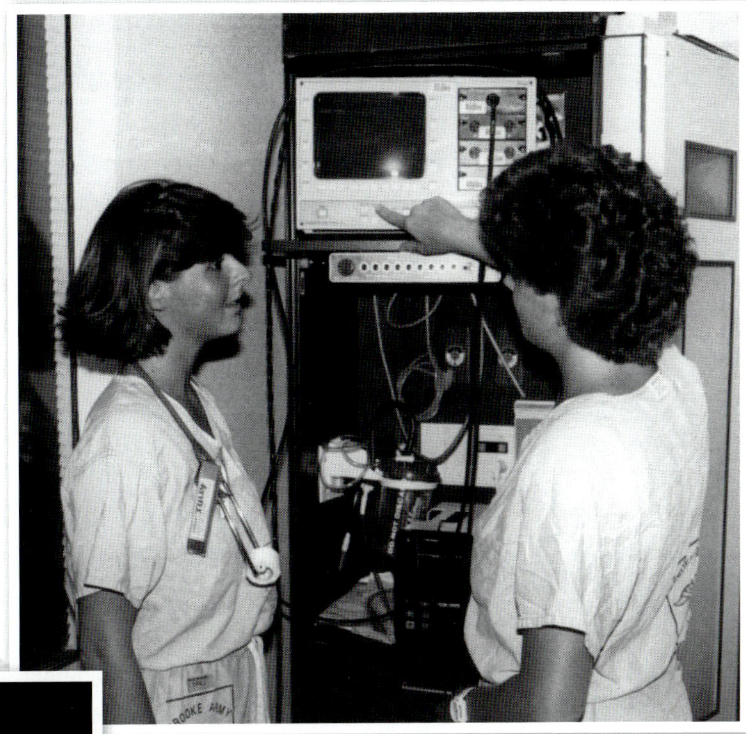

1LT Jean Andrysiak, right, explains the operation of a cardiac monitor to ROTC Nurse Cadet Tish Tully in the BAMC Cardiac Care Unit.

(U.S. Army Photo, AMEDD Museum Photo Collection)

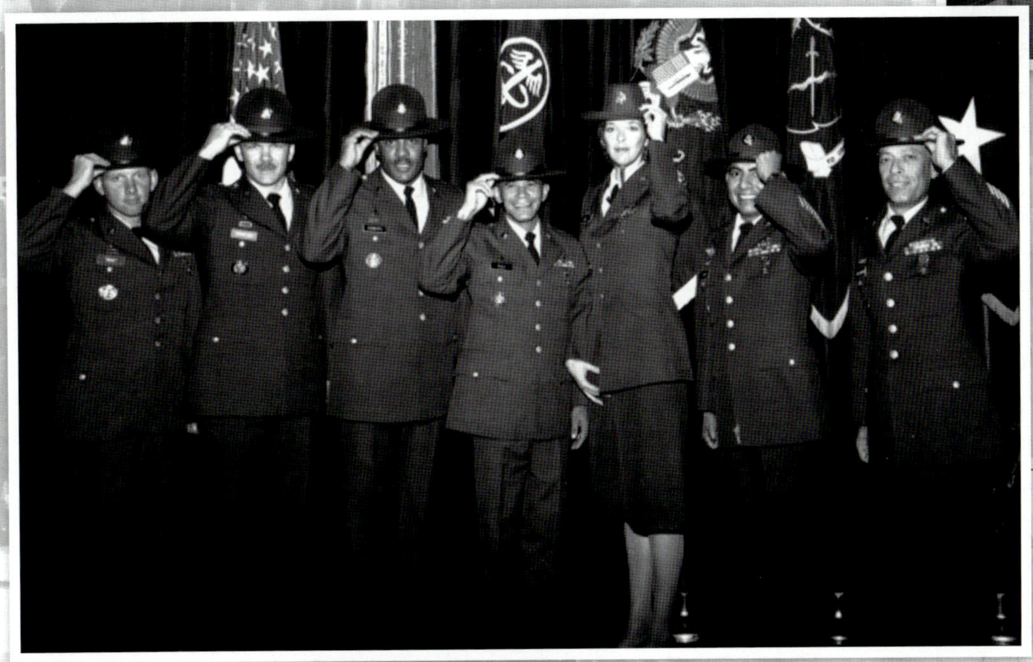

The first AHS Drill Sergeants don their caps in 1989.

(U.S. Army Photo, AMEDD Museum Photo Collection)

1990 - 1999

Operation Just Cause, the joint military incursion in the Republic of Panama, continued, although fighting throughout the country had subsided. Fort Sam Houston and San Antonio Joint Medical Command were alerted on 19 December to activate their contingency plans for support and prepare to receive large numbers of casualties. BAMC received 43 casualties during the conflict and, fortunately, all injuries were diagnosed as minor. All of FSH played a major role in ensuring soldiers in combat support readiness roles were prepared to respond in whatever capacity necessary.

("Panama: FSH Responds to Major Crisis," News Leader, 5 Jan 1990)

A new "tool" traveled with the 41st Combat Support Hospital during a week of training at Camp Bullis. The new tool was a computer program that became part of the Theater Army Medical Management Information System (TAMMIS). TAMMIS enhanced health care combat support hospitals by assisting medical personnel in the management and accountability of patients and logistics. It had an automated, on-line interactive microcomputer system that assisted units by providing accurate and timely medical information in blood management, patient accounting and reporting, supply maintenance, and optical fabrication.

("Computer Program Provides Army with Pertinent Soldier Information," News Leader, 9 Feb 1990)

A week-long Army medical evacuation conference was held at the Embassy Suites in San Antonio that focused on ways to better accommodate casualties in a hospital environment. More than 250 soldiers from all services attended. A major topic of discussion was tactics used in Operation Just Cause. A static display of a 1918 Ford WWI ambulance; a CASA 212 turbo prop series 300 used for light transportation and front line support; and the latest generation of ground ambulances, including the M1009 CUCV, were highlights of the conference.

("Medical Conference Highlights Past, Present Modes of Transportation," News Leader, 2 March 1990)

Students training on the new TAMMIS system

(U.S. ArmyPhoto)

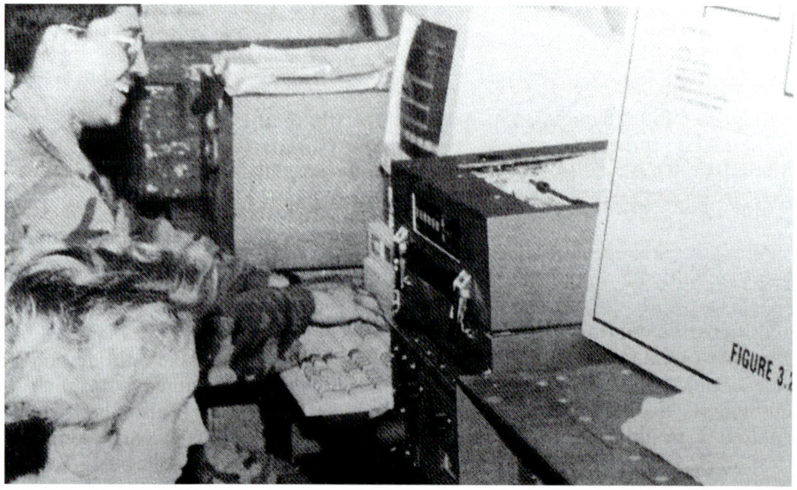

On June 15, a proposal was authorized to commission all warrant officers who served as active duty physicians assistants. Awaiting congressional approval, the legislative change allowed PAs to join the Army Medical Service Corps and to apply constructive service credits when converting to commissioning. The change was made in hopes of making the Army more competitive, and of recruiting and retaining quality physician assistants.

("Army Submits Proposals to Commission PAs," News Leader, 6 July 1990)

In 1990, the AHS maintained its stature as the largest health care training facility in the world. Approximately 67,000 students completed training annually (including 38,000 enrolled in correspondence courses) in more than 150 programs of instruction. In order to sustain a military and civilian academic balance, the Academy maintained its affiliation with several universities and colleges and more than 30 civilian and government agencies.

("AHS Teaches Medical Soldiers "World of Medicine," News Leader, July 1990)

With very little spare time during Initial Entry Training, a group of trainees from the Academy found time to serve God – with their voices. The "Voices of the Brigade" was a 65-member gospel group composed of soldiers from the 232nd Medical Battalion. SSG Bennett, a drill sergeant, formed the group and stated that his purpose was, "to provide a positive outlet for student soldiers and allow them to share their love of God and music with others."

("Trainees Sing Gospel," News Leader, 10 Aug 1990)

Army, Navy, and Air Force doctors, nurses and dentists learned to treat wounds in wartime conditions while attending the Joint Medical Readiness Training Center. The week-long course taught map reading, radio procedures, rappelling, and other squad-level necessary skills. The goal, according to COL John Mullen, was "medical readiness so they won't be a fish out of water if they ever treat in battlefield conditions."

("Medical Officers Develop Field Skills," News Leader, 24 Aug 1990)

Heat injuries were initially the biggest threat facing American soldiers deployed to Operation Desert Storm. Poisonous snakes, spiders and scorpions were later identified as potential threats to the health and well being of soldiers. A program of awareness and preventative training measures was offered by AHS as part of armed forces pre-deployment to the Middle East.

("Desert Demons: Snakes, Scorpions are Other Enemy to Operation Desert Shield Soldiers," News Leader, 16 Nov 1990)

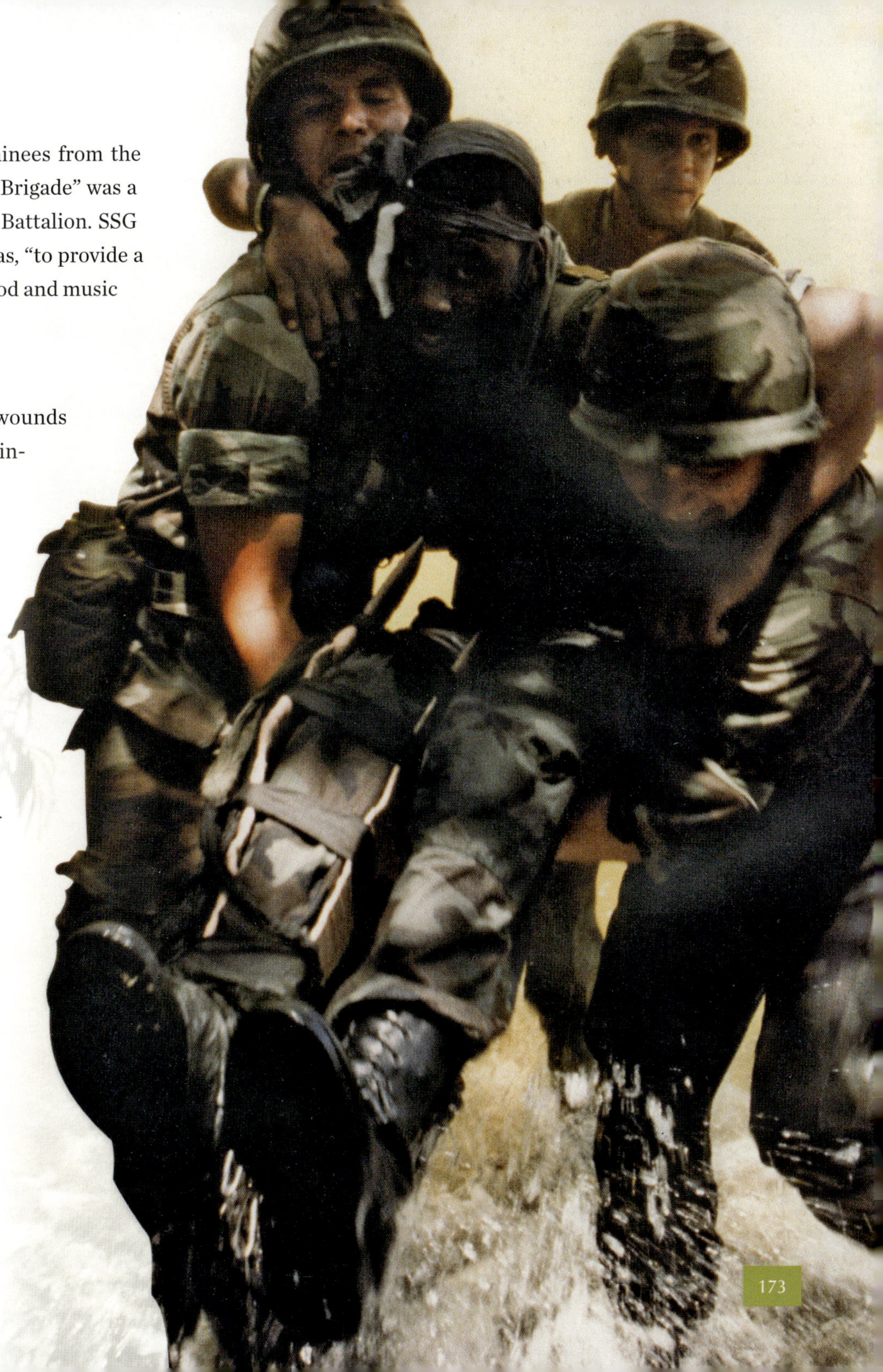

A "wounded" soldier is carried by Army medics during a training exercise for 91B students at Camp Bullis.

(U.S. Army Photo, AMEDD Museum Photo Collection)

1991

Army physician assistants (PAs) at the AHS were ranked best in the nation following an independent test administered annually by the University of Nebraska. The test measured the medical know-how of second year PAs nationwide. Students at AHS had an average score of 160.62 compared to a national mean of 139.63. The "intense instruction" the PAs received at AHS was credited for the high ranking.

("Army PAs Ranked Best in U.S.," News Leader, 4 Jan 1991, p 6)

MG Fredrick N. Bussey, departing AHS commandant, became the Army Deputy Surgeon General succeeding MG Alcide M. Lanoue, AHS Commander from 1986 to 1989.

("Farewell," News Leader, 11 Jan 1991, p 1)

The liberation of Kuwait began on 17 January 1991 as Allied planes bombed Iraq.

Camp Bullis served as the primary deployment site for medical reserve units deploying in support of Operation Desert Shield.

("94th Heads to Europe," by Terri Christensen, News Leader, 18 Jan 1991)

As a result of Operation Desert Storm, military requirements necessitated the call-up of certain members of the Individual Ready Reserve (IRR) for the first time in U.S. history. Once processed, the IRR went to BAMC and AHS for training in their MOS.

("New USAG Unit Activated," by John E. Juhaz, Jr., News Leader. 1 Feb 1991, p 1)

The Army's stop loss program went into effect in February 1991. It was expanded to include members of the IRR in medical specialties: AOC 60 through 68 for officers; MOS 600A, 640A and 670A for warrant officers; and any enlisted 91 series MOS.

("Stop Loss Program Expands Roster," Army News)

Team members of the Army Training and Evaluation Program Branch of the AHS, 1991.

(AMEDDC&S Photo)

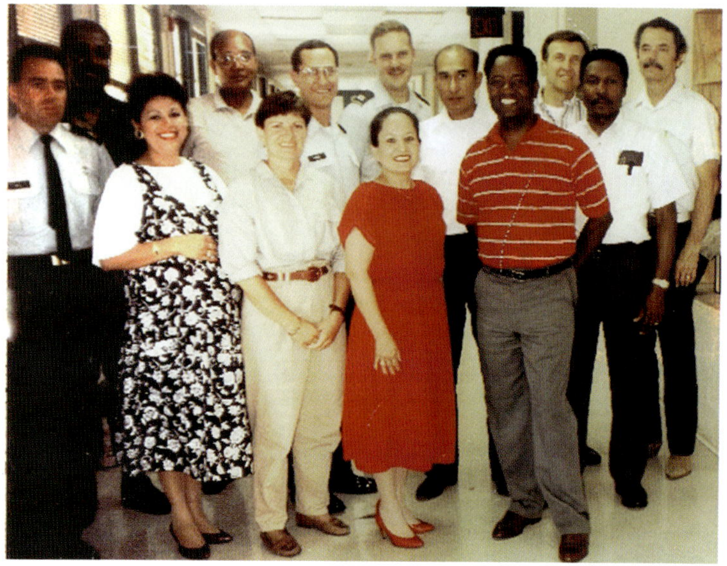

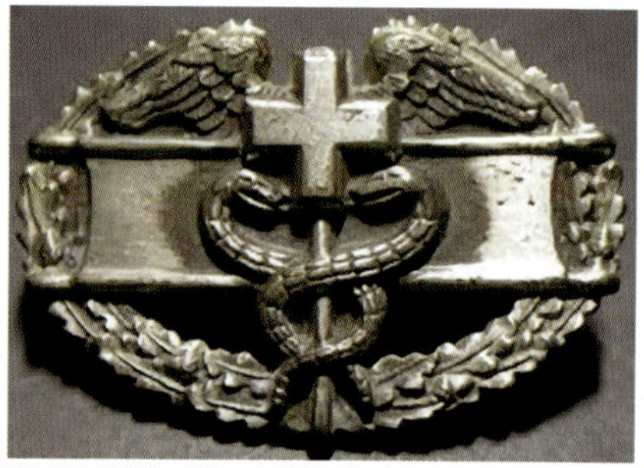

PFC Marissa Struland, 18 years old, becomes one of the first women and one of the youngest medics to earn the coveted Combat Medic Badge.

("Female Soldier Awarded Coveted Combat Medic Badge," News Leader, 15 Nov 1991)

Fiesta 1991 was the first year both female and male representatives were chosen as FSH military representatives. SGT Michael D. Church, a military policeman assigned to Company A, USAG, was elected as the male representative, while SGT Martha McCleland, an administrative specialist assigned to Company A, Academy Battalion, AHS, was chosen as the female representative. The two represented Fort Sam during Fiesta and other civilian and military activities throughout the year.

("1991 FSH Military Representative Chosen," News Leader, 8 Feb 1991)

SSG Henry L. Lackland, Company D, 232nd Medical Battalion, became the post's first Drill Sergeant of the Year.

("Post's First 'Drill Sergeant of the Year' Selected," by Lena K. Fisher, News Leader, 8 Feb 1991)

Ret. CWO 2 Louis R. Rocco—combat medic, physician assistant and Vietnam-era Medal of Honor recipient—joined 800 other physicians, nurses, dentists, and fellow PAs nationwide who voluntarily returned to active duty during Desert Shield.

("Medic Returns from Retirement: Chief Warrant Officer Gives Knowledge Back," LuAnne Fantasia, 22 Feb 1991) {incomplete reference, News Leader?}

The liberation of Kuwait was confirmed on 27 Feb 1991.

Military medical officers from major English-speaking countries met at the AHS the second week of April as part of a continuing program to provide medical standardization among the American, British, Canadian, and Australian armies. New Zealand was an associate at the time. Meeting sites for the program were rotated among the partners of the "Quadripartite" work groups that met every 18 months.

("Medical Officers Meet," News Leader, 12 April 1991)

Enrolled in the one-year Licensed Practical Nurse Course, 21 Reserve Component trainees volunteered to become CPR instructors. Later in the year, they went on to join nearly 250 other CPR instructors during CPR Day, teaching more than 800 students the life-saving skill of CPR.

("AHS Students Learn, Teach CPR," News Leader, 19 April 1991)

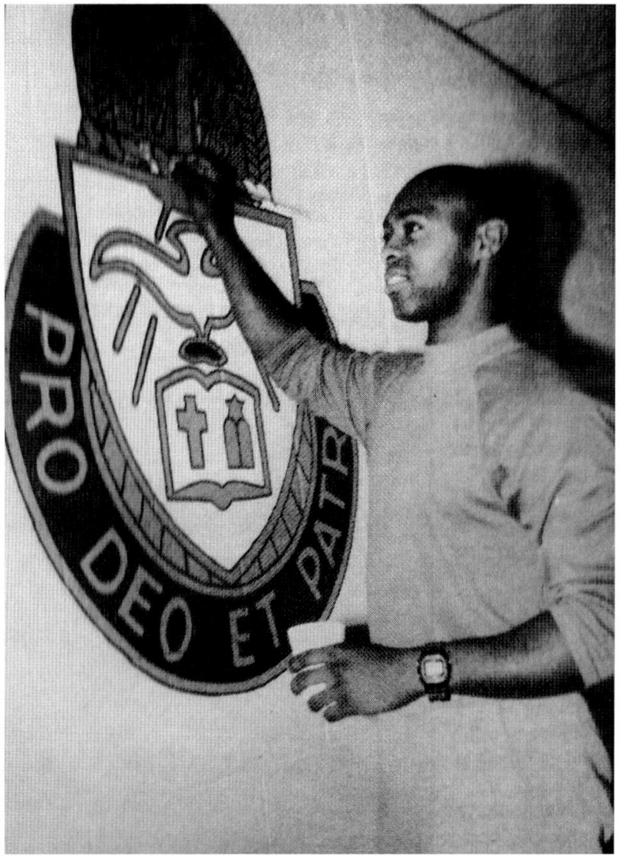

SSG Bruce Coleman adds a finishing touch to the Chaplain's Corps crest he painted on the Academy Chapel wall.

("Soldier Revives Artistic Skills to Enhance Academy Walls," by Remo M. Scarsella, News Leader, 22 Feb 1991)

1991

The AHS blew the doors off the competition in Army-wide selection for promotion to the top NCO grade in 1991. It scored an impressive 42% selection rate for promotion to command sergeant major and sergeant major. The Academy's CSM David S. Cahill reported that five of its twelve senior NCOs eligible for promotion were selected. Three of the five for the command sergeant major rank included 1SG James G. Catena, MSG Joseph M. Laynor, and MSG Paul W. Pfeifer.

("AHS NCOs Promoted, Beat Army-wide Ratio," News Leader, 14 June 1991)

The "Voices of the Brigade," a gospel choir of 140 AHS students, was selected Most Outstanding Gospel Choir in San Antonio by KCHL Radio 1480 during the station's Choirfest in June.

("AHS Gospel Choir Earns Honors, New Leader, 28 June 1991)

A team from the AHS Behavioral Sciences Department traveled the country teaching DoD families how to cope with problems associated with reunion after deployment.

("Behavior Experts Assist Families with Reunions," New Leader, 28 June 1991)

The AHS Physician Assistant Program began training Navy and Air Force students. The students completed their Phase I training at AHS and then were assigned to various military hospitals for a second year of hands-on training. The Army and Air Force students received their degrees from the University of Oklahoma, while the Navy students graduated from George Washington University.

("AHS Begins Special PA Class," News Leader, 6 Sep 1991)

The AHS became the Army Medical Department Center and School on 1 July 1991.

(DASG-HCO-P (525n) Memo for CMOR, U.S. Army Health Services Command, 12 July 1991.)

NCO and Soldier of the Year competitions took place at Camp Bullis 18-20 September.

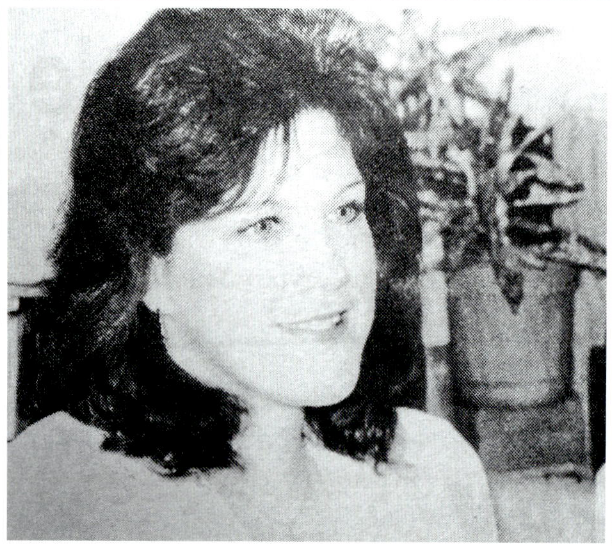

Roberta Booth, editorial assistant in the AHS's Directorate of Evaluations and Standardization, was named one of the Outstanding Young Women of America in 1991. Ms. Booth, nominated for the award by Neta Lesjak, her Academy supervisor, competed for the award against thousands of young women nationwide.

("AHS Employee Honored," News Leader, 7 June 1991, p 5)

The Phase I through Phase III concept plan for the newly designated Army Medical Department Center and School was announced during a press conference at the AMEDD Museum. 1991 was cited as a growth phase year. The Center and School had already begun receiving new employees and senior officers at AHS to fill new roles. Phase II—which included the implementation of Field Operating Activities (FOA) and the addition of the Joint Medical Readiness Training Center (JMRTC)—was scheduled for 1992. FOA activities included Patient Administration System and Biostatics, Health Care Management Engineering, and Health Care Studies and Clinical Investigation. Phase III, scheduled for 1993, planned to bring 209 more personnel, administrative and operations positions to the center.

("Medical Department Announces Plans for Center, School," News Leader, 25 October 1991)

The Combat Service Support Training Simulation System (CSSTSS) was demonstrated during the Campaigner's Conference 1-92, "Medical Force 2000," at Camp Bullis the third week of November. AMEDD commanders and staff from active-duty, Reserve, and National Guard units from Wiesbaden, Germany, to Fort Sam Houston had the opportunity to test the new CSSTSS software. Synchronization of asset management to provide effective heath service support to the solider in the field was the designed result.

("Bullis Hosts 'High-Tech' Computer Exercise," News Leader, 22 Nov 1991)

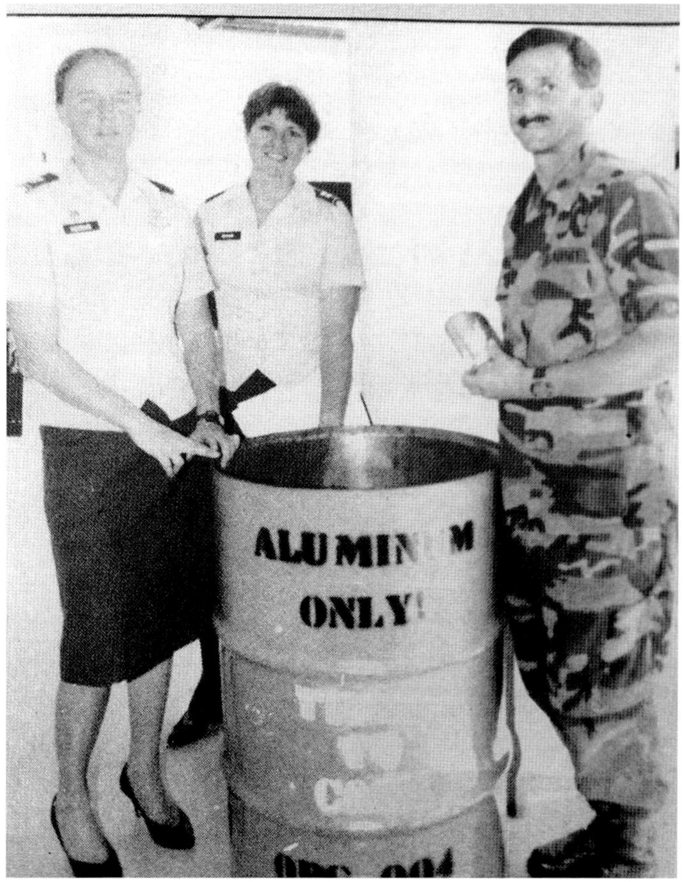

AHS students set up recycling cans in the hallways of Willis Hall for a fundraiser campaign to be used for projects to benefit both students and faculty. New seats for the "Pit Area," vegetation to beautify the area, and monies to pay for guest lecturers topped the wish list.

("Good Idea," News Leader, 27 Sep 1991)

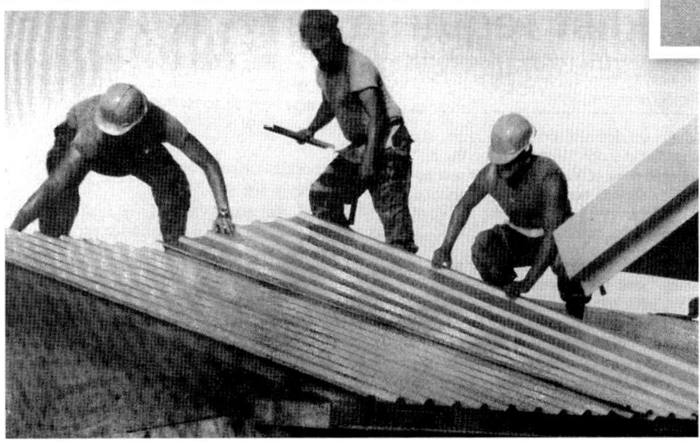

Soldiers refurbish billets at Camp Bullis. Billets used during WWI, WWII, and the mobilization stage of Operations Desert Storm and Shield at Camp Bullis are torn down and rebuilt using the same foundations.

("Soldiers Refurbish Billets," News Leader, 26 July 1991)

1992

Fort Sam Houston played numerous parts in supporting the Army's battle-focus theme, "Training the Forces," but of all the medical courses offered at the AMEDDC&S, none was as vigorous as the Special Operations Medical Sergeants Course. Thirty-one weeks of the 14-month course began here, with the remainder being completed at Ft Bragg, NC. The AMEDDC&S gave the combat medic essential training needed to react to the stress of battle and perform in a combat environment. Students learned how to jump into a heavy battle area with the proper medical equipment; quickly triage and evaluate the extent of an injury; and, most importantly, know what to do to prevent a wounded soldier from becoming a fatality.

("Course Challenges Toughest Soldiers," News Leader, 7 Feb 1992)

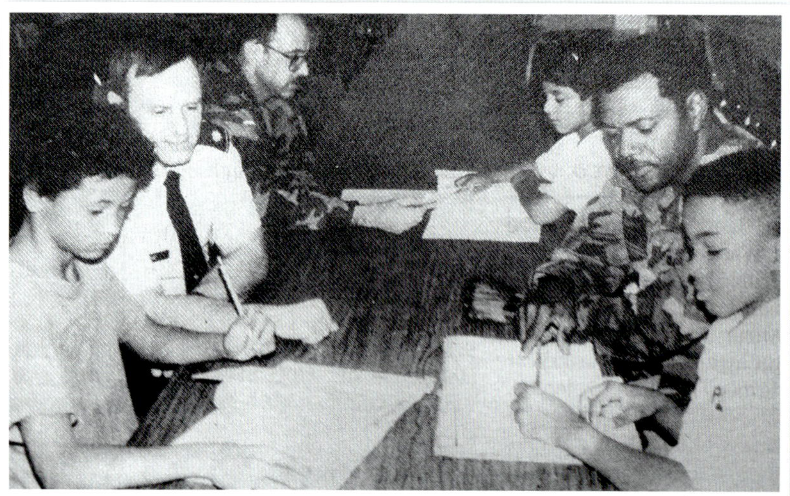

School commanders from the AMEDDC&S schedule "mentoring" as a priority when compiling their monthly calendars. All of them volunteered to mentor for one hour a week at Booker T. Washington Elementary School, and had nothing but great things to say about the mentorship program. While mentors used their own teaching techniques to help the children, all saw mentoring as a "golden opportunity to put to practice some of the things I have learned."

("School Commanders Take on Mentoring," News Leader, 14 Feb 1992)

Two medical officers from BAMC and AMEDDC&S were part of a 17-member medical team of U.S. military medical experts who visited war-ravaged Kuwait to help that country improve its military medical system. The experts found that the Kuwaiti military medical system had essentially shut down. Recommendations ranged from immediate actions, such as hiring advisers and workers, to long-term solutions such as increasing the number of Kuwaiti citizens in the military who had been trained either abroad or within their own university system.

("FSH Officers Help Kuwaitis Develop Medical System," News Leader, 10 April 1992)

CPT Amy Fitzgerald, a medical laboratory student at the AMEDDC&S, received the General Douglas MacArthur Leadership Award in May 1992. The award was presented to those soldiers who exemplify the leadership ideals of "Duty, Honor, Country." CPT Fitzgerald served as the chief of immunochemistry before deploying to the Gulf War, where she served with the 41st Combat Support Hospital, 24th Infantry Division. During the ground offensive, CPT Fitzgerald's laboratory was the focal point of forward blood supply. She was credited with being instrumental in establishing the 1st Medical Group's policy on the shipment, distribution, and recovery of blood products for forward medical treatment facilities.

("Desert Storm Vet Gains Recognition for Leadership," News Leader, 8 May 1992)

Military retirees and their families, as well as active duty military, were offered preventive dental care at the AMEDDC&S Preventative Dentistry Clinic. It provided cleaning and dental fillings as part of its support training mission. Students worked under the supervision of licensed dental hygienists and dentists and, because it was a teaching program, appointments were frequently two to three hours in length.

("AMEDD School Offers No-Cost Dental Care," News Leader, 28 Aug 1992)

The 187th Medical Battalion established a partnership with the Sexual Assault Crisis and Resource Center to bring sexual assault awareness and avoidance training to the AMEDDC&S in November 1992.

("Medical Battalion Takes Steps to Prevent Assaults," by Debra Dodds, News Leader, 7 April 1994)

CW5 William Johnson was the first soldier at FSH to be promoted to CWO5. The Warrant Officer Management Act established the new pay grade in 1992. CW5 Johnson was the chief, Consolidated Installation Property Book Division, Directorate of Logistics. "I was elated even just to make the first CWO5 list. As I look at it, I think it's the Army's reward for a sterling career."

("Johnson Becomes the First CWO5 Promotion at Fort Sam Houston," News Leader, 4 Dec 1992)

The Emergency Medical Treatment tent becomes a beehive of activity as "patients" are brought in for initial care. 320th Evacuation Hospital members team up to restrain a mock mental patient. The Army Reserve unit spent two weeks working in the Army's new Deployable Medical System (DEPMEDS) at Camp Bullis.

(U.S. Army Photo)

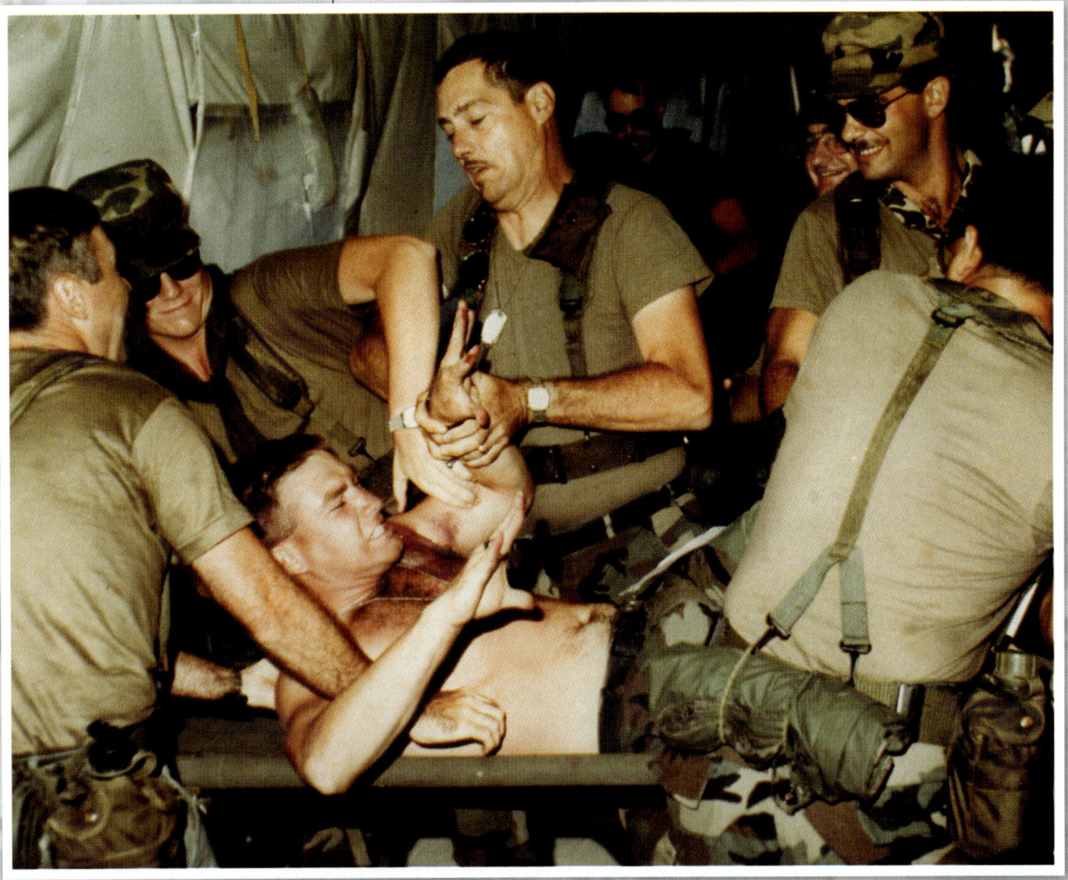

1993

Two AMEDDC&S officers participated in Operation Restore Hope Joint Task Force in Somalia. They returned to Fort Sam Houston with lessons learned in preventive medicine, setting up hospitals, and establishing a casualty-evacuation system in a country with little infrastructure and resources.

("Officers Return From Somalia – Medical Operations in Somalia Very Challenging," News Leader, 26 Feb 1993)

As part of the Army's streamlining and downsizing efforts, a nine-member task force was established by the Army Surgeon General to begin redesigning the Army Medical Department. Headed by MG Girard Seitter, former commander of Tripler Army Medical Center, the task force's primary objective was to re-organize the AMEDDC&S to eliminate duplication and achieve significant savings. The re-designation would eventually affect personnel, facilities and programs within the then current AMEDDC&S force structure.

("Task Force Proposes Changes for Army Medical Department," News Leader, 9 April 1993)

The Pharmaeconomic Center was assigned to the AMEDDC&S. The Commander of the AMEDDC&S was appointed as executive agent for implementing the Joint Medical Executive Skills Institute (JMESI).

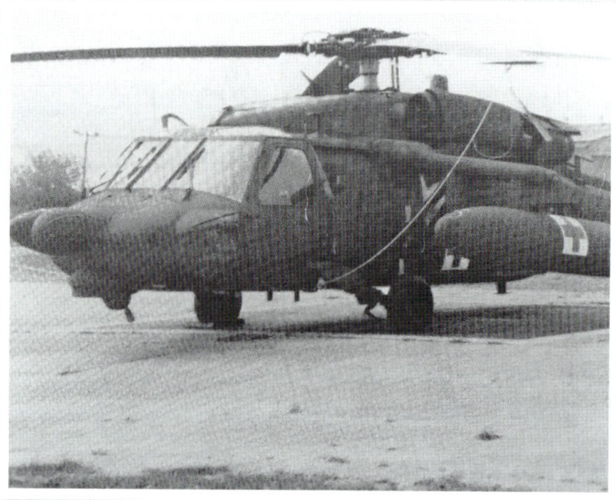

A "Proof of Concept," UH-60Q Blackhawk medical helicopter on display at MacArthur Field showed off advanced medical evacuation features. The improved MedEvac helicopter transported nine (ambulatory) litter patients. Its cockpit was the model for modernization of the entire Blackhawk fleet.

("Medical Blackhawk Visit," News Leader, 9 April 1993)

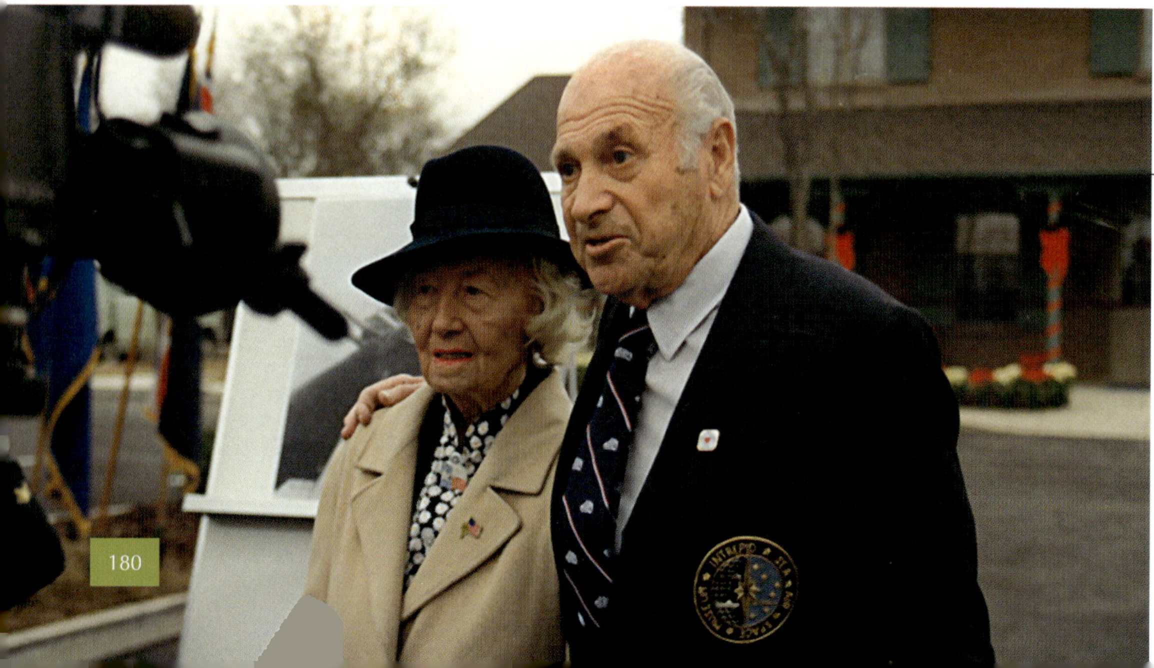

Zachary and Elizabeth Fisher dedicate the Fisher House for families sent here for hospitalization of a family member.
The house is located on George C. Beach Road, adjacent to the new Brooke Army Medical Center. "I consider myself the #1 patriot in the U.S.," Fisher said. "I was never in the military – I was 4F, so this is my way of paying back."

("Fisher Donates House Here Easing Burden for Families," News Leader, 8 Jan 1993)

"It is the Expert Field Medical Badge (EFMB), not the so-so medical badge," stated MSG Robert Turner, the NCO in charge of FSH's annual EFMB test. Conducted at Camp Bullis, the four-day event included students whose ranks stretched from PFC to LTC. How tough was the EFMB? A total of 113 soldiers started and only 8 received the badge.

("Expert Field Medical Badge–Many Try but Few Earn the Coveted Medical Award," News Leader, 5 June 1993)

More than 360 Advanced Individual Training soldiers from A Company, 232nd Medical Battalion, sent a touch of holiday cheer by sending Christmas cards and letters to over 400 U.S. troops serving in Somalia. Given a two-hour time period, the students completed their cards and letters in an effort to boost the morale and spirit of those deployed.

("Combat Medic Students Send Cheer to Troops in Somalia," News Leader, 17 Dec 1993)

The Animal Care Specialist Basic Course transferred from Walter Reed to the AMEDDC&S in December 1993.

("Animal Care Specialist Basic Course taught here," News Leader, 8 Sep 1994, p 6)

The 232nd Medical Battalion trained approximately 9,000 Combat Medic Specialists in 1993.

("Combat Medics endure grueling course," New Leader, 14 Jan 1994)

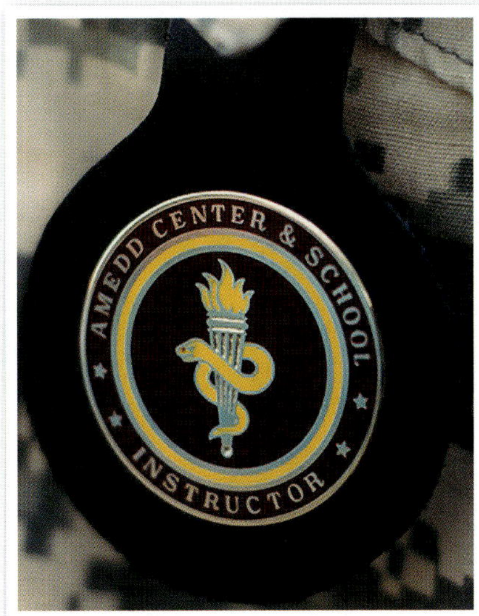

There's an old saying, "You can't tell the players without a program" but at the AMEDDC&S it was and still is, easy to tell the teachers from the students. Approximately 950 military and civilian instructors from various backgrounds and services began wearing a new "instructors" badge to set them apart. The badge was designed to serve as a symbol of professionalism of our instructor staff.

("Instructor Badge a Symbol of Professionalism," News Leader, 2 July 1993)

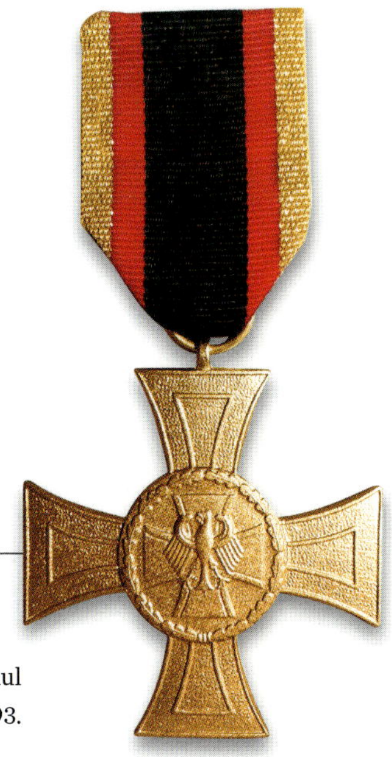

CDR Knut Reuter, MC, FRG Navy, German Exchange Officer, presented the Ehrenkreuz (Iron Cross of Honor) (Bronze) to CSM David C. Dunbar, CSM, 187th Medical Battalion, Center Brigade on 1 September 1993. The foreign award, normally awarded only to German military personnel, was presented to CSM Dunbar for his many contributions to German-American friendship, specifically for arranging many NCO-to-NCO gatherings and combined activities while stationed in Germany.

(Information for Hometown News Release 10 Sep 1993)

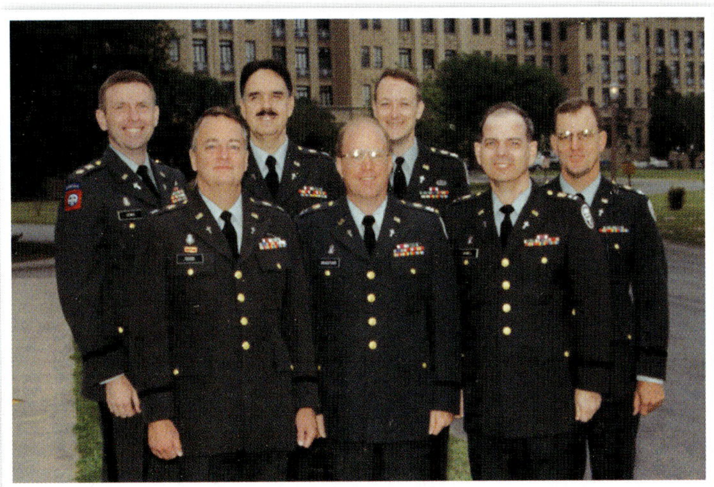

CPT Paul Bradford, CPT Charles Howell, CPT Benjamin Richardson, CPT David Norvell, MAJ James M. Lewis, LTC Robin Aplet, and COL Paul Dodd graduated from the Clinical Pastoral Education Class, 27 April 1993.

(U.S. Army Photo, AMEDD Museum Photo Collection)

1994

The barracks that housed soldiers from Companies A, B, C, and F of the 232nd Medical Battalion received new furniture as part of an ongoing Army-wide program designed to improve the quality of life for soldiers. Later in the year, the 187th Medical Battalion received $886,000 worth of year-end ACOE funding to upgrade billets to the "Better Opportunities for Single Soldiers Standards." The funds were used to completely refurbish the billets to include installation of comfortable furniture, microwave, stereos, color TVs and VCRs.

("187th Medical Battalion Achieves New Standard," News Leader, 28 April 1994; "New Furniture Adds to Quality of Life," News Leader, 14 Jan 1994)

Senior Drill Sergeant Jitendra Shukla of Company E, 187th Medical Battalion, led a team to instruct the people of Samoa in Basic Trauma Life Support by the request of the Office of the Surgeon General.

("Drill Sergeant Teaches Basic Trauma Life Support in Samoa, Finds Hospitals Half-Century Behind," News Leader, 18 Feb 1994)

The "Band Building," damaged by fire in 1980 and neglected for 12 years, was rehabilitated by a joint partnership team from the Army, Navy, Air Force, and National Park Service using DoD Legacy program funds. Restoration of the building revealed that 95% of its original woodwork was still intact.

("Joint Partnership Craftsmen Descend on Band Building," News Leader, 25 Feb 1994)

The 232nd Medical Battalion opened its own Learning Resource Center in Building 1449 in February 1994. The center served the needs of 220 instructors by providing reference books, interactive video disc systems; conference rooms; overhead projectors; TV/VCRs; slide projectors; learning modules; classrooms for small group work; journals and magazines; and correspondence course material.

("Resource Center for Instructors Opens," News Leader, 25 Feb 1994)

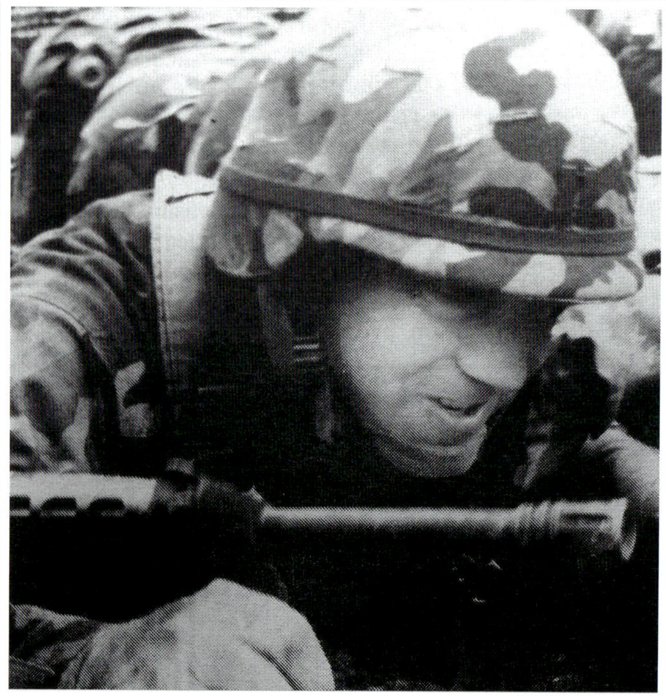

CPT Neal Woollen
Tries to stay low, crawl fast and lift, not drag, the patient on the litter. CPT Woollen and three others struggle under the barbed-wire portion of the Litter Obstacle Course during the March 1994 EFMB.

(Candidates willing to do what it takes for prestigious EFMB," by SPC. J. Paul Bruton, News Leader, 18 March 1994, pg 1)

The Preventive Dentistry Specialty Clinic at Willis Hall reopened in March 1994.

("Preventive Dentistry Medical Clinic Reopens," by PFC Sharon L. Stewart, News Leader, 11 March 1994)

Twenty-two Medical MOSs were restructured to assure better promotion potential for enlisted medical personnel. MOS 91B (Medical Specialist) became a prerequisite for most medical MOSs. After completing the 91B MOS, a soldier would go on to take additional skill identifiers (ASIs). Once they reached the rank of 1SG they would resume duties as 91Bs.

("Medical Occupational Specialties Revised," News Leader, 1 Apr 1994)

The 232nd Medical Battalion, along with the American College of Emergency Physicians, sponsored a three-day joint services symposium on emergency medicine at the Municipal Auditorium in downtown San Antonio.

("Medical Unit Hosts Symposium," by PFC Sharon L. Stewart, News Leader, 1 Apr 1994, p 6)

The 147th Medical Battalion conducted a four-day FTX at Camp Bullis. In addition to the Battalion's traditional FTX objectives of practicing rear-security, perimeter defense, and tactical convoy procedures, the 147th tested the capabilities of the relatively new INMARSAT Magnaphone Magnavox 20/20 with fax and transmission capabilities. The INMARSAT was a satellite system capable of ordering and tracking supplies around the world.

("147th Medical Battalion Heads for the Field," by PFC Sharon L. Stewart, News Leader, 19 May 1994)

MG William L. Moore, Jr., commander of the AMEDDC&S, retired after 28 years of Army service on 27 May 1994. MG Moore was instrumental in modernizing the Army's air ambulance. BG Jerome V. Foust replaced MG Moore as the commander of the AMEDDC&S.

("AMEDD Center and School Commander to Retire," News Leader, 26 May 1994, p 1)

AMEDDC&S hosted a three-day cross-cultural communications course. The course was instructed by a group of college and university professors from Hurlburt Air Force Base. The course primarily focused on Middle East, Africa, Asia, and Latin America.

("AMEDD Hosts Cross-Cultural Communications Course," News Leader, 14 July 1994, p 6)

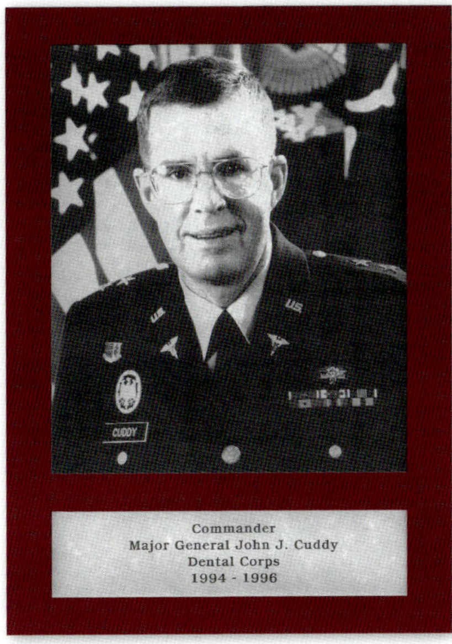
Commander
Major General John J. Cuddy
Dental Corps
1994 - 1996

BG John James Cuddy

In July 1994, BG Cuddy assumed command from BG Jerome V. Foust, who resumed his duties as deputy commander. BG Foust had served as commander since 27 March, when MG William L. Moore, Jr. retired.

("New Commander Named for U.S. Army Medical Department Center and School," News Leader, 14 July 1994, p 1)

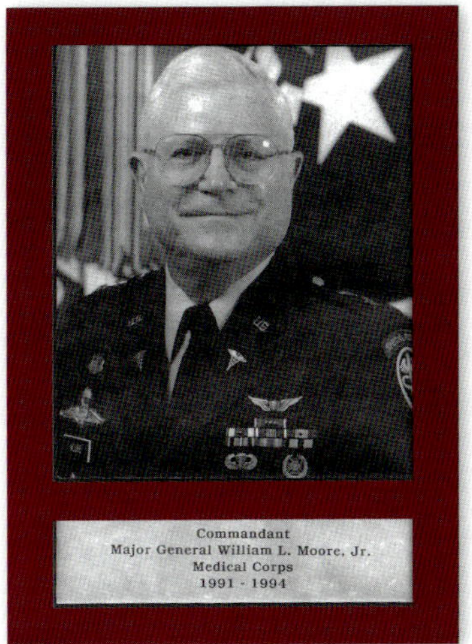
Commandant
Major General William L. Moore, Jr.
Medical Corps
1991 - 1994

MG William L. Moore, Jr.

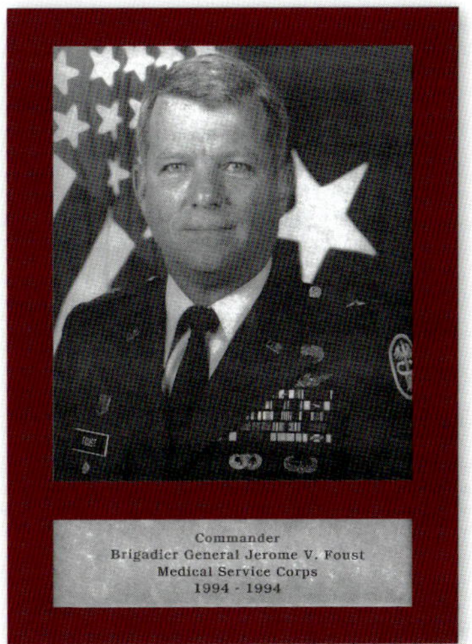
Commander
Brigadier General Jerome V. Foust
Medical Service Corps
1994 - 1994

BG Jerome V. Foust

1994

The 232nd Medical Battalion joined the Alpha, Bravo, and Delta Companies of the 1st Battalion, 141st Mechanized Infantry, Texas National Guard at Camp Bullis in an demonstration of combat medic readiness for MG Thomas W. Robinson, Commanding General U.S. Army Combined Arms Support Group, in August 1994.

("232nd Medical Battalion Gets a Taste of Reality," News Leader, 18 Aug 1994, p 14)

After a year as the provisional command, the U.S. Army Medical Command (MEDCOM) was officially activated in September 1994.

("Army Medical Command Activation Scheduled," News Leader, 29 Sept 1994)

Construction began on the new NCO Academy on the corner of Garden Avenue and White Road. The AMEDD NCO Academy was established in 1987 and received full accreditation from the Training and Doctrine Command in 1990.

("Construction Begins for New NCO Academy," News Leader, 1 Dec 1994)

The Medical Unit Staff In Operation exercise (MUSIO), part of the OAC, was a seven-day, semi-free play staff exercise, conducted on a 24-hour basis. Students were battle-rostered in support of a Corps Support Command position (COSCOM), Medical Brigade, Medical Group, CSH, Evacuation Battalion or Medical Logistics Battalion in a Korean-based scenario at the onset of a counter-offensive operation. The object of the MUSIO was to train AMEDD OAC students to better operate in staff position; to plan Health Service Support (HSS); increase problem-solving skills; work issues up and down the chain of command; and hone briefing skills.

("AMEDDC&S Students Experience Realistic Training," News Leader, 1 Dec 1994, p 3)

Communications Training
Soldiers from the 147th Medical Logistics Battalion improved skills associated with operating unit equipment such as the INMARSAT Magnavox/Magnaphone 20/20 satellite, which fed off of four other satellites worldwide.

("147th Heads for the Field," News Leader, 19 May 1994)

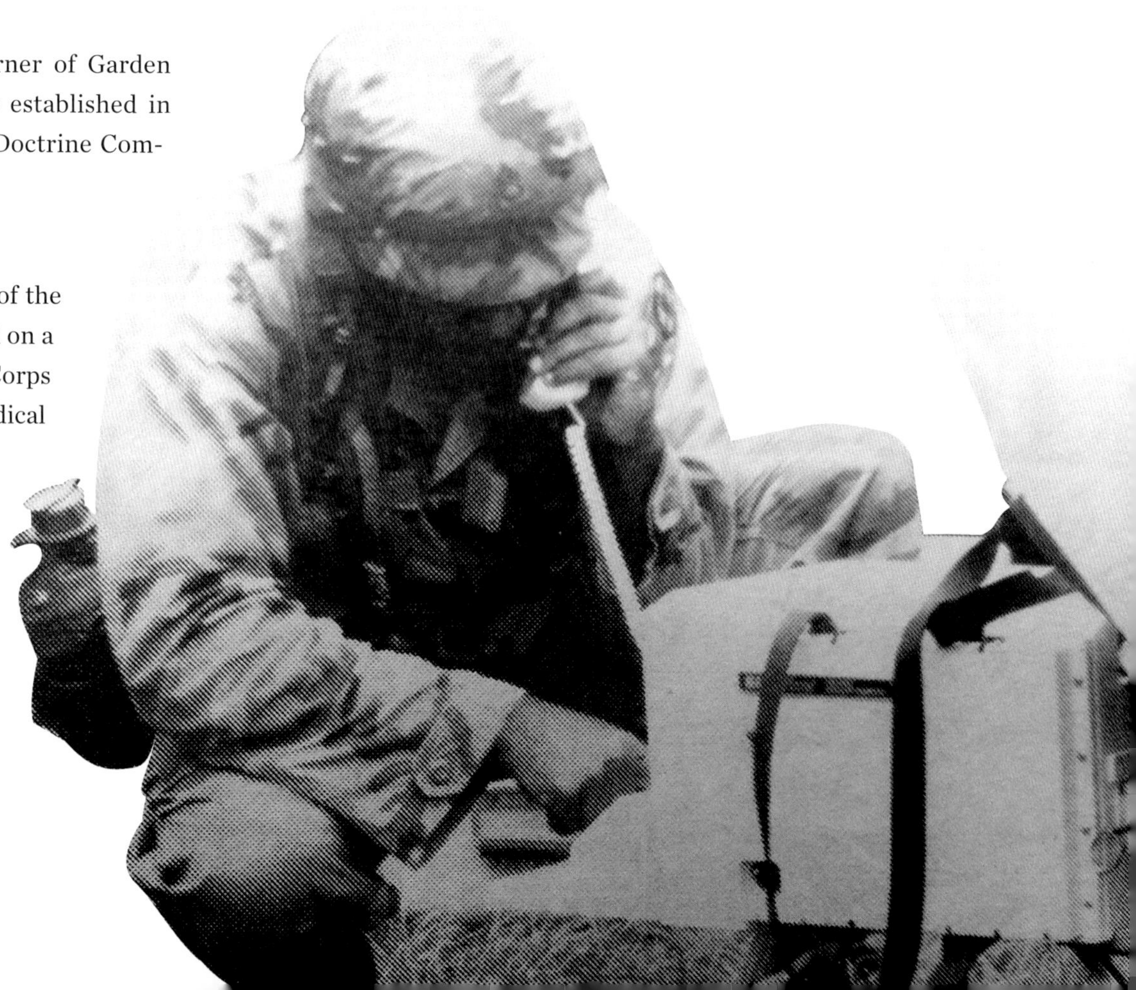

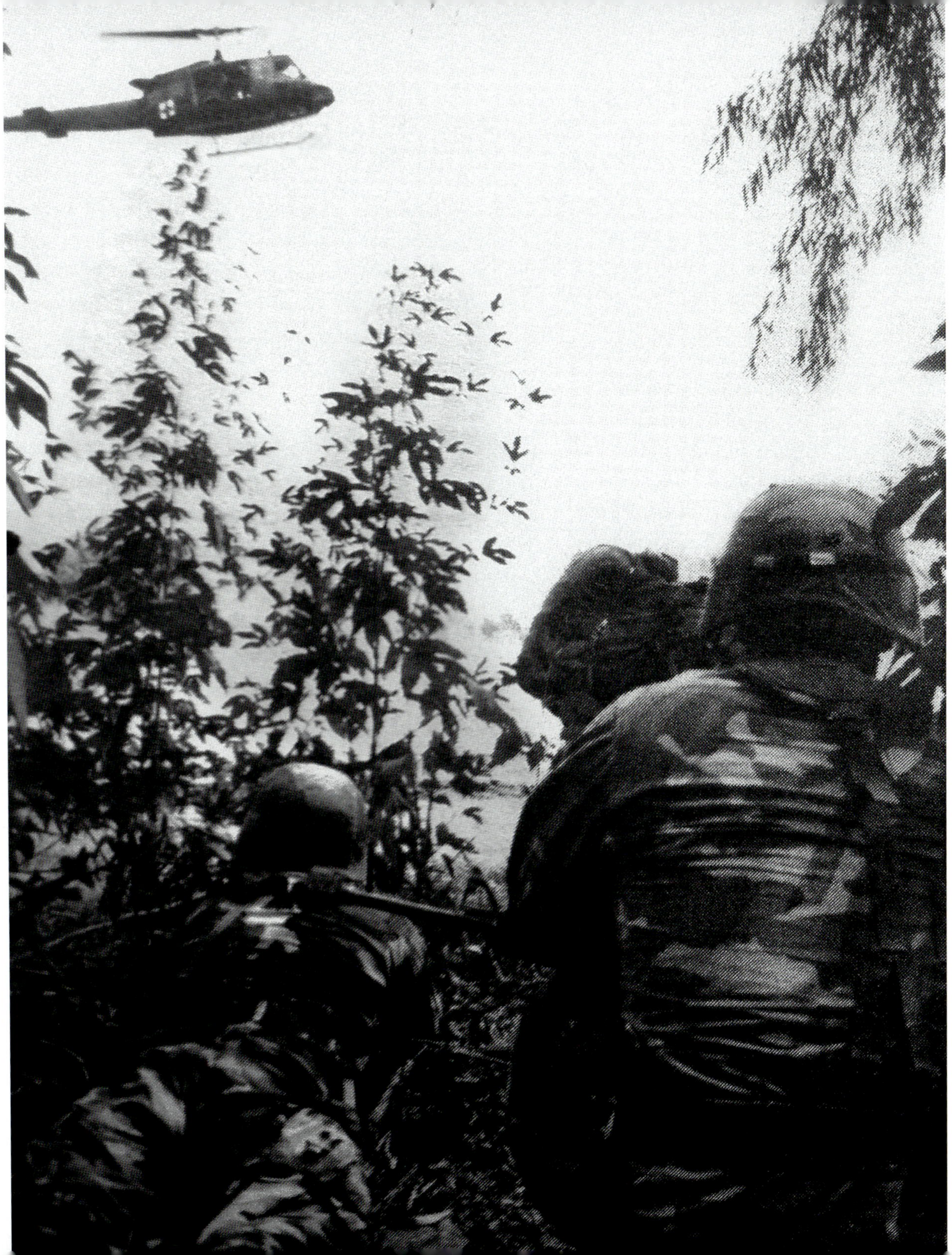

Soldiers take cover in the bush as they wait for air evacuation support during MG Robinson's visit

("147th Heads for the Field," News Leader, 19 May 1994)

1995

SSG Randy S. Ryan, drill instructor for Echo Company, 187th Medical Battalion, received the Soldier's Medal for Heroism in the face of catastrophic circumstances following the crash of an F-16 aircraft at Pope Air Force Base, N.C., 23 March 1994.

("187th Med Battalion Drill Instructor Receives Soldier Medal for Heroism," News Leader, 23 Feb 1995)

The AMEDDEX '95, a computer exercise to test medical units' mission skills, was held over a 12-day period at Camp Bullis. Army, Navy, and Air Force "players" joined in this joint exercise designed to train units in wartime combat health support missions; train unit staffs to overcome the challenges of the extended and integrated operations; train participants in the application of combat health support fundamentals; provide a forum for the exchange of information concerning procedures and techniques; and accommodate units' internal training objectives and Mission Essential Task Lists.

("Computer Exercise Sharpens Medical Units' Mission Skills," by SGT J. Paul Bruton, News Leader, 16 March 1995, p 5)

The 232nd Medical Battalion collaborated with the Wilderness Medical Associates to host a national level Wilderness Rescue/Extended Patient Management Course at Camp Bullis the week of 4-10 June. The course was the initiative of CPT Sandra Greider, an Army nurse with 25 years' experience outside of the Army. CPT Greider realized that other armed forces medical training centers, as well as state, local and federal agencies responsible for EMT and trauma care needing annual training and certification, were also experiencing severe budget cuts. The Wilderness Rescue/Extended Patient Management Course became one of the first Army-based shared training resources that the AMEDDC&S initiated. The course focused on training participants on key wilderness medicine principals when a rescue is undertaken far from the safety of hospital and emergency transportation.

("Wilderness Rescue, Patient Management Course Scheduled," News Leader, 11 May 1995, p 6; "New Training Management Initiative Saves Scarce Training Dollars," by Pat Davis, News Leader, 22 June 1995)

Company F (Airborne), Academy Battalion, underwent a change of command the first week of September 1995. The Special Forces unit commander, MAJ Billy W. Haydon, credited for decreasing attrition rate in the course from 40% to 25%, handed responsibility to MAJ Scott A. Burgess.

("Special Forces Unit Undergoes Change of Command," by PFC Sharon L. Stewart, News Leader, 7 Sept 1995)

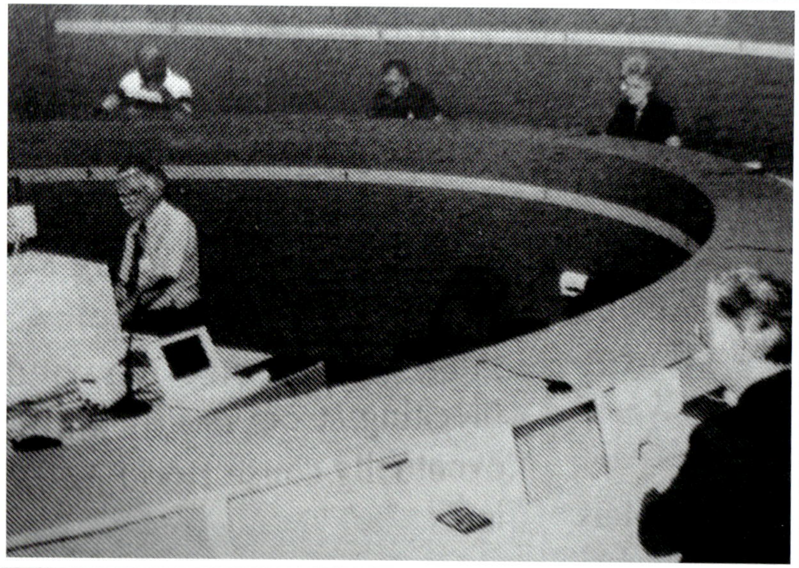

The AMEDDC&S opened the Army Medical Department Executive Skills Technology Center (AESTC) in April 1995. The AESTC was described as the "bridge of the Starship Enterprise," with two circles featuring 21 state-of-the-art computer terminals surrounding an instructor/facilitator computer-controlled terminal. The AESTC was developed for use by all medical service officers to develop executive skills needed to command and operate modern medical treatment facilities.

("Army Medical Department Opens Technology Center," News Leader, 13 April 1995, p 2)

The AMEDDC&S Chaplaincy hosted the 232nd Center Brigade Marriage Enrichment Conference at the historic Menger Hotel. The marriage retreat was one of the first funded by the Army Chief of Chaplains "Initiatives" grant program.

("232nd Hosts Center Brigade Marriage Enrichment Conference," News Leader, 5 Oct 1995)

Under permanent orders 261-1 dated 18 Sep 1995, the U.S. Army Garrison Fort Sam Houston was transferred to the U.S. Army Medical Command (MEDCOM), effective 12 Oct 1995. MG John J. Cuddy, commander, AMEDDC&S, became installation commander. At the same time the 323rd Army Band was activated, as the Fifth Army Band was inactivated.

("Fort Sam Houston Transfers to U.S. Army Medical Command," News Leader, 12 Oct 1995)

"Operation Bushmaster," the field training exercise portion of the Military Contingency Medicine Course at Camp Bullis, was held, once again, for the senior medical students in the Army, Navy, Air Force and Public Health Service medical students attending the Uniformed Services University of the Health Sciences.

("Volunteers, Soldier-Mentors Help Others Learn During Realistic Training," by LT Wilson Ariza, News Leader, 19 Oct 1995)

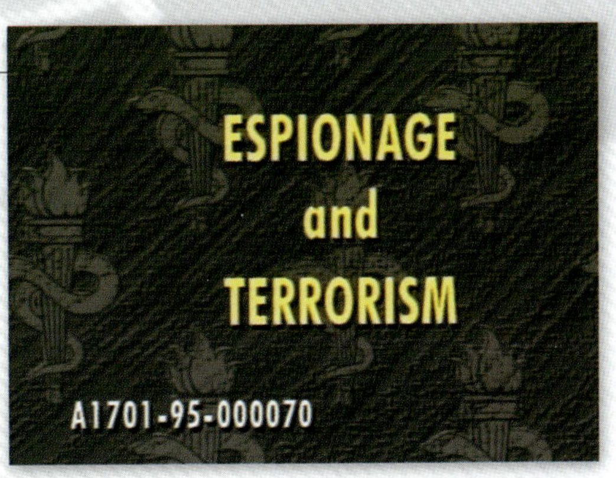

The Army Medical Department C&S Media Division released a video on "Subversion and Espionage Against the U.S. Army."

("Anti-terrorists Video-Teamwork Makes It Happen," News Leader, 22 June 1995)

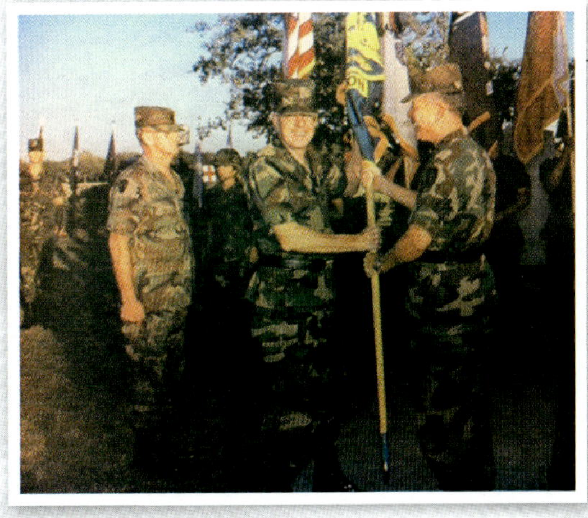

Fifth U.S. Army Commander, LTG Marc A. Cisneros (right) passes the Fort Sam Houston colors to MG John J. Cuddy, commander of the Army Medical Department Center and School.

(U.S. Army Photo, "Fort Sam Houston transfers to U.S. Army Medical Command," News Leader, 12 October 1995)

The AMEDDC&S begins using Teletraining Network (TNET) to train soldier medics in the Sinai. The TNET allowed classroom training to be conducted on a worldwide basis, with live two-way audio and two-way compressed video relaying digital images, audio, and data via satellite. The 10-day course taught to the medical units assigned to the 101st ABN DIV (Air Assault) enforcing the Camp David Accords in the Sinai included subjects such as Desert Medicine; Treatment of Shock and Burns; Orthopedic Principles; Principles of Rescue; Parasites; Dental Emergencies; Intro to Natural Disasters; Wilderness Trauma; Poisoning; Patient Handling; Snakes, Arthropods, and Spiders; Animal Bites; and the Psychological Aspects of Emergency Care.

("Video Teletraining Aids Army Medics in Sinai," by Pat Davis, News Leader, 7 Dec 1995)

Company F of the 232nd Medical Battalion set the new standard in the battalion history book when 100% of their eligible 91B10 students passed the NREMT exam.

("232nd Sets Highest Standard," SSG Ernest Estrada, News Leader, 14 Dec 1995)

The U.S. Army's 1st Armored Division began deploying to Bosnia in mid-December.

1996

The only the one of its kind, the AMEDDC&S Battle Simulation Center officially opened in 1996. The facility represented the first phase of incorporating battle simulation into the classroom in support of Distance Learning, the Classroom of the Future, On Demand Training/Mission Rehearsal, Automation/ Digitization, and the Total Army School System. It also provided AMEDDC&S with a Command Control, Communications, Computers, and Intelligence Command Post Exercise Program for the conduct of institutional and collective training.

("New Battle Simulation Center will Train 4,000 Soldiers," News Leader, 18 Jan 1996)

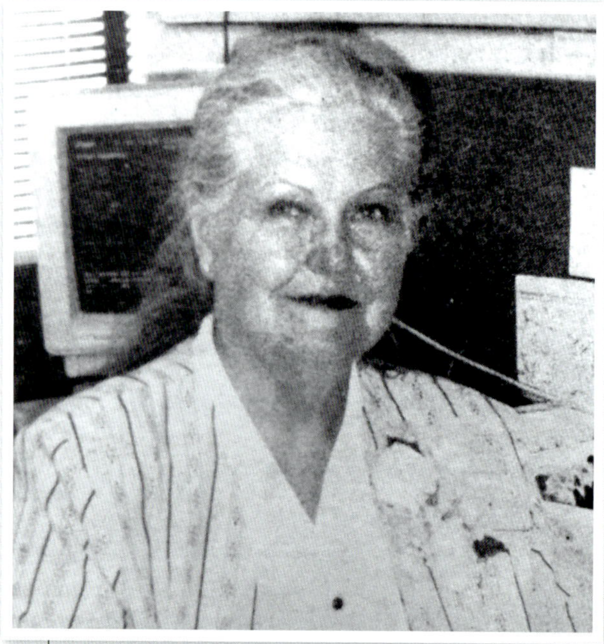

Emelyn Wolters
Emelyn Wolters portrays the grace that made her an institution at AMEDDC&S. For 38 years, Wolters was the Chief of the Training Input Branch, where she scheduled classes and annually placed more than 30,000 students from branches of the military into training classes. In addition, she also designed the AMEDDC&S course catalog.

(U.S. Army Photo, "AMEDD C&S Civilian Cherishes Every Lesson and Experience," News Leader, 25 July 1996)

Students in the Basic Non-Commissioned Officers Course Phase II Technical Training underwent a simulated mission to rescue and medically treat American soldiers trapped in an urban warfare setting. The medical NCOs were challenged to use only feeling and hearing to determine and treat injuries in a dark, noisy cement building, a setting they might encounter one day. The medical NCOs were also taught principles of wilderness medicine and ways of constructing improved litters and splinting devices.

("Medical NCOs Train in Urban Wilderness Environment," News Leader, 30 May 1996)

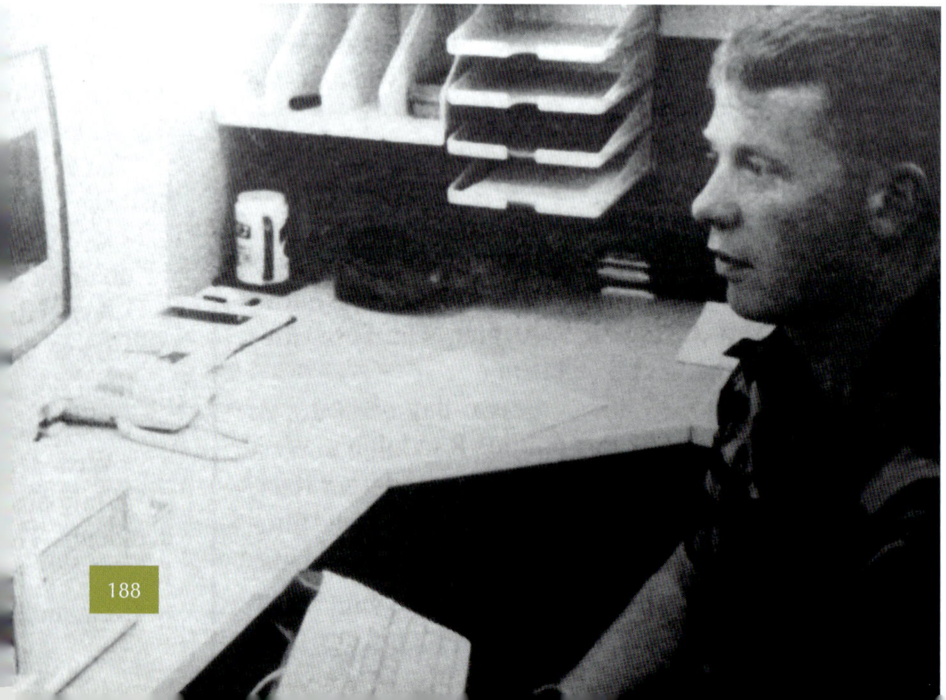

CW2 Robert Rallyea, an AMEDD C&S Veterinary Science instructor, completed his college degree in animal science from Kansas State University via long distance learning on the Internet. It took him about two and a half years to earn his bachelor's degree. Long distance learning became an ideal option for soldiers subject to multiple TDY assignments or deployments.

("Fort Sam Houston Soldier Completes His College Degree via Long-Distance Learning," News Leader, 30 July 1996)

In September 1996, members of the AMEDDC&S training support and force development department took their combat lifesaver course (CLS) to Panama City, Panama. The conference brought medical officer physicians from 19 Central and South American countries to share information on preventative medicine practice and different ways of treatment. The AMEDDC&S instructors explained the importance of the CLS course to the military and local civilian population.

("Combat Lifesaver Course Goes South of the Border," News Leader, 3 Oct 1996)

Two hundred fifty high school students visited the AMEDDC&S as part of Science '96. Science '96 was a cooperative community effort to reach high school science students. Displays explored both military science career options and scholarship opportunities. BG Simmons, installation deputy commander, addressed the students, telling them, "Education is a passport to the future. Your time is here and it is now. Each of us has something unique to contribute if we choose to work together. Be proud of who you are and what you want to be."

(The AMEDD C&S Hosts Science 96," News Leader, 7 Nov 1996)

Center Brigade was assigned to the AMEDDC&S in July of 1996.

(Permanent Order 96-1, 26 Jul 1996)

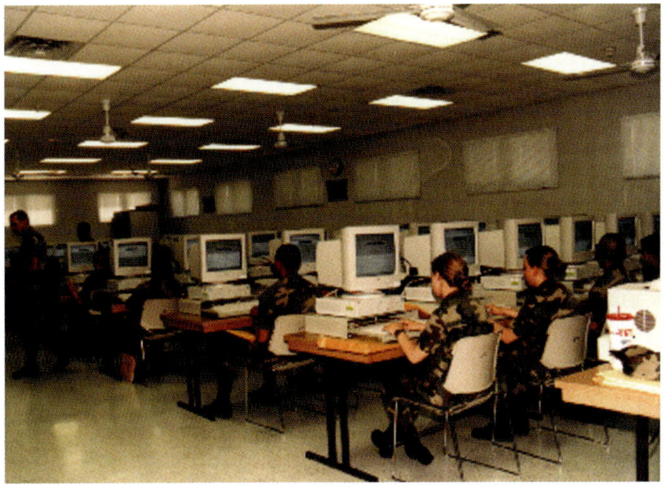

91W in the Battlefield Simulations Training Center

(U.S. Army Photos, "New Battle Simulation Center will Train 4,000 Soldiers," News Leader, 18 January 1996)

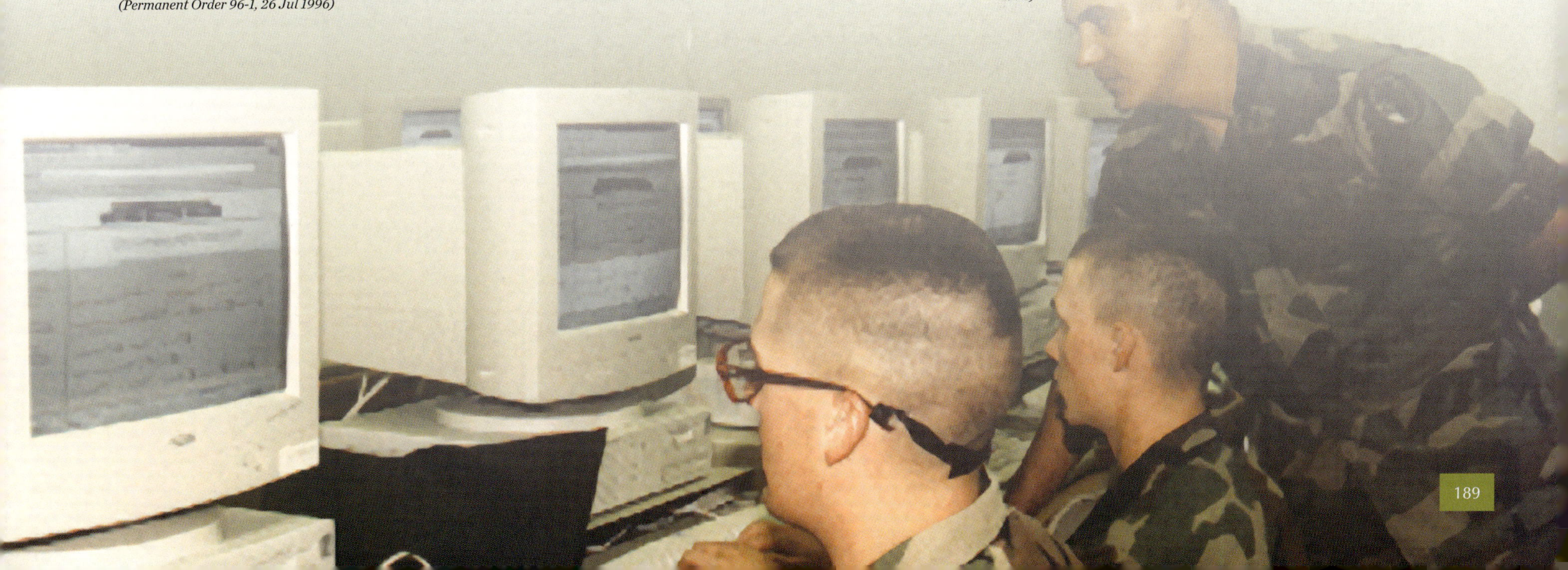

1997

The AMEDDC&S added a new building and computer lab for students in patient administration. The new facility, located at 4015 N. New Braunfels Avenue, was where students received training in health care organization and eligibility, medical terminology and diagnostic coding, Army medical records, behavioral sciences, patient administration, and automated hospital support systems.

("Patient Administrators Get a New School House," News Leader, 9 Jan 1997)

Interested in seeing the training of his future force, LTG Ronald Blanck, the Surgeon General, visited all three Center Brigade battalions to see ongoing operations firsthand. The Medical Command was responsible for providing the medical force for the total Army.

("Army Surgeon General Scopes Out Training," News Leader, 6 Jan 1997)

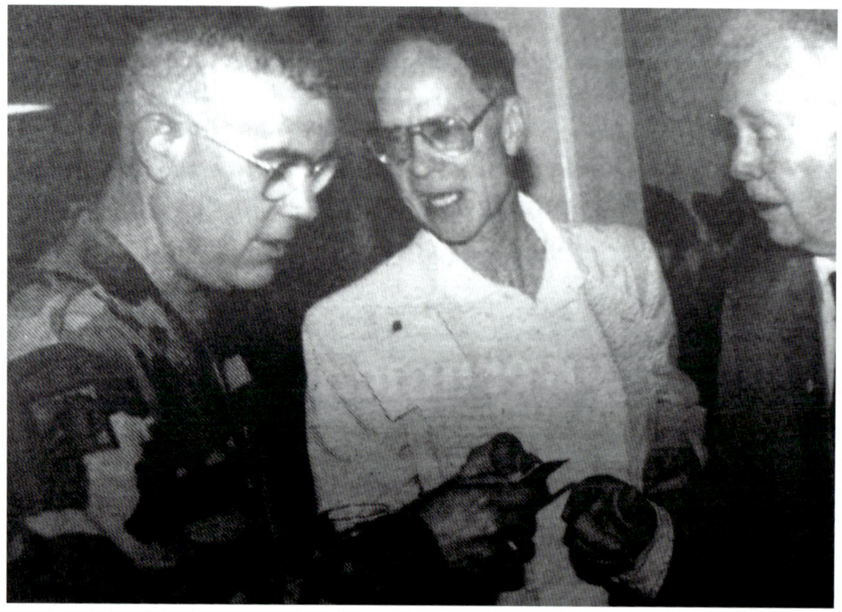

LTC Jay Harmon, Commander, 187th Medical Battalion
Exchanges unit insignia and commemorative medals with members of the Ukrainian delegation, which visited the Post in May of 1997.

("Post Hosts Ukrainian Delegation," News Leader, by Phil Reidinger, 8 May 1997, p 3)

A prototype of the new armored treatment vehicle went on display during the first week of February 1997. The vehicle was expected to move emergency treatment teams forward in the battlefield. Casualties were to be treated within because enough space was provided for the trauma treatment team and their equipment. The modifications in the new vehicle were expected to eliminate 30-minute treatment delays caused by the need to unload equipment in the then current M577 treatment team carrier.

("Army Medical Evacuation Looks at Next Century's Battlefield Equipment," News Leader, 27 Feb 1997)

The 232nd Medical Battalion remote tactical medicine class was designed to bridge the gap in the combat medic role between the high technology of distance learning and the tangible, tactical, and often isolated task of combat patient care in the dirt. The course was a combination of emergency medical treatment, wilderness medicine, and combat survival tactics. The lessons were applicable to situations ranging from the golf course to a traffic accident to remote reaches of the world.

("Unique Course Teaches Medic Broad Scope of Survival," News Leader, 7 Aug 1997)

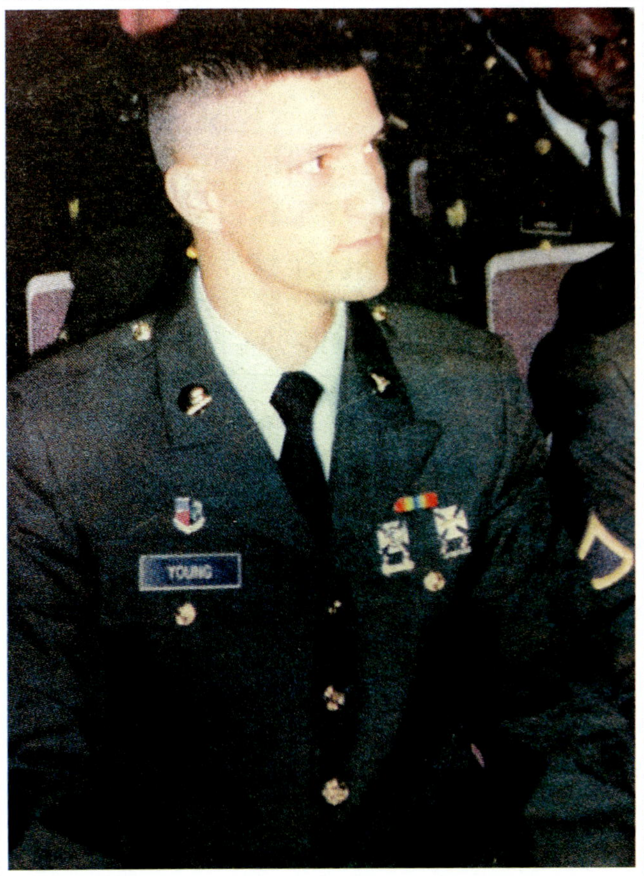

PVT Zachary Young, a student soldier medic, with E Company, 232nd Medical Battalion, became the first soldier in the known history of the AMEDDC&S and school training battalion to achieve a 100% grade point average on all academic and performance tests. A high school drop-out, PVT Young was the distinguished honor graduate of his class and credits many people who contributed to his success.

("Medic Maxes Course with First Recorded Perfect Score," News Leader, 8 May 1997)

SSG Jimmy Credo became the first instructor in the 22-year history of the AMEDDC&S course to achieve all professional certification licensure offered by the National Board of Respiratory Care in the United States. Credo became namesake of an award established by his colleagues and fellow instructors to recognize a level of unsurpassed achievement and expertise as a legacy to students and as a benchmark to other instructors.

("Retired AMEDD Instructor Gives New Name to Excellence," News Leader, 9 Oct 1997)

After 19 years of persistence and raising $6 million, the AMEDD Museum Foundation broke ground for an addition to the museum. The second phase of the museum included a second exhibit hall, glass-enclosed gallery, train station cover for the hospital train and a memorial garden. "The AMEDD Museum is a true asset to San Antonio's museum network. Many people are unaware of the Army's contributions to medicine in general – the artifacts tell the story," said Pat Lee, Public Affairs Chairman for the Museum Foundation.

("AMEDD Museum Breaks Ground Again," News Leader, 6 Nov 1997)

SSG Lynn Hale, a 91B instructor in F Company, 232nd Battalion, had been working on promoting the Women's Memorial since its approval by Congress in the mid-1980s. When the date for her last re-enlistment coincided with the dedication of the Women's Memorial in Arlington Cemetery, she actually re-enlisted at the site following its dedication. She was surprised and ecstatic when she found out that she would take the oath from Attorney General Janet Reno.

("232nd Soldier Re-enlists at the Women's Memorial Dedication," News Leader, 26 Nov 1997)

1998

The AMEDDC&S Department Board, "the conscience of the Army Medical Department," was involved, in 1998, in the field-testing of several new technologies and processes, including the Deployable Medical System, Telemedicine systems, a new wound bandage, a field medical oxygen generation system, a resuscitating fluid production system, and a combat medic vest to replace the combat medic bag.

("Medical Department Board Checks Out New Ideas and Equipment," News Leader, 15 Jan 1998, p 1)

The NCOA was awarded accreditation during an assessment visit by a team of evaluators from the Army's Sergeants Major Academy. The on-the-spot accreditation was a surprise. The team of evaluators was impressed with the leading-edge technology and recommended that the NCOA be used as the test bed for any and all NCO Classroom XXI initiatives.

("NCO Academy Cited as Classroom XXI Model," News Leader, 15 Jan 1998, p 3)

The 91 Mikes (MOS 91M Hospital Food Service Specialist) conducted field exercises at Camp Bullis the second week in January. The field exercise was part of the biannual 14-week NCO Course for hospital food service specialists.

("Hospital Food Service Specialists Conduct Field Exercise," by Nelia Schrum, News Leader, 15 Jan 1998)

A CD-ROM version of Phase I of the Officer Advanced Course (OAC) was debuted Army-wide at a video teletraining broadcast premier during the Training and Doctrine Command's Swap Shop in January 1998. The Swap Shop was a TRADOC program targeted to share lessons learned throughout the Army. The CD-ROM Advanced Course program was designed to allow students to set their own pace for mastering the material.

("Officer Advanced Course Goes High Tech," by Nelia Schrum, News Leader, 29 Jan 1998, p 4)

AMEDDC&S officers were offered early retirement as Personnel Command searched for a means of reaching the budgeted end strength voluntarily.

("AMEDD Officer Offered Early Retirement Option," News Leader, 19 Feb 1998, p 4)

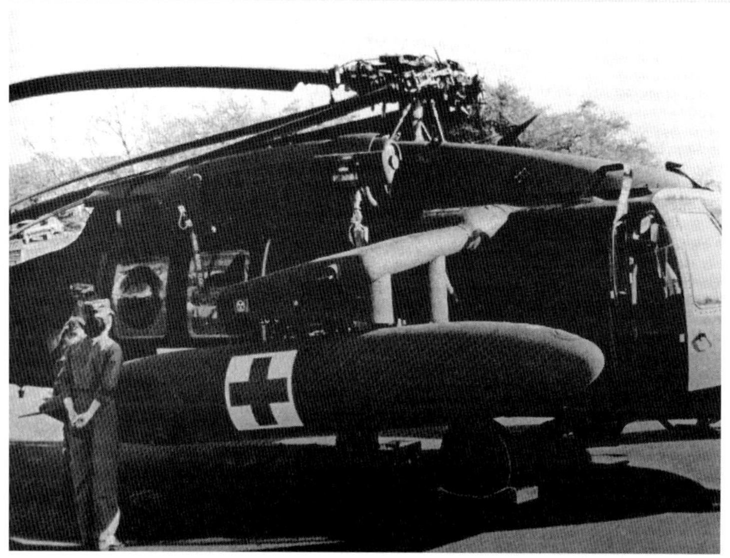

Two hundred Army evacuators gather in San Antonio for the annual Army Medical Evacuation Conference. The new Army air ambulance, the UH-60Q, a modified Blackhawk helicopter airframe with a state-of-the-art medical interior, could accommodate up to six patients. The conference also displayed the Armored Medical Evacuation Vehicle (AMEV) and Armored Medical Treatment Vehicle (M577).

("AMEDD Evacuation Personnel Converge on San Antonio," by Nelia Schrum, News Leader, 5 March 1998, p 1)

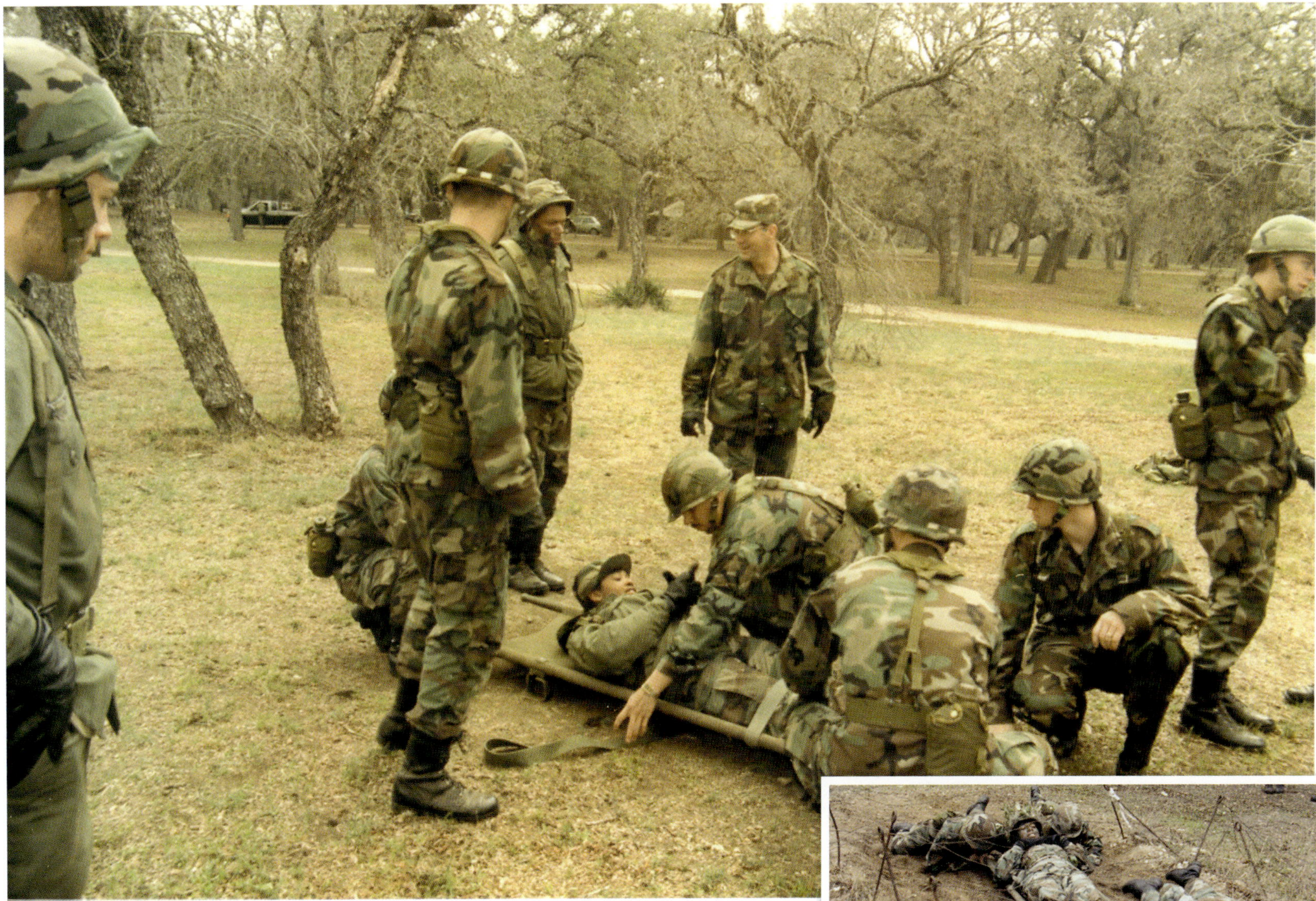

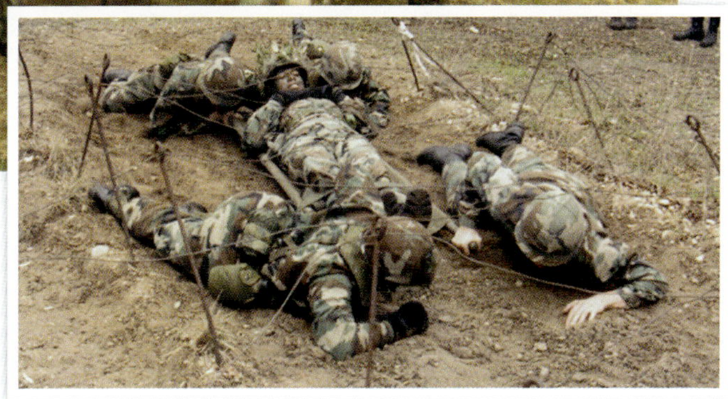

The Management of Combat Stress Casualties Course of the Occupational Therapy Branch ran simulations examining the full range of battle stresses at Camp Bullis in May 1998.

("Occupational Therapy Leads a Way to Manage Combat Stress," by COL Valerie Rice, News Leader, 7 May 1998, p 7; photos courtesy of COL (Ret) Valerie Rice)

1998

By bringing four South Carolina Army National Guard 91B MOS sustainment instructors via military air to train 73 Texas Army National Guard (TXARMG) soldiers at the AMEDDC&S, the Active Army and the TXARMG provided one of the lowest-cost training programs to date. The end cost per student and instructor was $18.50 per participant.

("MOS Sustainment Training for TXARMG," by Jeanette Devine, News Leader, 12 March 1998)

MG Peake, commander of the AMEDDC&S, announced an upcoming training program called "Consideration of Others." The new program, mandatory for both military and civilians alike, focused on decent treatment of people, a key value for a successful workplace.

("Facilitators Receive Consideration of Others Training," News Leader, 2 April 1998)

Creating computer literate NCOs was the top priority of the NCO Academy in 1998.

("Computer Literate NCO Top Priority of the Academy," by Nelia Schrum, News Leader, 23 April 1998, p 4)

The new Soldier Medic Training Site at Camp Bullis opened 29 May.

("232nd Relished New Training Site at Camp Bullis," by Mike Pollen, News Leader, 14 May 1998)

The Joint Field Nutrition Operation Course was held at Camp Bullis the third week in May.

("Nutrition Care Exercise Includes Training Challenges," News Leader, 21 May 1998)

The AMEDD Museum opened Phase II of its grounds on 30 July.

("AMEDD Museum Foundation Opens Phase II," by Phil Reidinger, News Leader, 30 July 1998, p 1)

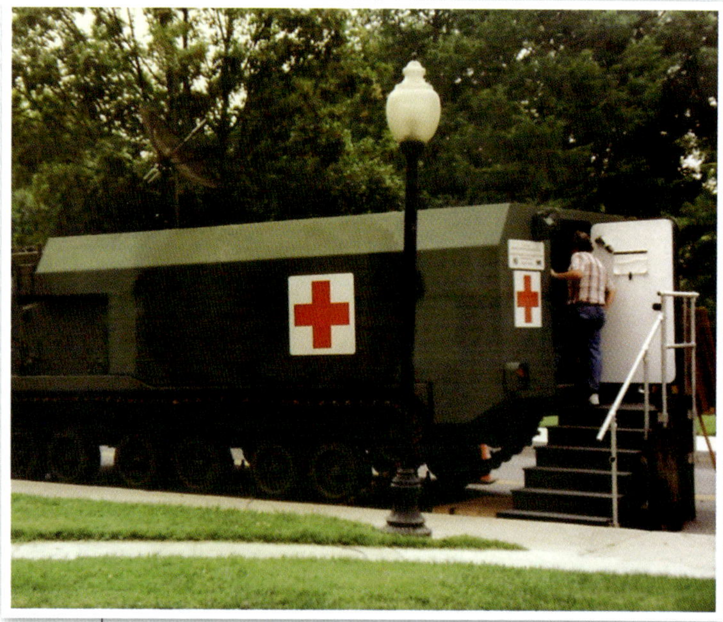

A prototype "21st Century" Armored Treatment and Transport Vehicle (ATTV) was used in the mid-1990s to develop support for the concept vehicle. The ATTV was designed as a platform to medically evacuate, while providing treatment, from the site of battlefield injury to the appropriate echelon of care. The vehicle was built on a Bradley chassis and touts satellite communication to provide "Digital Medicine," circa 1996.

(U.S. Army Photo, "21st Century," News Leader, 30 July 1998)

AAFES opened the bookstore in the old student club area of the basement of Willis Hall in August 1998.

("AAFES Opens Store for AMEDDC&S Students," News Leader, 6 Aug 1998)

In August 1998, the AMEDDC&S sent its first class of Army flight medics to attend Navy Physiology training at Naval Operational Medical Institute. Previously, this train-the-trainer instruction had been conducted by the Air Force.

(News Leader, 20 Aug 1998)

A pilot class of advanced course AMEDDC&S NCOs attended the first totally Internet-based distance learning program. The class of more than 90 medical sergeants completed courses on technology, logistics, command support, and information security online over a six-week period before arriving at FSH for the second phase of their course.

("Distance Learning Bridges Training Gap," by Cleo Brennan, News Leader, 10 Dec 1998)

The Animal Medicine Branch trained its students in animal CPR with the Resusci-pup, a dog-like training manikin.

("Resusci-pup Trains Dog's Best Friends," by Cleo Brennan, News Leader, 17 Dec 1998)

1999

SSG Milton Padua, aerospace physiology instructor at the U.S. Army School of Aviation Medicine, was named TRADOC Instructor of the Year — a first in AMEDDC&S history.

(AMEDD Fosters Top Instructor in TRADOC Competition," by Cleo Brennan, News Leader, 11 March 1999)

The AMEDDC&S, in cooperation with the DA Chief of Chaplain Office, completed the first iteration of the Combat Medical Ministry Course, to confer the new Additional Skill Identifier 7S.

("Bloody Boots Course Battle-Proofs Chaplains For New Skill Identifier," by Cleo Brennan, News Leader, 24 June 1999)

Under MG James Peake, the 91B and 91C MOSs combined to become the 91W, a more versatile combat medic and first responder.

("91W Is Combat Medic MOS of the Future," by Phil Reidinger, 8 July 1999, p 1)

The Veterinary Food Safety training received its own training site at Building 325 after 29 years of being at Ft. Sam Houston.

("Veterinary Food Safety Training Facility Nears Completion," by Daniel Holland, News Leader, 12 Aug 1999, p 1)

AMEDDEX 99 employed sophisticated training techniques in three simulation centers as well as the rock drill facility. The exercise was conducted using continuous, real-time computer driven operations based on a master list related to Corps-level offensive operation on the Korean peninsula.

("Three Simulation Centers and Rock Drill Facility Used," News Leader, 19 Aug 1999)

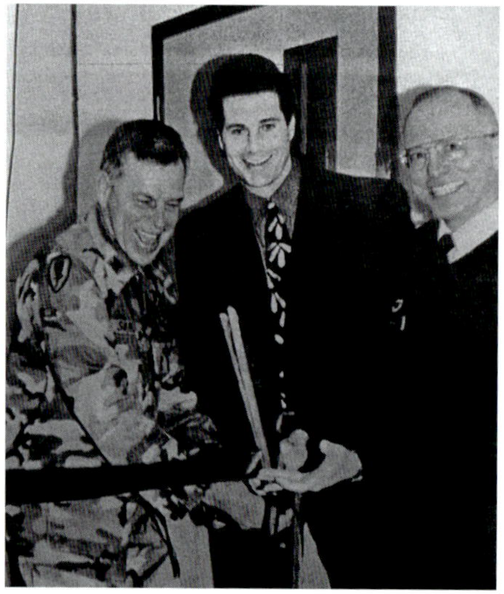

MG James Peake cut the ribbon for the opening of three distance learning classrooms in support of the Total Army Distance Learning Program. With MG Peake are Gary Winkler, Total Army Distance Learning Plan (TADLP) and COL Richard Shipley, Dean, AHS.

("Distance Learning Classrooms Open For New Generation In Training," by Cleo Brennan, News Leader, 21 Jan 1999)

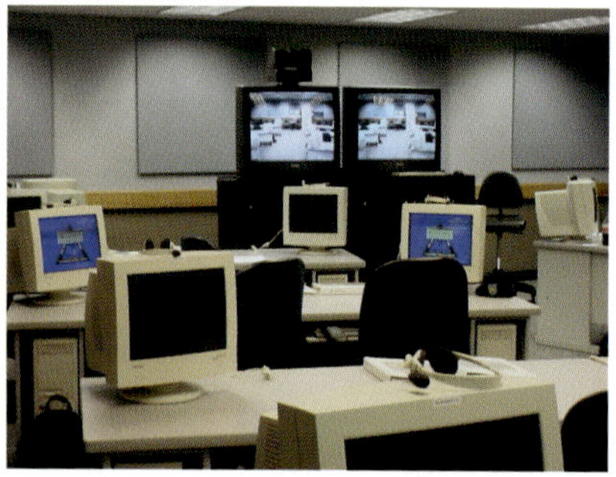

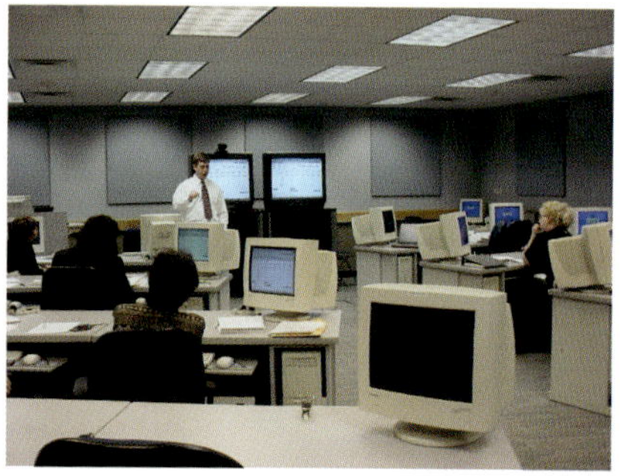

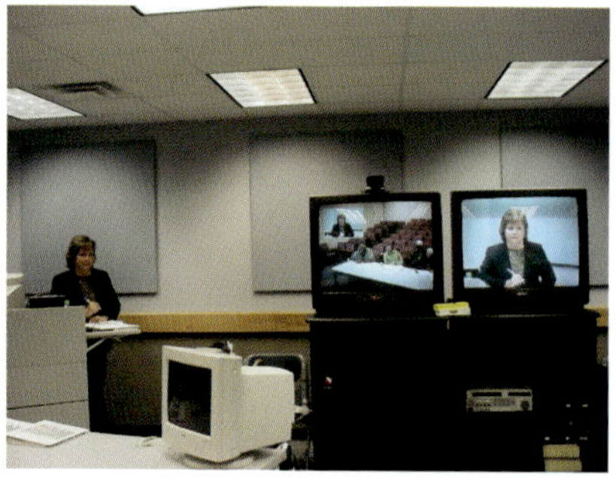

The new distance learning classrooms, circa 1999

(Photos courtesy of Dwayne H. Rogers, Ph.D., Director, Distributed Learning Division, Academy of Health Sciences, AMEDDC&S)

Leading medical suppliers from healthcare industries throughout the country displayed the latest in medical training devices at the Medical Training and Education Vendors Fair in Blesse Auditorium. The fair highlighted the latest in medical education and training technology simulation devices that are significant in AMEDDC&S's educational program for their quality, safety and cost.

("Medical Simulation Fair Exhibits Elaborate Training Techniques," News Leader, 16 Sept 1999)

In an effort to expand domestic violence prevention and intervention services for troubled Army families around the world, a mobile training team from the AMEDDC&S Family and Advocacy Program racked up many miles to bring an idea to life. Throughout the year, training sessions at more than a dozen installations brought local decision-makers new tools and a new approach to help families who had experienced domestic violence.

("Mobile Training Teams Keep Skills up to Date for Family Safety," News Leader, 21 Oct 1999)

The Military Health System met an aggressive timeline to identify, assess, renovate, validate and implement all of its Year 2000 (Y2K)-affected systems before 1 January 2000. If any problems related to Y2K were to occur, the "ace in the hole" Military Health System Y2K Automation Information System Contingency and Continuity of Operations Planning Guide had been developed to assist in addressing those problems. Needless to say, the new millennium came and went without a glitch.

("The Military Health System – Preparing for the New Millennium," News Leader, 16 Dec 1999)

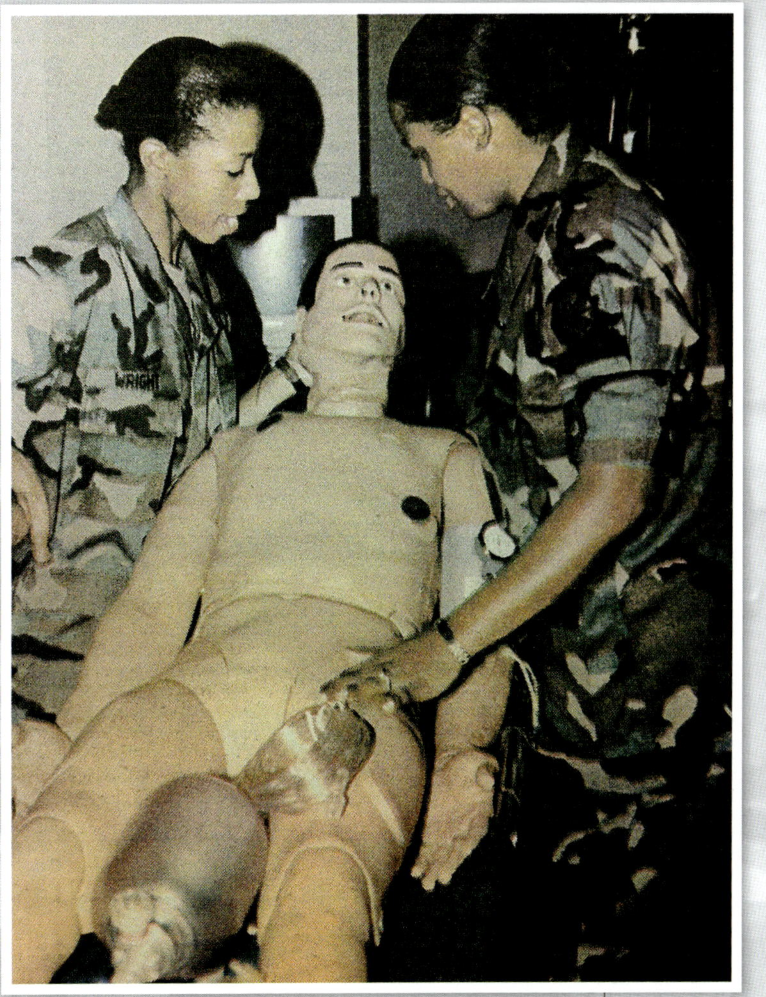

Patient Simulation

Faculty, staff, and students with the AMEDDC&S Noncommissioned Officer Course test the latest technology in patient simulation at Willis Hall the first week in May. The manikin simulated 25 different patient profiles representing various ages, physiology, medical history and gender. It replicated clinical signs such as heart and breath sounds, palpable pulses, chest excursion, and both normal and difficult airway modules.

("High Tech Patient Visits the Center and School," by Phil Reidinger, News Leader, 13 May 1999)

2000 - 2010

The Council on Occupational Education (COE) reaffirmed AMEDDC&S accreditation in September 1999 after evaluating 109 items addressing training support and conduct of training. AMEDDC&S prepped for their visit in advance by conducting its own, year-long self-assessment and intensive review led by the AMEDDC&S standardization and evaluation team. In 2000, AMEDDC&S had the largest and most active evaluation and quality assurance element in the Army, as many TRADOC schools eliminated their evaluation and QA programs in 1994.

("Credentials and Initiatives Keep C&S in the Lead," News Leader, 12 Jan 2000)

A total media platform debuted at the AMEDDC&S Officer Basic Course. An integrated unit that was both self-contained and easy to ship, the new platform was a multimedia device that could serve as a computer, TV, video player, and DVD player. The unit, which could be operated with a remote keyboard, could run PowerPoint presentations, access the Internet, and operate on the Knowledge Management Network.

("Portable Media Unit Provides Versatility in a Practical Package," by Cleo Brennan, News Leader, 27 Jan 2000, p 1)

Six hundred students from 34 high schools assembled at Willis Hall to test their health occupation, communication, and leadership skills in January for the Health Occupation Student of America competition. Thirty military and civilian instructors from the AMEDDC&S judged the contestants.

("Future Health Care Providers Test Their Knowledge and Skills at Willis Hall," by Yolanda Hagsberg, News Leader, 27 Jan 2000, p 16)

AAFES expanded its service at Willis Hall to include a laundry service, barber shop, and shoe shine stand.

("AAFES Expands Service at Willis Hall," News Leader, 27 Jan 2000, p 25)

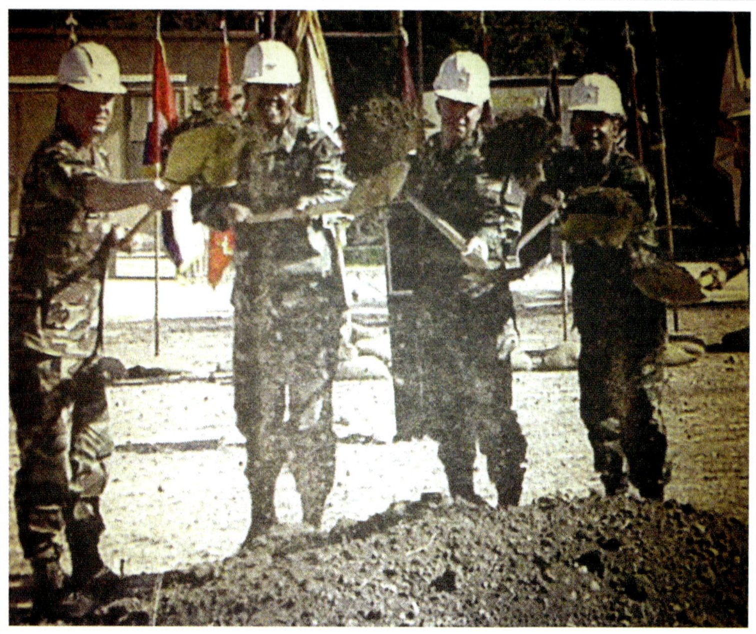

FSH Garrison Commander COL William Thresher, Center Brigade Commander COL Larry Campbell, Camp Bullis Commander LTC Timothy Williamson, and Academy Battalion Commader LTC Bede Ramcharan raise their shovels, marking the beginning of construction of E Company's new warehouse and one-stop issue facility at Camp Bullis on 10 January 2000.

("New Digs at Camp Bullis," News Leader, 27 Jan 2000)

After three years of development, the new Officer Basic Course (OBC) was introduced. A three-phase course of instruction, the first phase remained a general introduction to the Army and the AMEDDC&S. Curriculum was taught as a mixture of conferences and practical exercises, with a comprehensive exam at the end of the third week. Phase II transitioned students into "squad-level" training with an intensive five-day field training exercise that focused on development of basic leadership skills in a field setting through highly realistic situational training exercises. For the final phase, students returned to the classroom and were taught the fundamental doctrine that supports the AMEDD Mission.

("AMEDD OBC Redesigned," by MAJ Randy Story, News Leader, 17 Feb 2000, pp 1 & 7)

The AMEDDC&S Directorate of Combat and Doctrine Development established training requirements for chaplains as part of a medical team, which made it the only Army proponent school to train a career field outside its own branch. The AMEDDC&S, through the Clinical Pastoral Education program, offered chaplains the opportunity to get the same type of training within a medical setting.

("Fort Sam Duty Fulfills Chaplaincy's Breadth and Depth," by Cleo Brennan, News Leader, 24 Feb 2000, p 3)

The installation retention office was officially reopened after renovations in March 2000.

("Re-up!," News Leader, 2 March 2000, p 1)

In early February, three members of the 232nd Medical Battalion traveled to Quito, Ecuador, to teach basic first aid classes to U.S. embassy employees. The classes were taught in both English and Spanish.

("232nd Soldiers Train Ecuador Embassy Employees," by 1LT Kenneth Walters, News Leader, 2 March 2000, p 11)

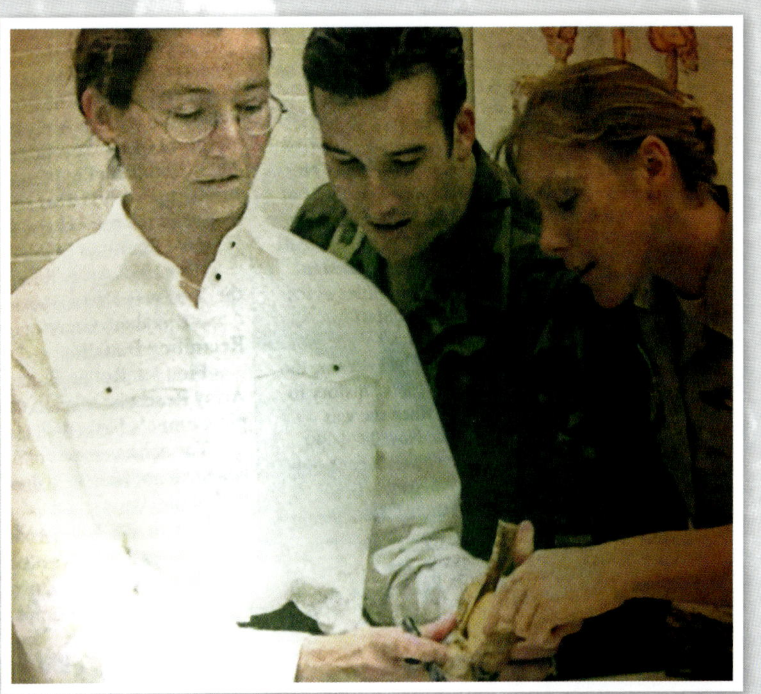

Deborah Egger (left) studies bone and joint structure with officer candidates Ian Stack and Tobijah Griffin in an AMEDDC&S anatomy class. Egger is a UT Health Science Center student enrolled in the Interservice PA Program (IPAP).

("IPA Program Strives for Highest Degree of Achievement," by Cleo Brennan, News Leader, 16 March 2000, p 1)

2000

The Patient Administration Branch of the AMEDDC&S opened the doors to its new facility in Building 1026 in April 2000.

("Improved Facility Anchors Cornerstone of Concerned Health Care," by Cleo Brennan, News Leader, 20 April 2000, p 4)

Nine instructors from the 232nd Medical assisted with the soldier medic training for the 8th Battalion, 5th Brigade, 100th Division, U.S. Army Reserve in Smyrna, Tennessee, strengthening the growing bond between reserve and active component.

After Building 4011 was assessed with Risk Assessment Codes (RAC) 1 and 2 conditions and deemed a "sick" building, it underwent a half-million dollar renovation to eliminate the health hazards.

("Sick Building Restored To Healthy, Attractive Work Environment," by Cleo Brennan, News Leader, 8 June 2000, p 3)

The AMEDD Museum broke ground on Phase III of its building program the second week of July. Phase III included an artifact conservation repository, Museum Foundation Office, a garden area with a walking path, a gazebo, and a variety of medicinal plants.

("AMEDD Museum Breaks Ground for Phase III," by Bruce Nelson, News Leader, 13 July 2000, p 2)

More than 500 hospital corpsmen of the U.S. Navy Reserve Dallas Fleet Hospital "Alamo Pride" trained at Camp Bullis for three days during their yearly medical refresher training. The training was arranged by the Joint Defense Medical Readiness Training Institute.

("Fleet Hospital Trains at Camp Bullis," by Phil Reidinger, News Leader, 17 Aug 2000, p 17)

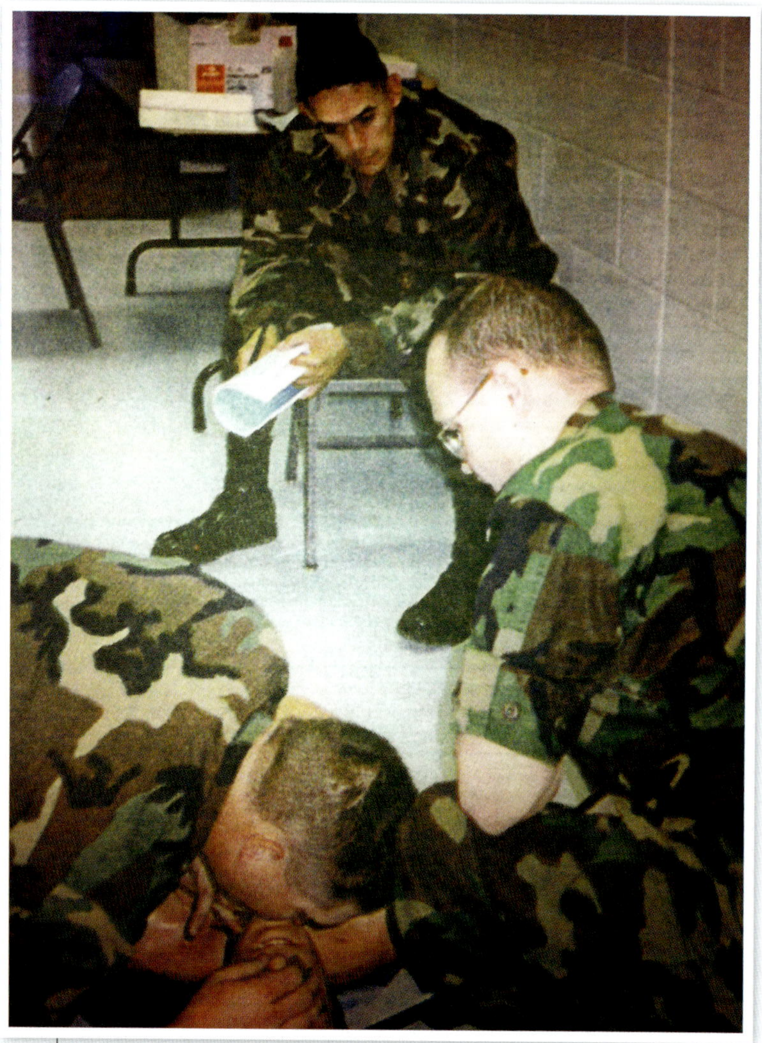

Training the National Guard
A Tennessee National Guardsman pinches the simulated patient's nostrils preparing to deliver breath to the training aid, practicing CPR under the supervision of instructor SSG Mark Cornejo (seated).

("232nd Instructors Extend Total Army Training," by Cleo Brennan, News Leader, 27 May 1999, p 1)

Camp Bullis was the site of the world's largest medical simulation exercise the last week of August. AMEDDEX 2000 drew units from around the world. The most complex tactical operation centers (TOCs), the TOC of the AMEDD, and the TOC of the 30th Medical Brigade, were field tested and validated for functionality as they simultaneously supported both the exercise and their soldiers in a real-world deployment. Another first was the use of the Very Small Aperture Terminal (VSAT), which enhanced communications capabilities during the exercise.

("Medical Units Get Money's Worth In Training," by Cleo Brennan, News Leader, 31 Aug 2000, p 1)

The 187th Medical Battalion released a new handbook for leaders designed to ensure the total readiness of its female soldiers. The handbook covered topics such as pre-deployment education information, pregnancy considerations, promiscuity, and perceptions and information on sexual assault. The handbook was designed after viewing a similar guide put together by the staff at Madigan Army Hospital in Fort Lewis, Washington.

("187th Med. Bn. Manual Speaks To Female Soldiers' Issues," by LT Kara Escajada, News Leader, 5 Oct 2000, p 13)

The AMEDDC&S began gearing up its modified POI for the Radiology Technologist Course. The AMEDDC&S was the first site to test the latest technology in radiographic equipment, and planned to train roughly 400 subject matter experts per year.

("High Speed Equipment Demands High Speed Techs," News Leader, 16 Nov 2000, p 19)

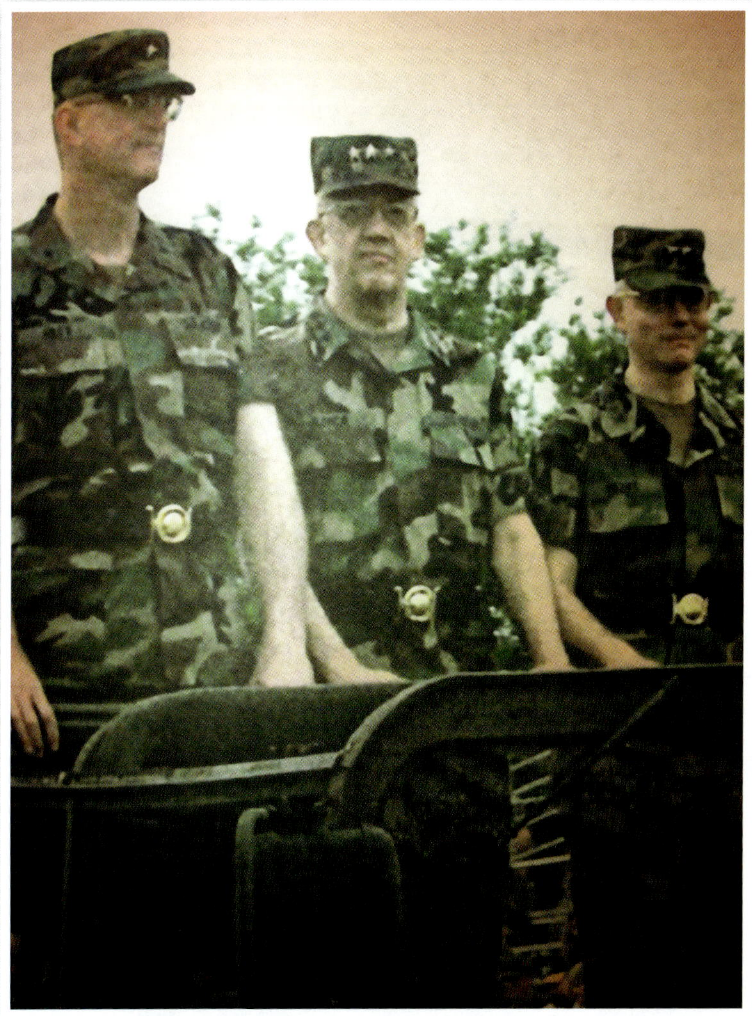

Change of command

BG Kevin Kiley (left), incoming commander of Fort Sam Houston and the AMEDDC&S, joins MEDCOM Commander LTG Ronald Blanck, and MG James Peake for a final inspection of troops before Peake surrendered his command.

("Kiley Assumes Command of the Installation and AMEDDC&S," by Cleo Brennan, News Leader, 8 June 2000, p 1)

2001

The new "Army of One" recruiting campaign kicked off in January 2001 and focused on Army strength and teamwork.

(News Leader, 18 Jan 2001)

Dr. John McCollum, an instructional systems developmental specialist for DoD, lectured on the influence of diet and learning to Brigade trainers, instructors, and leaders.

("Chicken Soup for the Classroom Supports Student Success," News Leader, 1 Feb 2001)

Nearly 75 dignitaries and visitors joined the AMEDDC&S staff for the opening of the new facility of the Occupational Therapy branch in April 2001. The new facility features a more realistic training setting, a better environment, and new equipment and resources to enhance learning.

("OT Branch Celebrates New Home, Professional Standing," News Leader, 19 April 2001)

In May, the program of instruction for the new 91W healthcare specialist MOS was completed and expected to supply medics trained in the skills and operational doctrine to support Army operations of the future.

("91W Training Program Ready," News Leader, 24 May 2001)

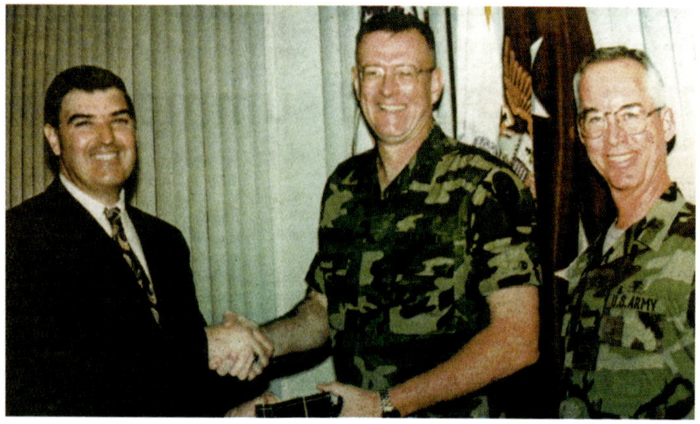

Paul Nadeua, Managing Director of KPMG Consulting Inc., and COL David Kirkpatrick, Dean of the AHS, presented the 91W Program of Instruction to AMEDDC&S Commander MG Kevin C. Kiley. The 91W Healthcare Specialist replaced the current 91B Combat Medic. The 91C Licensed Practical Nurse specialty was designated with the additional skill identifier 91WM6.

("91W Training Program Ready," News Leader, 24 May 2001)

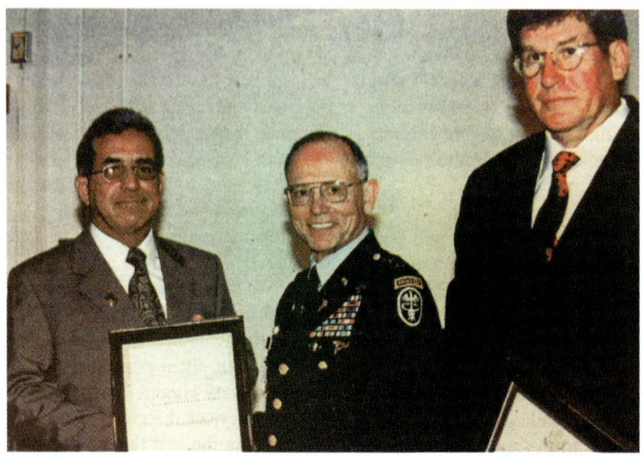

The U.S. Army Medical Regiment passed on the gauntlet of honor and duty to retired SGM Julius Bennet and SGM Oscar Ramos-Riveria in a ceremony presided over by the Surgeon General, LTG James Peake. The honorary positions of leadership are filled by appointment by the SG. The mission of the regiment is to enhance combat effectiveness by providing the opportunity for affiliation, developing loyalty and commitment, fostering a sense of belonging, improving unit spirit and institutionalizing the war fighter ethos.

("Transition of AMEDD Regiment Perpetuates Proud Legacy," News Leader, 25 Jan 2001)

Educators from America's heartland toured Fort Sam Houston and gave the Post high marks after taking a peek at what the Army does to prepare soldiers for the challenges of providing medical care to troops and families around the globe. Dr. Harold Hullemen, head of the Nevada Community School district in Iowa said, "I didn't conceive of the breadth of military training."

("Educators Tour Post For Up Close View of Medical Training," News Leader, 28 June 2001)

Contributing from their own recent experience as military medical students and at BAMC, members of the Post Graduate Medical Education Council gave 258 OBC students a day of insights, answers, and strategy. The program was designed to help future Army doctors attending the AMEDDC&S to be more successful in their military and medical service.

("BAMC Docs Add Personal Experience To AMEDD Training," News Leader, 5 July 2001)

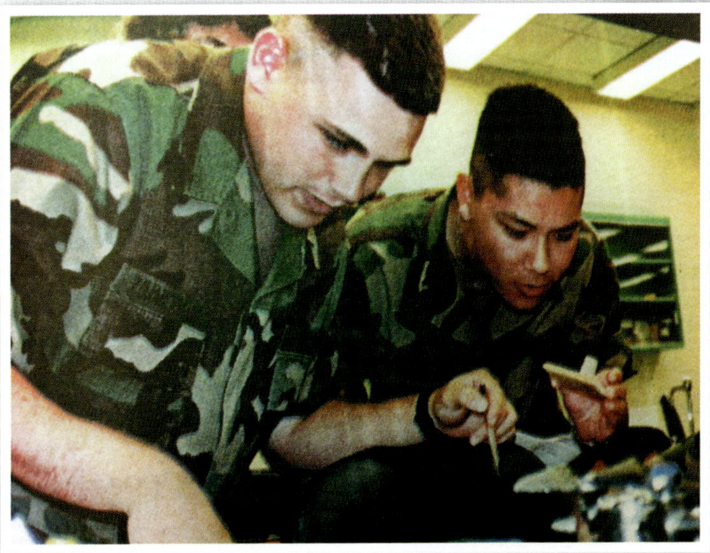

PVT James Zimmerman (left) and PVT Henry Weckesser identify bacteria as part of the Army training class on water quality.

("Educators Tour Post For a Close Up View of Medical Training," News Leader, 28 June 2001, p 8)

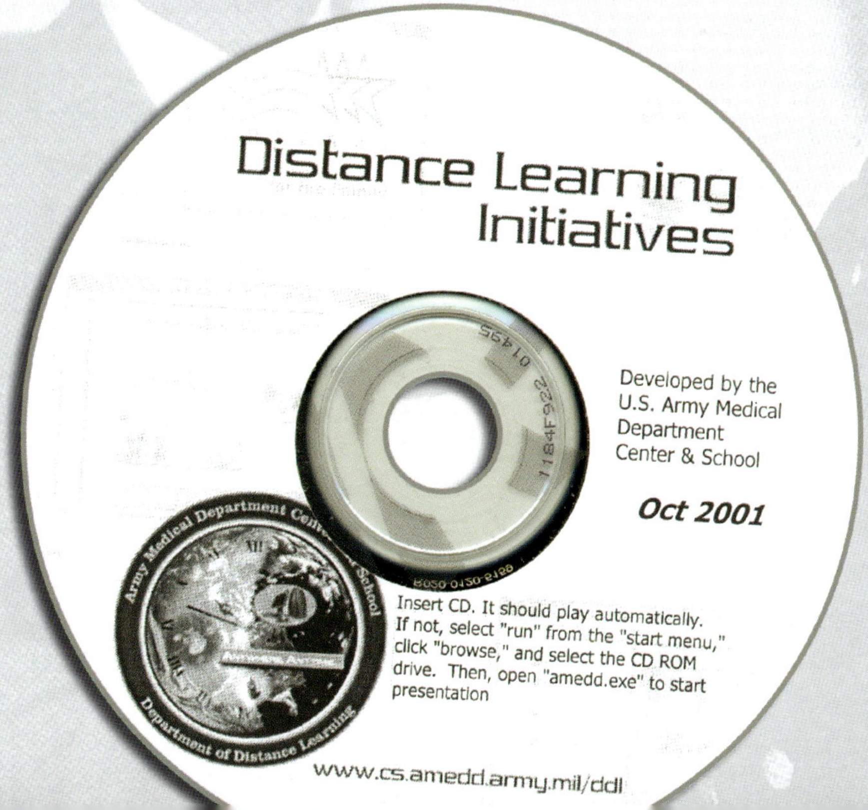

The Army's new black beret was introduced and became required headgear for soldiers on 23 Aug 2001.

The national anthrax scare was publicized and precautionary measures were published in a News Leader article entitled, "10 Things You Need To Know About Anthrax," 18 Oct 2001.

The Olympic Torch passed through San Antonio and Fort Sam Houston on 11 Dec 2001 as part of its travels across the United States on its way to the lighting ceremony at the Winter Games in Salt Lake City, Utah.

("Olympic Torch Gets Army Welcome at Fort Sam Houston," News Leader, 13 Dec 2001)

2002

The AMEDDC&S Clinical Pastoral Education Program received an accreditation certificate from the Association for Clinical Pastoral Education during a ceremony at the Fort Sam Houston's Officers Club. The Clinical Pastoral Education training program was unique in that it combined academic discipline with intensive first-hand trauma experience, which included in-depth pastoral supervision and theological integration.

("MedCom Pastoral Education Gets National Accreditation," News Leader, 17 Jan 2002)

For the third consecutive year, local high school students had the opportunity to observe medical and veterinary-oriented job disciplines and discuss Army medical career opportunities with AHS and 232nd Medical Battalion instructors during the annual Groundhog Shadowing Day.

("AMEDDC&S Instructors Welcome Students' Third Job Shadowing Day," News Leader, 17 Jan 2002)

The Medical Strategic Leadership Program began in February 2002.

("228th Combat Support Hospital Exercises Multi-Component Staff Realistic Training During MASCAL," News Leader, 14 March 2002)

COL William Tozier became the first PA to be promoted to colonel in the active Army. His son, Coast Guard PO3 Evan Tozier, pinned on his father's new rank at a ceremony held at the Stilwell House on 1 April.

("Tozier Is First Physician Assistant to Wear Eagles," News Leader, 4 April 2002)

To keep up the pace in the highly competitive world of recruiting, 70 recruiters and support staff members from the 3rd Army Medical Department's Recruiting spent a few days at Fort Sam Houston familiarizing themselves with the AMEDDC&S. "The main purpose of the trip was to give recruiters a better working knowledge of AMEDDC&S specialties, programs, and environments," said SFC John Bohmer, a recruiter trainer from Fort Knox, Kentucky.

("Recruiters Get the Low Down on Army Medical Department," News Leader, 18 July 2002)

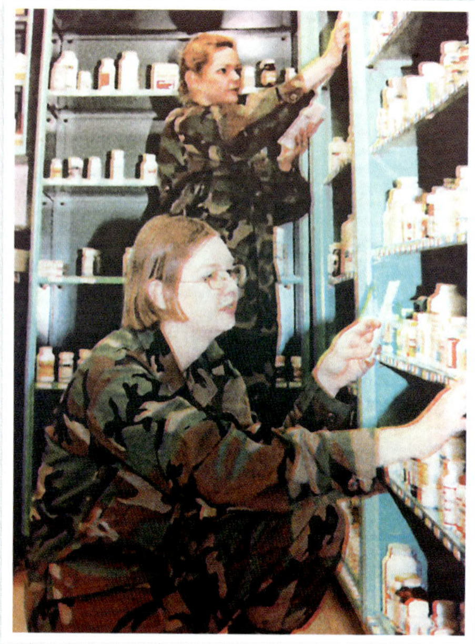

Blood is thicker than water for the family "buddy team" of PFC Joan Beaver and PVT Kimberly Beaver who were assigned to C Company, 187th Medical Battalion. Not only did this mother-daughter duo join the Army together, they completed basic training together, and continued through the 91Q Pharmacy Specialist School at the AMEDDC&S.

("From Birth To Basic Training... Soldiers Stick Together," News Leader, 7 March 2002)

Medical Aspects of Harsh Environments was released by the Borden Institute as part of its popular *Textbooks of Military Medicine* series. With soldiers deploying to mountainous places like Afghanistan and other countries with similar harsh environments, many agreed that the release of this particular book could not have come at a better time. It was believed that the textbooks should be mandatory reading and issued to every soldier.

("Military Medicine Textbook Helps Soldiers," News Leader, 3 Oct 2002)

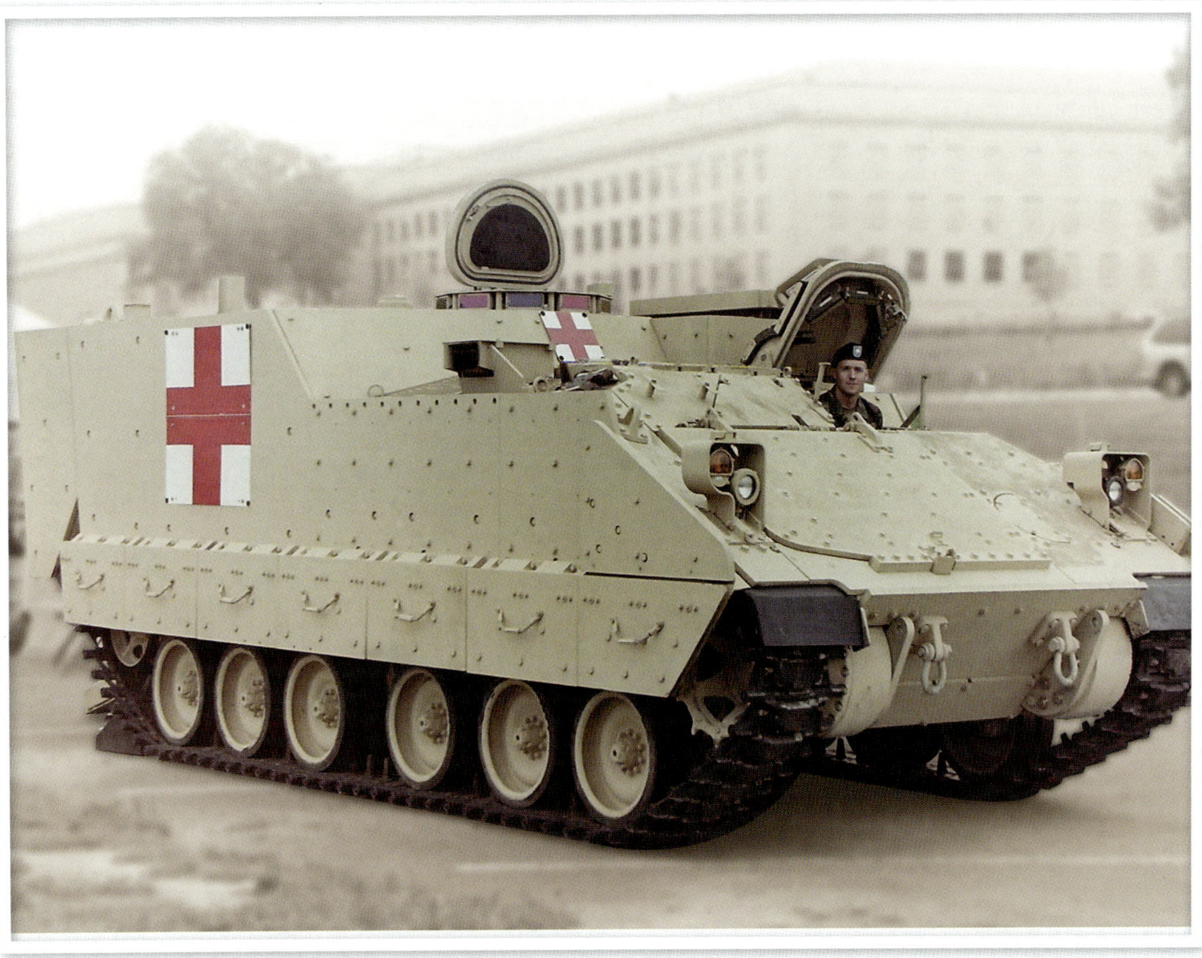

The AMEDDC&S worked with the Office of the Surgeon General and U.S. Army Medical Research and Materiel Command to bring the AMEV to the Pentagon. The purpose of this demonstration was to gain senior Army and Congressional support for a much needed vehicle to replace an aging fleet of M113 Armored Ambulances. Here, LTC Randall Anderson, Aviation Staff Officer to the Surgeon General, demonstrated the AMEV's maneuverability around the Pentagon north parking lot.

(Photo courtesy of COL Randall Anderson)

The Army Medical Board completed an evaluation of a new kitchen that replaced the modular field kitchen used by the nutrition care section in deployable hospitals. The two-day experiment, tested at Camp Bullis, utilized surveys and observations to determine if any changes needed to be made in doctrine, training, staffing, and equipment sets. The new kitchen with modifications was projected for fielding for operations with combat field hospitals in FY 04.

("Center and School Looks At New Containerized Kitchen During Camp Bullis Evaluation," News Leader, 24 Oct 2002)

The Center Brigade was redesignated as Headquarters and Headquarters Company, 32d Medical Brigade, effective 1 October 2002.

(Permanent Orders 274-001, 1 Oct 2002)

2003

Medical officers from Germany, Austria, Canada, and Japan joined medical officers from the Army, Air Force, and Navy for the Defense Medical Readiness Training Institute's (DMRTI) Joint Operations Medical Managers Course (JOMMC) in San Antonio. The JOMMC provided familiarization with joint care levels as well as with the medical capabilities available to maximize return-to-duty status, patient stabilization, and appropriate and timely evacuation of casualties.

("Allied Service Medics Join American Medics Attending DMRTI Course," by Edward Rivera, News Leader, 23 Jan 2003, p 1)

CPT James Craig, SGT Aaron Bishop, and SPC Rolex Mentore of the Academy Battalion, Company E, completed the challenging U.S. Army Air Assault Course at Fort Polk with record scores. Their accomplishments were noted in the News Leader in February 2003.

("Academy Battalion Trio Lead The Way at Fort Polk," by LT Alejandro Gonzales and MAJ Steve Middlecamp, News Leader, 20 Feb 2003, p 11)

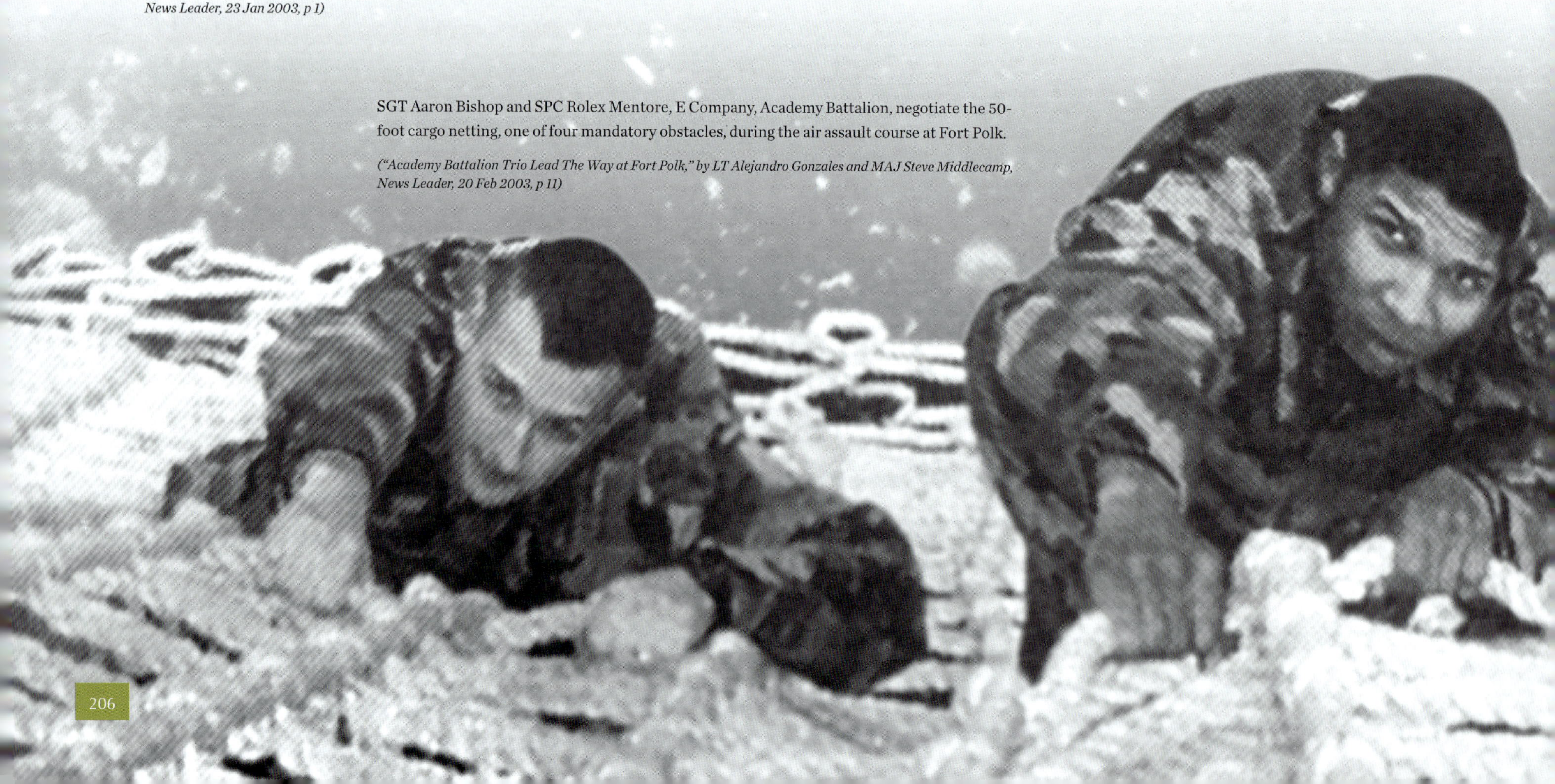

SGT Aaron Bishop and SPC Rolex Mentore, E Company, Academy Battalion, negotiate the 50-foot cargo netting, one of four mandatory obstacles, during the air assault course at Fort Polk.

("Academy Battalion Trio Lead The Way at Fort Polk," by LT Alejandro Gonzales and MAJ Steve Middlecamp, News Leader, 20 Feb 2003, p 11)

DMRTI hosted 12 iterations of its C4 at Camp Bullis in 2003. Most class participants, doctors, nurses, dentists, physician assistants, and forward medical officers from the U.S. Armed Forces Reserves, Active, Reserve, National Guard, and members of allied medical practitioners, received instruction in Advanced Trauma Life Support, Trauma Nurse Core Course, Basic Trauma Life Support, and War Skills Trauma Laboratory, as well as field skills such as litter carries, rappelling, entomology, preventive medicine, battlefield wounds, patient and personal decontamination, treatment of nuclear and chemical casualties, joint levels of care, and casualty evacuation.

("Care-Givers Learn Self Protection To Better Serve Wounded," by Edward Rivera, News Leader, 6 Feb 2003, pp 18-19)

The Stryker Medical Evacuation Vehicle (MEV) was displayed at Tavernier Circle on 20 Feb 2003. One of nine configurations of the Stryker vehicle, the MEV was designed to transport 4 litter or 6 ambulatory patients. Operated by a crew of three, driver, vehicle commander, and medic, it was equipped with standard ground medical ambulance equipment kit, chest, and life support systems. An improved mechanical lift system, similar to the one in the UH-60, allowed the NATO litter system to be loaded into the MEV.

("Stryker MEV, Army's Newest Field Ambulance Will Be On Display at Tavernier Circle Feb. 20," News Leader, 13 Feb 2003, p 17)

Thirty-seven soldiers from Company E of the Academy Battalion received water survival training at the Jimmy Brought Fitness Center Pool. The company planned to incorporate other types of survival training during the year.

("Soldiers from Academy Battalion Receive Water Training," by LT Alejandro Gonzales, News Leader, 27 Feb 2003, p 7)

The first new medical evacuation helicopter, the HH-60L, deployed to Afghanistan in February 2003.

("New MEDEVAC Helicopter Deploys to Afghanistan," News Leader, 23 March 2003, p 3)

A 35-member team at the Institute of Surgical Research (ISR) took on the responsibility of testing and approving a revolutionary chitosan-based bandage designed to halt bleeding, the leading cause of battlefield deaths. After positive initial tests on hand-made versions of the hemostatic bandage, the mass-produced version was tested and failed by the ISR. A rapid turn-around of test work and data collection on the bandage (four weeks completed in approximately 36 hours) by the ISR allowed the manufacturer to produce another set of dressings for testing which passed a second round. As soon as the dressing was approved, 1,000 were sent overseas and an order for an additional 20,000 was placed.

("ISR Team Steps Up Testing For New Bandage Approval," by Edward Rivera, News Leader, 3 April 2003, p 1)

Dieticians and Nutrition Care Specialists attended the Joint Field Nutrition Operations Course at Camp Bullis, 10-18 April. Through intense hands-on training, the dieticians set up and operated an Army Medical Field Feeding System. The course consisted of two phases, combat and humanitarian. The humanitarian phase focused on the feeding of enemy prisoners of war and civilians in military care, while the combat concentrated on feeding the troops and wounded.

("Is It Army of One, or 'A-1,'" by Edward Rivera, News Leader, 24 April 2003, p 17)

The U.S. Army Trauma Training Center was organized and assigned to the AMEDDC&S effective 1 Oct 2003. Its unit mission is to ensure clinical readiness of the Army Forward Surgery Teams by providing hands-on experience with the management of severely injured patients.

(Permanent Orders 052-004, 1 Oct 2003)

2003

Members of the Carmack family presented BG Richard Ursone and MG Darrel Porr an endowment fund donation to continue presentation of the Carmack Medal to the top Medical Service Corps graduate of the AMEDDC&S OBC. One of the first Medical Administrative Corps alumni promoted to the rank of colonel, Joseph Carmack established the Carmack Award in 1958 to honor the top MSC graduate of each OAC.

("Medal Honors Top Army Medical Service Corps Graduate," by SFC Doug Sample, News Leader, 15 May 2003, p 13)

DMRTI began training tri-service nursing personnel in the Trauma Nursing Core Course with advanced human patient simulators. The patient simulators facilitated a shift in the focus of the assessment process from instructor back to the patient.

E Company, Academy Battalion, held its first vehicle rodeo at Camp Bullis. Soldiers competed in a variety of driver skills test as both individuals and platoons.

("E Company, Academy Battalion Holds First Vehicle Rodeo," SPC Georgina Sawyer and SPC Stephanie Ramirez, News Leader, 2 Oct 2003, p 5)

Dell W. Rocco, grandson of Medal of Honor recipient Louis R. Rocco, enlisted in the Army on 29 October 2003 as a 91D, Operating Room Specialist. PVT Rocco said he hoped to carry on the family tradition.

("Private Rocco Hopes To Continue Grandfather's Legacy," by Stephen Noland, News Leader, 13 Nov 2003, p 11)

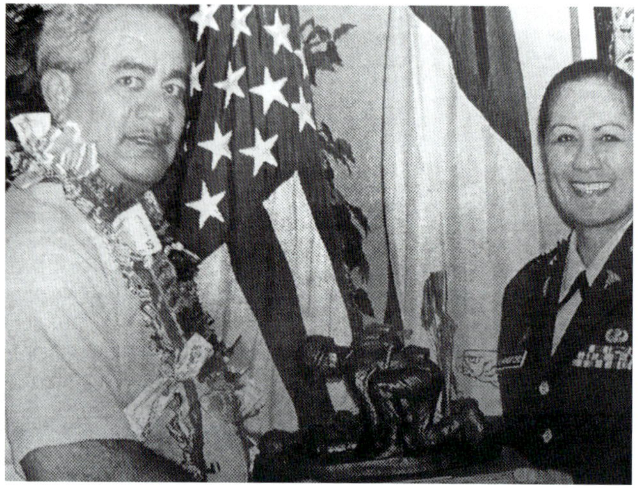

LTC Evelyn Langford

Langford is shown wearing her new rank proudly as the first American Samoan to achieve the rank of lieutenant colonel in the Army. LTC Langford was promoted in December 2003 while a member of the Active Guard and Reserve Program with the Headquarters, Dental Command.

("AMEDD Officer Is First Samoan To Achieve Lieutenant Colonel Rank," by Phil Reidinger, News Leader, 4 Dec 2003, p 4)

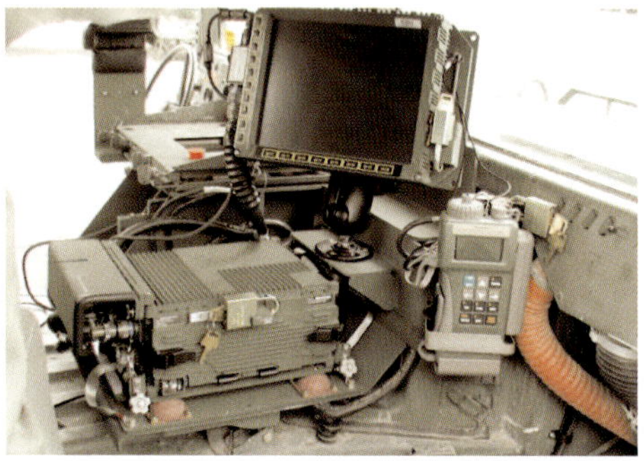

The AMEDDC&S became the first TRADOC school to issue the Force XXI Battle Command and Below (FBCBC) and Blue Force Tracker (BFT) Tactical Boxes. They were installed in the M996 and M997 Front Line Ambulances and the M998. The Tactical Boxes enabled both classroom and field environment training.

("Tactical Boxes Arrive," News Leader, 3 July 2003, p 13)

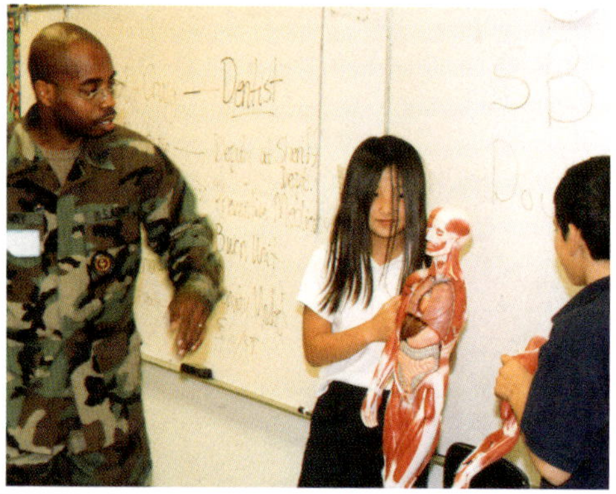

Soldiers inspire and educate young students during the 2003 Career Day

("Soldiers Inspire And Educate," by Esther Garcia, News Leader, 3 April 2003, p 19)

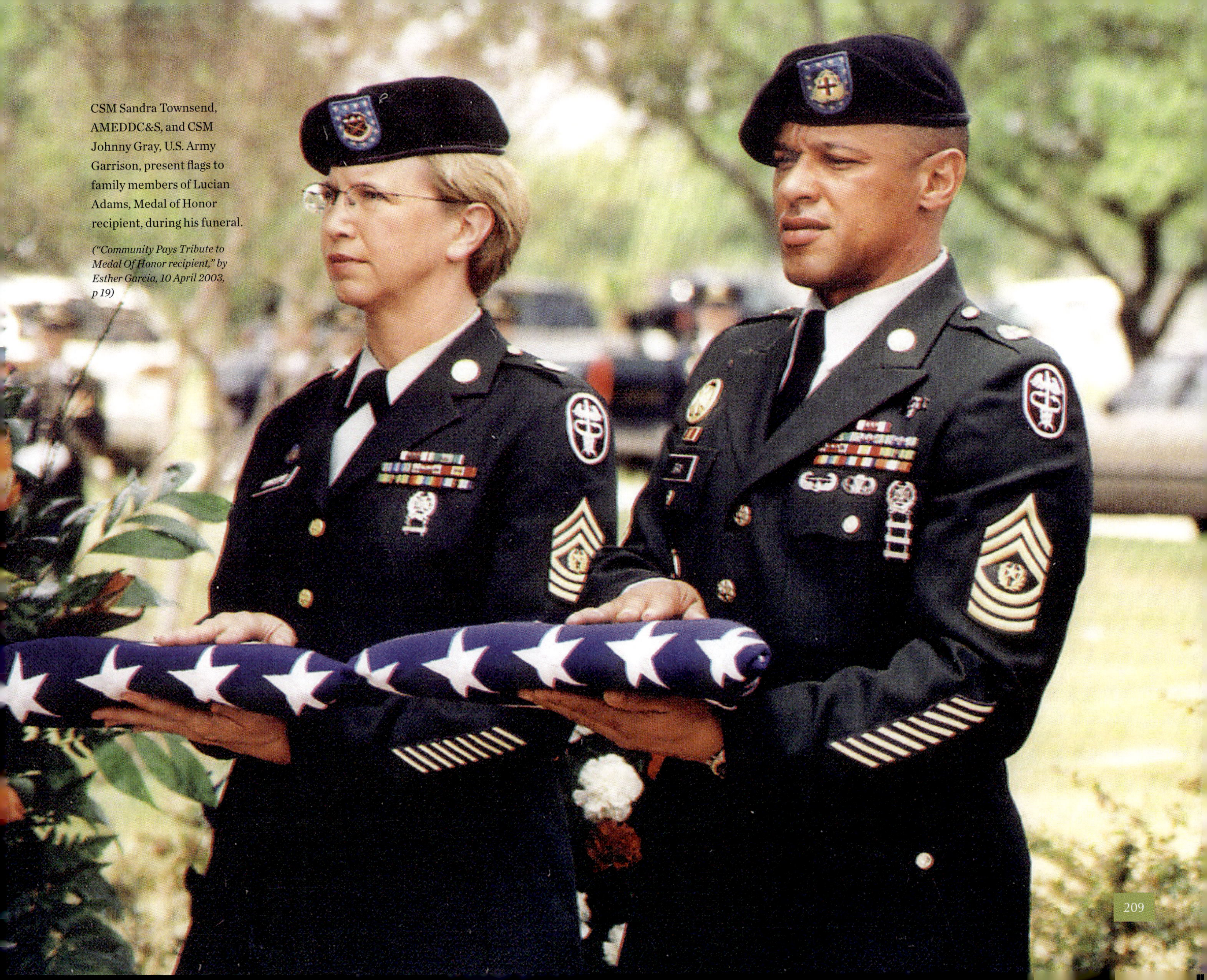

CSM Sandra Townsend, AMEDDC&S, and CSM Johnny Gray, U.S. Army Garrison, present flags to family members of Lucian Adams, Medal of Honor recipient, during his funeral.

("Community Pays Tribute to Medal Of Honor recipient," by Esther Garcia, 10 April 2003, p 19)

2004

Two AMEDDC&S AHS programs received top national rankings in the U.S. News and World Report annual rankings of top graduate school educational programs. The AHS U.S. Army Baylor University Doctoral Program in Physical Therapy ranked fifth in the nation in the 2 April 2004 edition of the magazine. The U.S. Army-Baylor graduate program in Health Services Administration was ranked 20th nationally.

("Center and School Faculty And Programs Receive National Recognition," News Leader, 22 April 2004)

The Army fielded a new combat uniform designed by NCOs and tested by Stryker Brigade Soldiers in Iraq. Three different versions of the ACU were developed, and more than 10,000 uniforms were produced and drug through the sand in Iraq and at Army training centers. Fielding to the total Army was completed in December 2007.

("Army Gets New Combat Uniform," News Leader, 17 June 2004)

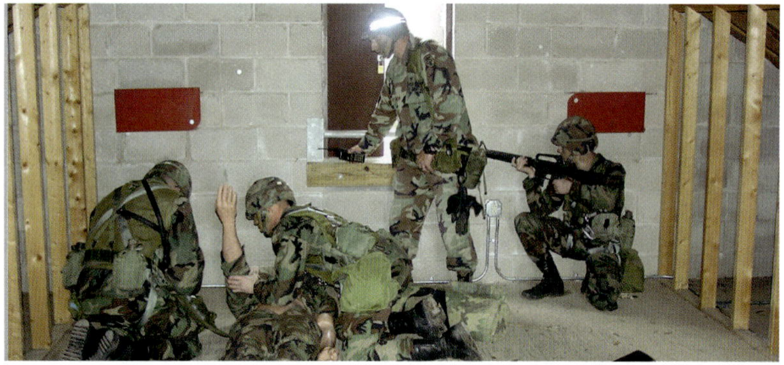

The 232nd Medical Battalion added Military Operations on Urban Terrain (MOUT) training as a new major task to the soldier's culminating FTX. Soldiers were placed in an urban setting where they received a patrol order provide security for their medical teams, and treat, stabilize, and evacuate patients out of buildings under combat conditions.

("232nd Medical Battalion Conducts MOUT Exercise in 91W Training," News Leader, 29 Jan 2004)

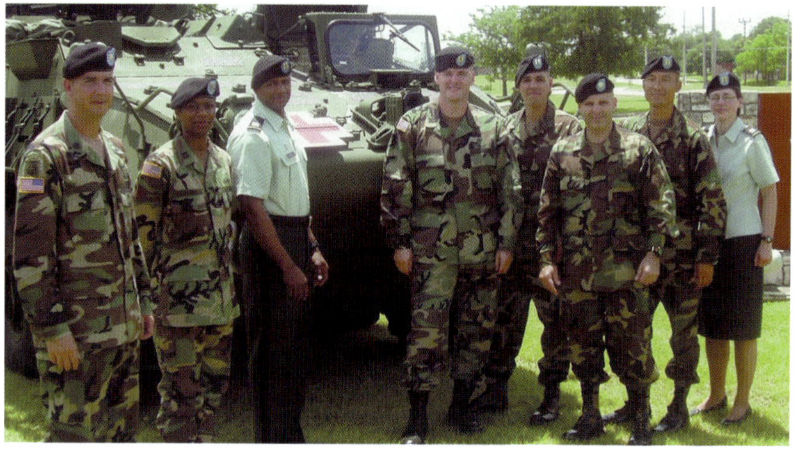

The 232nd Medical Battalion took possession of a Stryker MEV from a General Dynamics representative following the 5th Annual Association of the United States Army Medical Symposium & Exhibition held at the Henry B. Gonzalez Convention Center. The Stryker, the combat vehicle of choice for the Army's Interim Brigade Combat Teams, was a highly deployable-wheeled armored vehicle that combines firepower, battlefield mobility, survivability, and versatility with reduced logistics requirements. The MEV variation was used to instruct students in the 91W Healthcare Specialist Course.

("Stryker Medical Vehicle To Support 91W Training Here," News Leader, 27 May 2004)

Four former Army medics visited the 232nd Medical Battalion and the 91W program training areas in May 2004. The veterans, all assigned to the 8th Medical Detachment, 155th Assault Helicopter Company Kilo Vietnam enjoyed the opportunity to confer with Initial Entry Training Soldiers and the 91W staff instructors. The tour of the simulation training center left them spellbound as they observed soldiers training with human patient simulators that replicated wounds and reacted to treatment. They were astounded by the contents of the current medic aid bag and the skills of the soldiers, both of which are much improved since they trained at Fort Sam Houston more than 35 years ago.

("232nd Medical Battalion Hosts Former Vietnam Era Army Medics," News Leader, 20 May 2004)

AMEDDC&S and Webster University entered a cooperative degree program agreement allowing graduates of the OAC an opportunity to complete a Master of Arts Degree in Health Services Management or a Master of Business Administration through shared academic credits between the AHS and Webster University.

("AMEDDC&S and Webster University Establish Cooperative Agreement," News Leader, 15 April 2004)

Trinity University was the host site for 384 students from around the world completing the OAC the summer of 2004. Nine instructors, in addition to AMEDDC&S functional area subject matter experts, supported the two-week intensive training course. The students completed an aggressive schedule of classes and practical exercises including administration, logistics, combat stress control, preventive medicine, maneuver and tactical operations, medical force planning, medical organization structure, combat health service support, and echelons of care instruction. The students used the military decision making process (MDMP) to apply the most current doctrine including a detailed mission analysis component.

("Reserve Officers Take On The Challenge of Officer Advanced Course Compressed Schedule," News Leader, 15 July 2004)

With post and community leaders present, Fort Sam Houston unveiled its newest state-of-the-art training facility during a dedication ceremony 21 October. Jennings Hall, the new 30,000-square-foot home to the 91T Animal Care Specialist Course, was the culmination of several years of hard work and planning. "The students and instructors used to be in a bunch of temporary buildings that were cramped and improperly designed," said MG George Weightman, AMEDDC&S and Fort Sam Houston commander. The new school is vastly superior to the old one, with larger classrooms, cutting-edge technology and facility-wide equipment upgrades. "It sends the right message to the students," Weightman said. "It will be a model animal care teaching facility."

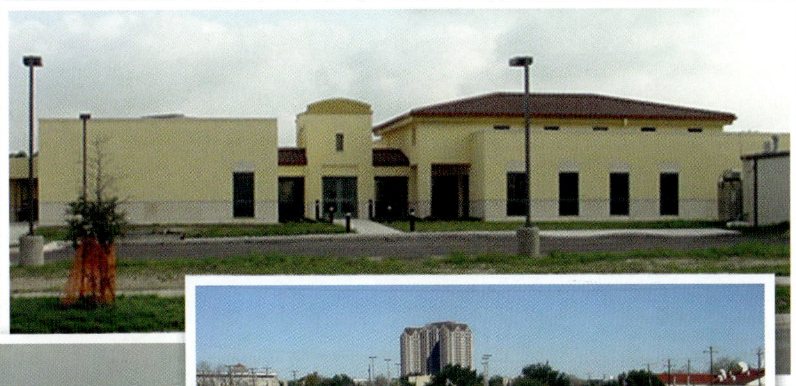

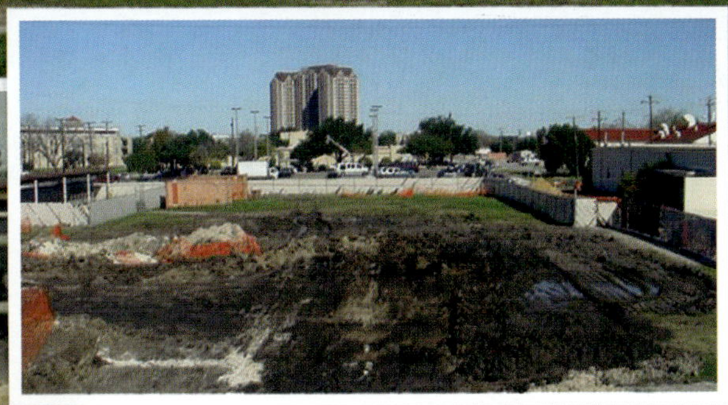

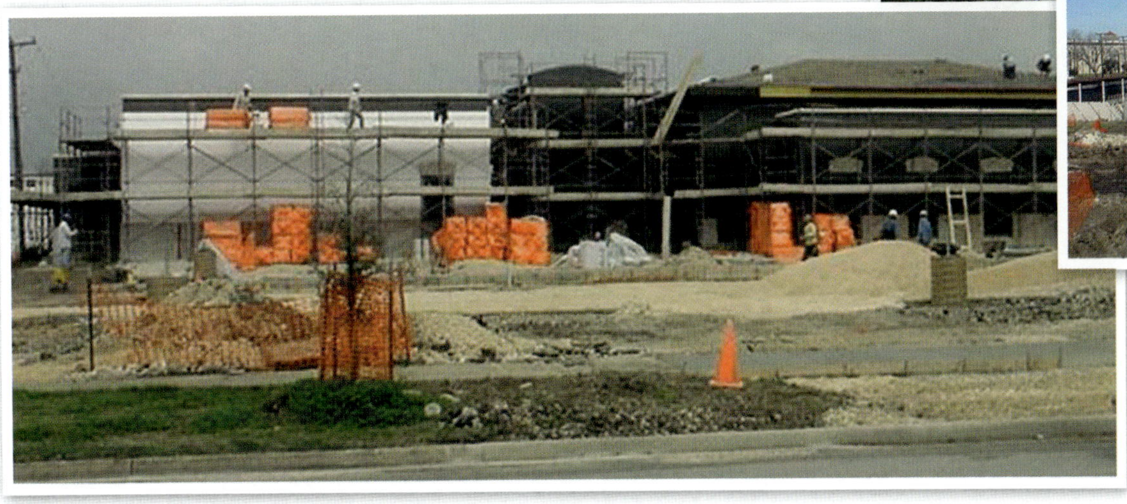

The groundbreaking, building and completion of Jennings Hall. Building dedication occurred on 21 Oct 2004.

(Courtesy Photo)

2005

A joint venture between BAMC, AMEDDC&S and a local Veterans Affairs hospital changed the face of Army operating room technician training. The Audie L. Murphy Memorial VA Hospital in San Antonio was the newest addition to the AMEDDC&S team and the first civilian hospital to join the 91D (operating room technician) roster. "This partnership marks a paradigm shift for us," said LTC Joseph Paulino, 91D Branch chief. The hospital, which offered care to veterans nationwide, was one of 23 training sites that provided Phase 2 training for OR technicians.

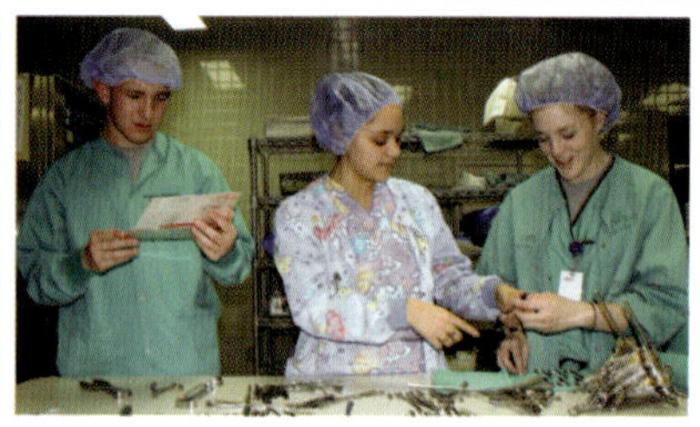

("Joint Venture - Military, Civilian Partnership Improves Training For OR Techs," News Leader, 17 Feb 2005)

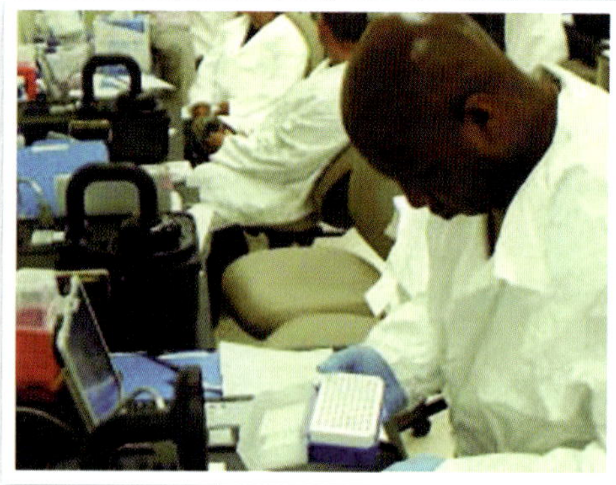

The AMEDDC&S's newest multi-service course teaches students the inner workings of a cutting-edge biological warfare identification device

The first formal Joint Biological Agent Identification and Diagnostic System (JBAIDS) Course, taught at Brooks City-Base, started mid-July with 24 military and civilian students from military installations throughout the world. JBAIDS was the latest weapon in the race to identify biological warfare agents quickly and accurately. It used to take the military two to four days in a microbiology laboratory far from the detection site to identify a biological warfare agent. JBAIDS was capable of doing it near the site in about an hour.

("AMEDD Launches Class For Bio Warfare Identification," News Leader, 28 July 2005)

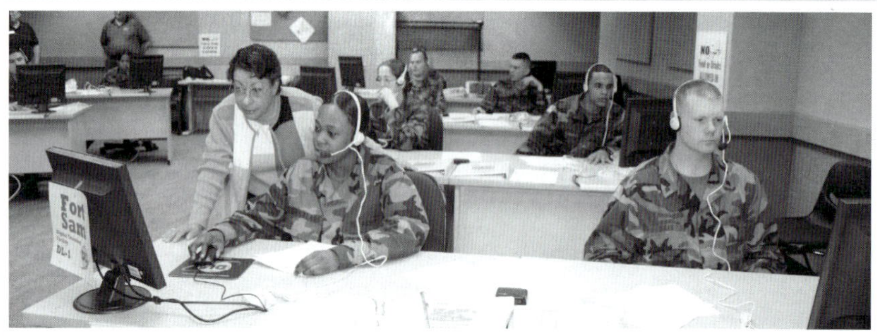

Soldiers and Department of the Army civilians at Ft. Sam Houston and the AMEDDC&S interested in taking courses to fulfill their training requirements or enhance their careers do so through the Army's Distributed Learning System (DLS). The DLS was a fully-funded Army initiative to assist soldiers and civilians to receive quality training in state-of-the-art facilities and to improve efficiency and flexibility. "It's a method of delivering training which helps avoid TDY costs and time out of the office," said David Glass, Installation Labor Relations officer at Fort Sam Houston Civilian Personnel Advisory Center.

("Distributed Learning Revolutionizes Army Training," News Leader, 24 Feb 2005)

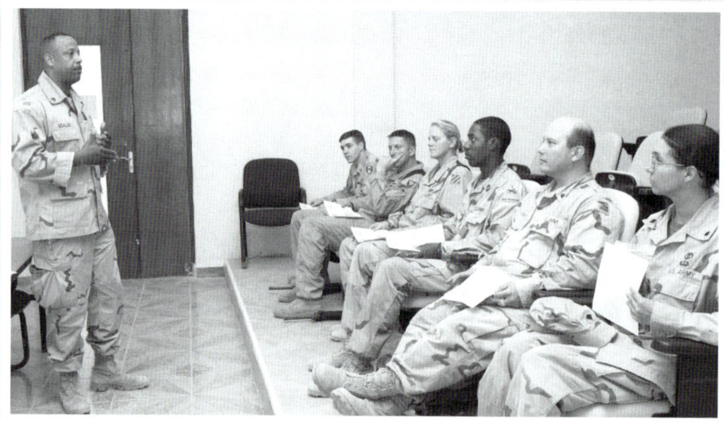

The CMTC 44th Medical Command at LSA Anaconda was the only medical training center of its kind in theater. Set up as a long distance learning site, medics and practical nurses could complete the 91W MOS transition while they were deployed through the center.

("Soldiers Conquer 91W Transition Training In Iraq," News Leader, 9 June 2005)

The Academy Battalion deactivated 23 August, then immediately reactivated as the 264th Medical Battalion, continuing a lineage started in 1943.

("Academy Bn. Assumes Proud Lineage as 264th Medical Battalion," News Leader, Aug 2005)

A trauma course based on real-world combat scenarios filled a gap in training for hundreds of medical officers preparing for deployments in support of Operations Iraqi Freedom and Enduring Freedom. The Tactical Combat Medical Care (TCMC) course, part of the Department of Medical Science at Fort Sam Houston, taught students the "tricks of the trade" for trauma medicine on the battlefield. "We've had an overwhelming response to the course," said CPT Jim Rice, a physician assistant and TCMC program manager. "People who have taken the course and deployed have been very grateful for the training."

("Trauma Course Preps Medical Officers For Battlefield," News Leader, 6 Oct 2005)

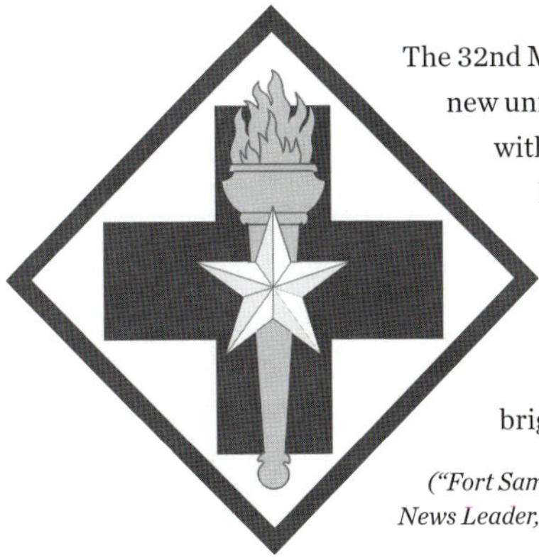

The 32nd Medical Brigade soldiers started displaying a new unit symbol on their uniforms in conjunction with a ceremony where the brigade's Academy Battalion was deactivated in line with the Army Chief of Staff's transformation and was reactivated as the 264th Medical Battalion. The new shoulder sleeve insignia replaced the Medical Command insignia worn by the brigade's soldiers for more than 13 years.

("Fort Sam Houston Unit Receives New Shoulder Sleeve Insignia," News Leader, Aug 2005)

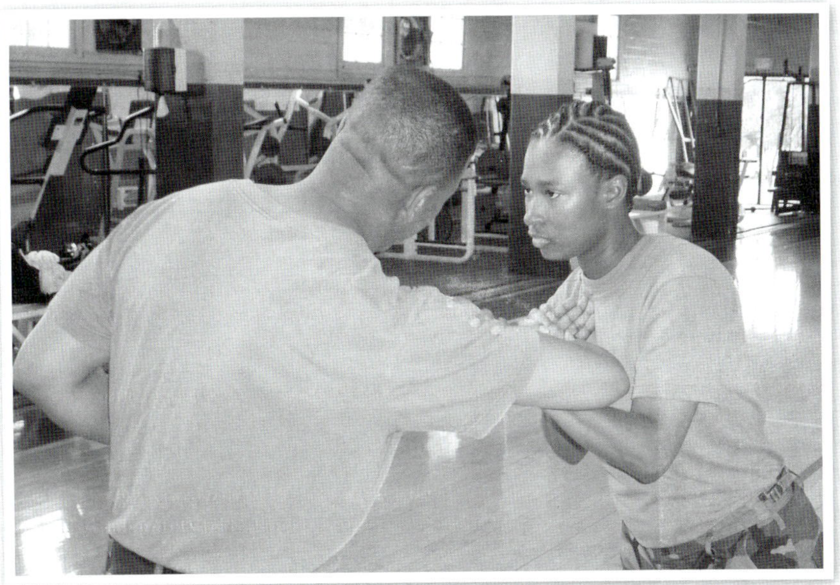

Drill sergeants and instructors from the 232nd Medical Battalion and Department of Combat Medic training began teaching the Combatives Program the beginning of 2007.

("232nd Med. Bn., DCMT Use Hand-To-Hand Combat In Training," News Leader, 11 Aug 2005)

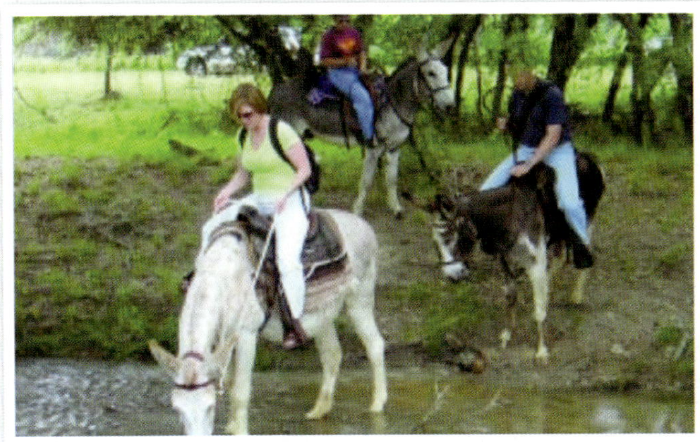

The horse cavalry made its return to Fort Sam Houston in Summer 2005, but in a different form. MAJ Howard Gobble, an instructor from the AMEDDC&S Leader Training Center, used donkeys for staff rides to impart leadership and decision-making skills to his captain's career course students. A staff ride is comprised of a classroom study of a designated battle followed by a visit to the actual site of the encounter. On site, student officers walk the ground, analyze the terrain as the combatants may have seen it, and derive lessons from the success or failure of the opposing commanders' decisions and actions.

("AMEDDC&S Student Officers Learn 'History On The Hoof,'" News Leader, 22 Sept 2005)

2006

The 70K Health Services Materiel Officer Course was an intense, 10-week training in medical logistics for junior AMEDDC&S officers, warrant officers, international officers and Department of the Army civilians. Training included hands-on exercises, warehouse and distribution tours, and a comprehensive logistics research project.

The 32nd Medical Brigade was reorganized into the following configuration:

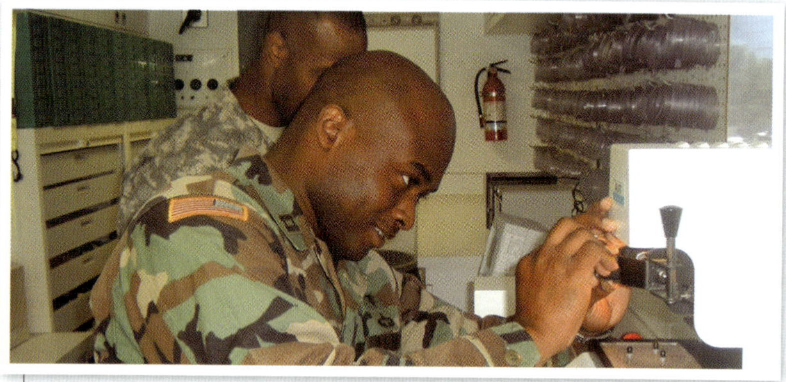

CPT Tellis Carr, from the 70K Health Services Materiel Officer Course, prepares prescription glasses during an optical exercise.

(U.S. Army Photo, "Behind the Scene, Medical Logistics Course Prepares Students For Theater," News Leader, 5 Jan 2006, p 15)

The 32nd Medical Brigade

Headquarters and Headquarters Company • Medical Command Band • E Company • D Company • NCO Academy

187th Medical Battalion

A Company
Leadership Training Center • Department of Pastoral Ministry Training

B Company
Department of Medical Science

D Company
Department of Dental Science • Department of Veterinary Science

E Company
Department of Preventive Health Services

232nd Medical Battalion

A Company
68W

B Company
68W

C Company
68W

D Company
68W

E Company
68W

F Company
68W

G Company
68W

264th Medical Battalion

A Company
Department of Health • Services Administration

B Company
Department of Clinical Support Services

C Company
Department of Nursing Science

D Company
DHSA • Department of Dental Science

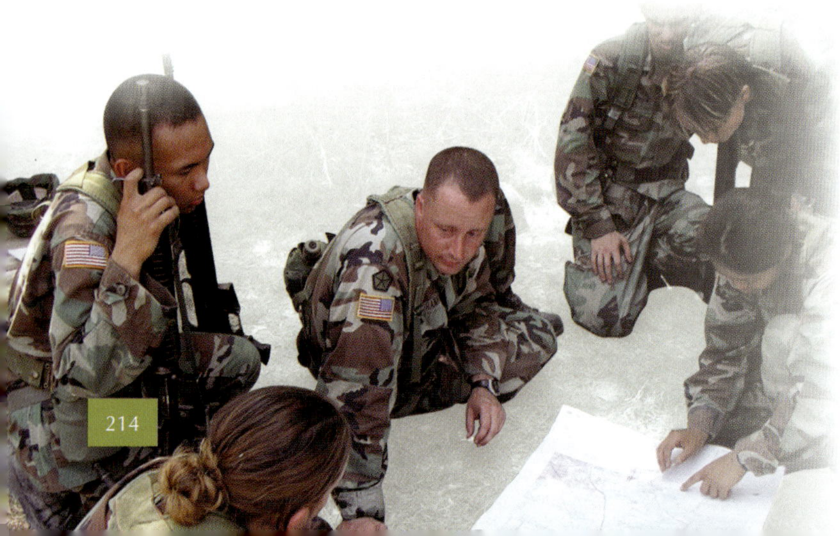

Students from the 91J Medical Logistics Specialist Course received navigation training during a field training exercise at Camp Bullis. The five-week 91J course provided enlisted soldiers formal training in medical materiel procedures and included several hands-on practical exercises.

(U.S. Army Photo, "Behind the Scene, Medical Logistics Course Prepares Students For Theater," News Leader, 5 Jan 2006, p 15)

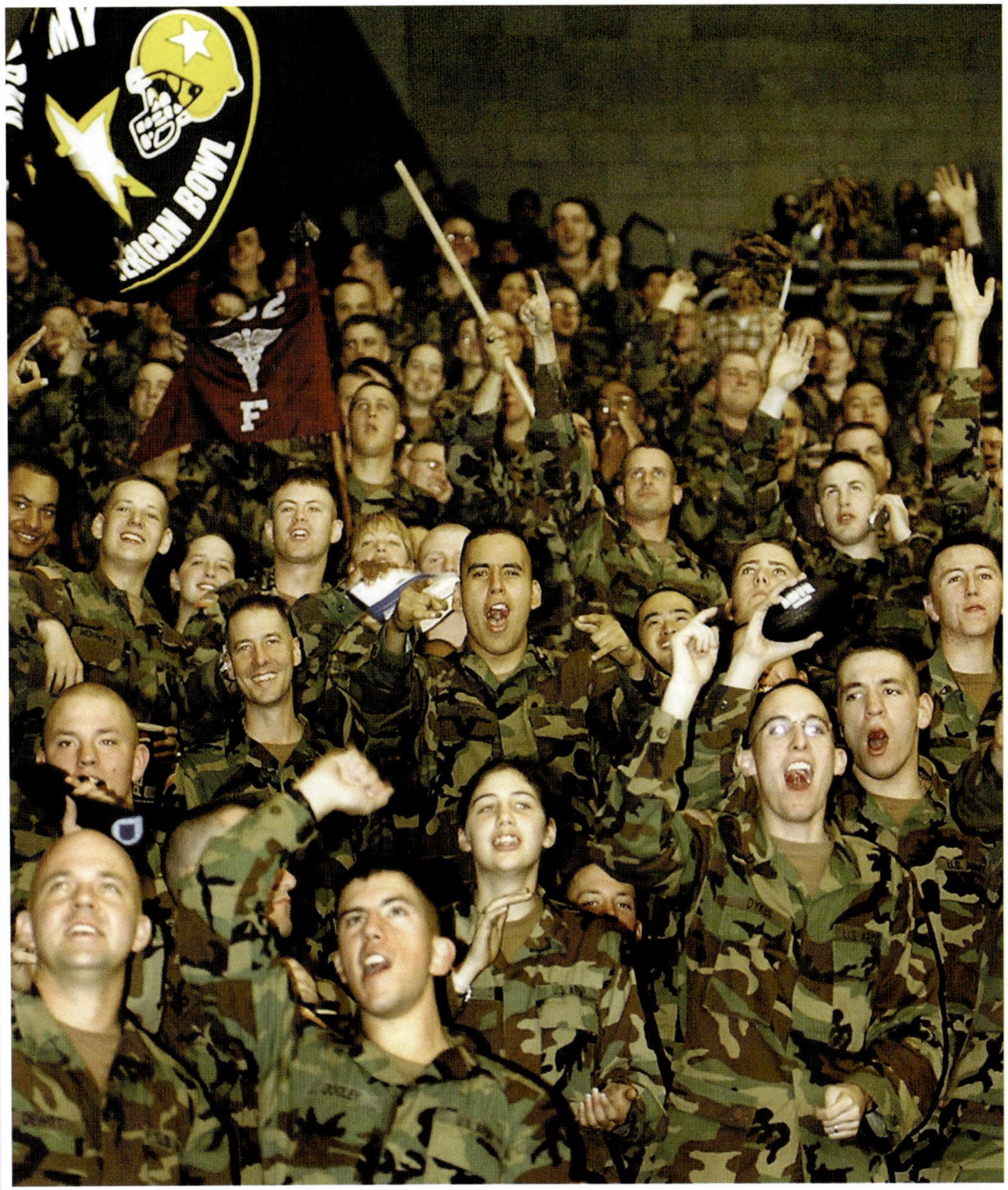

Student soldiers from the 232nd Medical Battalion enjoy the U.S. Army All-American All Star High School Bowl at the Alamodome in January 2006.

(Photo by Daren Reehl, "Showdown at the Alamodome," News Leader, 12 Jan 2006, p 1)

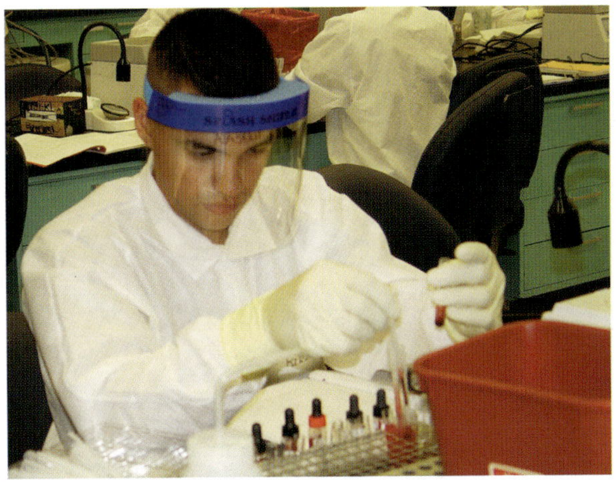

SPC Nikolay Kirilov, a student at the Blood Bank and Hematology Branch, tests donor blood. The blood bank and hematology course was part of the 52-week medical laboratory technician training.

("Seeing Red," News Leader, 26 Jan 2006, p 1)

2006

AMEDDC&S announced the inauguration of the Post's first high-speed wireless classroom. Three classrooms being used by the Army-Baylor University Graduate Program in Health and Business Administration and the Captains Career Course were wired for complete and full wireless capabilities.

("Army-Baylor Program Goes Wireless," by Cheryl Harrison, News Leader, 30 March 2006)

The first graduates of the Army-Baylor University Doctoral Program in Physical Therapy graduated April 2006.

("PT Program Confers First Doctoral Degree," by Yolanda Hagberg, News Leader, 13 April 2006)

The Combat Application Tourniquet (CAT), tested and recommended as essential equipment for every deployed soldier, was named one of the Army's 10 greatest inventions.

("New Tourniquet Named One of The Army's 10 Greatest Inventions," by Karen Fleming Michael, News Leader, 6 July 2006, p 11)

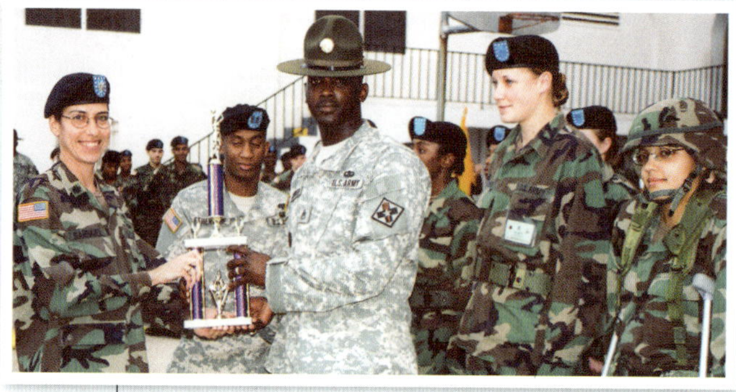

Drill SGT Sheldon Groover, E Company, 187th Medical Battalion, accepts the battalion women's basketball trophy from 187th Med. Bn. Commander LTC Patricia Darnauer. Groover coached the women's team.

("Basket Ball Champs," News Leader, 26 Jan 2006, p 10)

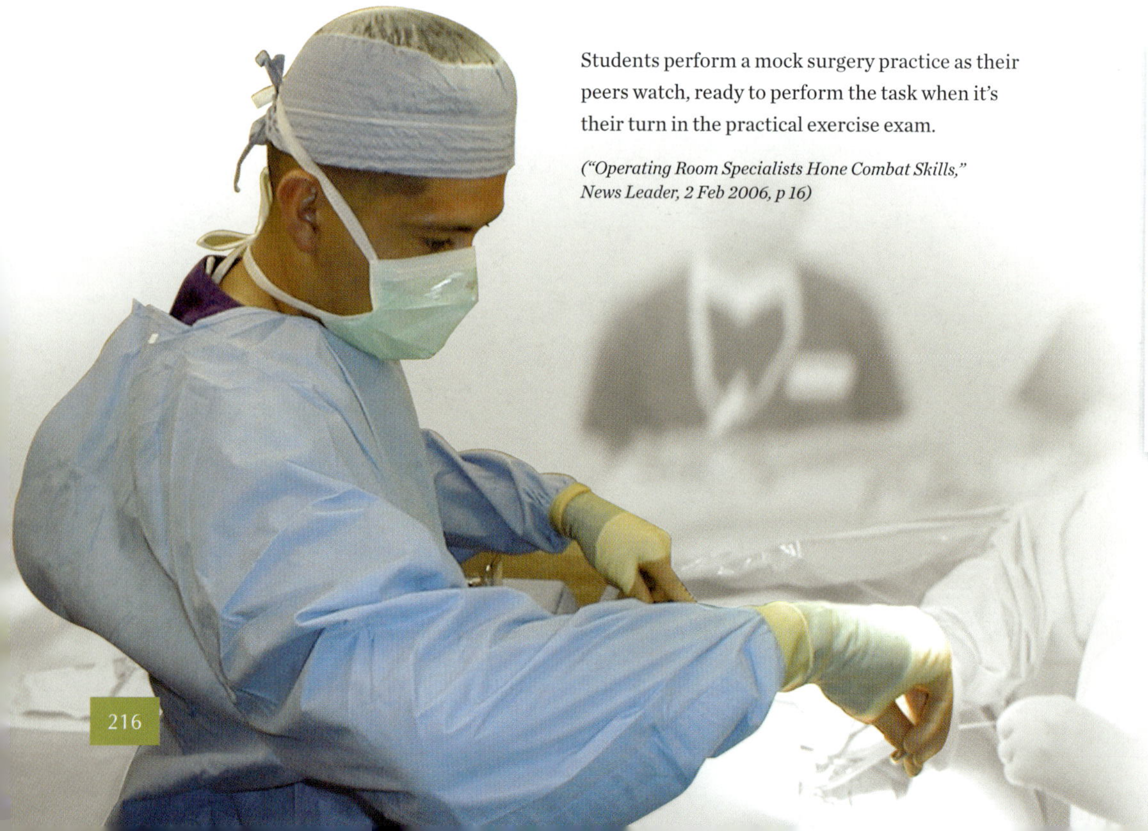

Students perform a mock surgery practice as their peers watch, ready to perform the task when it's their turn in the practical exercise exam.

("Operating Room Specialists Hone Combat Skills," News Leader, 2 Feb 2006, p 16)

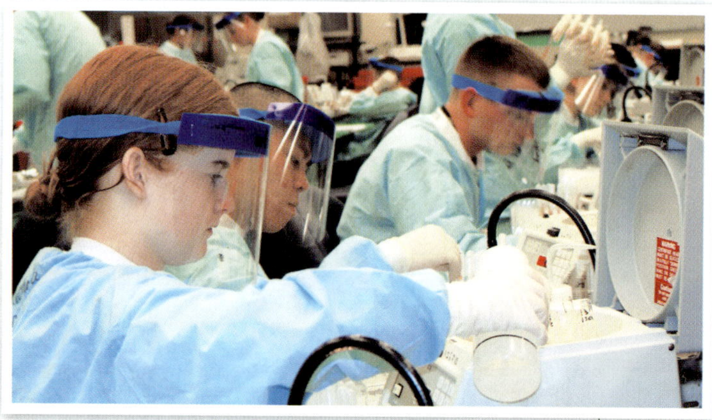

SPC Danielle Scagnelli washes cells to remove impurities and any interfering substances as part of blood donor processing during the blood bank portion of the blood bank and hematology course. Pre-transfusion testing is done prior to issue of a blood product, such as platelets.

("Analyze This," News Leader, 26 Jan 2006, p 18)

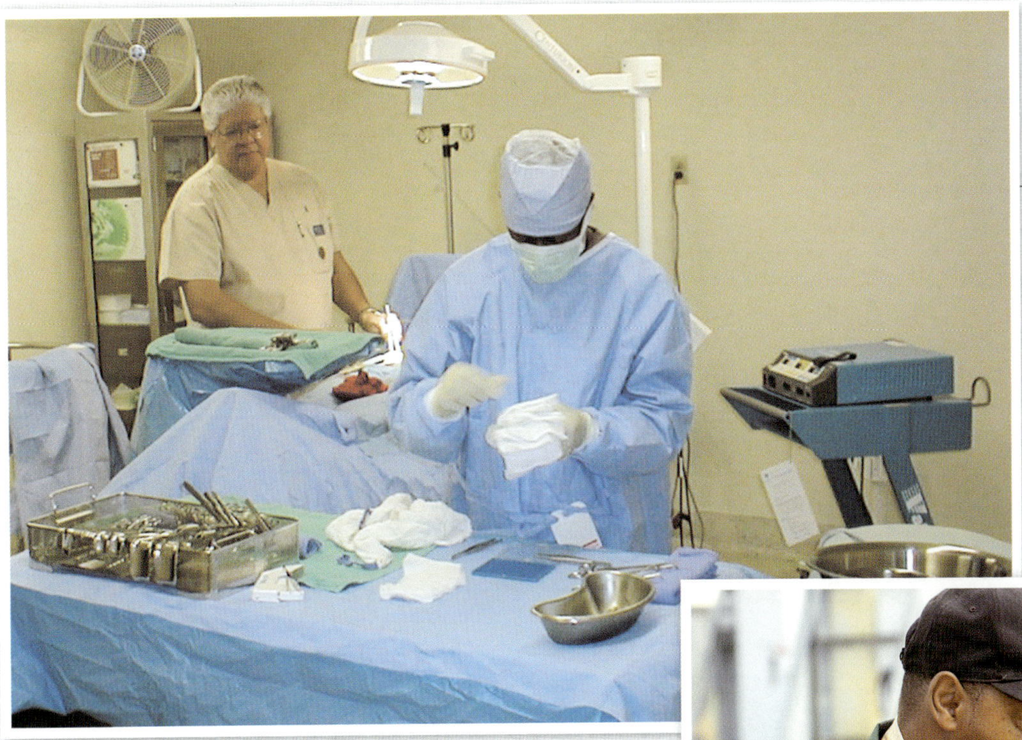

Students experience the sponge and sharps counting practical exercise in the classroom and use it prior to the mock surgery practical exercise exam. Instructor John Martinez keeps a watchful eye on a student as he counts sponges.

("Operating Room Specialists Hone Combat Skills," News Leader, 2 Feb 2006, p 16)

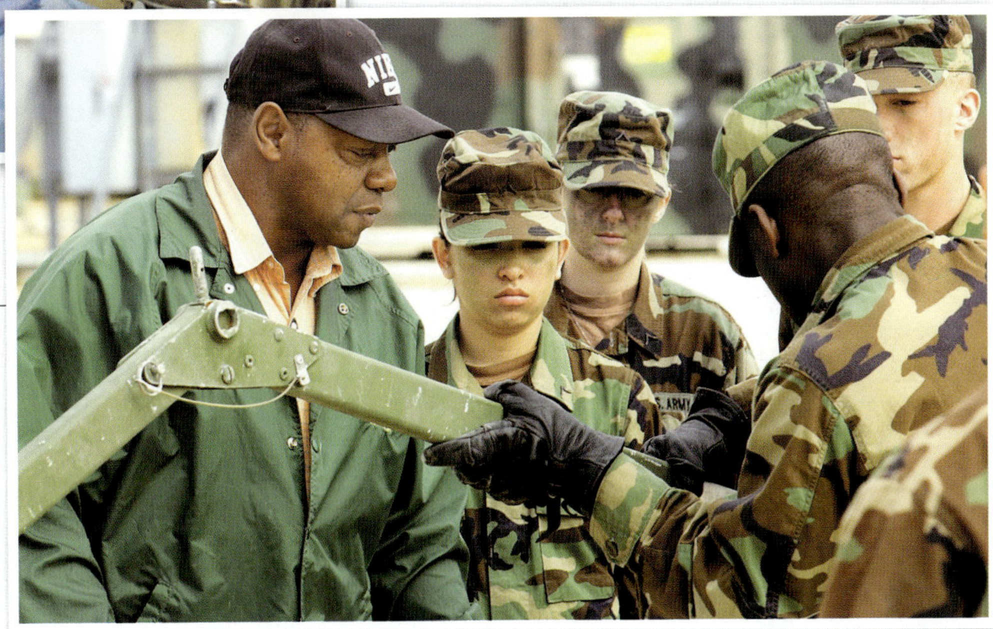

Soldiers of the 91D Operating Room Specialist Course, held at Camp Bullis, gather around instructor Donald Williams as he explains the way the tent poles are connected to construct a frame for a field hospital tent. From left: PVT Yessica Palma-Villanuena, PVT Chamaine Schlagel and PVT Dustin Crawford watch as PVT Joseph Amissah works on the tent frame.

(Photo by Daren Reehl, "Tent Building 101," News Leader, 2 Feb 2006, p 1)

2006

The Defense Medical Readiness Training Institute (DMRTI) hosted a new decontamination course at Fort Sam Houston. The Mass Casualty Decontamination Course trained participants on both civilian and military approaches to casualty decontamination. The focus was on field and hospital decontamination and the incorporation of site set-up and triage.

("Decontamination Course Prepares Soldiers For Today's Reality," by Cheryl Harrison, News Leader, 2 March 2006, p 17)

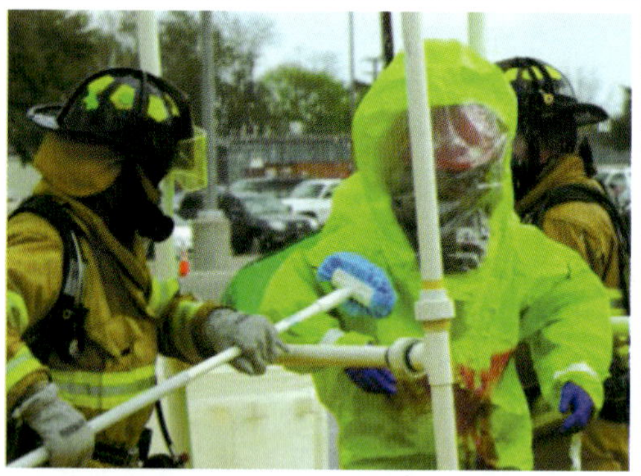

Emergency personnel scrub one of their own with warm water to prevent possible contaminants from spreading.

(U.S. Army Photo)

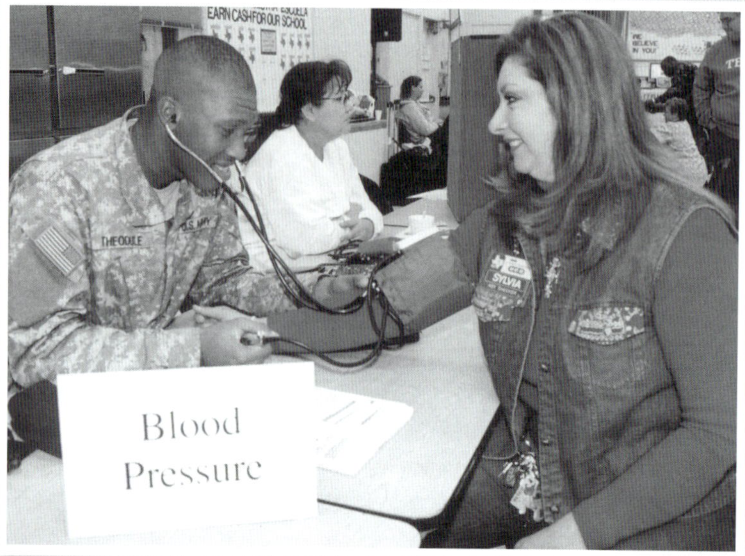

George Theodule, of G Company, 232nd Medical Battalion, checks blood pressure 11 February 2006 during a Health Fair for seniors in the community hosted by William Knox Elementary in San Antonio. The fair included booths that provided literature about nutrition programs, diabetes, drug plans, home health care, and assistance for those without transportation and for those who are homebound. "I am having a good time talking to members of the local community," said Theodule. "I think it's great that we are able to use the skills we have trained for."

("Soldiers Support Community," by Esther Garcia, 23 Feb 2006, p 3)

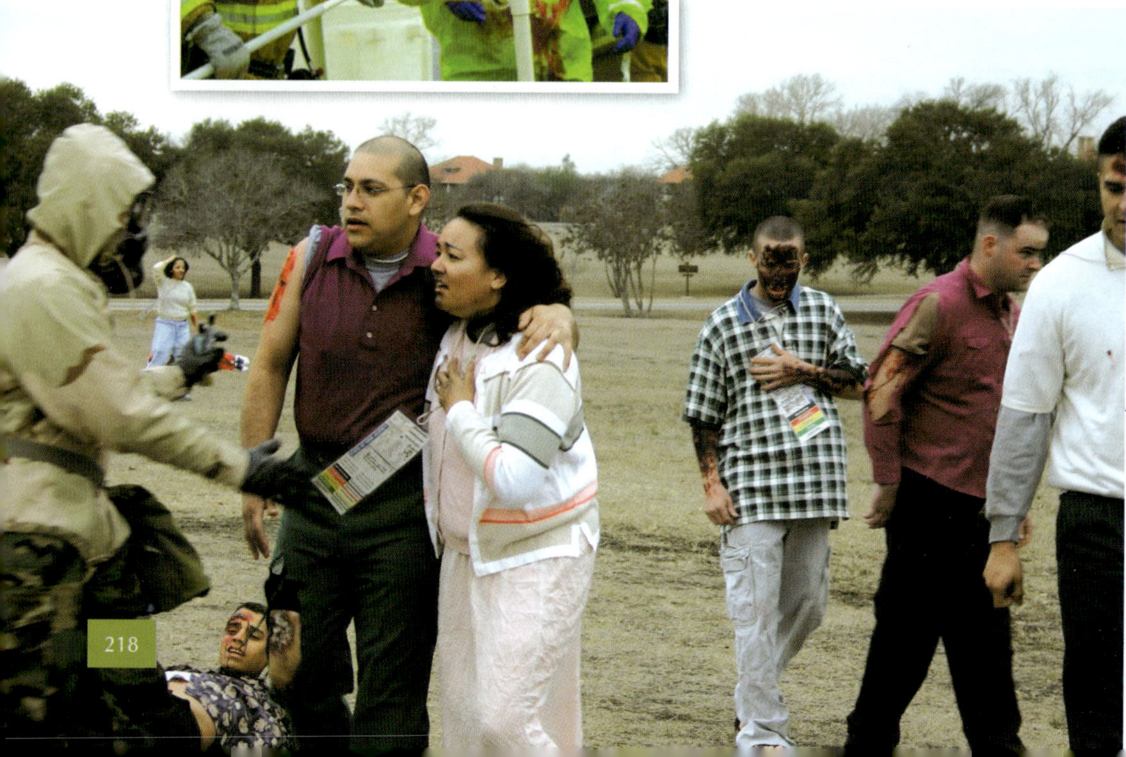

During the exercise, soldiers play one of two roles, either victim or responder. In this scenario, a soldier in chemical gear rushes to the aid of ambulatory victims, attempting to calm them and direct them to the decontamination tent. SGT Christopher Artiles, on the ground, waits for a gurney.

(U.S. Army Photo)

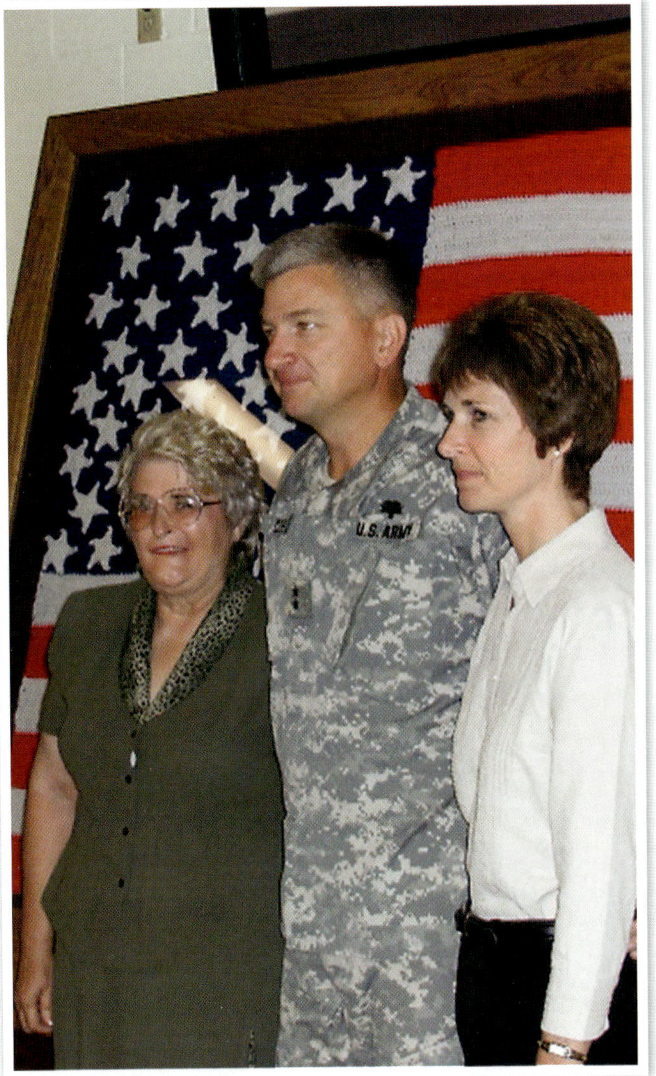

MG Russ Czerw, commander AMEDDC&S, stands between Ms. Ruthie E. Bartling (left) and his wife (right) in the corridor of Willis Hall after the unveiling of a crocheted American flag donated to the AMEDDC&S by Ms. Bartling.

(Photo courtesy of Ruthie E. Bartling, 14 September 2006)

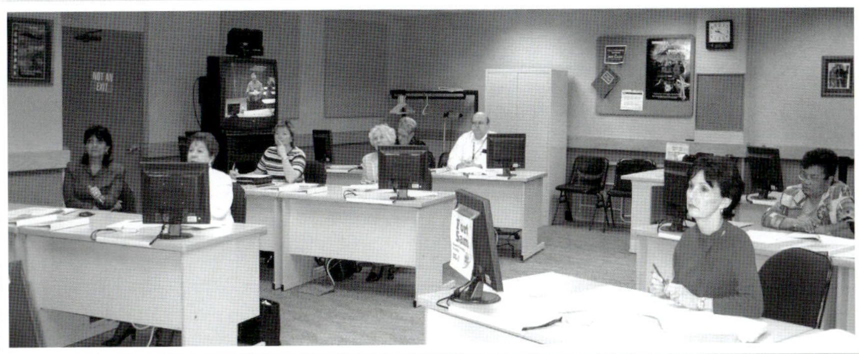

One of the new high-speed wireless classrooms introduced by the AMEDDC&S to the Army-Baylor University Program in Health and Business Administration in 2006.

(U.S. Army Photo)

The Rocco dining facility served an average of 3,200 meals a day in 2006.

("Dining facility offers up some 'food for thought'," by Minnie Jones, News Leader, 6 April 2006)

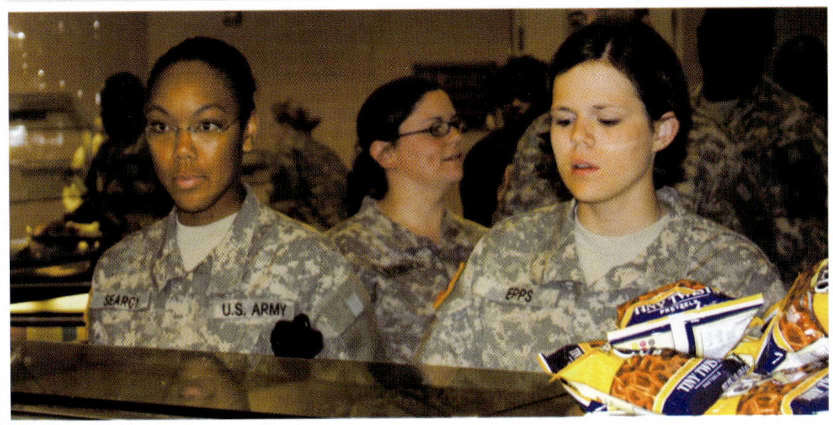

Soldiers from A Company, 264th Medical Battalion find a way to choose between delicious lunch options at the Rocco dining facility.

(U.S. Army Photo)

2007

To observe National Dental Health Month, interns from the AMEDDC&S's Preventive Dentistry Course visited Fort Sam Houston Elementary students. Not only did the students learn about their teeth, but they also had fun in the process. During the visit the students learned correct techniques to properly care for teeth and gums. Puppet productions, skits, plays, "dental rap" music, and demonstrations were used to teach children about good dental hygiene. All were high energy and humorous activities which kept even the kindergartners engaged and attentive.

("AMEDD Players Entertain, Teach," News Leader, 15 March 2007)

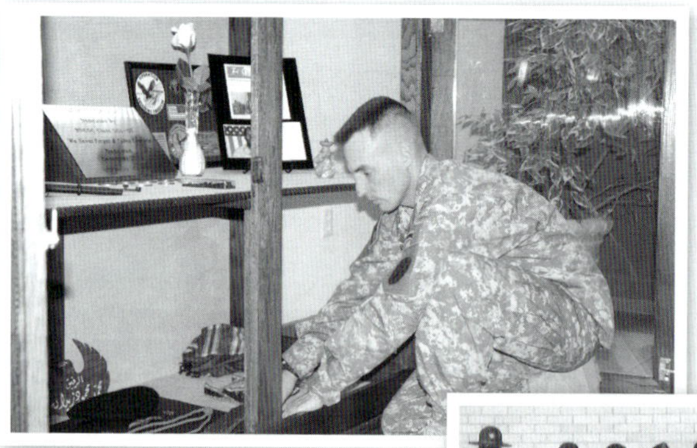

Two senior NCOs build a memorial in the NCOA lobby to honor fallen enlisted members of the AMEDDC&S.

("AMEDD Memorial Honors Fallen Heroes," News Leader, 15 Feb 2007)

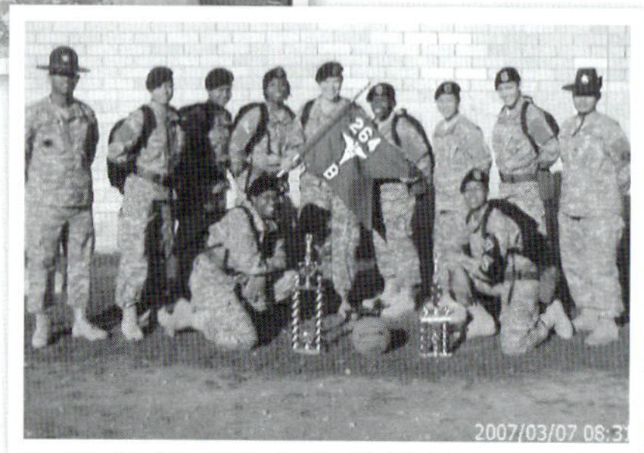

The Bravo 264th Medical Battalion women's basketball team defeated Delta 232nd and Bravo 187th women's teams to become 32nd Medical Brigade champions in March 2007.

("Lady Warriors Become Brigade Champions," News Leader, 15 March 2007)

The Captains' Career Common Core Course (C5) became a requirement for graduation from all branch Captain's Career Courses 1 June 2007. The C5 provides instruction in leadership, communication, composite risk management, critical reasoning and thinking skills, and developing a positive command climate. The skills better prepare officers for their next 10 years of service, and the program keeps the AMEDDC&S in step with the Army chief of staff's vision of continued transformation of the Army Officer Education System.

("Common Core Course To Be Requirement for Captain's Career Courses," News Leader, 29 March 2007)

U.S. Army Graduate Program in Anesthesia Nursing was ranked second in the nation by the U.S. News and World Report magazine in the 2007 edition of "America's Best Graduate Schools." The program missed top spot in the Nursing-Anesthesia category by only a tenth of a point with a score of 4.0 out of 5.0.

("Army Anesthesia Program Ranked Second in Nation," News Leader, 12 April 2007)

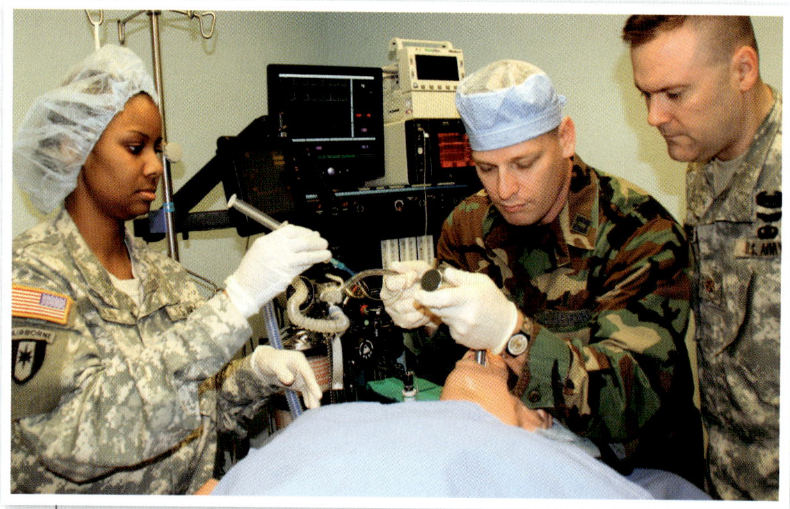

Nurse anesthesia students practicing on a simulated patient.

(U.S. Army Photo)

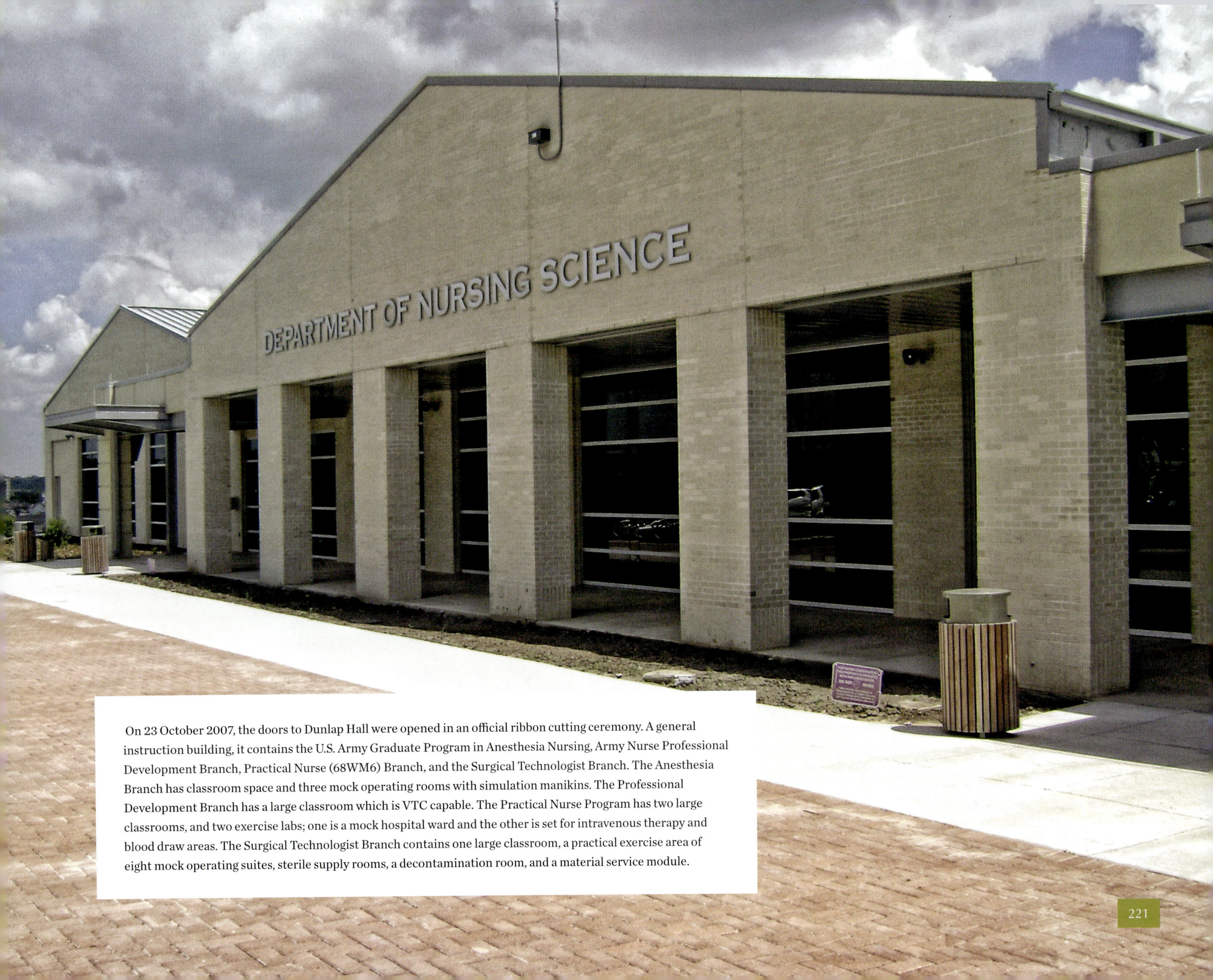

On 23 October 2007, the doors to Dunlap Hall were opened in an official ribbon cutting ceremony. A general instruction building, it contains the U.S. Army Graduate Program in Anesthesia Nursing, Army Nurse Professional Development Branch, Practical Nurse (68WM6) Branch, and the Surgical Technologist Branch. The Anesthesia Branch has classroom space and three mock operating rooms with simulation manikins. The Professional Development Branch has a large classroom which is VTC capable. The Practical Nurse Program has two large classrooms, and two exercise labs; one is a mock hospital ward and the other is set for intravenous therapy and blood draw areas. The Surgical Technologist Branch contains one large classroom, a practical exercise area of eight mock operating suites, sterile supply rooms, a decontamination room, and a material service module.

2007

AMEDDC&S took its first step in transforming the world-renowned facility for future excellence. The school's nine graduate programs, once scattered throughout four departments under the AHS, were aligned into one center, called the Center for Graduate Military Healthcare Education. "We are truly excited about this historic event," said COL Josef Moore, interim associate dean, at the center's opening ceremony in Blesse Auditorium.

("Eye On The Future: AMEDD Merges Graduate Programs," News Leader, 28 June 2007)

Fort Sam Houston's top leaders gathered at the AMEDDC&S to learn about the signature wounds of the war on terror – mild traumatic brain injury (mTBI) and posttraumatic stress disorder (PTSD). "TBI and PTSD are invisible wounds so they are not as easy to recognize as physical wounds," said COL Joseph Pecko, one of the program's authors and Chief, Soldier and Family Support Branch, Department of Preventive Health Services, AMEDDC&S. "This program is designed to heighten awareness among soldiers, battle buddies, leaders and families so our soldiers can receive the help they need and deserve. This program is by the soldier, for the soldier."

("Fort Sam Launches Army's PTSD, mTBI Training," News Leader, 2 Aug 2007)

Effective in October 2007, soldiers entering Basic Combat Training started receiving Combat Lifesaving Training (CLS) and became CLS certified before graduation. The change adds 7.5 hours to the current curriculum. Soldiers learned how to perform advanced first aid and conduct potentially lifesaving procedures—from controlling bleeding, conducting CPR, and reintroducing fluids into the body to keep a serious injury from worsening until professional medical help arrives.

("New Soldiers to Become Combat-Lifesaver Certified," News Leader, 11 Oct 2007)

"In a pig's eye" is a nonsensical phrase used to describe something that is highly unlikely. It is highly unlikely that a handful of Army Medical Department Center and School students would often be required to dissect pig eyes, but the task is a useful hands-on method of training. The 300-P3 Eye Specialty course trained and prepared soldiers in vision and ocular health. This enabled the future eye specialists to work in optometry, ophthalmology, and refractive surgery clinics and to deploy with optometry teams and ophthalmologists to provide ophthalmic care in theater. The course consisted of classes in anatomy and physiology, ocular pathology and disease, surgical assistance during ocular surgery, optics, spectacles, and contact lens prescriptions and fittings, optometry field set, and lessons learned from Operations Iraqi Freedom and Enduring Freedom.

("Students Go Eye To Eye in AMEDD Course," News Leader, 17 May 2007)

(U.S. Army Photo)

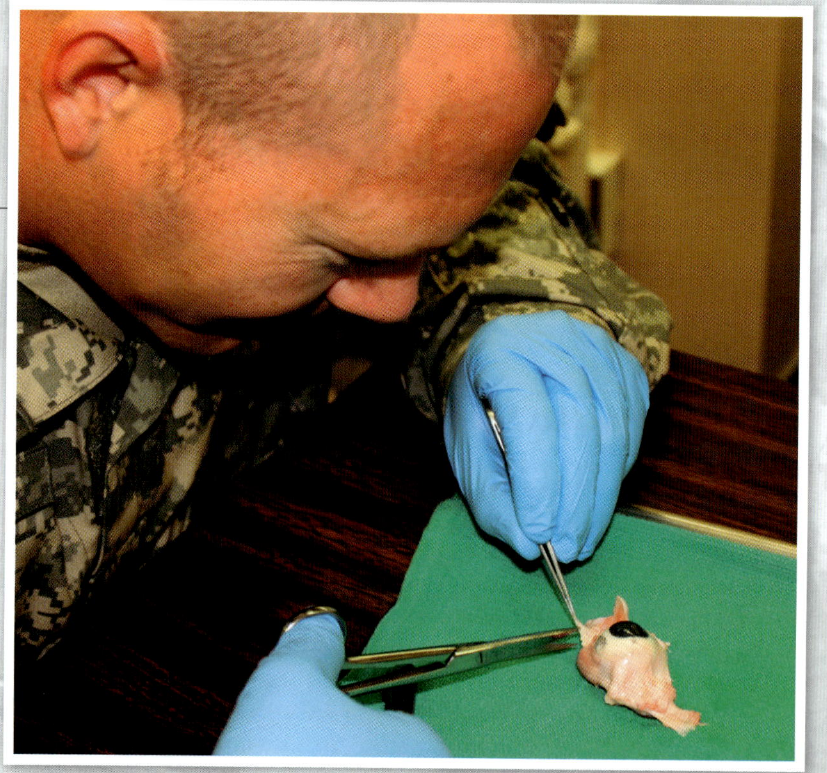

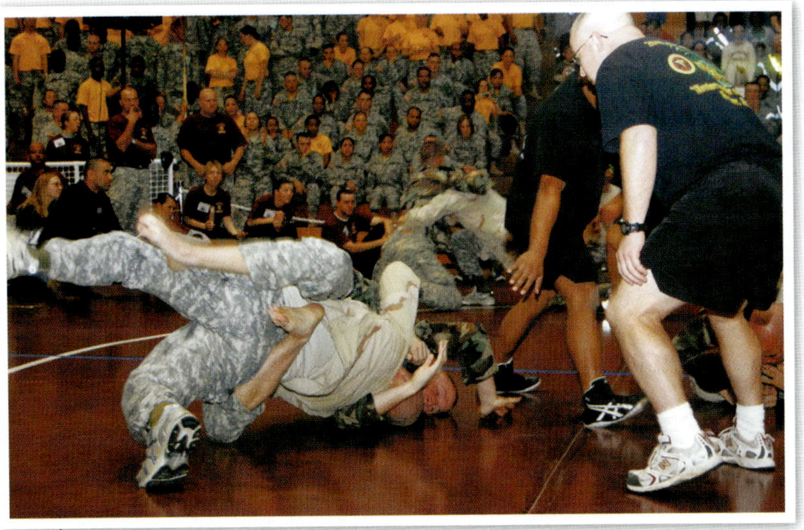

Students and cadre cheer on competitors during the November 2007 combative tournament.

(U.S. Army Photo)

Soldiers from the 32nd Medical Brigade spent the weekend competing in a combative tournament at Fort Sam Houston. "As you know, many of the soldiers you see here today will be joining combat units and deploy within weeks of finishing their training. In tandem with the medical skills they learn here, it is equally important that we provide them with the training, skills and experience that will help them personally survive the battlefields of today and tomorrow," said COL John Cook, 32nd Medical Brigade commander.

("Soldiers Compete For Best Combative Fighter," News Leader, 21 Nov 2007)

AMEDDC&S developed 18 distance-learning modules for Warrior Transition Unit (WTU) cadre to complete in areas like the medical board process and sensitivity training.

("Army Sets Training, Plans Next Steps For Medical Action," News Leader, 8 Nov 2007)

"Project Protégé was designed to produce not only better students, but better Americans."

— CPT Chadwick Fletcher
Project Protégé Lead

Twelve members of the Robert G. Cole High School Academic Decathlon Competitive Team visited the Fort Sam Houston AMEDDC&S to help to initiate a new and exciting program called Project Protégé.

Project Protégé represented an important and enduring partnership between Fort Sam Houston Independent School District and AMEDDC&S. The program provided career-related and educational opportunities and hands-on experiences between the students and the working professionals at Fort Sam Houston. Students from various grade and academic levels were introduced to a wide range of specific medical and technical courses and programs. "Project Protégé was designed to produce not only better students, but better Americans," said CPT Chadwick Fletcher, Project Protégé Lead.

("Cole Academic Decathlon Team Visits AMEDD," News Leader, 6 Dec 2007)

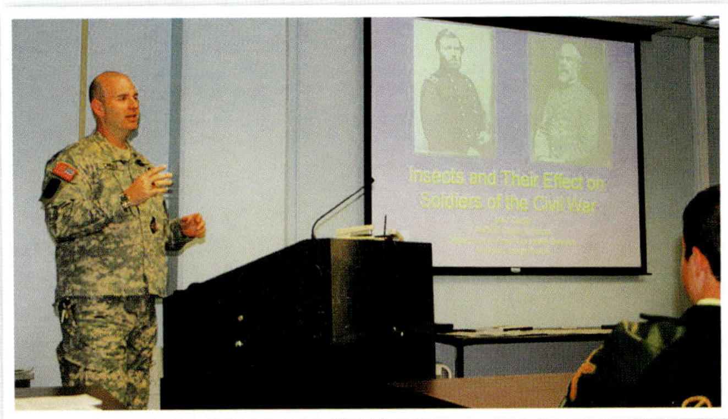

Project Protégé participants received a lecture on insects and their effects on soldiers of the Civil War.

(U.S. Army Photo)

2008

An instructor from AMEDDC&S received a Purple Heart medal for injuries sustained in Iraq during a ceremony at the Department of Combat Medic Training (DCMT). Installation Commander MG Russell Czerw presented the medal to SFC James Jeane, a tactical trauma instructor for DCMT. Jeane was wounded 26 Feb 2006 in Mosul, Iraq, when working with a scout platoon on a raid. After the raid, the platoon chased a suspected terrorist out of the mosque compound. As the platoon followed in a Stryker, they were struck by a vehicle-borne improvised explosive device, which exploded less than 10 feet from Jeane's position. He was hit in the head by shrapnel. "He had to learn how to walk and talk again, feed himself again. Think about that as a mission order," Czerw said.

("AMEDD Instructor Honored for Sacrifices," News Leader, 14 Feb 2008)

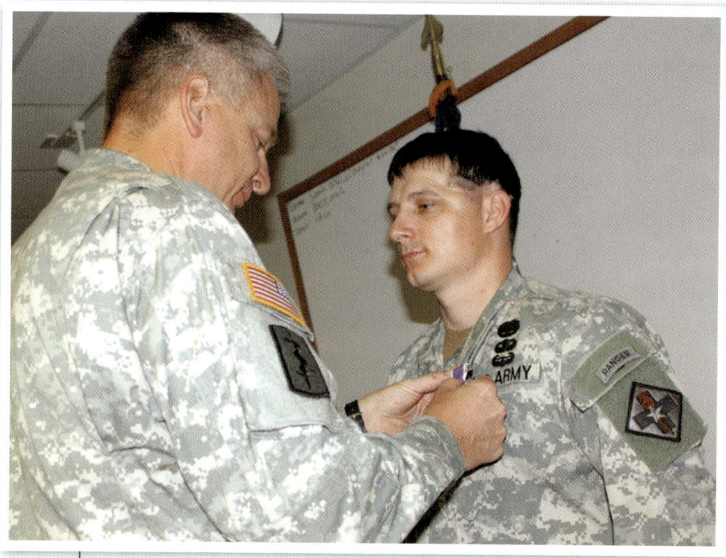

Commander MG Russell Czerw presenting SFC James Jeane his purple heart.

(U.S. Army Photo)

Nineteen students graduated from the post's first Army Lean Six Sigma (LSS) Black Belt course sponsored by the U.S. Army Medical Command at Fort Sam Houston in February. "It is very exciting to have the first group of Black Belts trained; now they can start improving processes and helping to coach Green Belts. It is our first step in becoming an independent program," said COL Donna Whittaker, director of the Office of Innovation, Initiatives and Improvement, AMEDDC&S, and LSS Master Black Belt. LSS is a business improvement methodology that maximizes shareholder value by achieving the fastest rate of improvement in customer satisfaction, cost, quality, process, speed, and invested capital. "LSS is an adventure and is a proven method of improving processes that can save money and get rid of waste. It will also change the way we look at all our processes," said COL Whittaker.

("Lean Six Sigma - MEDCOM sponsors first Black Belt course at Fort Sam," News Leader, 13 March 2008)

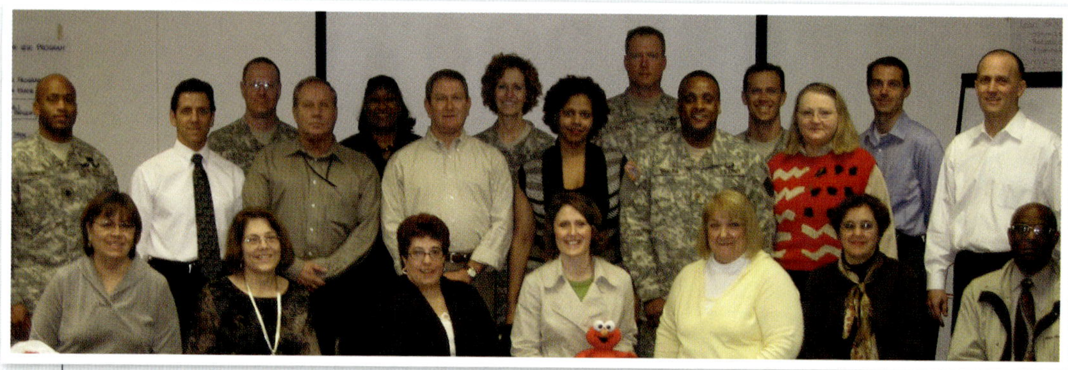

Graduates of the AMEDDC&S first Army Lean Six Sigma Black Belt course.

(U.S. Army Photo)

The film industry has the Oscar, television has the Emmy, the stage has the Tony Award and—not to be ignored—the Army has the Department of Army Visual Information Video Production Awards Program. The AMEDDC&S's "Army Medic: The Spirit of Courage" video was selected first place in the documentary category and first place overall in the 2008 Department of Army Visual Information Video Production Awards Program. The video documentary depicted the history of the Army medic, a battlefield job that has grown to become one of the most honored of military occupations. With a team effort of more than 100 soldiers, civilians, actors, and crew members, the video took more than a year to complete.

("Army Documentary Earns Video Award," News Leader, 20 March 2008)

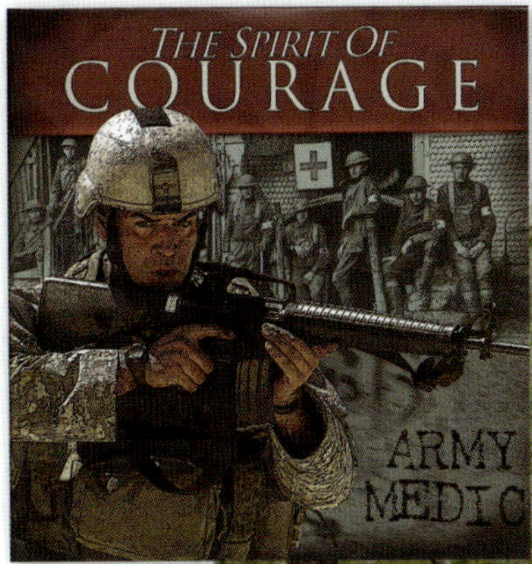

(U.S. Army photo)

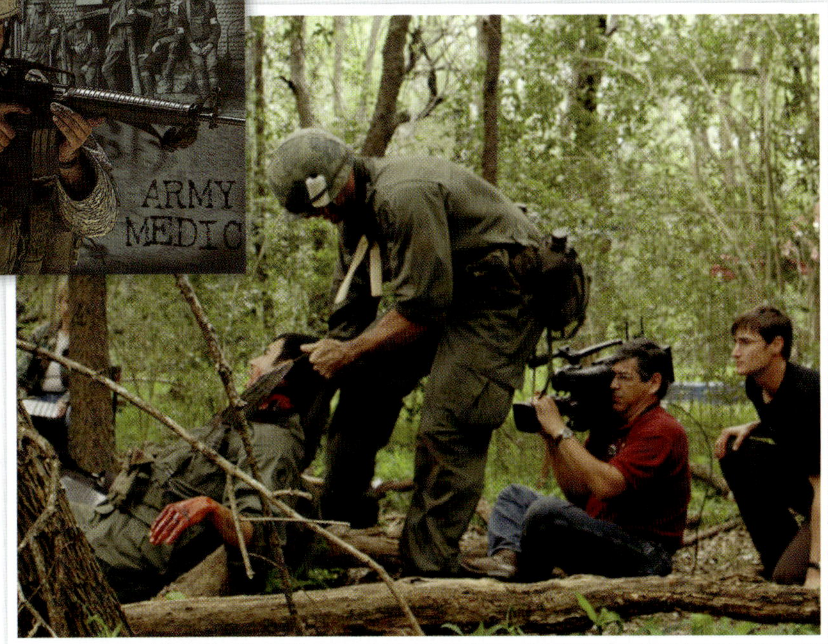

Enlisted physical therapy training has evolved significantly over the last six decades from its meager beginnings of on-the-job training. During World War II, the service commands presented growing needs for trained enlisted physical therapy technicians. As of 2004, the Physical Therapy Program conducted tri-service training for Army, Navy, and Coast Guard personnel.

("Army Strong, Army Limber - Soldiers Study To Become Physical Therapy Technicians," News Leader, 27 March 2008)

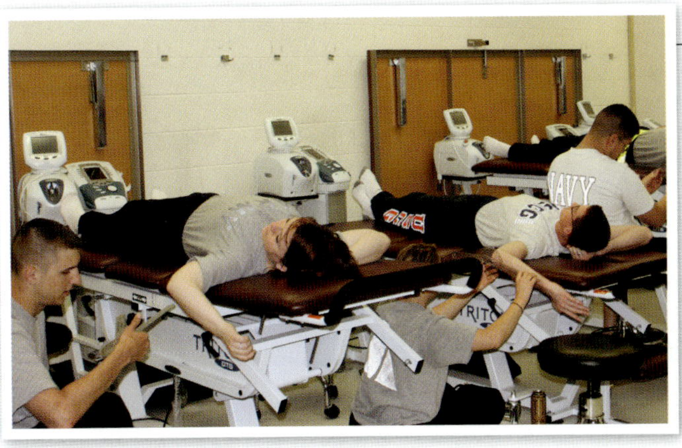

Navy, Coast Guard and Air Force students training alongside one another in the physical therapy course.

(U.S. Army Photo)

A new graduate program at the AMEDDC&S opened doors for aspiring social workers. Since June 2008, soldiers have had the opportunity to earn their master's degree in social work from an accredited university while still carrying out their active-duty military commitment. "My heart is still pounding," said COL Yvonne Tucker-Harris, social work consultant to the Army Surgeon General, of the program coming to fruition. "This is such a great investment for the Army." The program was made possible through an Army partnership with Fayetteville State University in North Carolina. As soldiers complete the graduate course at the AMEDDC&S, they will be awarded a master's degree from FSU.

("Soldiers Can Earn Master's Degree In Social Work," News Leader, 2 April 2008)

2008

The U.S. Army would soon have a new deployable platform to train soldiers in combat lifesaving skills through advanced simulation technologies. The Army's Research, Development and Engineering Command (RDECOM)'s Simulation & Training Technology Center unveiled its new Combat Medic Basic and Advanced Trauma Training (CoMBATT) unit at the Association of the U.S. Army Medical Symposium held in San Antonio. RDECOM delivered the first CoMBATT system during the summer to AMEDDC&S. CoMBATT created authentic battlefield environment scenarios through audio and visual programming, and provided real-life combat medical situations through the use of patient simulators. It created a training opportunity for combat medics unlike any other available.

("Cutting Edge - AMEDD To Receive New Medic Training System," News Leader, 12 June 2008)

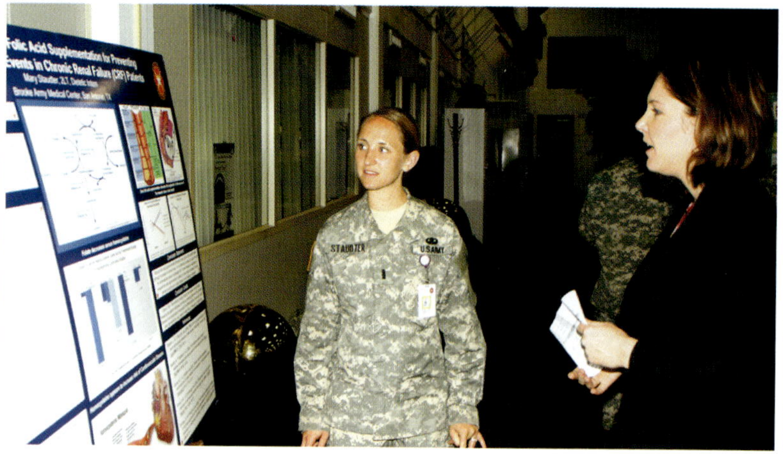

Open House
Close to 100 people participated in the AMEDDC&S AHS graduate school's inaugural Open House and Poster Session at the Army Community Service. The Open House and Poster Session provided the Fort Sam Houston community an opportunity to meet the staff and learn about the graduate programs at AHS. In addition to promoting relations and interaction among graduate program students, the open house provided a meeting opportunity for local universities, health care professionals, faculty and students, and the FSH community.

("Academy Showcases Graduate Programs at Open House," News Leader, 2 April 2008)

While most of the health care world was geared toward treating disease and illness, one Army medical specialty was solely in the business of prevention. Preventive medicine specialists worked to ensure their comrades, whether stateside or downrange, remained injury and disease-free. Soldiers learned their trade at AMEDDC&S during a 15-week Preventive Medicine Specialist Course that covered everything from giant stinging scorpions in the desert to syrupy soda dispensers at the dining facility. "It's a very challenging and comprehensive course," said 1SG Roye Patton, course class adviser. The course work included nine phases covering every aspect of sanitation and safety for soldiers in the field and at home.

("Keep It Clean: Students Learn To Keep Soldiers Safe, Disease-Free," News Leader, 5 June 2008)

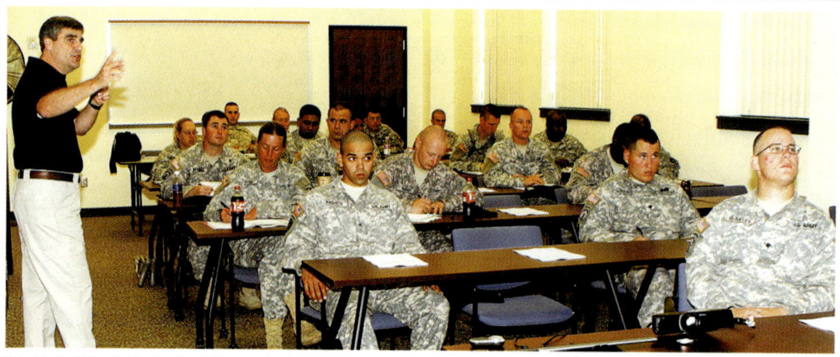

Preventive medicine students during the didactic portion of their program.

(U.S. Army Photo)

A ceremonial groundbreaking for the Medical Education and Training Campus (METC) on 10 July 2008 marked another step toward what leaders were calling the largest consolidation of training in the history of the DoD. Completed in 2011, the joint campus, led by tri-service leadership, centralized all Army, Navy and Air Force basic and specialty enlisted medical training at Fort Sam Houston. "With this institution becoming the largest in the world solely dedicated to medical training and education, San Antonio will be transformed into a national center for education and training," said keynote speaker Air Force MG Melissa Rank, chair, METC Flag Officer Steering Committee

("METC To Consolidate Enlisted Medical Training at Fort Sam," News Leader, 17 July 2008)

AMEDDC&S soldiers and students received training on one aspect of war that does not always take precedence: the battle of the mind. The training was integrated into the advanced individual training for health care specialists and AMEDD Officer Basic Leader Course/Basic Officer Leader Course curriculum in July. A mobile training team taught it to soldiers throughout the Army. Initially, the course intended to teach medics how to help themselves and others deal with stresses of military life. The medics' portion was a "train the trainer" segment to give them valuable information to take back and teach fellow medics and others. Warriors go to other warriors – someone they trust – when they have a problem. Some people are more able to cope than others, and even mild stressors can set people off.

("Medics Receive Battlemind Training to Help Fellow Soldiers," News Leader, 18 Sept 2008)

On 28 July 2008, the AMEDDC&S rolled out its new Balanced Scorecard to all employees. They learned of the Balanced Scorecard, saw where they fit in on the Strategy Map, and understood that they are valued both as an employee and as a person, and that their performance is critical to mission success. "For those who have not heard yet, we are welcoming the Balanced Scorecard as the management system and decision-making tool that we will use to align our vision and mission with customer requirements and day-to-day work. The new system will help us manage and evaluate business strategy; monitor operational efficiency; guide process improvements; build organizational capacity; and communicate progress to all employees," said MG Russell Czerw, Commander, Fort Sam Houston and AMEDDC&S.

("AMEDDC&S to Introduce New Balanced Scorecard," News Leader, 24 July 2008)

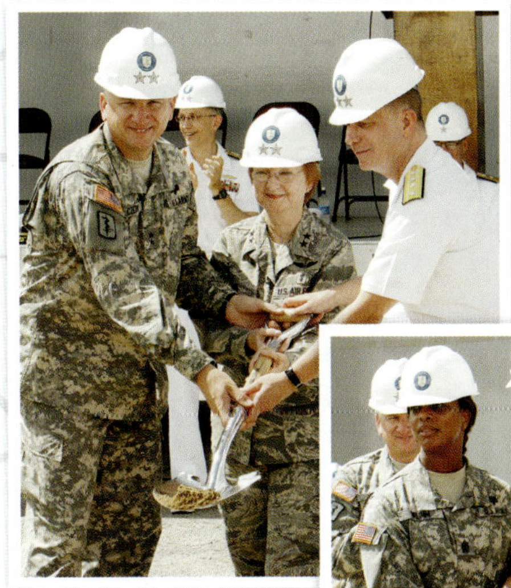

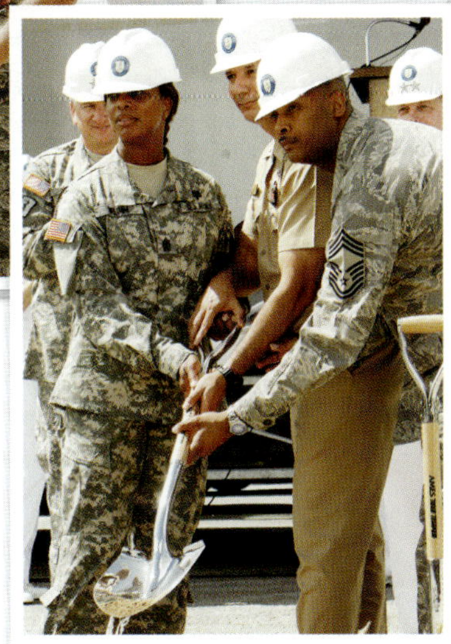

METC Groundbreaking Ceremony

(U.S. Army Photos)

The AMEDDC&S's first balanced scorecard

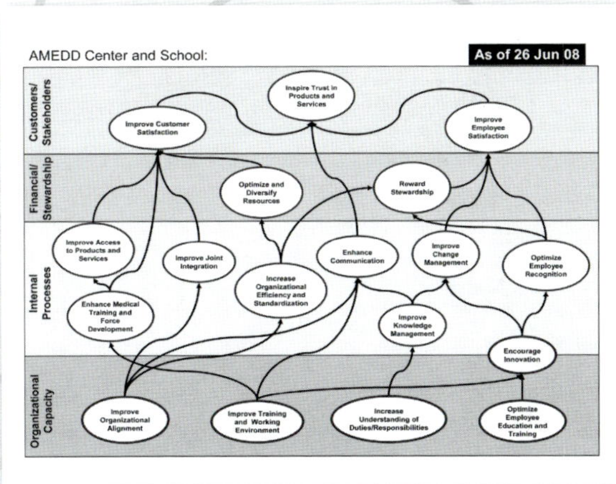

2009

The first Fort Sam Houston Community Information Forum was hosted by MG Russell Czerw and COL Mary Garr, U.S. Army Garrison Commander. COL Garr established the forum to give the diverse military agencies and activities at Fort Sam Houston an opportunity to showcase community events and programs and post operations that support mission readiness and quality of life activities.

("Forum Addresses Key Community Groups, Commanders," by Phil Reidinger, News Leader, 22 Jan 2009, p 1)

Army Reservist SPC Mark Pilar became the first recipient of the COL Brian D. Allgood 68W Distinguished Honor Graduate Award. Pilar was assigned to the 1984th DET 2, Tripler Army Medical Center, Honolulu, Hawaii, and a member of Soldier Medics graduating class number 17-08.

("32nd Medical Battalion Graduates Soldier Medics," by Minnie Jones, News Leader, 19 Feb, p 1)

The Interservice Physician's Assistant Program (IPAP), under pressure to expand its training capabilities to meet rising demands due to deployments and backfills, succeeded in expanding its enrollment capabilities in just one year.

("Interservice Physician's Assistant Program Successful in One-Year Expansion," by Martha Waldman, News Leader, 26 Feb 2009, p 4)

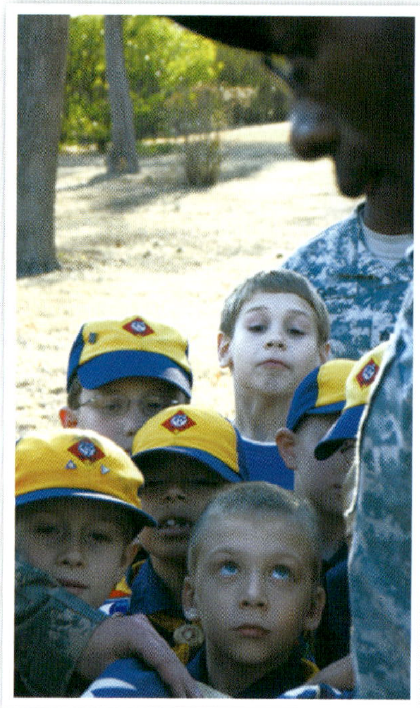

Cub Scouts of Pack 23, Den 7, watch carefully as soldiers from the AMEDDC&S Noncommissioned Officer Academy (NCOA) fold the American flag during retreat.

("NCOA Hosts Cub Scout Retreat," News Leader, 5 Feb 2009, p 15)

JROTC

More than 35 JROTC students from Jefferson High School spent the day visiting Fort Sam Houston on 27 February 2009. The trip included a visit to the Department of Combat Medic Training, Headquarters and Headquarters Company, U.S. Army Garrison and the Quadrangle.

("NCOs Visit With Jefferson High School JROTC," News Leader, 5 March 2009, p 4)

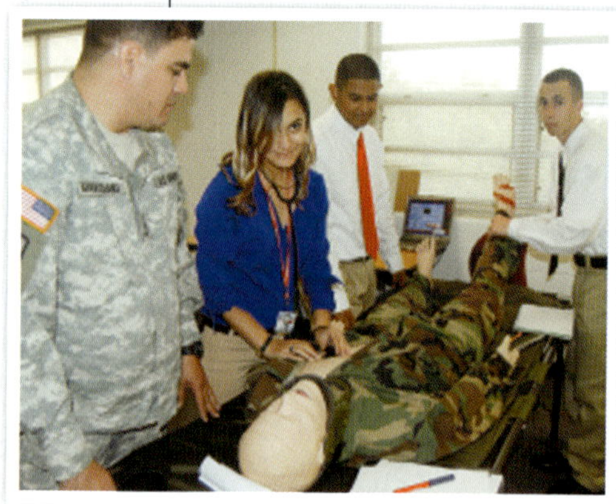

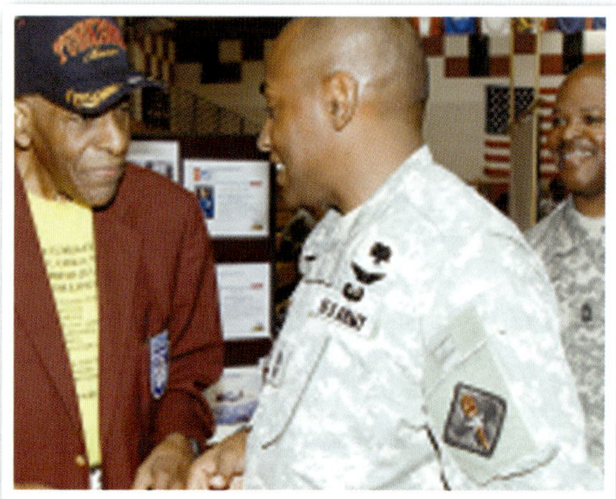

Dr. Granville Coggs, an original Tuskegee Airman and former staff radiologist at the BAMC, talks with MSG Anthony Stevens, AMEDD, during the 32nd Medical Brigade Black History Month celebration 27 Feb at the Jimmy Brought Fitness Center. This year's theme was "The Roots and Branches of Our Family Tree."

("32nd Medical Brigade Celebrates Black History Month," by Minnie Jones, News Leader, 5 March 2009, p 1)

The U.S. Army Emergency Medical Services (EMS) Office provided initial guidance and follow-on assistance to the U.S. Customs and Border Patrol in El Paso to create their first self-trained National Registry Emergency Medicine Technician Basic Course.

("AMEDDC&S Partners with U.S. Customs and Border Patrol," News Leader, 16 April 2009, p 1)

On 29 April 2009, leaders and training professionals from the AMEDDC&S attended the first Attrition Summit. Hosted by COL W. John Luciano, the Dean of the Academy of Health Sciences (AHS), the summit reviewed attition issues in AHS programs with the goal of producing initiatives and policies to prevent further attrition, reduce spending, and increase efficiency while continuing to provide top quality medical training for Army medical personnel.

("AMEDDC&S Holds Attrition Summit To Address Programs, Initiatives," News Leader, 7 May 2009, p 11)

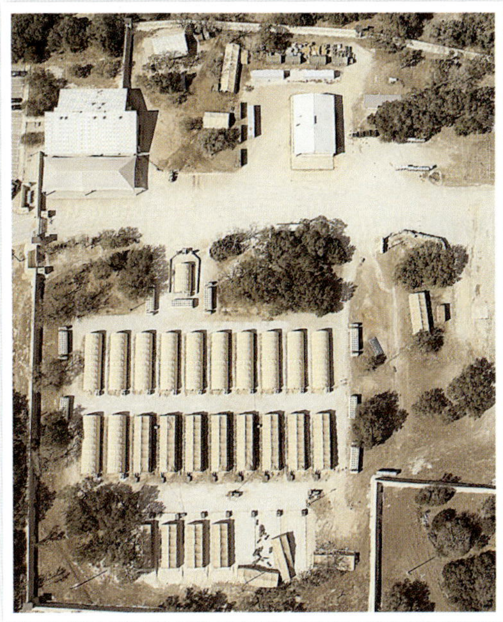

FOB Courage

A realistic, state-of-the-art training site designed and built to represent as accurately as possible forward operating bases throughout the world was unveiled on 20 March 2009 at Camp Bullis.

("FOB Courage Offers State-Of-The-Art Training For Combat Medics" by Lori Newman, News Leader, 26 March 2009, p 15)

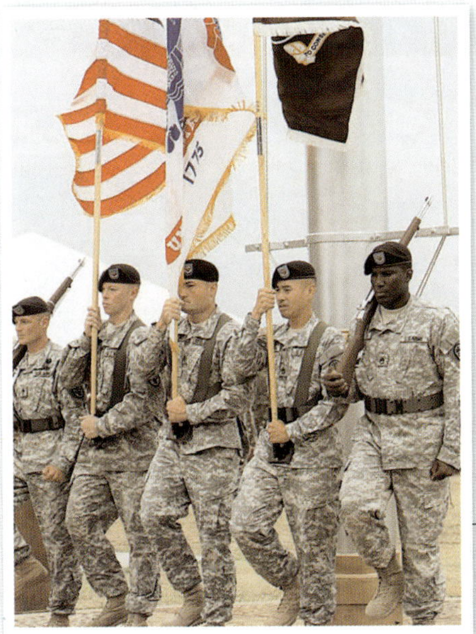

The NCO Academy Color Guard, led by 1SG Richard Patenia, presents the colors at the Army and Flag Day celebration at the post flagpole, 12 June 2009.

("Happy Birthday, Army!" by Esther Garcia, News Leader, 18 June 2009, p 13)

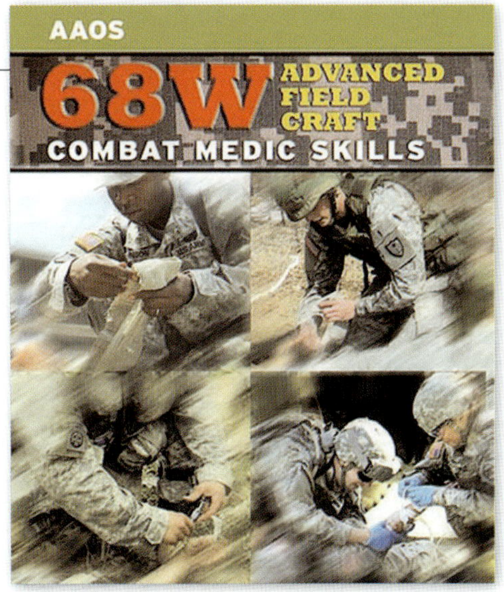

The AMEDDC&S "68W Advanced Field Craft: Combat Medic Skills," was named a "Hot Product" at the 27th Annual EMS Today Conference and Exposition, hosted by the Journal of Emergency Medical Services. The book placed in the top 30 of tens of thousands of EMS products submitted for being innovative, functional, potentially life-saving, and offering remarkable improvements to patient care and provider performance.

("AMEDD's New Medic Manual Considered Hot Product," News Leader, 25 June 2009, p 3)

2009

Local jurisdictions begin steps to apply recommendations of the 1995 Joint Land Use Study on Camp Bullis. Top priorities were: mitigating endangered species habitat; supporting an endangered species ordinance by the City of San Antonio; requiring real estate disclosure if a property or home is within the five-mile military influence area; managing dark skies through light ordinances; and ensuring land compatibility with fixed and rotary wing aviation, as determined by Fort Sam Houston.

("Local Jurisdictions Begin Steps To Apply Recommendations of 1995 Joint Land Use Study," by Neal Synder, News Leader, 16 July 2009, pp 16-17)

On 14 Aug 2009, AMEDDC&S graduated its inaugural class in the Master of Social Work Program. The program was designed to address unique challenges soldiers and their families face in a military culture during a time of war.

("Seeds, Trees Theme for AMEDDC&S Inaugural Master of Social Work," News Leader, 20 Aug 2009, p 1)

On 2 Oct 2009, Dr. James Kirkpatrick, senior clinical consultant, Directorate of Combat and Doctrine Development, AMEDDC&S, was awarded Capability Developer of the Year for redesigning the Combat Support Hospital and Hospital Augmentation teams and effecting significant improvements in the Army-wide Combat Lifesavers program.

("AMEDD's Kirkpatrick Named Capability Developer of the Year," News Leader, 22 Oct 2009, p 10)

The Department of Veterinary Science began its surveillance food laboratory managers course at the end of 2009.

By adding eight additional weeks to the Phase I program, 68 Victors were able to earn an associate degree from the Respiratory Specialist course.

("68 Victors to Earn Associate Degree from Respiratory Specialist Course," News Leader, 10 Dec 2009, p 1)

Thriller

Members of the U.S. Army Medical Command Band, dressed in scrubs, dance to the music of "Thriller," made famous by Michael Jackson, during Fright Night 25 Oct 2009 hosted by Fort Sam Houston Commanding General MG Russell Czerw, at the Staff Post Road gazebo. Many audience members arrived dressed in their favorite Halloween costumes.

(Photo by Esther Garcia, News Leader, 28 Oct 2009, p 1)

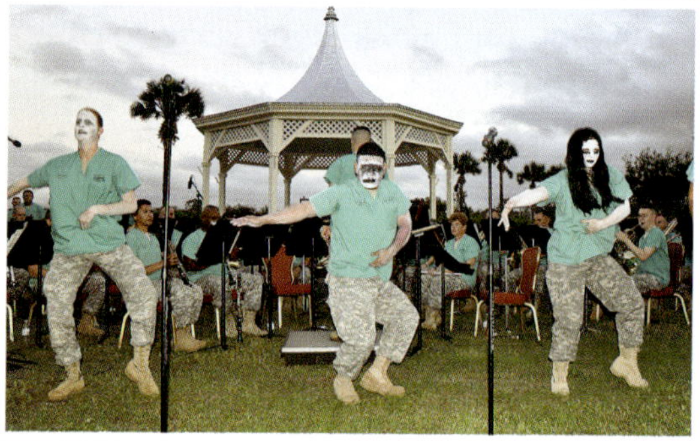

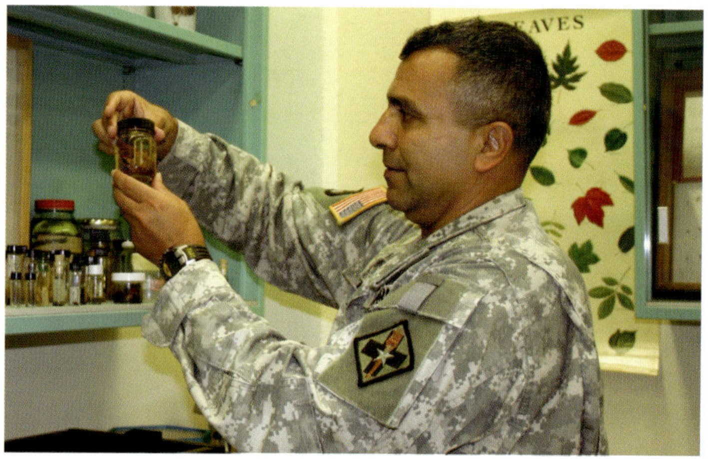

COL (Dr.) Mustapha Debboun

Chief of the AMEDDC&S Medical Zoology Branch, COL Debboun holds up one of several samples of various insects displayed in the Medical Zoology lab. COL Debboun is a co-author of Prevention of Bug Bites, Stings, and Disease, published in 2009.

("AMEDD Instructor Shares Insect Knowledge In New Book," by Lori Newman, News Leader, 20 Aug 2009, p 3)

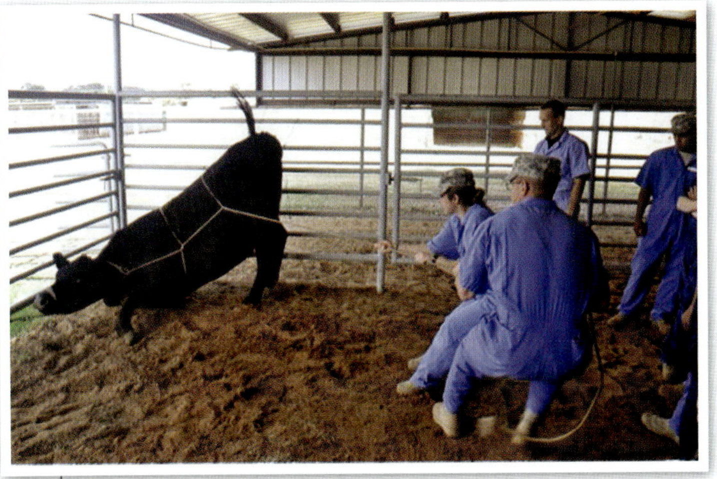

Animal Care Specialist Class 006-10 train at Texas A&M University on large animal management.

(AMEDDC&S Photo)

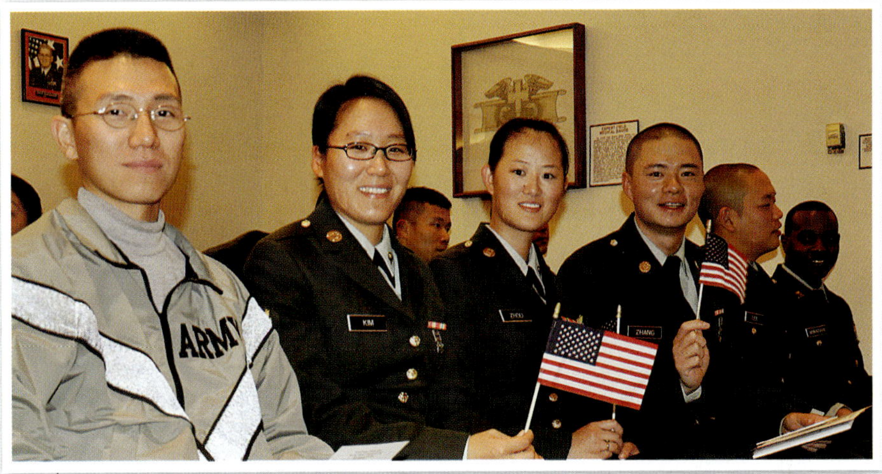

Soldiers assigned to the 232nd Medical Battalion hold U.S. flags after taking the U.S. Oath of Allegiance during a naturalization ceremony 20 Nov 2009 at the AMEDD Museum auditorium.

(News Leader, 26 Nov 2009, p 1)

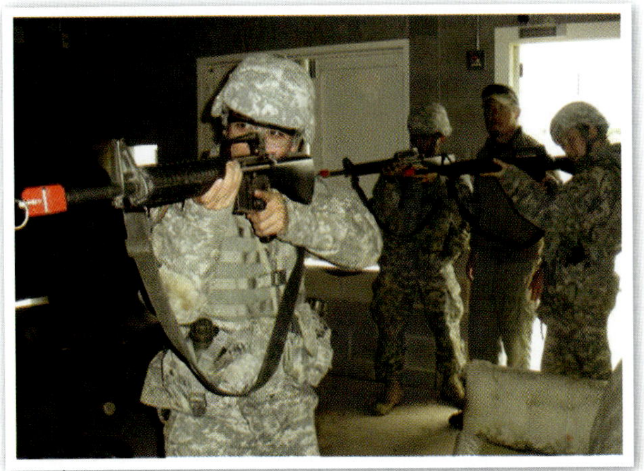

Animal Care Specialist Class 001-12 clears a building during their FTX at Camp Bullis.

(AMEDDC&S Photo)

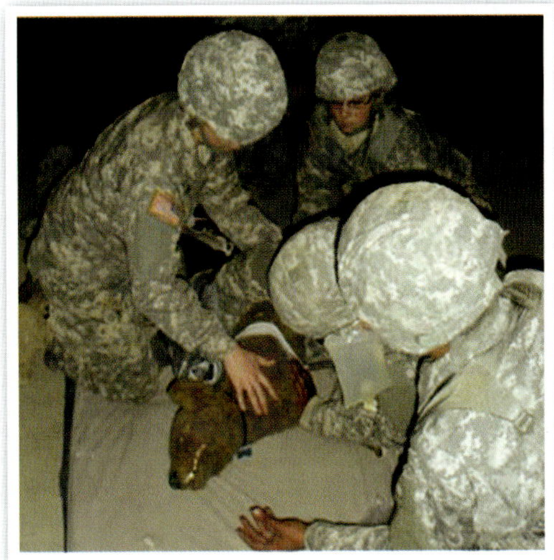

Animal Care Specialist Class 001-12 trains on emergency animal care during their FTX at Camp Bullis.

(AMEDDC&S Photo)

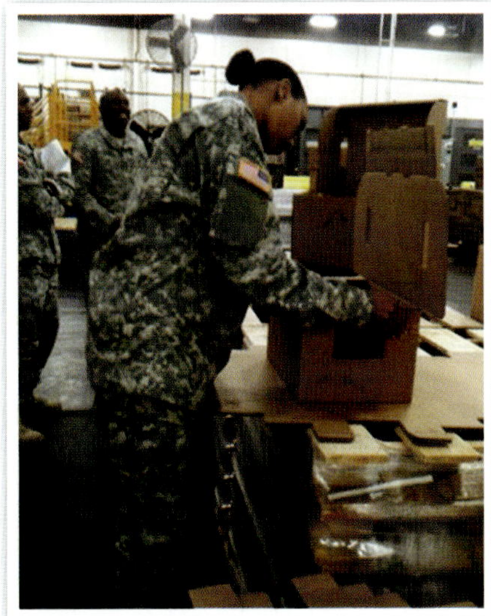

Instructor Rideoutt (with DVS) visits the Tracey Depot in California, where Unitized Group Rations (UGRs) are produced.

(AMEDDC&S Photo)

2010

AMEDDC&S did its part to promote international engagement, partnerships, and goodwill among accomplished international and U.S. senior level medical officers (0-5 and above) through a unique training opportunity called the Medical Strategic Leadership Program (MSLP). The MSLP, a course within the Leader Training Center at the AHS, was established in order to provide training support that focused on strategic-level military medical leadership health issues, working within coalitions and alliances, with an emphasis on combating terrorism and providing a networking environment for military professionals.

("AMEDDC&S Leadership Program Boosts International Relations," News Leader, 24 Jan 2010)

AMEDDC&S unveiled its new Deployable Medical Systems Equipment Training (DMSET) Site 25 January 2010 at Camp Bullis. The DMSET was made up of several Alaskan Shelter dome-shaped tents connected together to form a Combat Support Hospital with all the amenities of a brick and mortar hospital.

("New Site Offers Realistic Training for Student Soldiers," News Leader, 29 Jan 2010)

The AMEDDC&S offered a new two-week course in Surveillance Food Laboratory Techniques. The course was designed to train soldiers to recognize food and safety issues before they occur and to prevent food-borne illness.

("Capsules," The Mercury, Vol 37, No 4, Jan-March 2010, p 5)

AMEDDC&S was awarded the Army Distributed Learning (DL) Champion Award for 2009 during a ceremony at the 9th Annual Army Distributed Learning Conference at Newport News, Virginia, 15 March 2010. DL was a set of technology-supported methodologies that included interactive multimedia instruction using online lessons, games, simulations and learning scenarios. Lessons and instructional materials could also be used via iPod, video tele-training, or television broadcast. The Army Training Support Center awarded AMEDDC&S for distinguished leadership and outstanding achievements in the advancement of DL.

("AMEDDC&S Recognized as Army Leader in Distributed Learning," News Leader, 25 March 2010)

In April 2010, the AMEDDC&S received the award of excellence from the Balanced Scorecard Institute. The Medical Clinic at Camp Bullis was named in honor of SPC Taylor J. Burk, a medic killed in Iraq in 2005.

("Capsules," The Mercury, Vol 37, No 5, April 2010, p 5)

A four year study by the U.S. Army-Baylor University Doctoral Program in Physical Therapy at the AMEDDC&S and the University of Florida showed that strong core muscles make it easier to do most physical activities. The study showed that sit-ups, the traditional training exercise, only train the least important core component. The study led the way for a change in the core fitness training and testing standard.

("Study Prefers Core Training to Situps for AIT Students," by Minnie L. Jones, The Mercury, Vol 37, No 6, May 2010, p 9)

All active duty enlisted soldiers were invited to apply for the U.S. Army Master of Social Work program hosted by the AMEDDC&S and affiliated with Fayetteville State University. Upon completion enlisted soldiers received a direct commission in the Medical Service Corps and served on active duty as social work officers in a variety of clinical and operations settings including medical treatment facilities, brigade combat teams, combat and operational stress control units, and confinement facilities.

("Enlisted Soldiers Can Earn Master of Social Work," The Mercury, Vol 37, No 6, May 2010, p 9)

More than 600 soldiers stood in formation on MacArthur Parade Field, while cannons boomed and the band played during a ceremony 30 April 2010 to bid farewell to the commanding general of Fort Sam Houston and AMEDDC&S, MG Russell Czerw. MG Czerw turned over command of AMEDDC&S to MG David A. Rubenstein, as MG Czerw retired after more than 23 years of military service.

("Fort Sam Houston Bids Farewell to Czerw, Welcomes Rubenstein," News Leader, 6 May 2010)

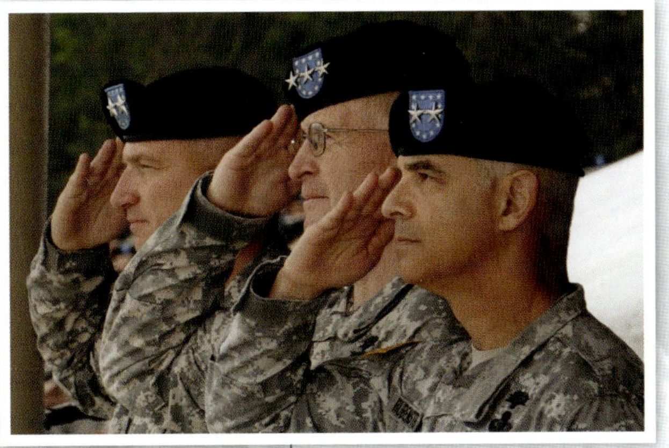

MG Russell J. Czerw, LTG Eric B. Schoomaker, and MG David A. Rubenstein salute the flag at the change of command ceremony.

(U.S. Army Photo)

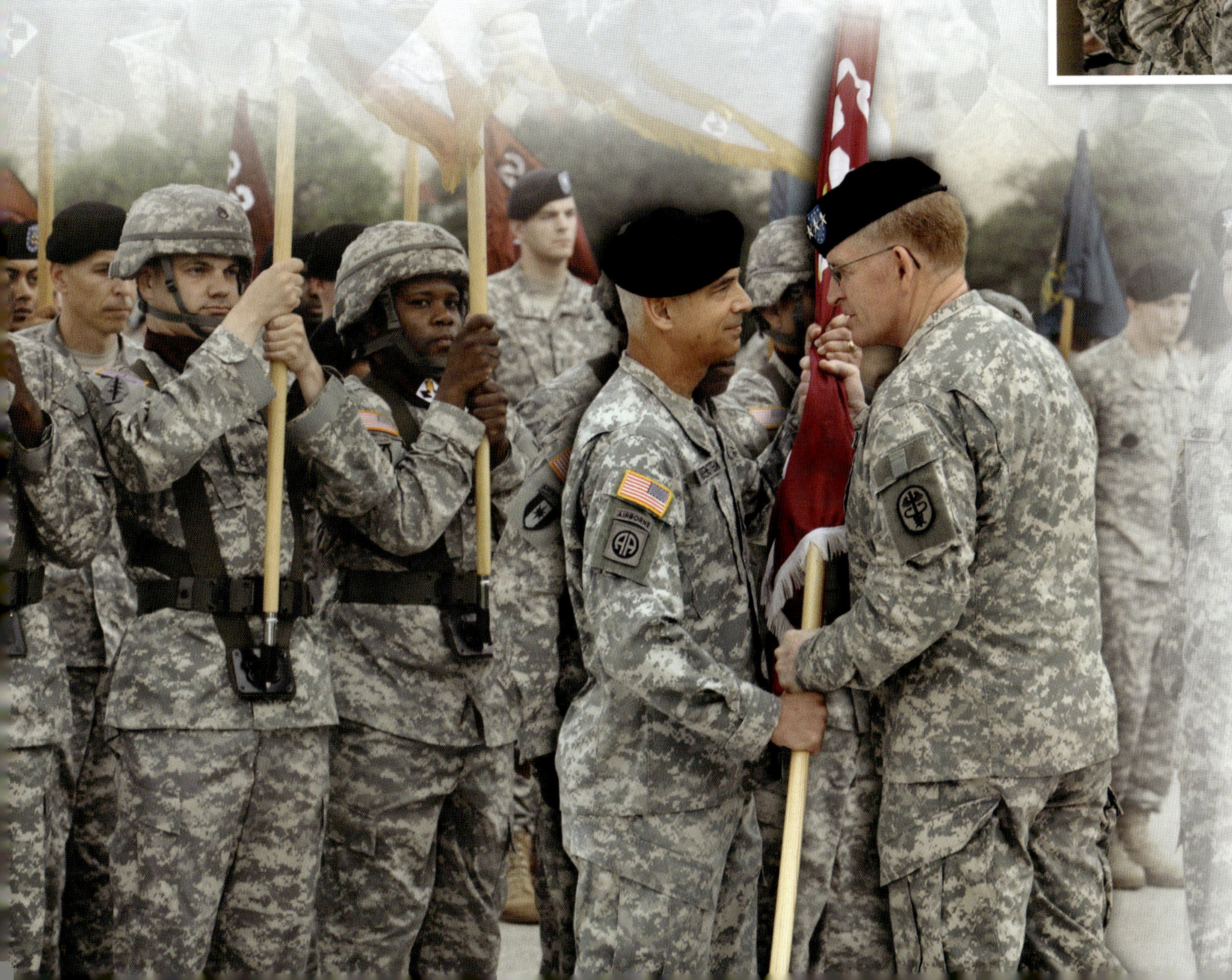

MG David A. Rubenstein (left) receives the command flag of the AMEDDC&S from MEDCOM Commander LTG Eric B. Schoomaker (right) during a change of command ceremony at Fort Sam Houston. Rubenstein replaced MG Russell J. Czerw, who retired.

(U.S. Army photo by Lori Newman)
(The Mercury, Vol 37, No 7, June 2010, p 6)

2010

The Medical Capabilities Integration Center launched its Medical Warfighter Forum (MedWfF) through the AMEDDC&S website. MedWfF was designed to provide information and knowledge to help personnel perform the job more effectively by giving access to clinical practice guidelines, up-to-date continuing medical education, Army enterprise subscription, lessons learned, deployment resources, and collaborative technology.

("Medical Warfighter Forum Offers Access to Information: Soldiers Collaborate Online, Share Lessons Learned," by COL Zach Wheeler, The Mercury, Vol 37, No 7, June 2010, p 2)

The future of military medical training arrived at Fort Sam Houston on 30 June 2010 with the opening of the sprawling Medical Education and Training Center. The METC, the crown jewel of the 2005 Base Realignment and Closure Commission's mandate for Fort Sam Houston, is an integrated campus under a single university-style administration, teaching more than 100 courses. RADM William R. Kiser, the METC's first commandant, said "Today marks a significant milestone in the ongoing story of military medicine. Everywhere our nation sends our finest to serve, our graduates will be there with them serving as a force for good because of the work done here."

("All Military Medical Training Roads Now Start at METC," News Leader, 1 July 2010)

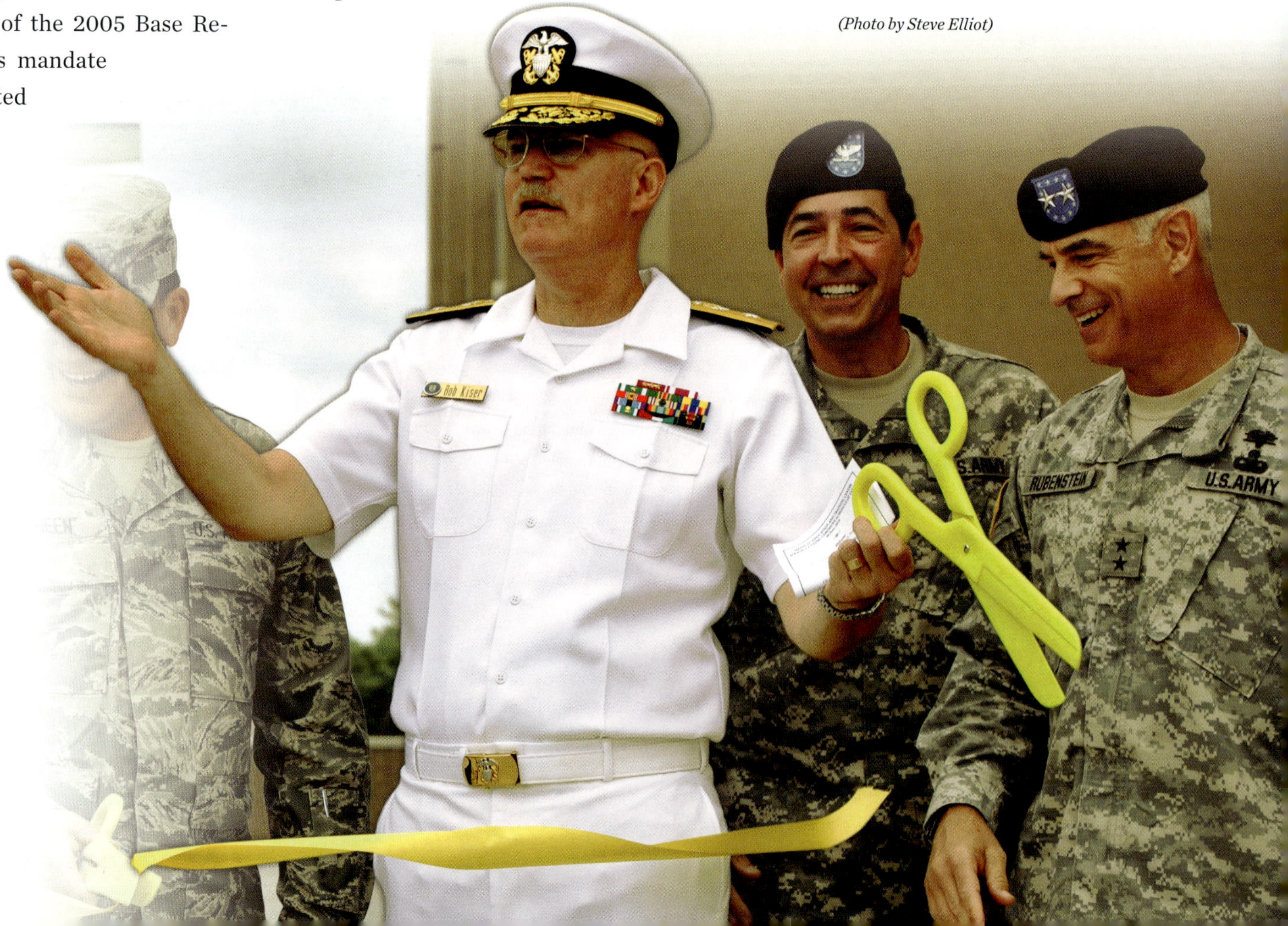

METC Commandant Navy RADM William R. Kiser (left), Army METC Transition Officer COL Don A. Gagliano (center), and AMEDDC&S Commander and Chief of the U.S. Army Medical Service Corps MG David A. Rubenstein (right) celebrate the opening of the Medical Education and Training Center with an official ribbon cutting ceremony.

(Photo by Steve Elliot)

The Army Training Support Center (ATSC) awarded the AMEDDC&S its distributed Learning (DL) Champion Award for 2009. The award was given for consistently championing DL, challenging existing practices, and developing new and innovative approaches to improve and expand delivery and training to soldiers in the field and schoolhouse.

("AMEDD Center and School Earns Award for Distributed Learning," The Mercury, Vol 37, No 7, June 2010, p 7)

The garrison at Fort Sam Houston, Texas, was redesignated the 502nd Mission Support Group. The Air Force assumed responsibility for garrison support of all military bases in San Antonio, Texas. Joint Base San Antonio became fully operational 1 October 2010.

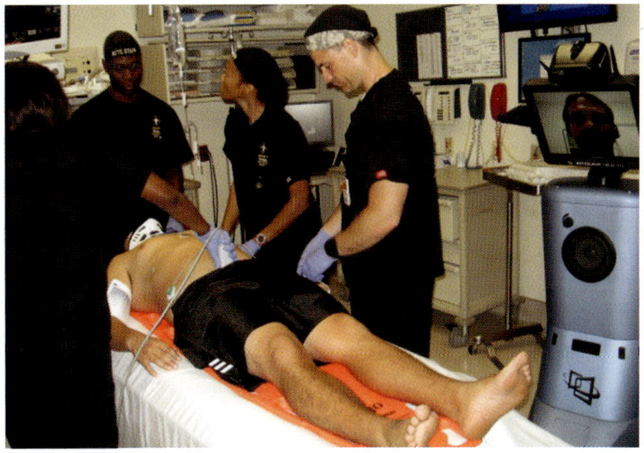

Training at the Army Trauma Training Center at the Miami Jackson Memorial Hospital, May 2010.

(U.S. Army Photo)

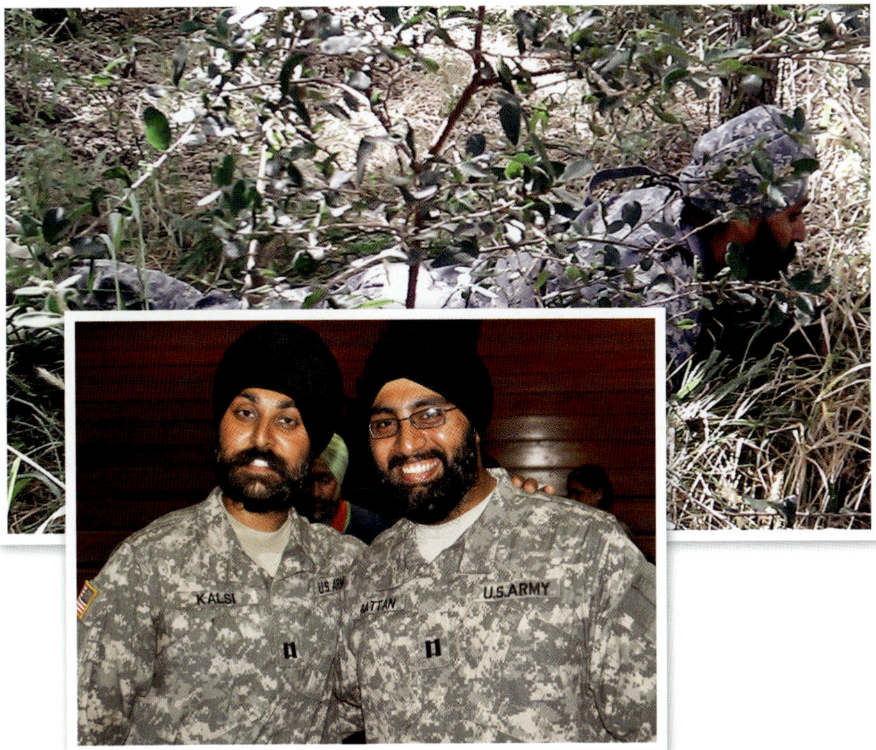

CPT Kamaljeet Kalsi, a practicing Sikh, during field exercises during his BOLC course (class 10-105). CPT Kalsi became the second Sikh in 2010 in a generation allowed to complete Army BAC without sacrificing his articles of faith. Earlier in the year CPT Tejdeep Singh Rattan became the first, a historic step by the Army in accepting practicing Sikhs into the Army.

("Second Sikh Doctor Allowed to Wear Articles of Faith; Enlisted Soldier in Training," News Leader, 9 Sept 2010)

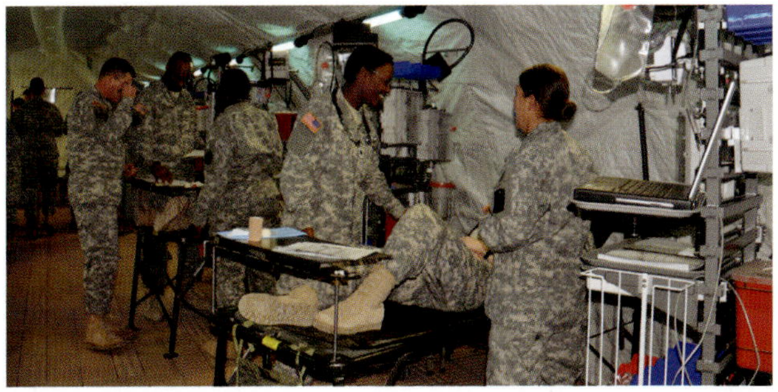

A combat support hospital during field exercises at Camp Bullis.

(U.S. Army Photo)

2010

COL Donna Whittaker, first female dean of the Academy of Health Sciences, managed 14 teaching departments providing 315 programs of instruction to officers, enlisted and foreign students with a total staff and faculty of 1,860, and an average daily student load of 4,900.

("Academy of Health Sciences - AMEDD Readiness Starts Here," News Leader, 12 Aug 2010)

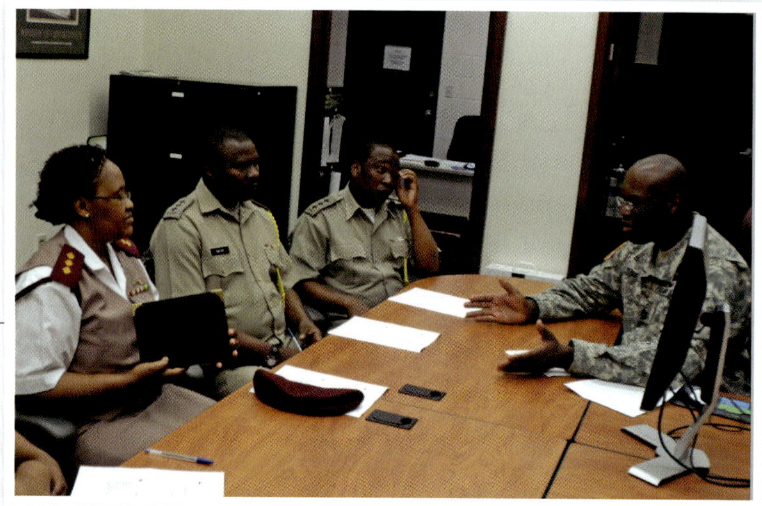

MSG John D. Perdue briefs Lesotho and Swaziland officers on Department of Medical Sciences and Army Trauma Training Center academic and functional programs in August 2010.

(Photo courtesy of the Department of Medical Sciences, AMEDDC&S, FSH, TX)

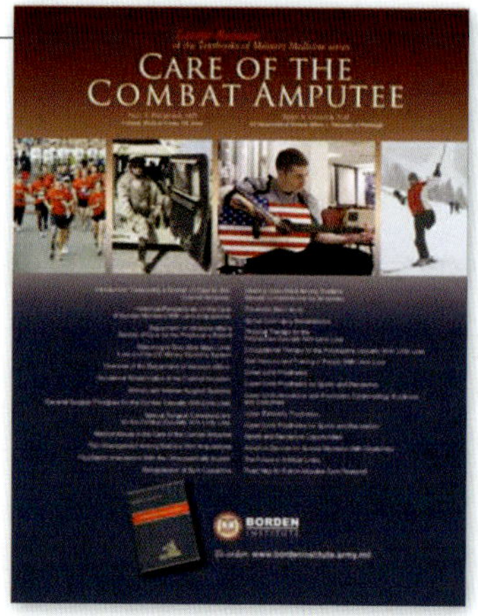

The Borden Institute published *Care of the Combat Amputee*, a significant update to the field of rehabilitation, covering emerging approaches, technologies and techniques for amputee care.

("New Borden Book Studies Amputee Care," The Mercury, Vol 37, No 5, April 2010, p 6)

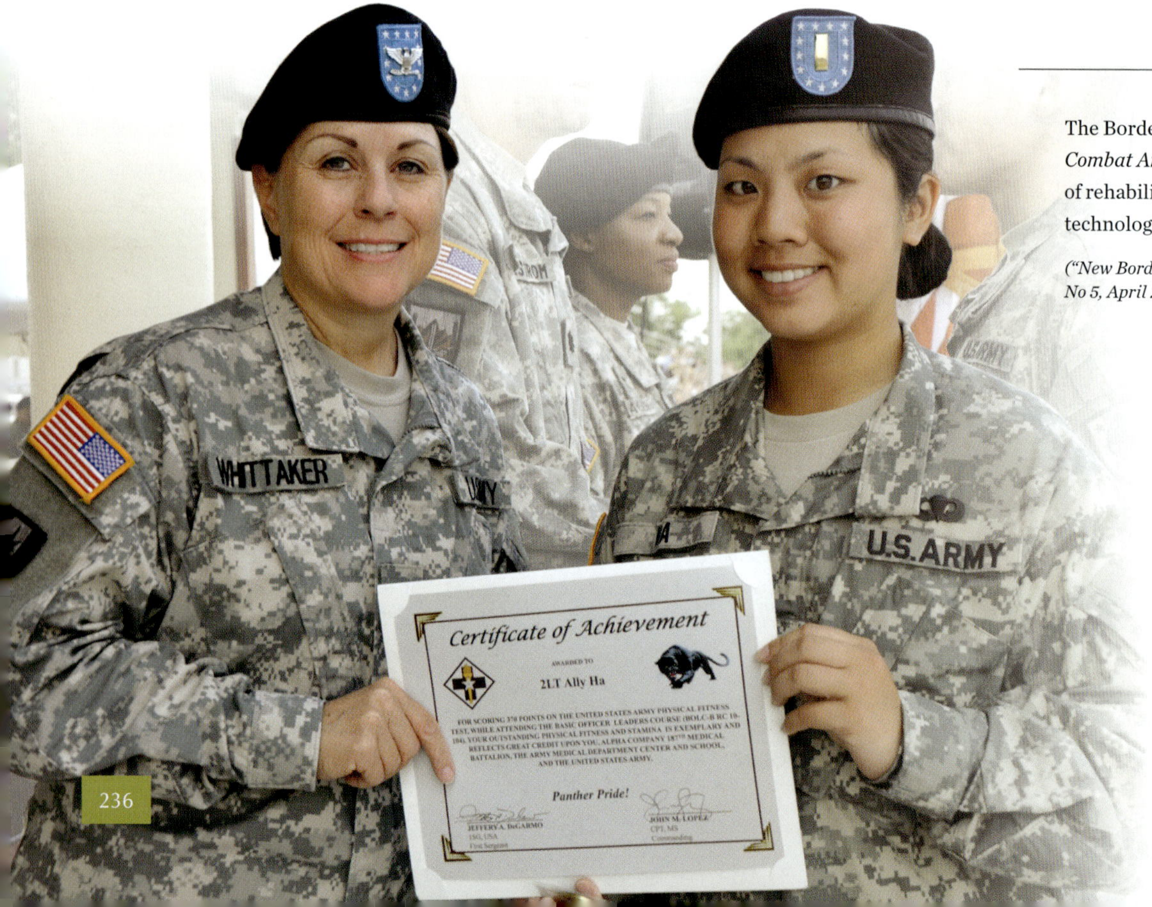

COL Donna Whittaker, Dean of AHS, presenting 2LT Ally Ha with a certificate of achievement.

(U.S. Army Photo)

After an eight-year process, the 91B MOS transformed into the 68W Health Care Specialist MOS. The new MOS qualified medics as EMTs trained in advanced skills, hemorrhage control techniques, shock management, and evacuation. The new MOS required 68W Medics to re-certify their skills every two years and earn 72 hours of continuing education credit during two years. LTG James B. Peake, Commander of the AMEDDC&S from 1996 to 2000, was responsible for initiating the conversion of the 91B MOS to 68W MOS.

("Leaders Celebrate Transition of 68W MOS," by Jerry Harben, The Mercury, May 2010, p 4)

A small group of airmen graduated at the METC 4 November 2010, making a huge historical impact as the first course to complete training at the billion-dollar joint training campus that opened in June 2010. The quartet of Air Force staff sergeants attended a two-week Pharmacy Craftsman course from 25 October to 4 November. "These four airmen training with us have provided a model for others to follow," said Navy Rear ADM William R. Kiser, METC commandant. "They were trained not only by Air Force, but by Army and Navy faculty as well. That will be the norm here at METC. This is the future of military medicine."

("First METC Grads Make History," News Leader, 4 Nov 2010)

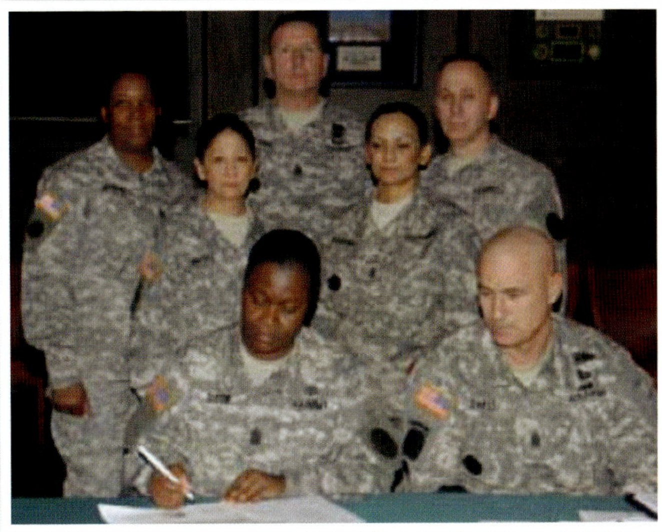

CSM Althea Dixon, the top noncommissioned officer of the Army Medical Command, signs a proclamation recognizing the transition of combat medics into the 68W MOS.

The first METC graduates.

(U.S. Army Photo)

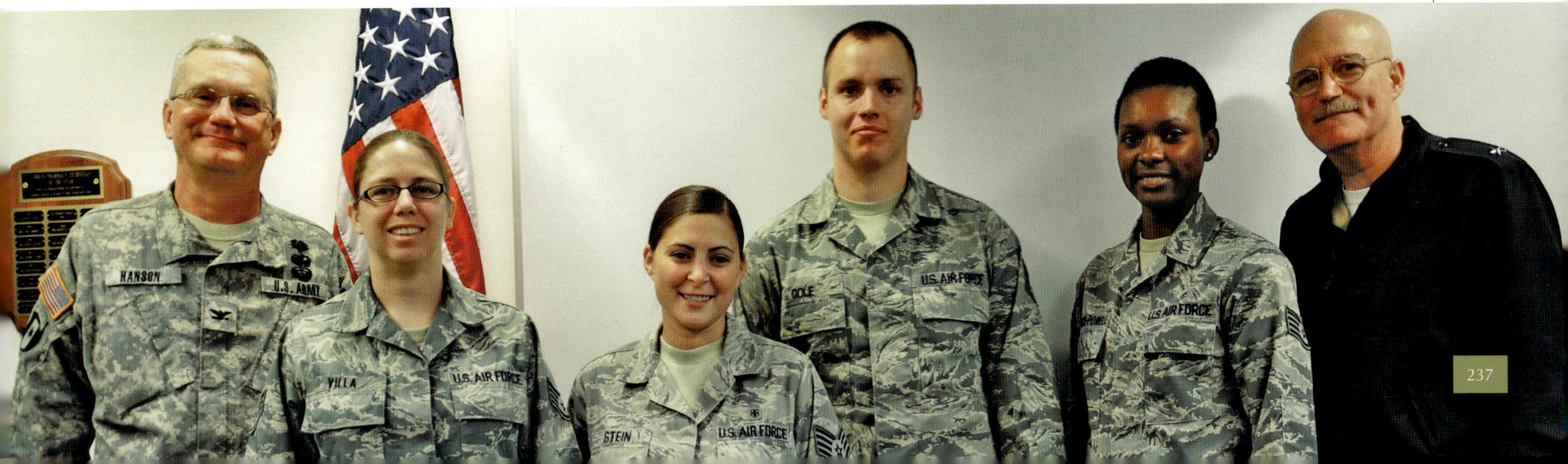

Appendix A

Commanding Generals (1920 – Present)

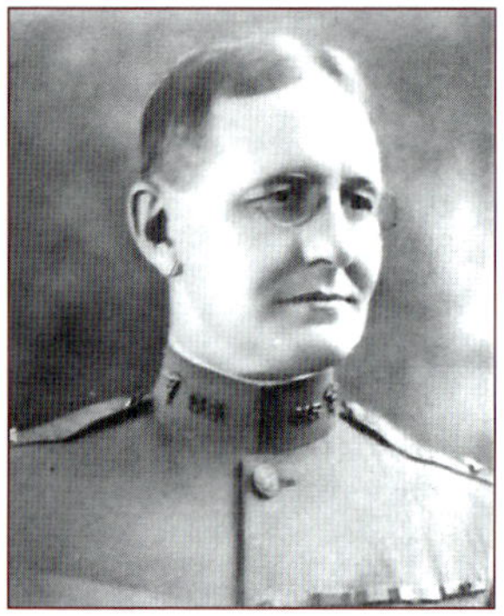

1920 – 1923
Colonel Percy M. Ashburn

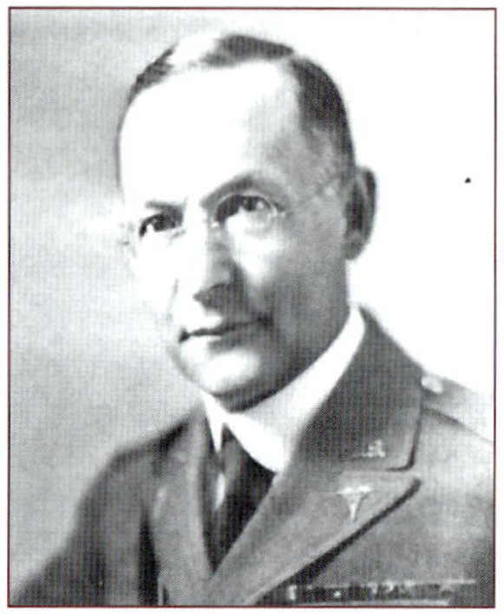

1923 – 1931
Colonel Charles R. Reynolds

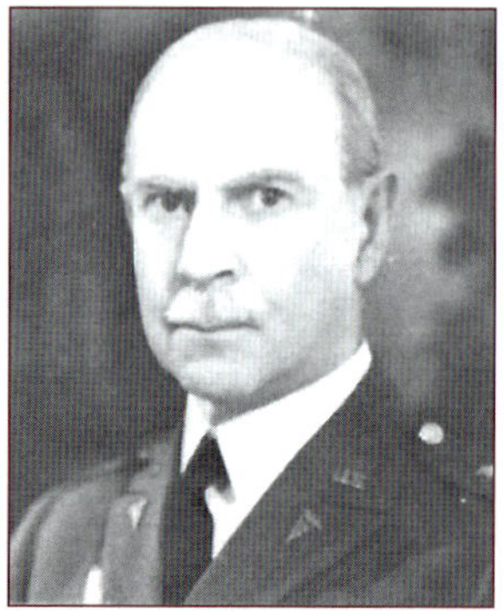

1931 – 1932
BG Edward L. Munson

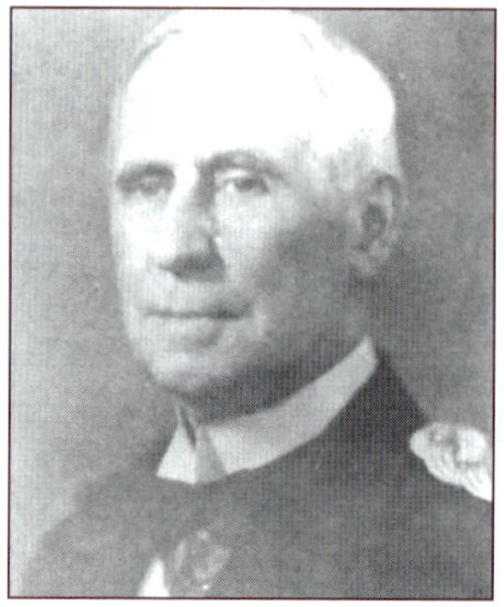

1932 – 1935
BG Matthew A. DeLaney

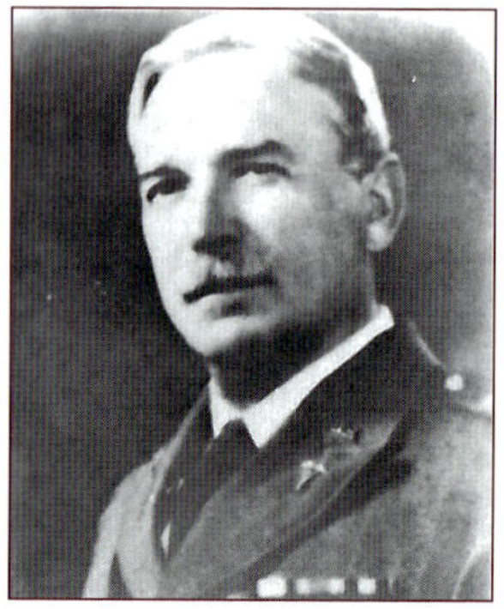

1935 – 1937
BG M.A.W. Shockley

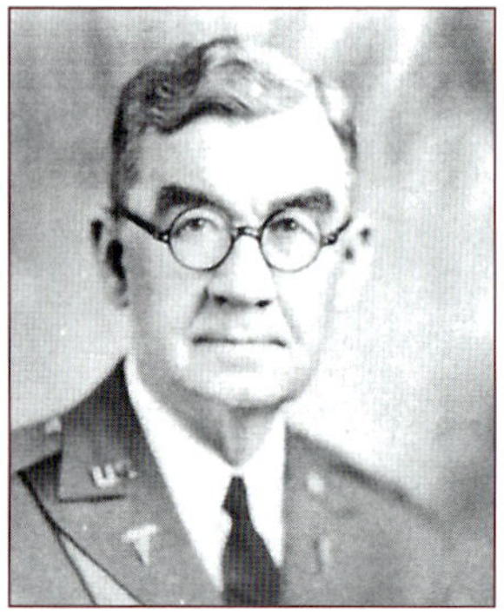

1937 – 1940
BG Roger Brooke

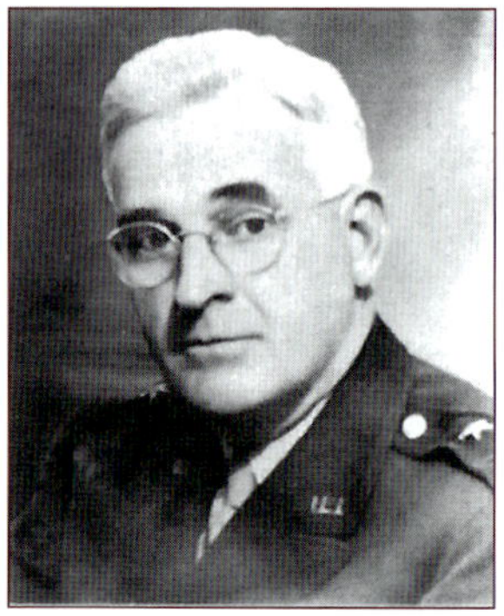

1941 – 1941
BG John M. Willis

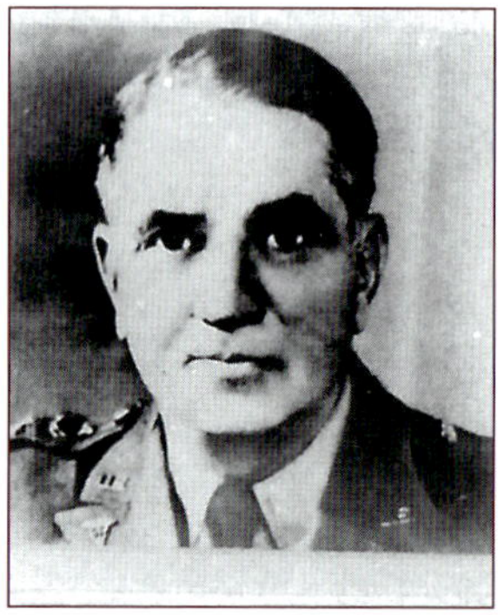

1941 – 1946
BG Addison D. Davis

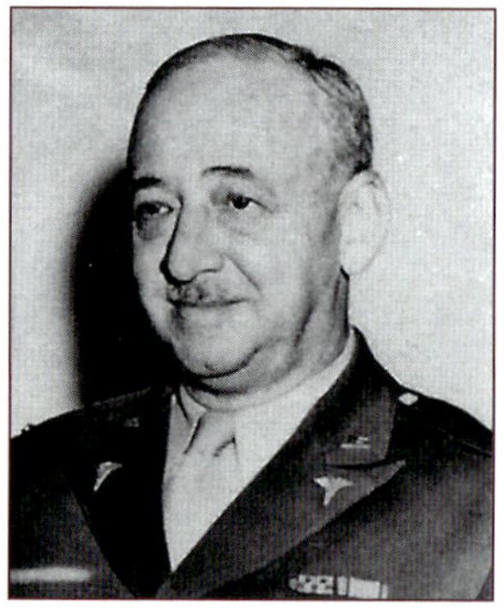

1946 – 1946
Colonel Howard T. Wickert

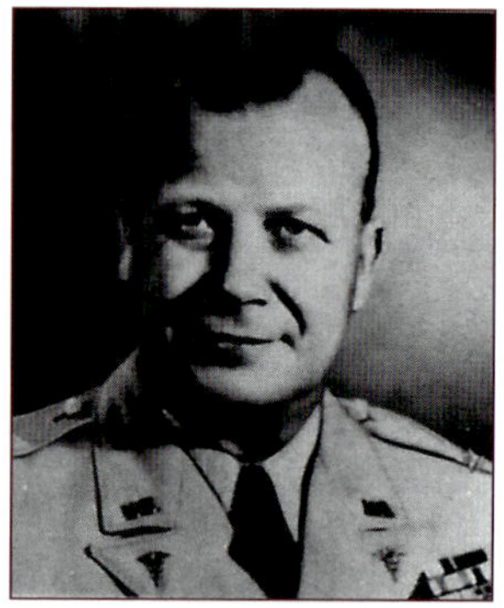

1946 – 1947
Colonel William E. Shambora

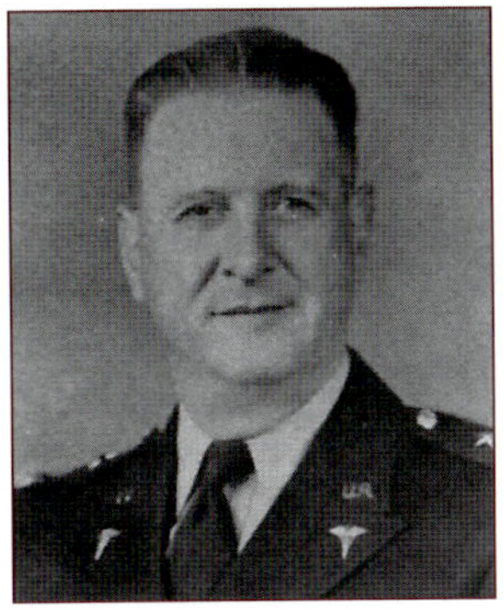

1947 – 1953
MG Joseph I. Martin

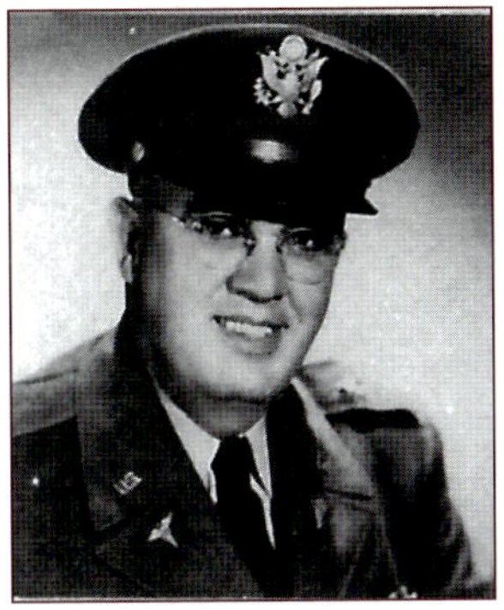

1953 – 1955
BG James P. Cooney

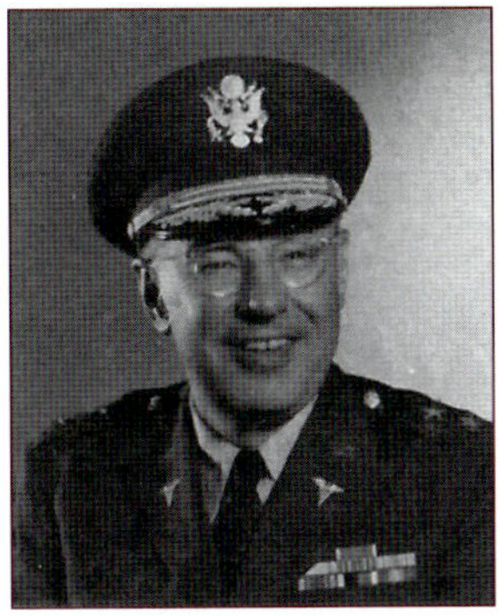

1955 – 1959
MG Elbert DeCoursey

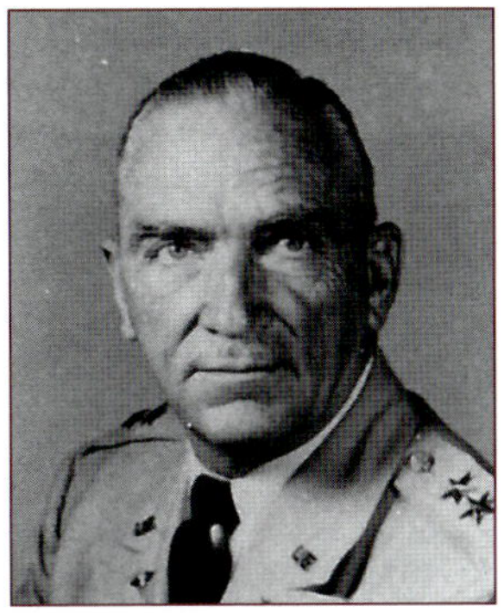

1959 – 1961
MG James L. Snyder

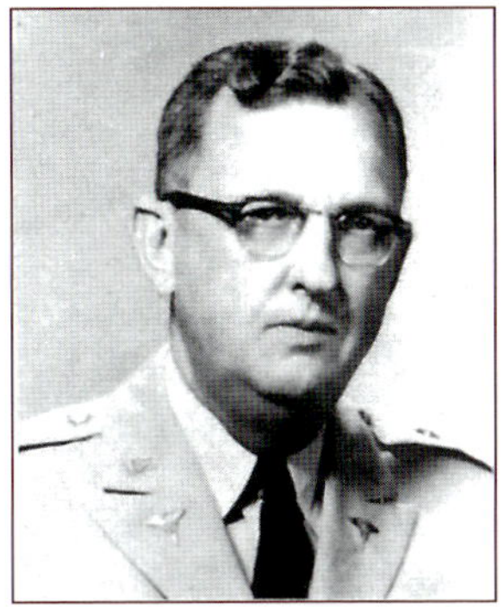

1962 – 1965
BG James T. McGibony

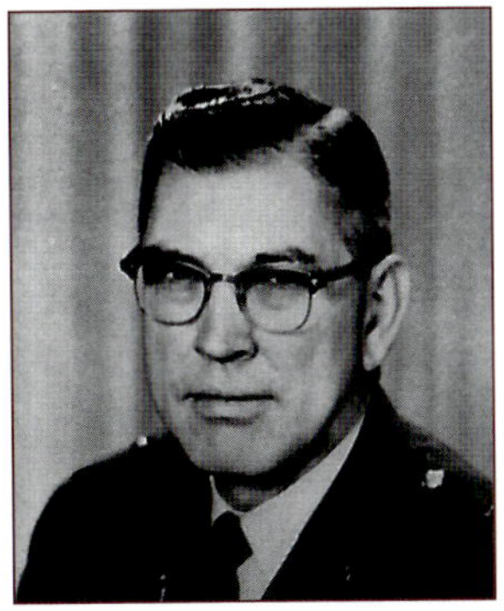

1965 – 1967
MG Glenn J. Collins

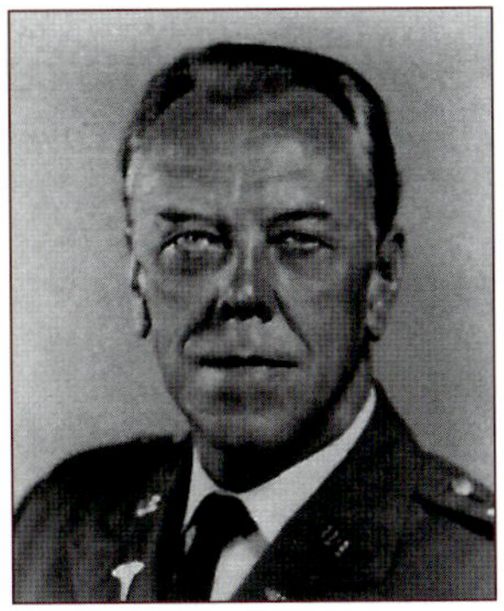

1967 – 1969
MG O. Elliott Ursin

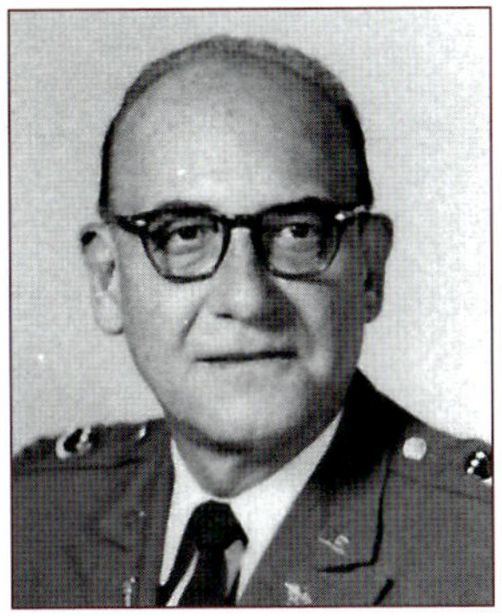

1969 – 1970
Colonel Frank A. Neuman

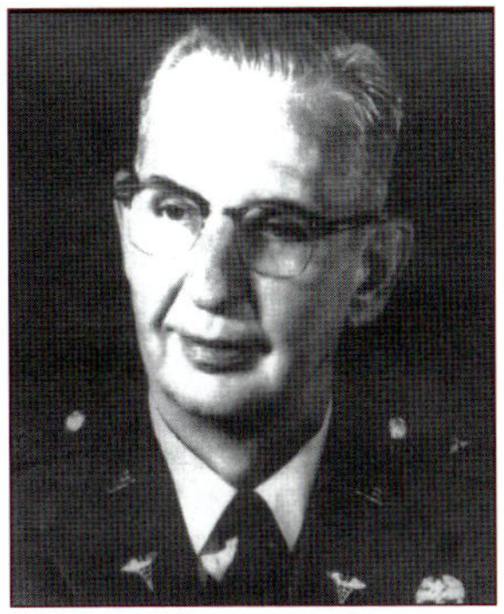

1970 – 1973
MG Kenneth D. Orr, MC
SUPERINTENDENT

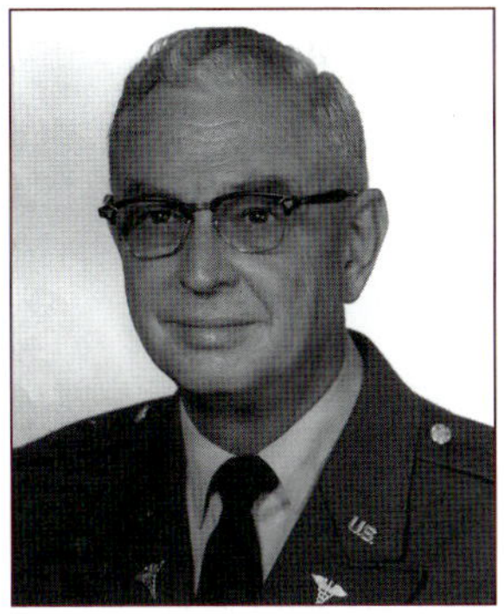

1973 – 1976
MG Edward H. Vogel, Jr., MC
SUPERINTENDENT

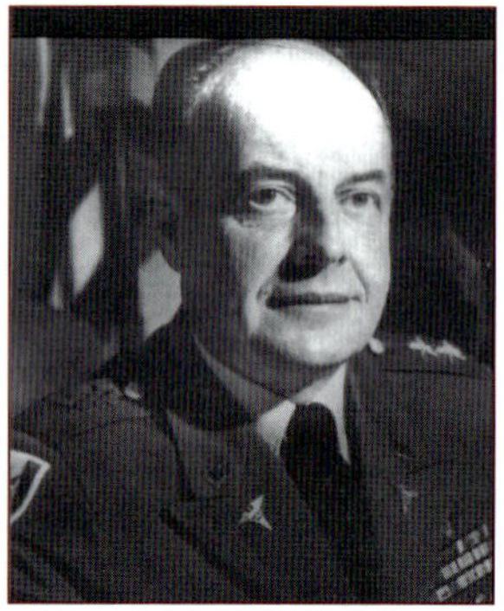

1977 – 1977
MG Charles C. Pixley, MC
SUPERINTENDENT

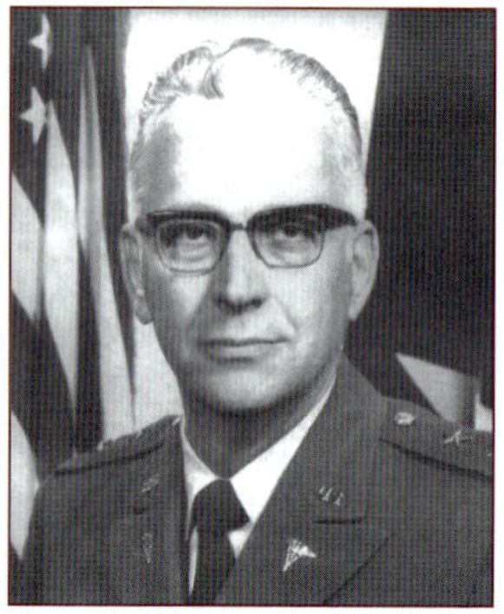

1977 – 1980
MG Kenneth R. Dirks, MC
SUPERINTENDENT

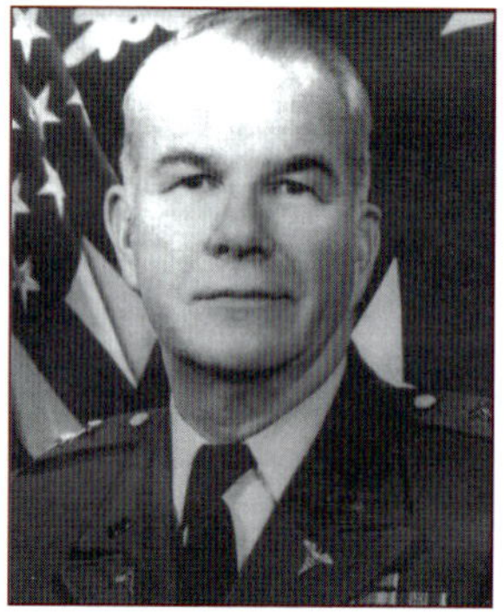

1980 – 1980
MG Raymond H. Bishop, Jr., MC
SUPERINTENDENT

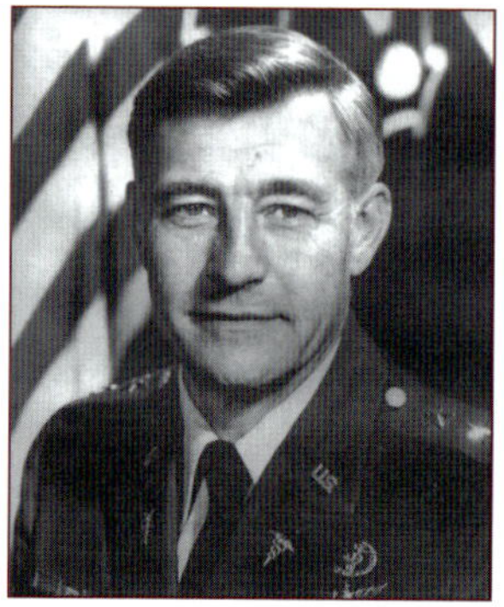

1980 – 1981
MG Quinn H. Becker, MC
SUPERINTENDENT/COMMANDANT

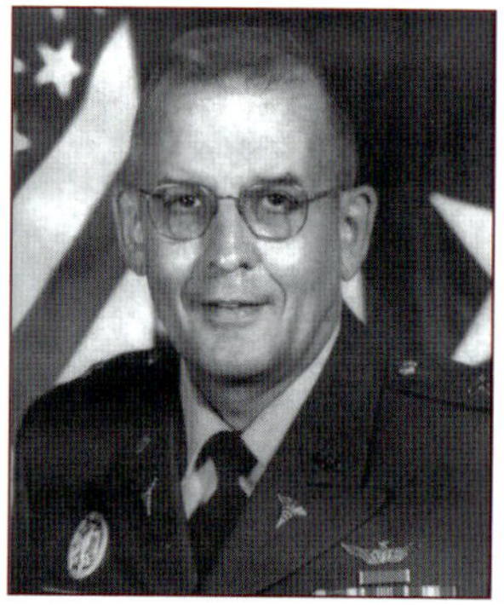

1981 – 1983
BG Robert H. Buker, MC
COMMANDANT

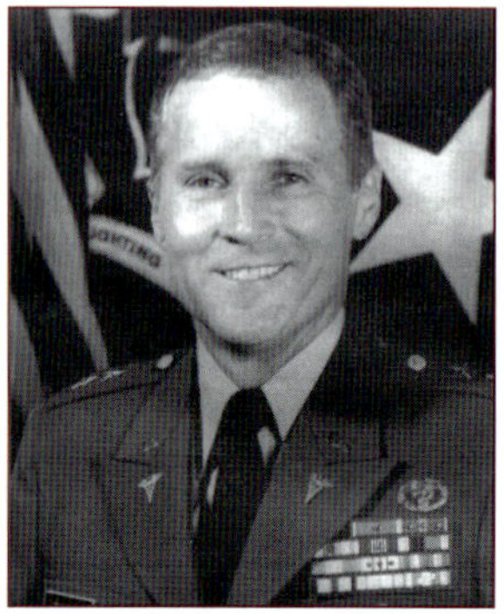

1983 – 1986
MG William P. Winkler, Jr., MC
COMMANDANT

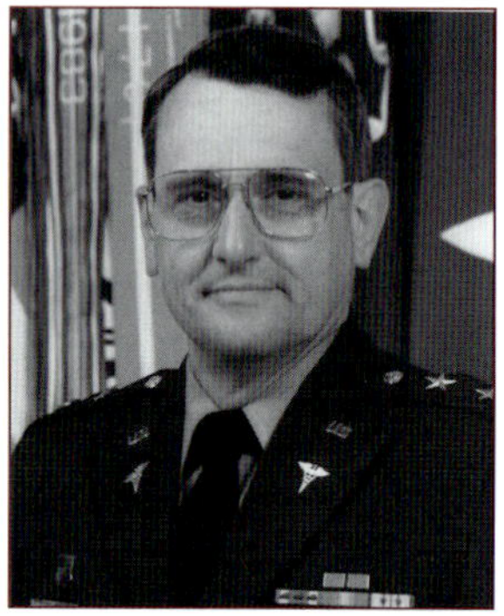

1986 – 1989
MG Alcide M. LaNoue, MC
COMMANDANT

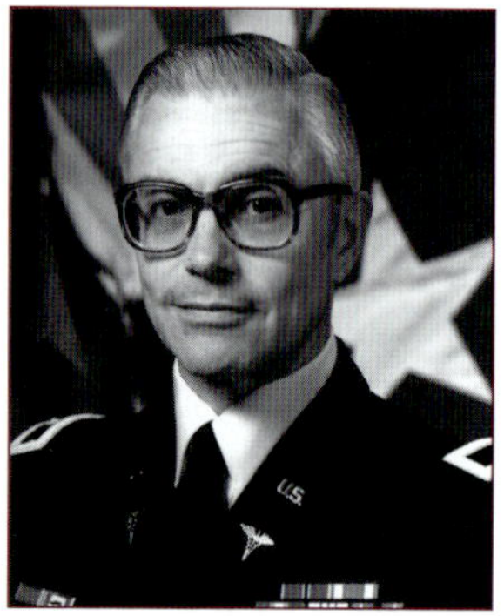

1989 – 1991
MG Frederick N. Bussey, MC
COMMANDANT

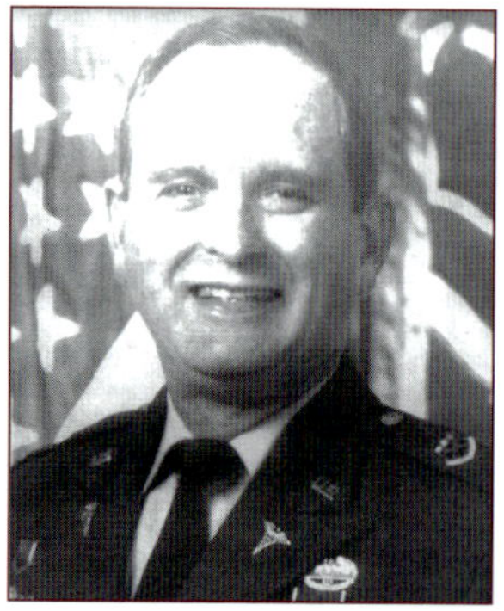

1991 – 1991
COL Paul L. Shelter, MC
COMMANDANT

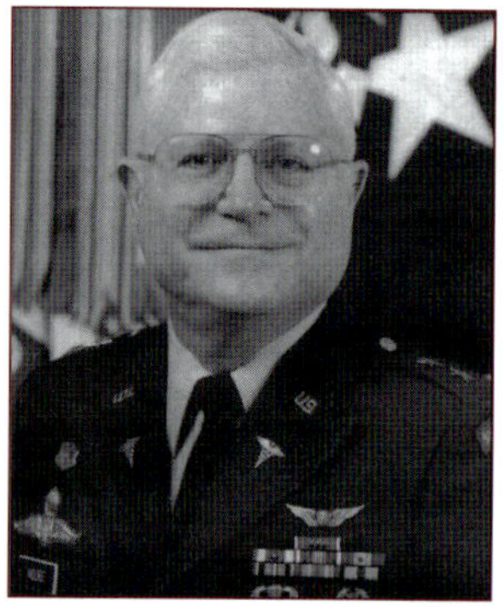

1991 – 1994
MG William L. Moore, Jr., MC
COMMANDANT

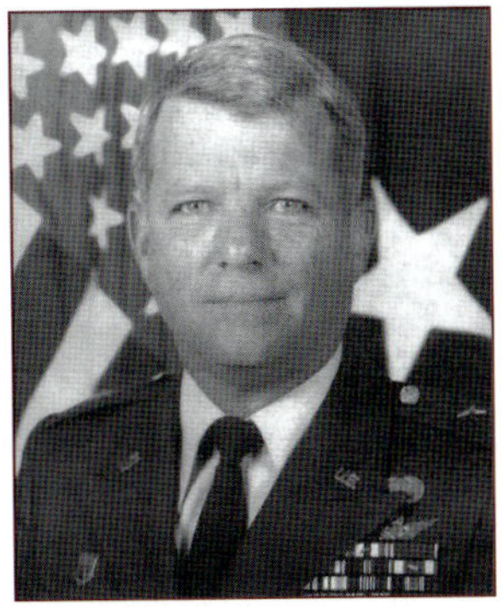

1994 – 1994
BG Jerome V. Foust, MSC
COMMANDER

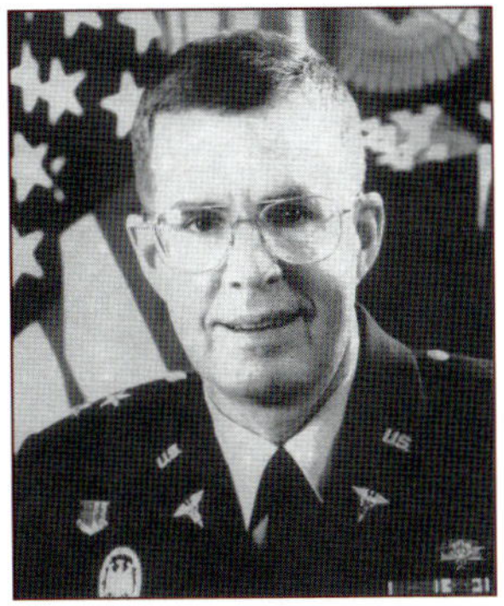

1994 – 1996
MG John J. Cuddy, DC
COMMANDER

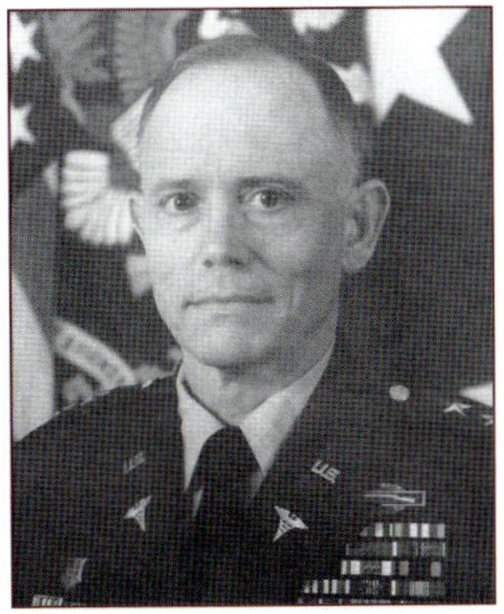

1996 – 2000
MG James B. Peake, MC
COMMANDER

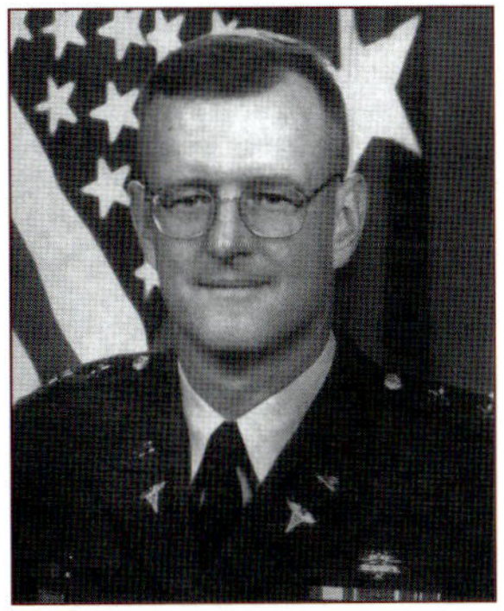

2000 – 2002
MG Kevin C. Kiley, MC
COMMANDER

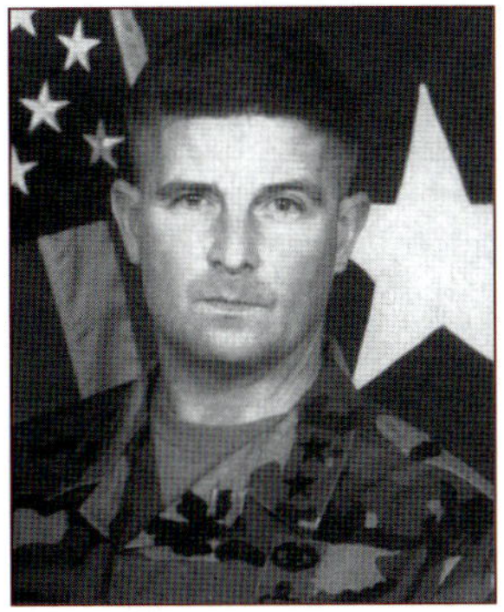

2002 – 2003
MG Darrel R. Porr, MC
COMMANDER

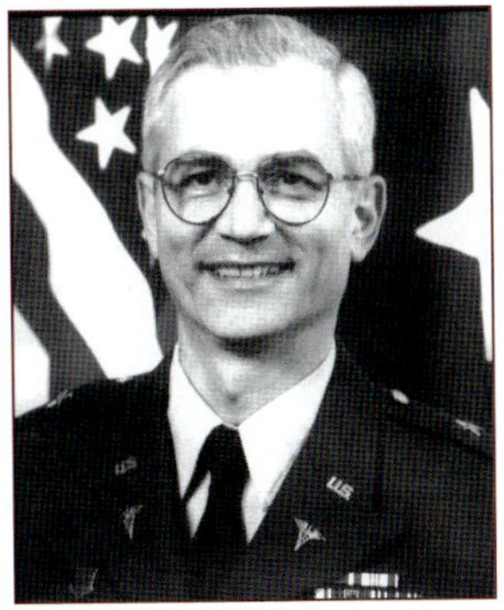

2003 – 2004
BG Daniel F. Perugini, MC
COMMANDER

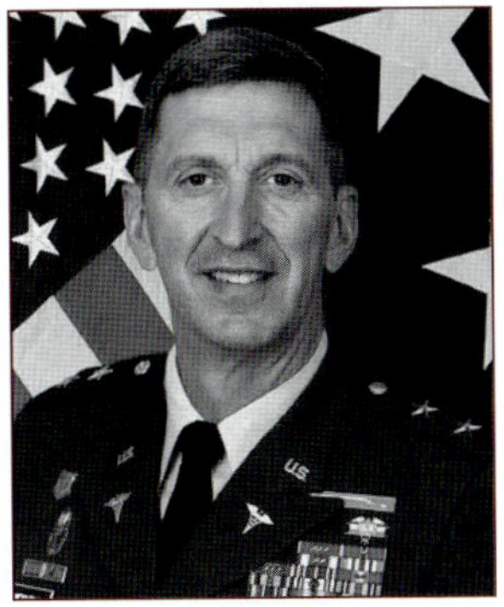

2004 – 2006
MG George W. Weightman, MC
COMMANDER

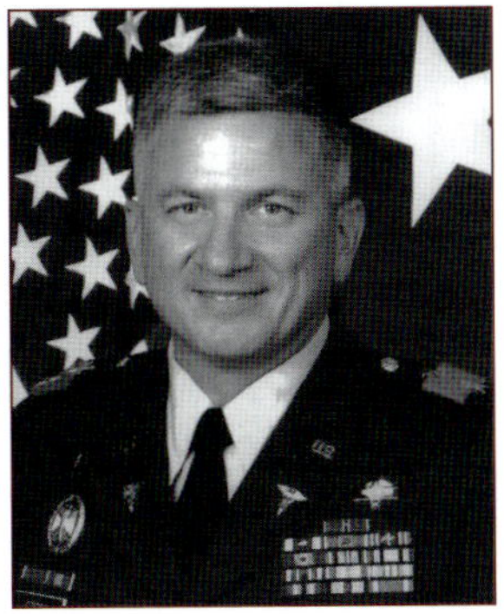

2006 – 2010
MG Russell J. Czerw, DC
COMMANDER

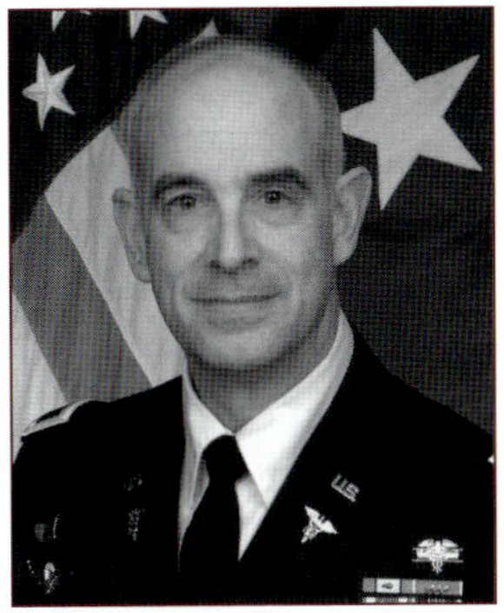

2010 – 2012
MG David A. Rubenstein, MSC
COMMANDER

Appendix B

Command Sergeants Major (1967 – Present)

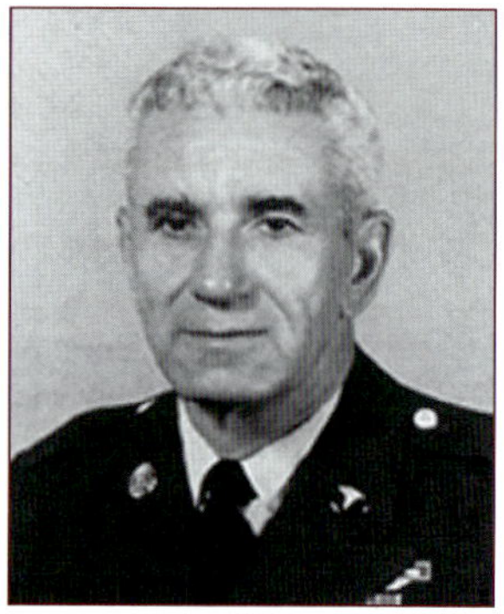

1967-1969
CSM Howard A. Tavernier

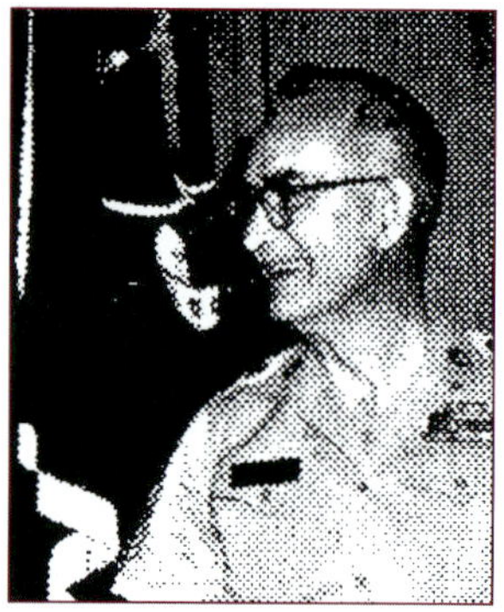

Jul 1970
CSM Robert C. Witt

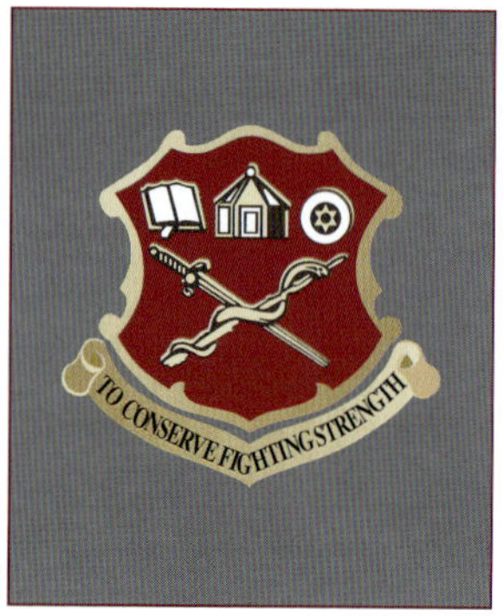

Oct 1972
CSM Melvin E. Huggins

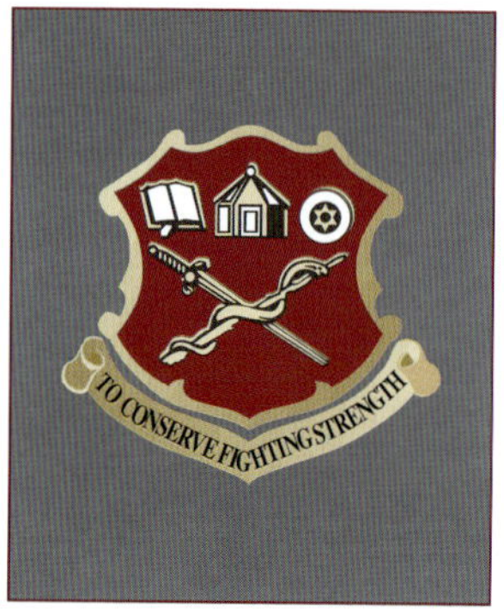

Mar 1973
CSM James A. King

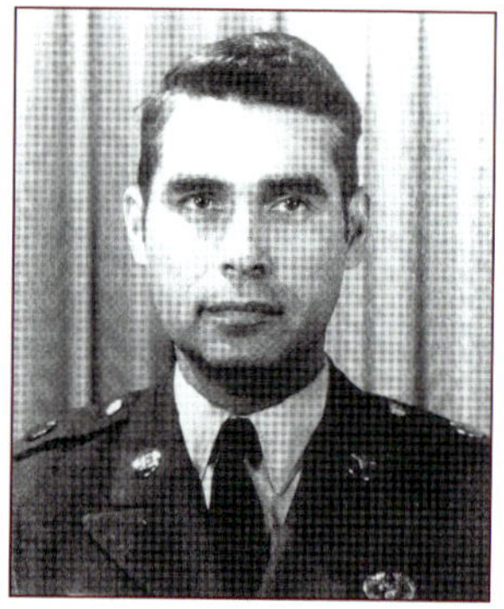

Aug 1975
CSM David O. Sandoval

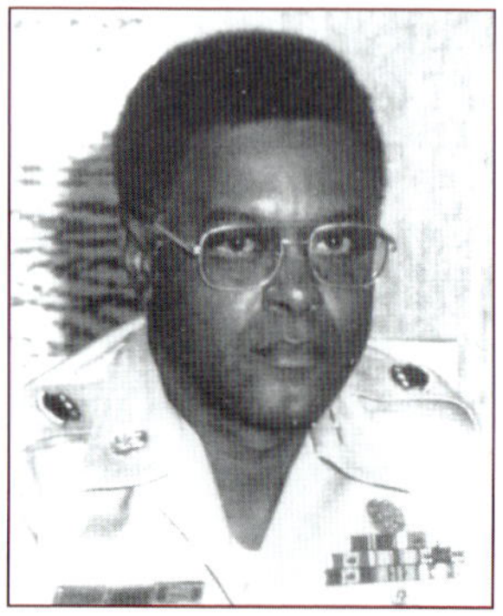

Oct 1976
CSM George J. Pierce

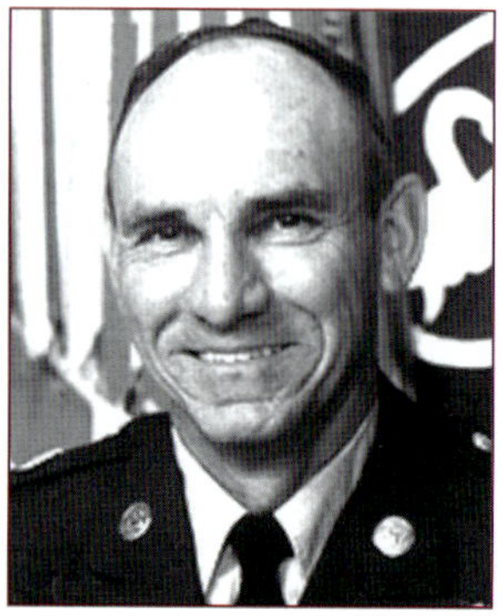

Jul 1980
CSM Howard R. Harrell

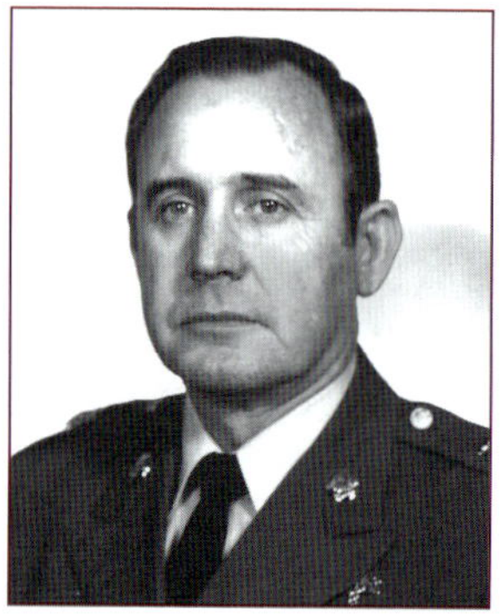

Apr 1985
CSM Joseph D. McLain

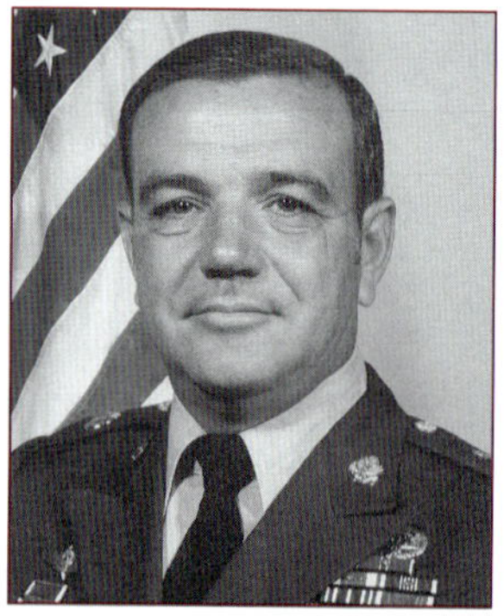

Jun 1986
CSM Kramer D. Regan

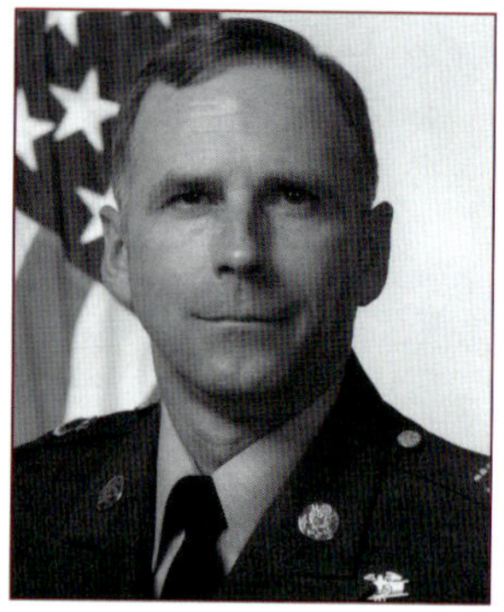

Jan 1990
CSM David S. Cahill

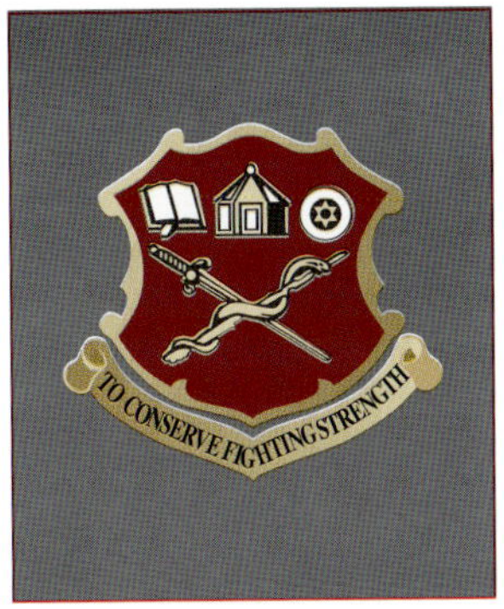

Feb 1993
CSM Roy Needham

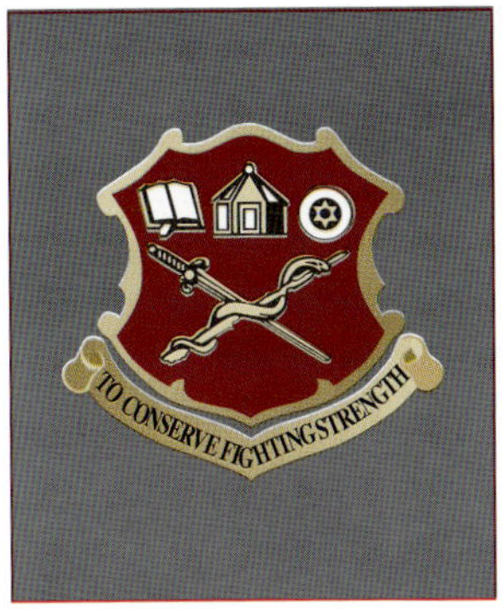

Oct 1996
CSM James Hosborough

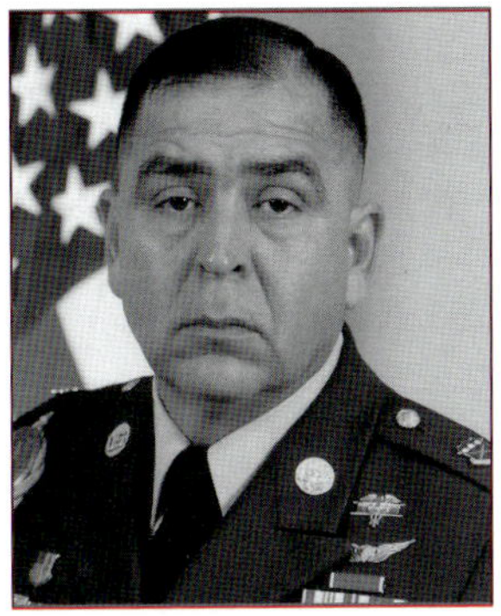

Jan 1999
CSM Adolph M. Arista

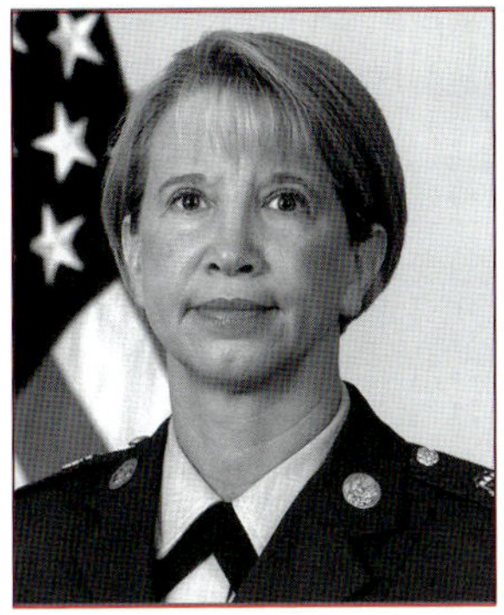

Sept 2002
CSM Sandra K. Townsend

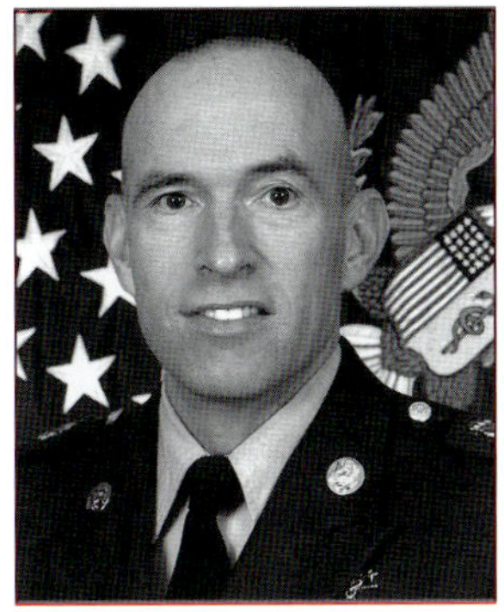

Aug 2004
CSM Timothy Burke

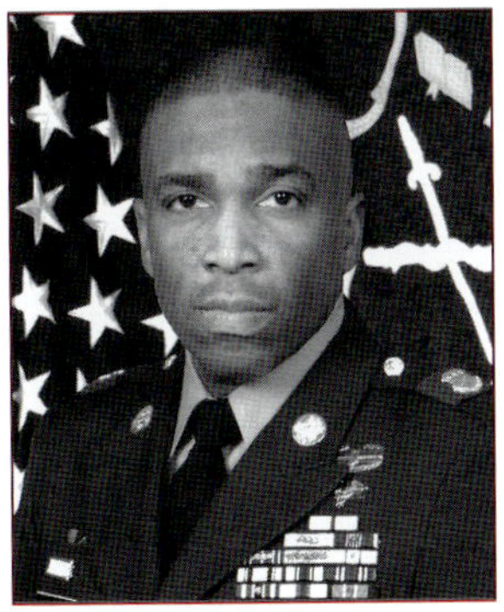

Aug 2007
CSM Howard R. Riles

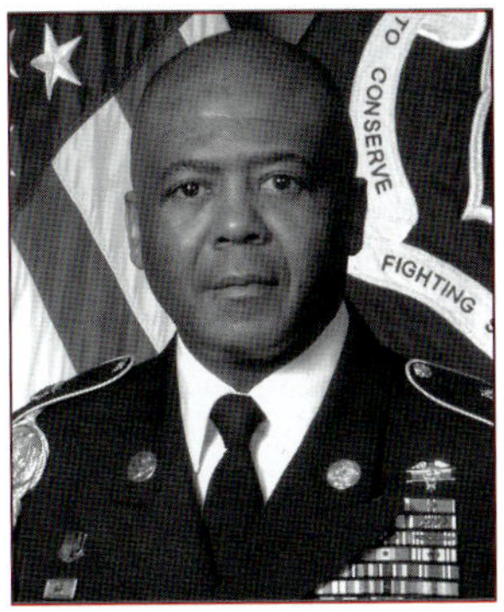

May 2010
CSM James E. Diggs